THE
PHARMACY
TECHNICIAN

A COMPREHENSIVE APPROACH

FOURTH EDITION

JAHANGIR MOINI, MD, MPH, CPHT

Professor of Science and Health, Retired,

Eastern Florida State College, Palm Bay, Florida

Former Professor and

Director of Pharmacy Technician Program

at Everest University, Melbourne, Florida

✳ Cengage

Australia • Brazil • Canada • Mexico • Singapore • United Kingdom • United States

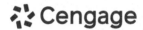

The Pharmacy Technician: A Comprehensive Approach, **Fourth Edition**
Jahangir Moini

SVP, Higher Education & Skills Product: Erin Joyner

Product Director: Matthew Seeley

Product Manager: Lauren Whalen

Product Assistant: Dallas Wilkes

Director, Learning Design: Rebecca von Gillern

Senior Manager, Learning Design: Leigh Hefferon

Learning Designer: Deborah Bordeaux

Marketing Director: Sean Chamberland

Marketing Manager: Jonathan Sheehan

Director, Content Creation: Juliet Steiner

Content Creation Manager: Stacey Lamodi

Content Manager: Tamara Starr

Digital Delivery Lead: David O'Connor

Senior Designer: Angela Sheehan

Cover Images: © iStockPhoto.com/Steve Debenport, © iStockPhoto.com/Ivan-balvan, © iStockPhoto.com/stevecoleimages, © iStockPhoto.com/JohnnyGreig, © iStockPhoto.com/Tom Merton, © iStockPhoto.com/gradyreese, © iStockPhoto.com/guruXOOX, © iStockPhoto.com/Kritchanut, © iStockPhoto.com/MJ_Prototype, © iStockPhoto.com/Moyo Studio, © iStockPhoto.com/PeopleImages, © Venus Angel/ShutterStock.com

For product information and technology assistance, contact us at
**Cengage Customer & Sales Support, 1-800-354-9706
or support.cengage.com.**

For permission to use material from this text or product, submit all requests online at **www.copyright.com.**

Library of Congress Control Number: 2019953841

ISBN: 978-0-357-37135-0

Cengage
200 Pier 4 Boulevard
Boston, MA 02210
USA

Cengage is a leading provider of customized learning solutions with employees residing in nearly 40 different countries and sales in more than 125 countries around the world. Find your local representative at: **www.cengage.com.**

To learn more about Cengage platforms and services, register or access your online learning solution, or purchase materials for your course, visit **www.cengage.com.**

Printed Number: 14   Print Year: 2024
Printed in Mexico

Dedication

*This book is dedicated
to my wonderful wife and
my two daughters Mahkameh
and Morvarid, and my two precious
granddaughters, Laila Jade,
and Anabelle Jasmine Mabry.*

CONTENTS

SECTION I
Pharmacy Practice 1

SECTION II
Pharmacy Practice Settings 189

SECTION III
Administrative Skills

SECTION IV
Medication Effects on Body Systems 411

CONTRIBUTORS

MICHAEL EDWARDS, PHARMD
Corporate Director of Pharmacy
Health First
Melbourne, Florida

MAHKAMEH MABRY, DMD
General Dentist
Mabry Dental Care
Melbourne, Florida

LEE ANNA OBOS, RPH
Pharmacy Skills Laboratory Instructor
Albany College of Pharmacy and Health Sciences
Albany, New York

NORMAN TOMAKA, CRPH, LHCRM
Pharmacist Consultant
Health First
Melbourne, Florida

VINCENT E. TRUNZO, RPH, MSM
Senior Pharmacy Operations Manager
Florida Hospital
Orlando, Florida

GREG VADIMSKY, PHARMTECH
Pharmacy Technician
Melbourne, Florida

KEITH M. BINION, BS, CPHT
Program Director, Pharmacy Technician Program
Henry Ford College
Dearborn, Michigan

RICHARD P. D'AMBRISI, AA, CPHT
Pharmacy Technician, Adjunct Faculty Allied Health
Hagerstown Community College
Hagerstown, Maryland

WILLIAM J. HAVINS, BUS, CPHT
Program Director, Pharmacy Technology
Central New Mexico Community College
Albuquerque, New Mexico

CARLA HOUSE JACOBS, RN, BSN, M.ED
Health Science Teacher
Claudia Taylor Johnson High School/NEISD
San Antonio, Texas

TOY LONG, RN, BSN, CCHP
Pharmacology and Health Science Instructor
Plainview High School
Plainview, Texas

BREANNE MARSHBURN, MHA, AAS, CPHT
Pharmacy Technician Instructor
Randolph Community College
Asheboro, North Carolina

MARCUS MASON, CPHT, RPHT, M.ED
Health Science Lead Instructor, Adjunct Instructor, Pharmacology and Pharmacy Tech
Singley Academy IISD, Dallas County Community College
Dallas, Texas

SHELLY R. MCCOWEN, CPHT, CSPT
Pharmacy Technician Instructor
Rend Lake College
Ina, Illinois

SHEENA MILLS, RPHT, CPHT, MHA
Academic Manager
Jacksonville Job Corps Center
Jacksonville, Florida

BRITTANY PATTESON, CPHT, CTE
Pharmacy Technician Instructor
Regional Occupational Center (ROC)
Bakersfield, California

TERRI S. REISINGER, RPHT, CPHT
Instructor
Cape Coral Technical College
Cape Coral, Florida

LORETTA RICHARDSON, MPA, CPHT
Program Coordinator
Ayers Career College
Shreveport, Louisiana

ANGELA RILEY, RMA, CPHT, MSBC
Associate Professor, Academic Program Coordinator
Jefferson Community and Technical College
Louisville, Kentucky

AISHA THOMAS, PHARM.D, CPHT, CMAC
Pharmacy Technician Instructor
Jacksonville Job Corps Center
Jacksonville, Florida

TRACY TUTTLE, RN
Health Professions Instructor
Boise School District
Boise, Idaho

RENEE ACOSTA, RPH, MS
Pharmacy Technician Department Chair
Austin Community College
Austin, Texas

DENISE ANDERSON, CPHT
International Education Corporation
Ontario, Canada

ETHAN ANDERSON, PHD
East Carolina University
Greenville, North Carolina

JEANIE BARKETT, BS PHARM
Professor
Clark College
Vancouver, Washington

JACQUELINE BONNER, MS, BS, RPH
Rasmussen College
St. Cloud, Minnesota

GAIL BROWN, BS, RPHT, CPHT
Pharmacy Educator, Consultant, CE/Healthcare/Pharmacy Technician Textbook Reviewer and National Speaker

LARRY CHAN, PHD, CCHP
Hospice and Home Health Consultant
Danville, Connecticut

NORA CHAN, PHARMD
Pharmacy Technician Program Coordinator
San Francisco Community College
San Francisco, California

LEZLEE FRANKE, PHARMD, RPH
Rasmussen College
Bloomington, Indiana

STEPHANIE GARTHRITE, CPHT
Polaris Career Center
Middleburg Heights, Ohio

ANTHONY GUERRA, PHARMD
Des Moines Area Community College
Ankeny, Iowa

CHRISTOPHER DEREK HARRIS, RPHT, CPHT, CDR
WellDyne
Lakeland, Florida

ANNE P. LAVANCE, BS, CPHT
Delgado Community College
New Orleans, Louisiana

MICHELE R. LINGO, RPHT, CPHT
Anthem College – Orlando West
Orlando, Florida

MICHELLE MCCRANIE, CPHT
Pharmacy Technology Instructor
Ogeechee Technical College
Statesboro, Georgia

CHRISTOPHER W. MILLER, PHARMD, BCPP
Director of Pharmacy Services
Circles of Care Inc.
Melbourne, Florida

MICHELLE MILLER, PHARMD, RPH
Pharmacy Technician Instructor
Kirkwood Community College
Cedar Rapids, Iowa

JAMES MIZNER, RPH, MBA
Pharmacy Technician Program Director
Applied Career Training
Arlington, Virginia

STEPHANIE MULLEN, RN, MSN, CPNP
Pediatric Nurse Practitioner
Medical College of Wisconsin, Children's Hospital of Wisconsin
Milwaukee, Wisconsin

SHERRI DOLA OJIKUTU, MS, PHARMD
Rasmussen College
Mokena/Tinley Park, Illinois

JAYSON PARSHALL, CPHT, RPHT
Sanford-Brown Institute – Jacksonville
Jacksonville, Florida

AGNES PUCILLO, BSN, ACHI, RHE
Educational Supervisor for Allied Health
The Cittone Institute
Edison, New Jersey

CRYSTAL A. RILEY, PHARMD, RPH, MSHCA, CPHQ, CPHIT
Baxter Healthcare Corporation
Washington, DC

ASHANTI LA ROCHE, AS, CTS, CPHT
Delgado Community College
New Orleans, Louisiana

LAURA SKINNER, CPHT
Wayne Community College
Goldsboro, North Carolina

JOHN SMITH, EDD
Associate Dean, Health Sciences
Corinthian Colleges, Inc.
Santa Ana, California

KAREN SNIPE, CPHT, AS, BA, MAED
Pharmacy Technician Program Coordinator
Trident Technical College
Charleston, South Carolina

STEVEN CLARK STONER, PHARMD, BCPP
Clinical Associate Professor of Pharmacy Practice
University of Missouri – Kansas City
St. Joseph, Missouri

MARY CATHERINE VONGARLEM, RN, BSN, MHA
Rasmussen College
Appleton, Wisconsin

STEPHANIE WEISKIND, RPH
Pharmacy Technician Instructor
Cuyahoga Community College
Cleveland, Ohio

TAMMY WILDER, RN, MSN, CMSRN, BC
Ivy Tech Community College
Evansville, Indiana

PAMELA S. WOOTEN, RN, MSN, EDDC
Rasmussen College

LORRAINE ZENTZ, CPHT, PHD
Pharmacy Instructor
GES/Cengage Learning
Mesa, Colorado

JENNIFER ZIMNICKI, CPHT
Wayne State University
Ross Medical Education, LLC

This fourth edition was written for pharmacy technician students and practicing pharmacy technicians. It expands upon the previous editions with an improved chapter order and more concise organization. Instructors will find this edition to be even more consistent in its learning flow, giving students needed information in an order that is more readily absorbed. The text is designed to give a comprehensive body of information and tools to pharmacy technicians and their educators. There are various chapters that are either new, relocated, or separated out of different chapters from the previous edition. The reason behind these updates is based on how revolutionary changes in the field of pharmacy have altered the duties of pharmacy technicians. All pharmacy technicians must be more knowledgeable and skillful about preparing and dispensing medications, whether they work in institutional or community pharmacy settings. Preparing medications involves using sterile and nonsterile techniques, compounding drugs, packaging, and labeling. However, the most important role for pharmacy technicians is to be able to assist pharmacists in preventing medication errors. Today, medication errors happen often and result in severe patient harm and even death.

Features

The fourth edition consists of 4 sections and 31 chapters, each containing many questions and exercises that help ensure a better understanding of the text. Each chapter begins with an outline, a list of objectives, and key terms. *What Would You Do* features consist of real-life scenarios that pharmacy technicians can contemplate regarding the proper reactions to authentic situations. *Medication Error Alert* boxes highlight important information that must be retained in order to provide the best possible patient outcomes. *Medical Terminology Review* boxes are designed for practice in understanding terminology and how words are divided into prefixes, roots, combining forms, and suffixes. *Tables* summarize important information and organize it into memorable formats, helping increase retention. *Figures* consist of drawings and photos that illustrate key components of the text. At the end of each chapter is a set of *Review Questions*, plus a *Critical Thinking* exercise in a case study format. The *Appendices* in this edition have been expanded to include additional and updated information in many areas of pharmacy practice. In the "body systems" chapters, the text has been reorganized to include brief structures and functions, common disorders, and their treatments. The book is printed in full color, which helps to illustrate important concepts in the text. There is updated information about laws and ethics, newly marketed medications, information about new diseases and conditions, updates on safety in the workplace, complementary and alternative medicine, and the ever-growing roles of pharmacy technicians.

New to This Edition

- Revised outline, objectives, and key terms throughout

CHAPTER 1

- Added content about the transition from the ancient to the post-classical world, involving the formalization of the pharmacy profession.

CHAPTER 3

- Changed title of this chapter from "Pharmacy Law and Ethics for Technicians" to "Pharmacy Law, Ethics, and Regulatory Agencies."

CHAPTER 4

- This chapter was Chapter 36, "Communications" in the Third Edition. The chapter has now been retitled to "Communication with Patients and Customers" and renumbered to Chapter 4.

CHAPTER 5

- This chapter is totally new to this Fourth Edition and provides details on many sources of drug information.
- It includes printed and online sources used in the practice of pharmacy, and also includes pharmacy journals and magazines.

CHAPTER 6

- This chapter was created by using information from the Third Edition's Chapter 27 (Community Pharmacy), which was specific to its title, "Prescriptions and Processing."

CHAPTER 7

- This was formerly Chapter 5 in the Third Edition.
- All information was verified and updated to reflect changes in available medications.

CHAPTER 8

- This was formerly Chapter 24 in the Third Edition.
- Added text about the conversion of time between the 24-hour and 12-hour clock systems.

CHAPTER 9

- This was created by using information from the Third Edition's Chapter 25 (Calculation of Dosages), which was specific to its title, "Conversion and Calculations."
- Some equations were revised and reconfigured.
- Certain portions of text were omitted for clarity.

CHAPTER 10

- This was formerly Chapter 8 in the Third Edition.
- The latest information concerning safety in the workplace was added to make it up to date with current OSHA requirements.

CHAPTER 11

- This was formerly Chapter 26, "Hospital Pharmacy Practice," in the Third Edition. In this edition, the chapter has been titled as "Hospital Pharmacy."
- New sections include "Policies and Procedures," "Hospital Protocol," "Point-of-Entry Systems," "Computerized Physician Order Entry," "Barcode Point-of-Entry," "Computerized Monitoring for Adverse Drug Reactions," and "Unit-Dose Liquids."
- Revised sections include "Unit-Dose Medications" and "The Roles and Duties of Pharmacy Technicians in Hospitals," which now features sub-headings on all of the items in its bulleted list.
- Updated summary, review questions, medication error alert boxes, and figures.

CHAPTER 12

- This was formerly Chapter 27 in the Third Edition.

- New sections include "Community Pharmacy," "The Role of the Pharmacy Technician," "Prescription Processing," "Pharmacy Stock Area," "Nonsterile Compounding Area," "Sterile Compounding Area," "Interacting with the Pharmacist," "Interacting with the Patient," "Elderly Patients," "Patients with Mental Disorders," "Patients with Health Literacy Issues," "Immunizations," "Durable and Nondurable Supplies and Equipment," "Long-Term Care Services," and "Disease Prevention."

- Revised sections include "Storage," "Controlled Substance Prescriptions," "Purchasing and Inventory Control," and "Ability to Handle a Busy Work Environment and Stress."

- Revised summary, review questions, points to remember boxes, and medication error alert boxes.

CHAPTER 13

- This was formerly Chapter 28 in the Third Edition.

- Revised sections include "Long-Term Care Pharmacy Services," "Unit-Dose System," and "Mail-Order Pharmacy."

- Revised figures.

CHAPTER 14

- This was formerly Chapter 29 in the Third Edition.

- Revised figures.

- New sections include "Electronic Mortars and Pestles," "Tongs," "Ultrasonic Cleaners," "Pipettes and Pipette Fillers," "Spray Bottles," and "Stirring Rods."

- Revised review questions.

CHAPTER 15

- This was formerly Chapter 30 in the Third Edition (Sterile Compounding). In this edition, it has been retitled as "Aseptic Technique and Sterile Compounding."

- New sections include "Storage and Stability" and "United States Pharmacopeia (USP) Chapter <800>."

- Tables added.

- Revised sections include "Large-Volume Parenteral Preparations," "United States Pharmacopeia (USP) Chapter <797>," and summary.

- Revised review questions and critical thinking.

CHAPTER 16

- This has been derived from Chapter 32 (Health Insurance) and Chapter 33 (Documentation, Billing, and Collections) in the Third Edition. In this edition, the chapter has been titled as "Insurance and Billing."

- Revised sections include "Individual Contract," "Types of Health Insurance," "Private Health Insurance," "Blue Cross®-Blue Shield® Association," "Medicare Part A," "Medicare Part B," "Medicare Part C," "Medicare Part D," "Medicaid," "Prior Authorization," "Claims Processing," and "Billing Secondary Payers."

- New sections include "Claim Rejections," "Days Supply Exceeded Rejection," "Refill Too Soon Rejection," "Plan Limitations Exceeded Rejection," "Patient Not Covered Rejection," "Provider Not Covered Rejection," "Coverage Terminated Rejection," "Special Billing," "Immunizations," "Durable Medical Supplies," "Clinic and Inpatient Billing," "Medication Therapy Management," "Healthcare Common Procedure Coding System," "Third Party Audits," "Dispensed Quantity Exceeds Authorized Quantity," "Higher Than Expected Usage," "Inconsistent Days Supply," "Wrong Package Size," "Inappropriate Dispense-as-Written-Code," and "Missing or Incomplete Original Prescription."

- Revised summary, review questions, critical thinking, and "What Would You Do?" boxes.

CHAPTER 17

- This was derived from Chapter 34 (Inventory Control) and Chapter 31 (Financial Management of Pharmacy Operations) from the Third Edition; it has been retitled as "Inventory Control and Management."

- Revised sections include "Inventory Control," "Inventory Management," "Computerized Inventory System," "Inventory of Controlled Substances," "Point-of-Sale System," "Ordering Process," "Receiving New Stock," "Medication Returns," and "Expired Stock."

- New sections include "Inventory Stock," "Duties of Pharmacy Technicians," "Bar Coding," "Manual Ordering," "Automated Dispensing System," "Posting," "Storage," "Return of Declined Drugs," "Drug Recalls," "Damaged Stock," "Purchasing Procedures," "Independent Purchasing," "Group Purchasing," "Wholesale Purchasing," "Prime Suppliers," "Special Purchasing of Controlled Substances," "Schedule II Purchasing," "Schedule III, IV, and V Purchasing," and "Controlled Substance Disposal."

- Revised summary, review questions, points to remember boxes, "What Would You Do?" boxes.

CHAPTER 18

- This was formerly Chapter 11 in the Third Edition, but in this edition it has been retitled as "Medication Errors and Safety."

- Revised sections include "Occurrence of Medication Errors," "Prescribing Errors," "Dispensing Errors," "Administration Errors," "Wrong Drug," "Wrong Dose," "The Patient's Role in Medication Errors," "Human Factors," "Inadequate Patient Monitoring," "Dangerous Abbreviations and Numerical Terms," "Avoiding Medication Errors," "Medication Error Reporting," "FDA MedWatch Program," and "ISMP-Medication Error Reporting Program."

- New sections include "Medication Safety for Children," "Medication Safety for the Elderly," "Vaccine Adverse Event Reporting System," and "Liability of Medication Errors."

- Revised summary, review questions, medication error alert boxes, and tables.

CHAPTER 19

- This was formerly Chapter 10 in the Third Edition.

- Revised sections include "Pharmacokinetics," "Drug Absorption," "Drug Distribution," "Drug Metabolism," "Drug Excretion," "Drug Half-Life," "Mechanism of Drug Interaction," "Synergism," "Antagonism," "Multiple Pharmacological Effects," and "Genetic Factors."

- Revised summary, review questions, and points to remember boxes.

CHAPTER 20

- This was formerly Chapter 14 in the Third Edition; it has been retitled as "Therapeutic Drugs for the Nervous System."

- Revised sections include "Peripheral Nervous System," "Neurons," "Disorders of the Nervous System and Their Treatments," "Migraine Headache," "Epilepsy," "Parkinson's Disease," "Multiple Sclerosis," "Alzheimer's Disease," "Bipolar Disease," "Major Depressive Disorder," "Anxiety Disorders," and "Narcotic Analgesics."

- New sections include "Stroke," "Attention Deficit and Hyperactivity Disorder," and "Naloxone."

- Revised summary, critical thinking, points to remember boxes, and tables.

CHAPTER 21

- This was Chapter 13 in the Third Edition; it has been retitled as "Therapeutic Drugs for the Musculoskeletal System" in this edition.

- Revised sections include "Skeletal System," "Musculoskeletal System Disorders," "Osteoarthritis," "Osteoporosis," "Osteomalacia and Rickets," "Other Medications Used to Treat Musculoskeletal System Disorders," "Muscle Relaxants," and "Neuromuscular Blocking Agents."

- A new section has been added entitled "Spasmolytics."

- Revised review questions, medication error alert boxes, tables.

CHAPTER 22

- This was formerly Chapter 16 in the Third Edition; it has been retitled as "Therapeutic Drugs for the Endocrine System."

- Revised sections include "Thyroid Gland," "Pancreas," "Disorders of the Endocrine System and Their Treatments," "Diabetes Insipidus," "Simple Goiter," "Hyperthyroidism," "Cushing's Syndrome," "Addison's Disease," "Diabetes Mellitus," and "Selected Drugs for Diabetes Mellitus."

- New sections include "Hypopituitarism," "Hyperpituitarism," "Hyperparathyroidism," "Hypoparathyroidism," "Hyperaldosteronism," and "Obesity."

- Revised summary, review questions, tables, and figures.

CHAPTER 23

- This was formerly Chapter 17 in the Third Edition; it has been retitled as "Therapeutic Drugs for the Cardiovascular System."

- Revised sections include "Valves of the Heart," "Blood Vessels," "Arteriosclerosis and Atherosclerosis," "Angina Pectoris," "Myocardial Infarction," "Cardiac Arrhythmias," "Heart Failure," "Folic Acid Deficiency Anemia," "Iron Deficiency Anemia," "Pernicious Anemia," "Thrombocytopenia," "Thrombophlebitis," and "Pulmonary Embolism"

- New sections include "Hyperlipidemia," and "Hypertension."

- Revised summary, review questions, points to remember boxes, and tables.

CHAPTER 24

- This was formerly Chapter 18 (Lymphatic System) in the Third Edition; it has been retitled as "Therapeutic Drugs for the Immune System."

- New sections include "Anatomy and Physiology of the Immune System," "Lymph Nodes," "Thymus Gland," "Spleen," "Innate Immunity," "Disorders of the Immune System," "Lymphoma," "Hodgkin's Disease," "Non-Hodgkin's Lymphoma," "Cancer and the Lymph Nodes," and "Autoimmune Disorders."

- Revised sections include "Types of Immunity," "Antibodies," "Immune Responses," "Hypersensitivity," "Vaccination," "Adverse Reactions," and "Current Vaccines in the United States"

- Revised summary, review questions, medical terminology review boxes, points to remember boxes, medication error alert boxes, "What Would You Do?" boxes, tables, and figures.

CHAPTER 25

- This was formerly Chapter 19 (Respiratory System) in the Third Edition; it has been retitled as "Therapeutic Drugs for the Respiratory System."

- Revised sections include "Anatomy and Physiology of the Respiratory System," "Lungs," "Disorders of the Respiratory System," "Common Cold," "Allergic Rhinitis," "Influenza," "Pneumonia," "Asthma," and "Chronic Obstructive Pulmonary Disease."

- There is one new section, entitled "Tuberculosis."

- Revised summary, review questions, points to remember boxes, medication error alert boxes, tables, and figures.

CHAPTER 26

- This was formerly Chapter 20 (Urinary System) in the Third Edition; it has been retitled as "Therapeutic Drugs for the Urinary System."

- Revised sections include "Kidneys," "Nephrons," "Functions of the Kidneys," "Urine Control," "Disorders of the Urinary System," "Glomerulonephritis," "Renal Failure," and "Diabetic Nephropathy."

- New sections include "Micturition" and "Urinary Tract Infections."

- Revised summary, review questions, and tables.

CHAPTER 27

- This was formerly Chapter 21 (Digestive System) in the Third Edition; it has been retitled as "Therapeutic Drugs for the Digestive System."

- Revised sections include "Small Intestine," "Large Intestine," "Gallbladder," "Disorders of the Digestive System," "Gastroesophageal Reflux Disease," "Peptic Ulcers," "Ulcerative Colitis," "Pancreatitis," and "Viral Hepatitis."

- New sections include "Antacids," "Histamine Receptor Antagonists," "Proton Pump Inhibitors," "Crohn's Disease," "Diarrhea," "Constipation," and "Colorectal Cancer."

- Revised summary, review questions, medication error alert boxes, points to remember boxes, tables, and figures.

CHAPTER 28

- This was formerly Chapter 22 (Reproductive System) in the Third Edition; it has been retitled as "Therapeutic Drugs for the Reproductive System."

- Revised sections include "Female Reproductive System," "Male Reproductive System," "Disorders of the Reproductive System," "Chlamydia," "Gonorrhea," "Trichomoniasis," "Genital Herpes," "Primary Syphilis," "Secondary Syphilis," "Tertiary Syphilis," and "Neurosyphilis."

- New sections include "Infertility," "Pelvic Inflammatory Disease," "Dysfunctional Uterine Bleeding," "Menopause," "Hypogonadism," "Benign Prostatic Hyperplasia," "Prostate Cancer," "Erectile Dysfunction," "Viral Hepatitis," "Hepatitis B," "Hepatitis C," "Human Papillomavirus," "Genital Warts," "Special Topic—Contraceptives," "Long-Term Contraceptives," and "Emergency Contraceptives."

- Revised summary, review questions, medical terminology review boxes, points to remember boxes, "What Would You Do?" boxes, medication error alert boxes, and tables.

CHAPTER 29

- This was formerly Chapter 15 (Sight and Hearing) in the Third Edition; it has been retitled as "Therapeutic Drugs for the Eyes, Ears, and Nose."

- Revised sections include "Anatomy and Physiology of the Eyes," "Sclera," "Choroid," "Retina," "Disorders of the Ears," and "Otitis Media."

- New sections include "Disorders of the Eyes," "Conjunctivitis," "Allergic Conjunctivitis," "Glaucoma," "Open-Angle Glaucoma," "Angle-Closure Glaucoma," "Macular Degeneration," "Diabetic Retinopathy," "Retinal Detachment," "Dry Eyes," "Artificial Tears," "Ototoxicity," "Anatomy and Physiology of the Nose and Sinuses," "Disorders of the Nose and Sinuses," "Allergic Rhinitis," and "Bacterial Sinusitis."

- Revised summary, review questions, and tables.

CHAPTER 30

- This was formerly Chapter 12 (Integumentary System) in the Third Edition; it has been retitled as "Therapeutic Drugs for the Integumentary System."

- Revised sections include "Accessory Structures," "Atopic Dermatitis (Eczema)," "Psoriasis," "Acne Vulgaris," and "Dermatophytosis."

- One new section was added, entitled "Nail Disorders."

- Revised review questions, tables, and figures.

CHAPTER 31

- This is a completely new chapter focusing on complementary and alternative medicine.

- It focuses on the history of supplements, dietary supplement regulation, herbal supplements, safety and efficacy of dietary supplements, and alternative therapies.

WORKBOOK TO ACCOMPANY *THE PHARMACY TECHNICIAN: A COMPREHENSIVE APPROACH, FOURTH EDITION*

ISBN: 978-0-3573-7136-7

The workbook focuses on application of key concepts and principles. Emphasis is placed on critical thinking and problem solving. Review of the objectives of each chapter and key terms are also incorporated.

MINDTAP

ISBN: 978-0-357-37198-5

MindTap is a personalized teaching experience with relevant assignments that guide students to analyze, apply, and improve thinking, allowing you to measure skills and outcomes with ease.

- MindTap features a complete integrated course combining additional quizzing and assignments, and application activities along with the enhanced e-book to further facilitate learning.

- Personalized Teaching: Becomes yours with a Learning Path that is built with key student objectives. Control what students see and when they see it. Use it as is or match to your syllabus exactly—hide, rearrange, add, and create your own content.

- Guide Students: A unique learning path of relevant readings and activities that move students up the learning taxonomy from basic knowledge and comprehension to analysis and application.

- Promote Better Outcomes: Empower instructors and motivate students with analytics and reports that provide a snapshot of class progress, time in course, engagement and completion rates.

INSTRUCTOR COMPANION WEBSITE

An Instructor Companion Website is available to facilitate classroom preparation, presentation, and testing. This content can be accessed through your Instructor account at **login.cengage.com**.

Components available on the Instructor Companion site include a(n):

- Instructor's Manual—includes lecture outlines, teaching strategies, and the answers to the end-of-chapter questions for each chapter.

- Computerized Testbank powered by Cognero—includes more than 2500 questions. Question types include multiple choice, completion, problem, and matching.

- Instructor Presentations on Microsoft™ PowerPoint™—correlate to the chapters in the book.

- Customizable syllabus.

- Customizable lesson plans.

- Correlation guide from the Third Edition to the Fourth Edition.

- Answer key for the Workbook.

- MindTap Educator Guide—provides an overview of the activities in the MindTap.

STUDENT COMPANION WEBSITE

A Student Companion Website provides additional resources. This content can be accessed through your Student account at **login.cengage.com**.

Components available on the Student Companion site include the following:

- Answer keys to the Practice Exams for the PTCB Examination (Appendices E and F).

- Online-only appendices:

  - Appendix G: Professional Organizations

  - Appendix H: Professional Journals

  - Appendix I: State Boards of Pharmacy

  - Appendix J: Top Drugs by Prescriptions Dispensed

  - Appendix K: Top 40 Herbal Remedies

Also Available

Laboratory Procedures for Pharmacy Technicians

By Jahangir Moini

ISBN: 978-1-4180-7394-7

Fundamental Pharmacology for Pharmacy Technicians, Second Edition

By Jahangir Moini

ISBN: 978-1-305-08735-4

Law & Ethics for Pharmacy Technicians, Third Edition

By Jahangir Moini

ISBN: 978-1-337-79662-0

Pharmacy Terminology

By Jahangir Moini

ISBN: 978-1-4283-1787-1

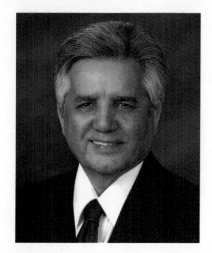

Dr. Moini was an assistant professor at Tehran University School of Medicine for nine years teaching medical and allied health students. He is a retired professor of science and health at Eastern Florida State College. He was also a professor and former director (for 24 years) of allied health programs at Everest University. Dr. Moini established, for the first time, the associate degree program for pharmacy technicians in 2000 at EU's Melbourne campus. For five years, he was also the director of the Pharmacy Technician Program. He also established several other new allied health programs for EU. As a physician and instructor for the past 39 years, he believes that pharmacy technicians should be skillful with various types of compounding and have confidence in their duties and responsibilities in order to prevent medication errors.

Dr. Moini is actively involved in teaching and helping students to prepare for service in various health professions, including the roles of pharmacy technicians, medical assistants, and nurses. He worked with the Brevard County Health Department as an epidemiologist and health educator consultant for 18 years, offering continuing education courses and keeping nurses up to date on the latest developments related to pharmacology, medication errors, immunizations, and other important topics. He has been an internationally published author of 40 allied health books since 1999.

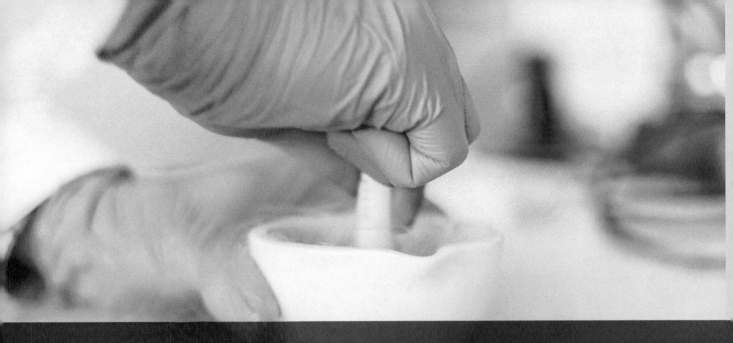

PHARMACY PRACTICE

SECTION

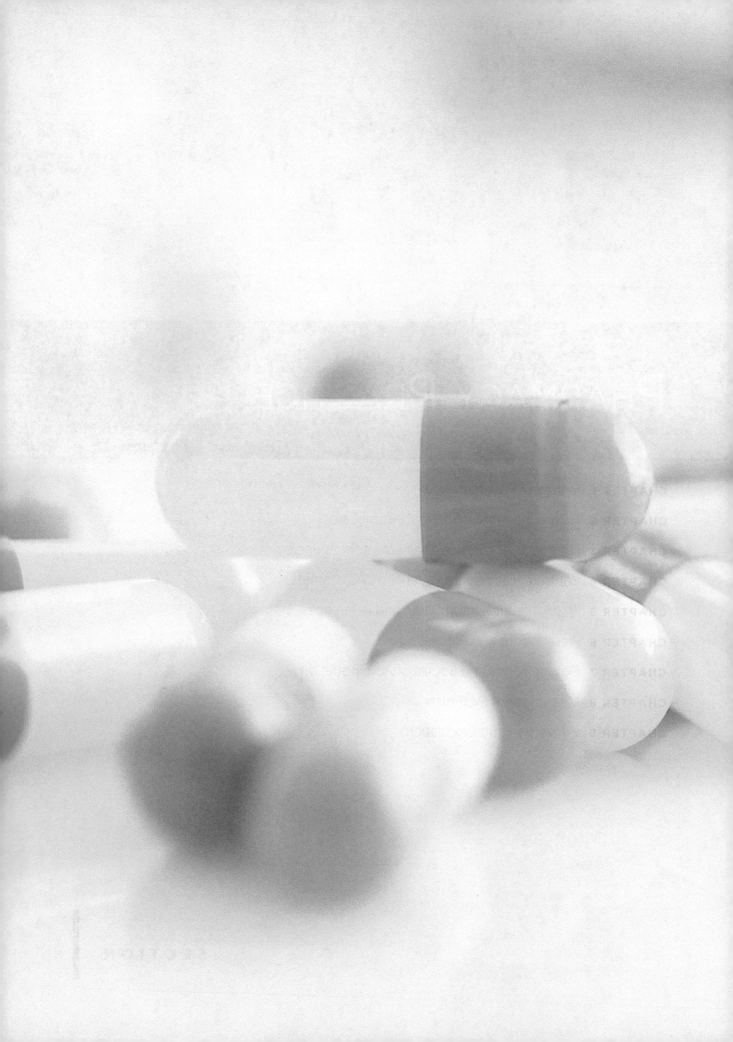

History of Pharmacy

OUTLINE

OBJECTIVES

Upon completion of this chapter, the reader should be able to:

1. Describe the historical evolution of the profession of pharmacy.
2. Discuss Hippocrates, the "father of medicine," and his role in the history of medicine.
3. Name the "father of botany" and the "father of toxicology."
4. Explain the establishment of the "pharmacy shop" operated by a pharmacist.
5. Describe the first attempts to regulate pharmacy.
6. Discuss the period of the Renaissance as it relates to the field of pharmacy.
7. Describe the Empiric Era and its impact on the field of pharmacy.
8. Explain the Industrialization Era and its impact on the field of pharmacy.
9. Describe the Patient Care Era and its impact on the field of pharmacy.
10. Discuss the future of the field of pharmacy.

KEY TERMS

biotechnology	genetic engineering	pharmacopeias	prescriptions
dosage form	immunity	pharmacy shop	vaccinations
formulary	pharmaceutical care		

Overview

Pharmacy is an ancient and intriguing profession that was once cloaked in mystery and reliant on closely guarded methods. The field of pharmacy is as old as humankind; yet it is ever changing and evolving. In studying the history of pharmacy, we find that its evolution parallels the evolution of humankind. Its history reflects the progress of societies based on their people and culture, religious beliefs, scientific abilities, geographic location, and participation in the events of war. Throughout time, pharmacy has evolved to meet the changing needs of the world's societies in their quest to treat and prevent disease. The development of the profession of pharmacy can be divided into five historical periods:

1. Ancient Through Early Modern Era—Human prehistory to AD 1500s
2. Empiric Era—1600 to 1940
3. Industrialization Era—1940 to 1970
4. Patient Care Era—1970 to present
5. Biotechnology and Genetic Engineering Era—The new horizon

Ancient Through Early Modern Era

One can make the case that ancient humans were the first pharmacists. Acting through natural instinct, they would have sought remedies for injuries and illnesses, using the materials that were available in their surroundings, such as leaves, mud, and cool water. Observing injured animals, they might have discovered many of the uses of natural materials. The methods used by animals to treat their injuries could thus have become the methods of early humans as well, such as using mud to pack wounds. Through trial, error, and observation, early humans would have learned which items were effective. For example, clay could be dried and used to splint broken bones.

As early humans evolved, they began to form larger social and cultural groups, such as tribes, that interacted with other well-organized groups. Many early cultures, like more recent indigenous people, likely believed that bad spirits caused diseases and that the cure for disease was to drive off the bad spirit from the sick person. One member of the tribe or group might have gained a reputation for possessing the ability to control spirits through spiritual rituals and the use of natural materials as techniques of healing. This person would have been held in high regard within the tribe or group—the equivalent of a religious leader, pharmacist, and physician all in one. These healers would have passed their knowledge of the healing rituals and techniques as well as the properties of medicinal plants and materials down to younger members.

CONTRIBUTIONS FROM EGYPT, MESOPOTAMIA, AND CHINA

Thousands of years ago, people in these early groups began to form larger, settled communities. They documented their knowledge of the world around them, including healing materials and methods, on clay tablets. In the region of ancient Mesopotamia in the city of Babylonia, the earliest known record of the practice of pharmacy was kept (around 2600 BC). From this Babylonian city, the science of drugs, organized pharmacy, and medicine had its beginnings. One of the earliest written records, known as the Ebers Papyrus (after Georg Ebers, who purchased it in 1872), was written in Egypt around 1500 BC. It contained formulas for more than 800 remedies (Figure 1-1).

In this same time period (about 2000 BC), the Chinese were developing an interest in herbs as having value in the cure of diseases. Shen Nung is reported (although not confirmed) to have written the first Pen T'sao, a native herbal treatise recording 365 drugs.

CONTRIBUTIONS FROM GREECE AND ROME

The first attempts to approach medicine and medicinal drugs scientifically were made in Greece around 600 BC. The Greeks began thinking logically about diseases rather than relying on spiritual explanations for physical phenomena. Hippocrates (about 460 to 377 BC), the "father of medicine," was a philosopher, physician, and pharmacist (Figure 1-2). He is credited with the separation of medicine from a religious context; he argued that disease was not a punishment but instead was caused by environmental factors. He is also known for authoring the Oath of Hippocrates; however, some feel that it was actually written after his death. This code of ethics is still used today.

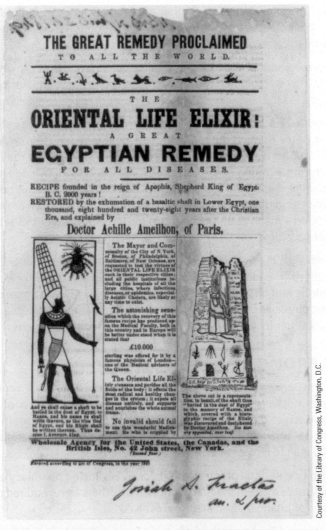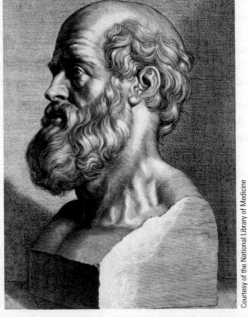

Figure 1-1 An advertisement of the discovery of an ancient Egyptian remedy in a New York newspaper in the early 1800s.

Figure 1-2 Hippocrates.

Theophrastus (about 371 to 287 BC), called the "father of botany," was an early Greek philosopher and scientist. He recorded observations about plants, classifying them by their various parts as well as their properties and uses. Much of his research and writing catalogued the medicinal properties of plants.

As the use of plants increased, some were found to produce adverse effects or to be poisons that could be used for murders. Mithridates (120 to 63 BC) studied the adverse effects of plants and later became known as the "father of toxicology." His experiments led to the discovery that small doses of toxins can help build an immunity to them.

As the ancient world began to expand its horizons, different groups came into conflict, beginning a period of frequent wars and conquest. As the Roman Empire expanded, it conquered the territory once held by the Greeks and adopted much of their culture. This was especially true in case of medicine. What the Romans added to the Greek system of knowledge was the organization of medical and pharmaceutical knowledge and the conversion of theory into rules and policies. Sometime during the first century AD, Dioscorides began this transition of the Greek system of knowledge to the Roman system of science. His written herbal treatise is known as *De Materia Medica* (*Of Medical Substances*) and was considered a major authority on drugs for 16 centuries. For this reason, some have considered him to be the "father of pharmacology."

Dioscorides' efforts to advance medical knowledge were followed by those of Galen (about AD 129 to 210), a Greek physician, who produced the great work *De Methodo Medendi* (*On the Art of Healing*). Galen's work further advanced the fields of medicine and pharmacy, and he became a highly revered figure in the history of these fields. Galen strongly believed that physicians should prepare their own remedies for treating disease and illness. Galen's preparations included natural organic substances prepared as various forms of liquids and ointments.

CONTRIBUTIONS FROM THE ARAB WORLD

The twin brothers Cosmos and Damien, the patron saints of pharmacy and medicine, represent the close relationship of these two fields. Both were Christians who practiced pharmacy and medicine in about AD 300. Cosmos and Damien did not charge for their services, yet they successfully cured many different illnesses in humans and animals. Their achievements included surgery, pharmaceutical preparations, compounding, urinalysis, and even the grafting of a leg from a recently deceased man to replace another man's cancerous leg.

After the fall of the Roman Empire, little progress was made in advancing pharmacy and medicine in the Western world. It was through the advances made in the Arab world, where others were required to perform the tasks relating to pharmacy, that the division of pharmacy and medicine evolved.

Three major advances occurred in pharmacy at this time: formularies, dosage forms, and pharmacy shops. The **formulary** was a continuation of the documentation of the knowledge of specific drug information intended for use by pharmacists and other preparers of medicine. The **dosage form** was introduced to the Western world. No longer were drugs harvested from the herb garden. They were now incorporated into sweetened dosage forms, such as syrups, conserves, confections, and juleps, all of which were mixed with sugar and honey. Thus, the myth that only bitter medicines were effective was disproved. The most significant advance was the establishment of the pharmacy shop operated by a pharmacist. The first **pharmacy shop** appeared in Baghdad in about AD 762. This is the earliest documentation of the existence and operation of a privately owned pharmacy shop.

The development of hospitals also played a role in the separation of pharmacy from medicine. In about 1190, a hospital in Marrakech had a room designated as a pharmacy. In the Arab world, once pharmacies were established, the duties, character, and responsibilities of a pharmacist were defined.

Transition from the Ancient to the Post-Classical World—Formalization of the Pharmacy Profession

A great change in attitudes occurred in the Western world during the transition from the classical period of Greece and Rome to the early Middle Ages. There was a greater interest in pharmacy and drug therapy, but the advances and knowledge of the Greek and the Arabic worlds had first to be transferred and then preserved for the Western world to advance. The monasteries of the Christian world were repositories of learning during this post-classical period, and the monks are credited with preserving much ancient knowledge that would otherwise have been lost.

The change in attitude toward this previously accumulated knowledge also resulted in the establishment of two centers of learning, one at Salerno, in southern Italy, and a second in Toledo, Spain. Salerno had a medical center that attracted students and patients. The school at Salerno, one of Europe's first universities, was responsible for major contributions to pharmacy and medicine.

The first attempts to regulate pharmacy appear to have occurred in southern Italy around the school in Salerno. In about the 12th century, guilds of pharmacists came into existence. The guilds provided pharmacists with an organization of their own in local towns. A very important event occurred between AD 1231 and 1240 when the Holy Roman Emperor Frederick II issued an edict regulating medicine. It contained the Magna Carta of Pharmacy, and it separated pharmacy from medicine. For the first time, an edict legally recognized pharmacy as a separate profession in Western Europe.

Beginning in the late Middle Ages, a period of accelerating societal change swept across Europe. These changes, which gave rise to the beginnings of modern science, culminated in the Renaissance, from AD 1400 to 1600. It was a period of rebirth of interest in the classical world, art, literature, philosophy, education, religion, and science that was characterized by the rise of secularism, individualism, and humanism. Theophrastus Philippus Aureolus Bombastus von Hohenheim, also known as Paracelsus, stimulated a revolution in pharmacy. He was a Swiss-born physician who emphasized a chemical rather than botanical orientation to medicine and contradicted the Galenic theories of the past (Figure 1-3). He believed that disease was a chemical manifestation and should be treated chemically.

During this time, monasteries remained important centers of learning for pharmacy. The monasteries maintained their own pharmacies to treat the poor. As a political unit, the city-state structure of the early Middle Ages began to decline in power and larger country/nation-states began to evolve, with increased governing power. Along with these changes, the practice of pharmacy began to vary from country to country. The guilds assumed the power of

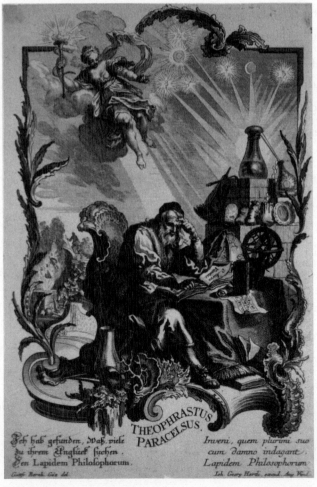

Figure 1-3 Paracelsus.

self-regulation, serving as the governing body of the profession of pharmacy. They gained in strength over time and set educational standards and experiential requirements that had to be met before an individual could practice pharmacy.

In many cases, the pharmacist did not have a friendly relationship with physicians. The pharmacist was often associated with "spicers" (those dealing in spices). In small towns, the pharmacist was forced into the same guild as the spicers. Physicians contended that pharmacists were ignorant of the medical profession, diagnosed and prescribed though they were unqualified, and were constantly making errors in compounding and dispensing. This conflict continued well into the 18th century. The Germans more tightly controlled the practice of pharmacy. While the rest of the world controlled the practice of pharmacy through the self-governing of the guilds, Germany used governmental controls to regulate the profession of pharmacy.

The royalty of various countries created another role for the pharmacist, that of Court Apothecary or Royal Apothecary, who provided pharmacy and other services to the royal family. This was a prestigious and honored position, and such court-sponsored pharmacists were usually quite wealthy.

The Renaissance was also a period in which new areas of the world were explored. During this exploration, new medicinal herbal substances from plants, trees, and seeds were sought and found. With these discoveries came a desire to document and preserve this new knowledge in herbal treatises, called **pharmacopeias**, and handbooks.

In summary, beginning in the late Middle Ages and continuing into the Renaissance and beyond, pharmacy went through many changes:

- Pharmacy became an independent profession separated from the physician.
- The profession of pharmacy achieved greater status and became socially accepted.
- Regulations increased the integrity and performance of the profession.
- An extensive pharmaceutical literature was created.
- University education of pharmacists was required.
- Importation of larger quantities of known drugs occurred.
- Importation of new drugs from the New World and Asia occurred.
- New chemical medicines were introduced that gave pharmacists broader expertise.

POINTS TO REMEMBER

The early development pharmacy can be summarized as follows:

- 2600 BC—The earliest known written documentation of pharmaceutical information is made on clay tablets.
- 2000 BC—Chinese Pen T'sao records 365 herbal drugs.
- 1500 BC—A papyrus containing more than 800 remedies is written in Egypt—it is later purchased by Georg Ebers; it becomes known as "The Ebers Papyrus."
- 460 to 377 BC—Lifespan of Hippocrates, the "father of medicine."
- 371 to 287 BC—Lifespan of Theophrastus, the "father of botany."
- 120 to 63 BC—Lifespan of Mithridates, the "father of toxicology."
- AD 50 to 70—Dioscorides pens *De Materia Medica* (*Of Medical Substances*).
- AD 129 to 210—Lifespan of Galen, who wrote *De Methodo Medendi* (*On the Art of Healing*).
- AD 762—The first pharmacy shop appears, in Baghdad.
- AD 1190—A hospital in Marrakech has a room designated as a pharmacy.

- AD 1231 to 1240—Holy Roman Emperor Frederick II issues an edict regulating medicine that contains the Magna Carta of Pharmacy.
- AD 1400 to 1600—The Renaissance, and the beginnings of modern science.

Empiric Era

During the Renaissance, pharmacists in Continental Europe had attained impressive social status and recognition as health care providers. Their actions were, however, still tightly controlled through self-regulation, quasi-governmental control, and governmental control. The medical profession also carefully watched them. The pharmacopeias became a regulatory tool used by governments to protect public health through standardization of medicines. Governmental control also guaranteed that pharmacists compounded and dispensed medicine.

Scientific knowledge had not yet become highly developed during this time. Knowledge of anatomy, physiology, and biochemistry was extremely limited or nonexistent. Nonetheless, the effectiveness of many of the medicines included in the popular pharmacopeias began to be questioned. A typical pharmacopeia contained three sections, as listed in Table 1-1.

Table 1-1 A Typical Pharmacopeia		
Section I	**Section II**	**Section III**
Vegetables	Composita galencia (galenicals)	Chemical compositions
Roots	Distilled waters	Mercury
Barks	Spirits	Antimony (a toxic metallic element)
Herbs	Distilled vinegars	Sulfur
Leaves	Tinctures	
Flowers	Elixirs	
Fruits	Decoctions (which utilize boiling to extract water-soluble substances and flavors)	
Seeds	Simple syrups	
Gums	Compound syrups	
Resins	Purging compound syrups	
Balsams	Aromatic powders	
Fungi	Extracts	
	Troches	
Animalia	Expressed oils	
	Distilled oils	
Mineralia	Balsams	
	Unguents	
Metalla	Plasters	
	Cerates (hard ointments or medicated pastes)	
Lapides et salia terrae (salt of the earth and stones)		
Marina		

Eventually, many medicines of questionable benefit were purged from these texts. This questioning also created an interest in testing of drugs and especially an interest in the toxicological effects of drugs and how medicines worked in the human body.

PHARMACY IN THE NEW WORLD

Pharmacy in the New World was a reflection of pharmacy in Europe (e.g., France, Spain, Italy, and England). Pharmacists did not participate in the colonization of the New World; thus it fell to physicians in these new lands to prepare their own remedies. The practice of pharmacy did not begin to develop in the British colonies until the 18th century. Benjamin Franklin organized the first American hospital in Philadelphia in 1751. It had a pharmacy, and the first hospital pharmacist was Jonathan Roberts. During the early colonial period in America, there was little control over the practice of pharmacy. In 1789, the College of Philadelphia employed a "professor of material medica and pharmacy." In 1821, the Philadelphia College of Pharmacy was founded.

William Procter, Jr. (1817 to 1874), who later became known as the "father of American pharmacy," was the greatest influence on the practice of pharmacy during this time (Figure 1-4). He devoted his time and attention to the advancement of pharmacy. He was the owner of an apothecary shop, an editor, a leader in organizing the profession of pharmacy, a teacher, and scientist. Procter was elected in 1846 to the newly formed chair of Professorship of Pharmacy at the Philadelphia College of Pharmacy. As a leader in organizing the profession of pharmacy, Procter introduced control into the practice of pharmacy in America.

POINTS TO REMEMBER

- 1751—Benjamin Franklin started the first hospital in America.
- 1817 to 1874—The lifespan of William Procter, Jr., the "father of American pharmacy."

The development of the modern drugstore in the United States can be traced to the four options available to people in the 18th century who wanted to purchase medications:

- The "dispensing doctor"
- The apothecary shop
- The general store
- The wholesale druggist

In the late 1800s, a mixture of opium and alcohol (usually *sherry*) known as *laudanum* was extremely popular. It was used widely as a tonic in both Europe and the United States, regardless of its actual potential to heal, and

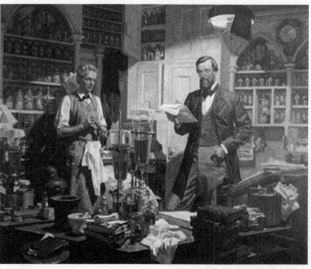

Courtesy of Walter Reed Army Institute of Research

Figure 1-4 William Procter, Jr.

many people became addicted. Conditions for which laudanum was used included insomnia, pain, anxiety, diabetes, diarrhea, gastrointestinal problems, menstrual pain, and morning sickness. The mixture was sometimes given to babies in an attempt to reduce crying episodes. Opium is a by-product of the poppy plant (*Papaver somniferum*). From this plant, opiates are made.

Monastic pharmacies began to decline in number toward the end of the 18th century as a result of competition with secular pharmacists. Continuing conflict between religion and political systems also led some monarchs to close pharmacies in the monasteries.

In the 19th century, Philadelphia became the center of the growing pharmaceutical industry, and in the middle of the century, the compounding of medications began to be a competitive activity between community pharmacists and the industry. Early manufacturers pioneered many medications, and some of these such as Merck and Squibb are still in business today. Medications began to be patented by their manufacturers.

Early in the 20th century, there was an emergence of research and development in the pharmaceutical industry, and industry-related pharmaceutical associations were created. Academic institutions and pharmaceutical companies began to collaborate on research. In the middle of this century, the generic pharmaceutical industry started. Near the end of the century, and into the 21st century, globalization occurred, with new biotechnologies being developed. The first *blockbuster drugs* were marketed, which were so named because they generated annual sales of at least $1 billion for their manufacturers. There began to be new business models in the industry. *Horizontal integration* is the process of a manufacturer increasing production of drug products at the same part of the supply chain, via internal expansions, acquisitions, or mergers with other companies. *Vertical integration* occurs when a company's supply chain is actually owned by the company. Both of these forms of integration became common in the pharmaceutical industry early in the 21st century.

Traditionally, there has been a "divide" between physicians and pharmacists, but their accepted roles have been redefined over time. Historically, the Bachelor of Science in Pharmacy degree was sufficient to start a career as a pharmacist. As of 2004, however, the PharmD degree became the new "entry-level" degree for all practicing pharmacists in the United States. The PharmD is a professional doctorate in pharmacy. The degree offers opportunities in research, clinical practice, teaching, industry, judicial, manufacturing, and many other areas. Generally, the total duration of college study to become an entry-level pharmacist is six to eight years. This combines three to four years of undergraduate prerequisite work as part of the bachelor degree and then three to four years of professional doctorate work.

EMERGENCE OF PHARMACY TECHNICIANS

During the Empiric Era, the first pharmacy technicians emerged as *pharmacy clerks*. Some of these clerks were individuals who had enlisted in the military. Because of great demand for medications related to war, they received on-the-job training and were allowed to fill **prescriptions** and perform some of the more basic duties of pharmacists. Other pharmacy clerks worked in drugstores owned by pharmacists. Standardized training for pharmacy technicians came about only in the 1960s.

DISCOVERY OF CHEMICALS AND MEDICINES

During the 17th and 18th centuries, pharmacists made major contributions to science in the area of chemistry. It was at this time that many chemicals were discovered and identified. Among these were sodium sulfate, ammonium sulfate, zinc chloride, oxygen, nitrogen, chlorine, glycerin, manganese, ammonia, some organic and inorganic acids, calomel, phosphorus, and ether. During the 18th century, the following medicines were identified: quinine, caffeine, morphine, hyoscyamine, codeine, atropine, niacin, diphtheria antitoxin, prontosil, adrenalin, penicillin, arsphenamine, phenobarbital, thyroxine, estrone, and testosterone. The 19th century brought with it the first sustained investigations in the field of organic chemistry. No major changes in pharmacy practice occurred in this period, but advances in chemistry paved the way for **vaccinations** against a variety of diseases, as well as the additional developments that would occur in the Industrialization Era (1940 to 1970).

HISTORY OF VACCINATIONS

The first established vaccination, against smallpox, was developed in 1796 by the English physician Edward Jenner. He took pus from a cowpox pustule and inserted it into an incision on an 8-year-old boy, basing this act on knowledge that people who developed the mild disease called *cowpox* never contracted the more serious disease *smallpox*.

Jenner proved that inoculation with cowpox resulted in **immunity** against smallpox. It took four years for the "experts" of the time to acknowledge that what Jenner had done was actually effective. Jenner is commonly referred to as "the father of immunology."

Beginning in 1877, French chemist and microbiologist Louis Pasteur made significant contributions to the history of vaccinations. Also known for his invention of pasteurization, in which bacteria are destroyed by heating foods (most often beverages) and then allowing them to cool, Pasteur's studies of germ theory led to the development of vaccinations against rabies and anthrax. Pasteur also pioneered the study of molecular asymmetry and helped to save the beer, wine, and silk industries in France from economic losses incurred through spoilage and disease.

In Germany, Emil Adolf von Behring discovered the antitoxins for tetanus, diphtheria, and typhoid fever. He identified both whooping cough and influenza and was instrumental in the development of the DPT (diphtheria, pertussis, and tetanus) and influenza vaccines. His significant works occurred between 1890 and 1945. The Nobel Prize was awarded to von Behring in 1901 for his contributions to medicine.

In the United States, Jonas Salk and Albert Sabin developed two different vaccines that have been widely used against polio. Vaccination programs using the Salk injectable and Sabin oral vaccines have led to near-eradication of polio in most of the world. Beginning in the 1970s, vaccine development came under the control of large pharmaceutical companies instead of individual researchers. Table 1-2 lists significant vaccine developments throughout history.

Table 1-2 Significant Vaccine Developments

Year of Establishment	Vaccine	Discoverer/Inventor
1796 (acknowledged in 1800)	Smallpox	Edward Jenner
1881	Anthrax	Louis Pasteur
1885	Rabies	Louis Pasteur, Emile Roux
1890	Tetanus	Emil Adolf von Behring
1892 to 1893	Cholera	Waldemar Haffkine
1896	Diphtheria, pertussis, tetanus (DPT)	Emil Adolf von Behring
1896	Typhoid	Almroth Edward Wright
1897	Bubonic plague	Waldemar Haffkine
1933	Influenza	Wilson Smith, Christopher Andrewes, Patrick Laidlaw
1955	Polio	Jonas Salk (inactivated, injectable vaccine)
1962	Polio	Albert Sabin (live, oral vaccine)
1970	Measles, mumps, rubella (MMR)	Maurice Hilleman
1974	Varicella (chickenpox)	Michiaki Takahashi
1977	Pneumonia	Robert Austrian
1978	Meningitis	Various scientists working at Sanofi Pasteur
1981	Hepatitis B	Various scientists working at GlaxoSmithKline
1992	Hepatitis A	Various scientists working at GlaxoSmithKline
1998	Lyme disease	Various scientists working at SmithKline Beecham
2006	Human papillomavirus	Various scientists at the University of Queensland, Australia
2006	Varicella-zoster virus (shingles)	Various scientists working at Merck

(Continued)

Table 1-2 Significant Vaccine Developments *(Continued)*		
Year of Establishment	**Vaccine**	**Discoverer/Inventor**
2009	Swine flu (H1N1)	Various scientists working at CSL Limited, MedImmune, Novartis, and Sanofi Pasteur
2009	Cervical cancer	Various scientists working at GlaxoSmithKline
2010	Influenza H3N2	Various scientists working at Protein Sciences Corporation
2010	Streptococcus pneumoniae	Various scientists working at Wyeth Pharmaceuticals
2011	Meningococcal disease (in infants and toddlers)	Various scientists working at Sanofi Pasteur
2012	Combination meningococcal and Hib (for infants)	Various scientists working at GlaxoSmithKline
2013	Hand-foot-mouth disease	Various scientists working at Sinovac Biotech
2014	HPV, meningococcal influenza	Various scientists working at Merck
2015	Meningitis	Various scientists working at GlaxoSmithKline
2016	Cholera	Various scientists working at Pax Vax Bermuda

Industrialization Era

Industrialization contributed to the practice of pharmacy in the United States in the setting of three major wars: the Civil War, World War I, and World War II. These conflicts led to the development of weapons capable of causing increasingly numerous casualties. This, in turn, led to greater demand for medicines and medical procedures to treat the injured. The demand was so great that the processes in place at the time for producing medications were inadequate to meet the need. Industrial manufacturing processes were developed to produce the quantities of drugs required during a major war.

In an article presented to the American Pharmacy Association at its annual convention in Detroit in 1914, Dr. Frank O. Taylor stated that "[u]p to the time of the early sixties [1860] it had been the almost universal custom for each pharmacist to prepare for himself such *galenical* preparations as he needed, but about this time several firms began manufacturing work on a small scale, developing this in most cases in retail drugstores that had been established for some years. The idea of centralized manufacture of medicinal preparations was just in its infancy and was probably not recognized as such at that time. ..." He then described four periods in the development of manufacturing (i.e., industrial) pharmacy, which were later expanded to eight periods (see Table 1-3).

POINTS TO REMEMBER

The most important manufacturing advance in the industrialization of the practice of pharmacy was the development of new machines for rapid mass production of medicines.

Although the roots of industrial pharmacy practice can be found in the retail pharmacy, its development did not proceed without opposition. Many retail pharmacists protested against what they viewed as an encroachment upon their professional practice. Ironically, both types of pharmacy practice (industrial and retail) survived and still have a role in the profession of pharmacy. The new scientific discoveries of the Industrialization Era contributed the following advancements to the practice of pharmacy: standardization, biologically prepared products, complex chemical

Table 1-3 Periods in the Development of Industrial Pharmacy

Original four	Formative Period (1867 to 1874)
	Botanical Research Period (1875 to 1882)
	Standardization Period (1882 to 1894)
	Biological Period (1895 to present)
Added at later date	Organic Chemical Synthesis, beginning in 1883
	Hormones, beginning in 1901
	Vitamins, beginning in 1909
	Antibiotics, beginning in 1940

synthesis, and the increasing use of parenteral medications. There was also a greater acceptance by the public of the attractive products that were mass-produced. Retail pharmacists became more accepting of the ease and convenience of dispensing the products of mass production. They also realized that industry-prepared products were new creations or specialties and that preparation of these products was not within the means of the average retail pharmacy. In the end, retail pharmacy not only survived the growth of the pharmaceutical industry but also experienced increased sales volumes itself. There were two reasons for this:

1. The pharmaceutical industry created new needs that were advantageous to the retail pharmacy.
2. The retail pharmacy had proved to be indispensable and irreplaceable as the fitting and distributing agency of medicinal products. Even today, there is a limit to the centralization, mechanization, and standardization that is possible in medicine and pharmacy.

Research, another focus of industry, began to proliferate during this period. Investigation into medicines and their effects occurred in some form throughout all the eras of pharmaceutical development. However, advances in the basic sciences—biology, chemistry, and physics—had to occur before systematic research focused on identifying medicines could realize substantial success. The phenomenal expansion of research that resulted was supported financially by the pharmaceutical industry.

One of the most important discoveries of the 20th century occurred in 1928 when Scottish bacteriologist and physician Alexander Fleming mistakenly contaminated a bacteria sample with penicillium mold. The active substance that Fleming named "penicillin" slowed growth of the bacteria. In 1938, mass-produced penicillin became available, resulting in effective treatment of many bacteriological diseases worldwide. This revolutionary antibiotic is still used today.

The 20th century also saw increased regulation of the pharmaceutical industry. These laws and their impact on the field of pharmacy are discussed in Chapter 3.

Patient Care Era

The beginning of the Patient Care Era was marked by increased concentration on the development of new medicines, especially by pharmaceutical manufacturers. This focus produced an expanding collection of medicines with a greater number of pharmacological activities. Well-coordinated teams of scientists (biologists, chemists, engineers, physicians, pharmacists, and toxicologists) and other professionals (statisticians and financial managers) now performed research. Pharmaceutical research moved from the empirical and intuitive identification of drugs to a rational, targeted approach. This new approach facilitated development of ideal drugs to meet specific needs using computerized methods. Through these efforts, many new drugs have been developed, making major contributions to the health and well-being of humankind.

With the plethora of new drugs came many complications. Multiple drug therapy led to adverse drug reactions, drug interactions (with other drugs, foods, and laboratory tests), and different outcomes with sub- or supertherapeutic doses. As a result of these complications, the public's expectations of the profession of pharmacy changed. A more demanding and educated public now expected the pharmacist to be a therapeutic advisor and patient advocate when pharmaceutical services were provided. The patient advocacy role creates an expectation among patients that the pharmacist will ensure that the maximal outcome is achieved with minimal harmful effects from their drug therapy. This patient-focused approach to drug therapy, which concentrated on the drug, was thought of as "drug review" or "drug monitoring." However, the new role did not relieve the pharmacist of the responsibility of dispensing medications. To incorporate the dispensing role with the patient care role, C. D. Hepler established the concept of **pharmaceutical care** in the late 1980s. This concept expands the role of the profession from that of dispensing drugs to include all aspects of drug therapy. As the role of the pharmacist continues to evolve, pharmacy education will need to be not only be scientifically based but also focused on human behavior as it relates to the provision of patient-focused care.

POINTS TO REMEMBER

Education in human behavior, communication management, and problem-solving skills is essential to prepare pharmacists to practice in the new environment.

Biotechnology and Genetic Engineering—The New Horizon

We are at the beginning of a new era in the field of pharmacy. Extensive research in the area of gene therapy is being conducted with the goal of developing new treatments for diseases related to genetic defects. The hope is that by modifying the genetic makeup of a patient with such a disease, a total or partial cure may be achieved. **Genetic engineering** is the scientific alteration of the structure of genetic material in a living organism.

Biotechnology is the use of microorganisms to produce specific drugs, synthetic hormones, and other medical products. Limited numbers of medications are being produced through recombinant DNA technology. Some of today's medications are available from natural sources, but these tend to produce allergic reactions in patients due to naturally occurring proteins. An early product produced by this method was insulin. Some other products produced by this method are used as therapies for cancer, anemia, and hepatitis.

Summary

Pharmacy is a profession with roots in human prehistory. It has evolved in parallel with the evolution of humans. The earliest "drugs" were products taken from nature. Human curiosity sparked a basic desire to determine why and how these drugs worked and to develop more drugs to treat more illnesses. Thus, in the evolution of pharmacy, the focus was first on botanical drugs and then on chemicals. Galen was a Greek physician who greatly influenced the practices of medicine and pharmacy and was critical of physicians who did not prepare their own remedies.

During the Renaissance, the profession of pharmacy went through many changes. In the 1700s and 1800s, throughout Europe and America, opium was commonly mixed with alcohol and used as a tonic; as a result, many people became addicted to the drug. The first established vaccination, against smallpox, was developed by the English physician Edward Jenner. The first pharmacy technicians emerged during the Empiric Era as pharmacy clerks, but standardized training for pharmacy technicians came about only in the 1960s. One of the most important discoveries of the 20th century occurred in 1928, when Alexander Fleming isolated penicillin.

Future therapies may come from the biotechnological processes or from the gene modification process. Genetic engineering is the scientific alteration of the structure of genetic material in a living organism. Chemicals yet to be discovered and synthesized may change the way a disease is treated, or even produce a cure for cancer or the common cold. The future of pharmacy lies in the new forms of research yet to come.

1. Jonathan Roberts is known as the:

    A. father of pharmacology.
    B. father of toxicology.
    C. first American hospital pharmacist.
    D. father of botany.

2. Benjamin Franklin is known as the:

    A. father of American pharmacy.
    B. patron saint of pharmacy.
    C. father of medicine.
    D. founder of the first American hospital.

3. Hippocrates is known as the:

    A. father of American pharmacy.
    B. patron saint of pharmacy.
    C. father of medicine.
    D. founder of the first American hospital.

4. Cosmos and Damien are known as the:

    A. fathers of American pharmacy.
    B. patron saints of pharmacy and medicine.
    C. fathers of medicine.
    D. founders of the first American hospital.

5. Who was the "father of toxicology"?

    A. Mithridates
    B. Cosmos
    C. Benjamin Franklin
    D. William Procter

6. William Procter is known as the:

    A. father of pharmacology.
    B. father of toxicology.
    C. father of American pharmacy.
    D. father of botany.

7. The establishment of the "pharmacy shop," operated by a pharmacist, first occurred in:

    A. Baghdad.
    B. Rome.
    C. Salerno.
    D. Spain.

8. The "father of pharmacology" was:

    A. Benjamin Franklin.
    B. Mithridates.
    C. Dioscorides.
    D. William Procter.

9. Industrial pharmacy found its roots in:

    A. medicine.
    B. biology.
    C. the monastery.
    D. retail pharmacy.

10. In which of the following civilizations did people first begin thinking logically about diseases rather than relying on spiritual explanations for physical phenomena?

   A. Greece
   B. Egypt
   C. Persia
   D. China

11. The historical era that heralded the beginnings of modern science is known as:

   A. the Industrialization Era.
   B. the Iron Age.
   C. the Renaissance.
   D. the New Age.

12. Hippocrates was a:

   A. physician.
   B. pharmacist.
   C. philosopher.
   D. All of the above.

13. Who of the following was a highly revered figure in the history of medicine and pharmacy whose great work was called *On the Art of Healing*?

   A. Galen
   B. Mithridates
   C. Hippocrates
   D. Shen Nung

14. A great change in attitudes, with greater interest in pharmacy and drug therapy, occurred in which part of the world?

   A. European
   B. Far Eastern
   C. Western
   D. Middle Eastern

15. The use of microorganisms to produce drugs, synthetic hormones, or other medical products is called:

   A. genetic engineering.
   B. bioengineering.
   C. biotechnology.
   D. genetic technology.

CRITICAL THINKING

1. Create a timeline establishing the history of pharmacy through each era. Be sure to name the key events that shaped the profession as well as the key individuals who contributed to it.

2. Research the early attempts to regulate pharmacy. What were the reasons for establishing such regulations? What were the advantages and disadvantages of regulation to pharmacy as a profession?

3. What are the goals of biotechnology and gene research? How do you think this will change pharmacy as it is known today?

4. When was the concept of pharmaceutical care developed? How did it affect the roles of the pharmacist?

WEB LINKS

American Institute of the History of Pharmacy: pharmacy.wisc.edu/aihp/

Ebers Papyrus: www.crystalinks.com/egyptmedicine.html

Genetic Engineering & Biotechnology News: www.genengnews.com

History of Vaccines: www.historyofvaccines.org

History of Vaccines and Immunization: www.healthaffairs.org/doi/full/10.1377/hlthaff.24.3.611

Kentucky Renaissance Pharmacy Museum: pharmacymuseumky.org

MedicineNet.com: www.medicinenet.com

READING LIST

Anderson, S. (2013). *Making Medicines: A Brief History of Pharmacy and Pharmaceuticals*. Chicago: Pharmaceutical Press.

Flannery, M. A., and Humphreys, M. (2017). *Civil War Pharmacy: A History*, 2nd ed. Carbondale: Southern Illinois University Press.

Gerald, M. C. (2013). *The Drug Book: From Arsenic to Xanax, 250 Milestones in the History of Drugs*. New York: Sterling.

Zebroski, B. (2015). *A Brief History of Pharmacy: Humanity's Search for Wellness*. Abingdon-on-Thames, England: Routledge.

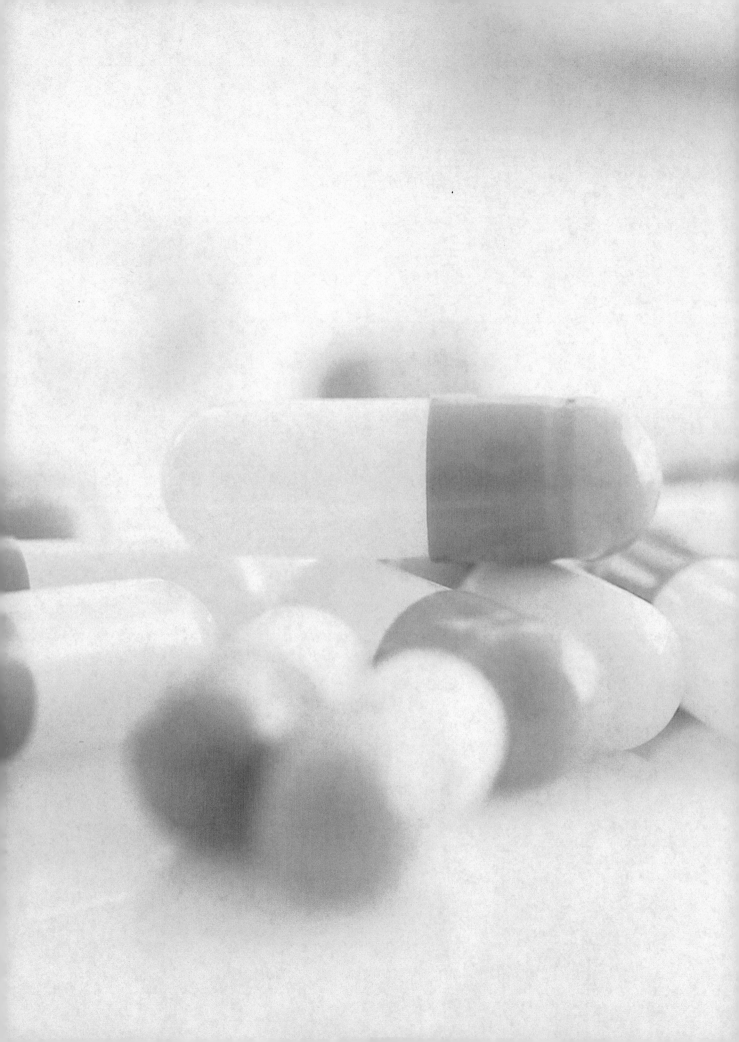

CHAPTER 2

The Foundation of Pharmaceutical Care

OUTLINE

The Profession of Pharmacy

Educational Requirements

The Pharmacist

The Pharmacy Technician

The Role of the Pharmacy

Providing Services to the Community

Responsibility to Those Being Served

Professional Organizations

American Association of Colleges of Pharmacy

American Association of Pharmaceutical Scientists

American Association of Pharmacy Technicians

American College of Clinical Pharmacy

Accreditation Council for Pharmacy Education

American Pharmacists Association

American Society of Health-System Pharmacists

National Pharmacy Technician Association

Pharmacy Technician Certification Board

Pharmacy Technician Educators Council

United States Pharmacopeia

Code of Ethics

Job Opportunities

OBJECTIVES

Upon completion of this chapter, the reader should be able to:

1. Discuss the characteristics that make the practice of the pharmacy technician a profession.
2. Identify the nine general areas in which skills will be measured on the Pharmacy Technician Certification Exam.
3. Identify the three general areas in which skills are measured on the ExCPT exam.
4. Explain why continuing education is important for the pharmacy technician.
5. Explain quality control of drugs and define the term "quality control unit."
6. Name five professional organizations related to the field of pharmacy.
7. Explain the United States Pharmacopeia (USP).

8. Explain the role of the American Society of Health System Pharmacists (ASHP).

9. Describe job opportunities for pharmacy technicians.

KEY TERMS

assay and control unit	drug control	licensed	profession
certified	ethics	nondiscretionary	quality control
competencies	externships	outpatient	quality control unit
confidentiality	inpatient	pharmacy	registered
continuing education	internships	preceptor	United States Pharmacopeia (USP)

Overview

A **profession** is an occupation or career that requires specialized education, ongoing training, and knowledge. Professionals have a specialized knowledge base that others do not possess but of which they are in need. Those who provide professional services thus fulfill a societal need. Therefore, professionals have certain social and societal obligations to apply their knowledge for the good of the communities in which they work. The following are examples of several characteristics that classify particular fields as professions:

- A specialized body of knowledge based upon advanced education that continues to expand throughout a person's career

- Provision of a unique service to society

- Responsibility to those being provided the service

- Membership that shares a common identity, values, and belief system

- A code of **ethics** (set of standards)

Pharmacy professionals are concerned with matters that are vital to the health or well-being of their patients. This chapter examines the characteristics of the field of pharmacy that make it a profession.

The Profession of Pharmacy

Pharmacy is the art and science of dispensing and preparing medications and providing drug-related information to the public. It involves interpreting prescription orders; compounding, labeling, and dispensing drugs and devices; selecting drug products and conducting drug utilization reviews; monitoring patients; and providing educational services related to the use of medications and devices. Today, pharmaceutical care is a necessary element of total health care. Pharmacists and pharmacy technicians perform highly useful social and health care–related functions. They improve the quality of life of patients by assisting in the prevention and cure of diseases and disease processes. They share common identities, values, and belief systems with the other members of the medical community with whom they interact. The pharmacist and pharmacy technician should value the provision of truthful, accurate, understandable information to ensure minimal patient risk. All pharmacy personnel should also take care to treat everyone equally, without prejudice toward race, religion, social or marital status, sex, sexual orientation, age, or health. The wishes of competent patients who refuse medication, treatments, or services should be observed, and the dignity of patients with diminished competence should be respected.

POINTS TO REMEMBER

The profession of pharmacy focuses on ensuring that patients receive the proper medication for their specific medical conditions.

Educational Requirements

As stated earlier, one of the characteristics of a profession is a specialized body of knowledge. This begins with furthering one's education beyond high school. There are two career paths in the field of pharmacy: pharmacist and pharmacy technician. Each of these careers has specific educational requirements and skill sets.

THE PHARMACIST

As reported by the American Association of Colleges of Pharmacy (AACP), as of 2012, overall enrollment at pharmacy schools totaled over 61,000 people, with women's enrollment numbers exceeding those of men. Enrollment in colleges of pharmacy has been increasing steadily since 1984. In 1992, a majority of pharmacy colleges voted to change the type of professional degree awarded from the bachelor of pharmacy (BS Pharm) degree to the doctor of pharmacy (PharmD) degree. The BS Pharm degree is no longer awarded. According to the AACP, a PharmD degree requires two years of undergraduate study followed by four years of graduate study. Either the Pharm D or the BS Pharm degree fulfills the requirements for taking the licensure examination of a state board of pharmacy (BOP) to practice pharmacy. The boards of pharmacy found in the United States and the National Association of Boards of Pharmacy (NABP) oversees its territories. The organization's website is www.nabp.net.

The Role of the Pharmacist

Pharmacists are professionals who have had advanced training in the pharmaceutical sciences. In all states, pharmacists must be **licensed** by their state's BOP before they can practice pharmacy and must follow the BOP's regulations when they practice. A license is permission granted by a government agency to practice in a particular field. As in the profession of medicine, pharmacy practice has become much more specialized in the past 25 years. Specialties in pharmacy may include ambulatory care, pharmacy administration, drug information, community practice, geriatrics, industry, managed care, long-term care, home health care, oncology, pediatrics, psychiatric pharmacy, nuclear pharmacy, and nutritional support. Table 2-1 lists the basic duties of the pharmacist.

THE PHARMACY TECHNICIAN

There are several degree options for individuals interested in becoming pharmacy technicians: certificate programs, diploma programs, and associate degree programs.

The certificate program can be completed in less than a year of study. It provides education in the fundamental skills needed to work in retail and clinical environments. A high school diploma is the basic requirement for this program.

A diploma program is generally a year-long program of study. This type of program focuses on application of skills in addition to foundational knowledge. Individuals pursuing this option of study may already have had a health background acquired through study of another allied health field such as medical assisting; however, this is not a requirement.

Table 2-1 The Basic Duties of the Pharmacist
Initiating, adjusting, or renewing medication orders/prescriptions based on knowledge and expertise
Using a drug list recommended by the Pharmacy and Therapeutics Committee
Monitoring dosages for continuing patients
Assisting consumers to choose the most appropriate over-the-counter medications
If required, assisting in administration of oral and parenteral (administered by a route other than through the gastrointestinal system) medications, performing venipunctures, and administering intravenous fluids
Signing all entries in the medical records
Ordering tests and laboratory studies appropriate for the medications they are approved to initiate, adjust, or renew
Offering consultation as required on the substances they control

The core requirements included in the two-year associate degree program for pharmacy technicians are the following: administrative and professional aspects of pharmacy, medical terminology, pharmaceutical calculations, anatomy, pathophysiology, pharmacology, drug distribution systems, intravenous admixture procedures, medication packaging techniques, customer relations, study of health care delivery systems, and current issues in the practice of pharmacy. The training at this level is more broadly based and generally includes externships in the field.

POINTS TO REMEMBER

In all states, licensed pharmacists supervise the activities of pharmacy technicians and are held accountable for the technicians' performance.

The Role of the Pharmacy Technician

Pharmacy technicians assist licensed pharmacists by completing tasks that do not require the professional judgment of a pharmacist to ensure accuracy. The role of the pharmacy technician has been expanding in recent years, and the number of pharmacy technicians is increasing. Pharmacy technicians now perform many clerical and technical tasks that were previously performed by pharmacists. The training and certification of pharmacy technicians expands their role within the profession, which ultimately allows the pharmacist to spend more time delivering pharmaceutical care services that require his or her professional judgment. All pharmacy technicians perform many different **nondiscretionary** (tasks required by an employer) duties in the pharmacy setting. A pharmacy technician's duties are *all* considered to be nondiscretionary, since they are required to be performed in an *exact* manner, following the guidelines of the supervising pharmacist or the pharmacy manager.

Recent studies indicate that pharmacy technicians are now involved in wider areas of pharmacy practice. These studies show that in addition to assisting with prescription preparation and dispensing, many pharmacy technicians participate in purchasing, inventory control, billing, filling hospital unit-dose medication carts, compounding (mixing) intravenous (IV) solutions, labeling and filling prescriptions, reviewing insurance information, and repackaging products. Educational requirements for pharmacy technicians include preparation for work in any number of health care facilities and retail establishments. These include hospitals, medical centers, teaching facilities, **outpatient** (outside of the hospital) clinics, urgent care centers, health maintenance organizations (HMOs), and retail and wholesale pharmacies.

Most hospital pharmacy technicians assist with **inpatient** (care within the hospital) medication dispensing and may also prepare intravenous admixtures and engage in compounding of nonsterile preparations, repackaging, purchasing, and billing. The basic duties of the pharmacy technician in institutional and community pharmacies are discussed in detail in Chapters 11 and 12.

Obtaining Experience

For pharmacy technicians, many colleges offer **externships**, which are short-term student work programs. Usually, each student completes one community pharmacy externship in an ambulatory or outpatient pharmacy and one at a hospital or other type of institutional pharmacy. When each of these begins, the student is assigned to an experienced practitioner called the **preceptor**, who offers instruction and supervision at the externship location. A variety of practical, hands-on learning experiences are given. The best externships offer instruction to students in tasks that are based on American Society of Health-System Pharmacists (ASHP) objectives, which are then assessed as to each student's strengths and weakness over a variety of skills.

Areas of assessment include communication, dispensing, documentation, error prevention, inventory, quality control, storage and drug product control, and work ethics. In community pharmacy settings, skills in billing and insurance are also assessed. Ambulatory pharmacy settings also assess skills in community dispensing and retail practice. Institutional pharmacies also assess medication orders and unit-dose cart filling skills. When the college does not offer externships, students can seek out to pharmacists and facilities to arrange externships on their own, which can be scheduled to work around their classes.

There are also **internships** that are official positions in which trained or semitrained individuals are hired to handle duties considered "entry-level" and work as apprentices under the guidance of experienced supervisors. Internships may be paid or unpaid. For pharmacy technicians, internships are usually paid and are intended for students in pharmacist programs. These positions are highly competitive. The individual interested in an internship has to apply as for any other job. Often, pharmacy technicians enter unofficial internships and work part-time. This may be in a community pharmacy's retail area. It can also be in a hospital, in nursing assistant, volunteer, or maintenance positions. Though considered "unskilled," these positions provide solid experience in the pharmacy setting. As students interact with staff members, they can develop potential references and contacts that will lead to full employment upon completion of their studies.

Certification Exam Preparation

Every state has unique requirements for the registration, licensure, and certification of pharmacy technicians. Most of the United States requires national certification or prefers pharmacy technicians to be nationally certified in order to become licensed and practice. Every year, more states require national certification. In states that have less requirements, many companies are deciding to require national certification for pharmacy technicians. This helps them improve their businesses and increase medication efficiency and safety. Most hospitals, since they need ongoing accreditation, are requiring national certification.

The ASHP has created a *model curriculum* as well as standards for accredited pharmacy technician education and training. It requires no less than 600 hours of work. This includes 360 or more hours of hands-on practice site experience, 160 hours of classroom work, and 80 hours of laboratory training. One task force of the NABP recommends that all state boards of pharmacy register or license pharmacy technicians. This requires standardized education and training guidelines.

Obtaining Certification as a Pharmacy Technician

Pharmacy technicians can choose to become **certified** in their profession. Taking and passing a standardized national exam one can obtain the certification. There are currently two national examination options: the Pharmacy Technician Certification Exam (PTCE) and the Exam for the Certification of Pharmacy Technicians (ExCPT). Certification is a valuable component for the pharmacy technician's career. More and more states are requiring certification for pharmacy technicians.

The Pharmacy Technician Certification Exam   The PTCE is prepared by the Pharmacy Technician Certification Board (PTCB) and tests competency in basic functions of the pharmacy and its activity. The exam blueprint was revised in 2013. In the new exam blueprint, content is organized into nine general knowledge areas:

1. Pharmacology for Technicians (13.75%)
2. Pharmacy Law and Regulations (12.5%)
3. Sterile and Nonsterile Compounding (8.75%)
4. Medication Safety (12.5%)
5. Pharmacy Quality Assurance (7.5%)
6. Medication Order Entry and Fill Process (17.5%)
7. Pharmacy Inventory Management (8.75%)
8. Pharmacy Billing and Reimbursement (8.75%)
9. Pharmacy Information Systems Usage and Application (10%)

The exam contains 90 multiple-choice questions, 10 of which are not actually scored. The nonscored questions are used for statistical purposes only. A score of at least 650 (of a possible 900) is required to pass. Once the pharmacy technician passes the exam, he or she is able to use the designation CPhT. Candidates can apply to take the exam online or by phone. The exam is offered year-round at test centers across the country for general applicants. Exams can also be completed at military test centers for people in the armed services and their families. In 2017, the PTCB expanded their eligibility parameters to allow high school students who are within 60 days of acquiring their high school diploma, or equivalent educational diploma, to take the PTCE. A graduation date must be provided when submitting an application for certification. The PTCB then requires proof of high school completion (or equivalent) to be provided before PTCB certification is granted.

National Healthcareer Association's ExCPT Exam   The ExCPT is also recognized by many states in America. Completion of the exam is required to become certified with the National Healthcareer Association (NHA) Pharmacy Technician Certification Program. This computerized exam is overseen and administered by the Institute for the Certification of Pharmacy Technicians (ICPT), a part of the NHA. The ExCPT is offered at various test centers across the

United States and can be scheduled online at www.nhanow.com. This exam contains 120 questions; 100 questions are scored and there are 20 pretest questions. The ExCPT exam is divided into three sections:

1. Regulations and Pharmacy Duties
2. Drugs and Drug Therapy
3. Dispensing Process

Most of the questions (52%) focus on dispensing of medications. Additional questions relate to pharmacy regulation and technician duties (25%) and drugs and drug products (23%).

The Dispensing Process section includes prescription information, preparing and dispensing prescriptions, pharmacy calculations, sterile products, unit doses, and repackaging. The Regulations and Pharmacy Duties section includes general technician duties, controlled substances, federal and state law, and federal/state/agency rules and regulations. The Drugs and Drug Therapy section includes drug classification, most frequently prescribed medications, dosage forms, and brand and generic drug names.

Comparing the PTCE and ExCPT Exams   The National Commission accredits both the ExCPT and the PTCE for Certifying Agencies (NCCA). Candidates for both exams must be at least 18 years of age. Costs for both exams are similar, with the PTCE usually costing slightly more. The exams are equally challenging but have different structures, and the ExCPT is more focused on community retail pharmacy. The PTCE is more aligned with the standards of the ASHP, requires background checks, and is accepted by all 50 states as a legitimate certification to practice. In nearly half of the United States, it is the only test described as a *practice standard*, and it is *required* by a few states, and also favored by hospitals and other institutional pharmacy settings. The questions in each exam assess similar **competencies** (skill sets). All questions for both exams are multiple choice, and the exams are 2 hours in duration. For both exams, pharmacy technicians must complete 20 continuing education credits within two years to remain certified. This must include one unit of continuing education in related law topics. Recertification costs $40 and is the same for both exams. To retake the PTCE, the candidate must wait 90 days, and to retake the ExCPT, 30 days. Both exams offer an online practice exam at similar costs. The PTCE is endorsed by the NABP. The National Association of Chain Drug Stores and the National Community Pharmacists Association (NCPA) endorse the ExCPT.

POINTS TO REMEMBER

Before deciding which exam to take, individuals must determine which organization is recognized by the BOP in their state. The PTCE is more widely recognized by states across the country because it has been in existence longer. Regardless of which exam you take, certification assures employers that you are qualified to work safely and effectively with medications and prescriptions, with licensed pharmacists, and in a pharmacy setting. The completion of either exam may improve your chances of employment and promotion.

POINTS TO REMEMBER

Certification is valid for two years. After this time, certification must be renewed with the fulfillment of 20 continuing education credits and must then be renewed.

WHAT WOULD YOU DO?

When you graduate from an accredited pharmacy technician program, what steps do you need to take in order to become certified?

Continuing Education

The practicing pharmacy technician must keep up with the changes that are occurring rapidly within the profession. Education does not end with the completion of formal training. The traditional roles of the pharmacist and the pharmacy technician are changing, and new services are being identified as functions for both. Therefore, a personal commitment to continue education is essential. Pharmacy technicians need to have a specialized body of knowledge about aspects of their job, including the various types of pharmacy practices they may work in (e.g., community or hospital settings), the constantly changing medications they may work with, and recognition of adverse effects and interactions of drugs. They will regularly assist the pharmacist in providing patient support, giving information to patients, attending to special needs of patients (especially of geriatric patients), and overseeing the use of nutritional supplements, in addition to being involved in packaging control, pharmacoeconomics, and even poison control.

Lifelong learning is becoming part of the philosophy of professional education, and, through it, a sustaining influence for nurturing of the profession is being supplied. The amount of medical knowledge is said to double every five years. By reading or reviewing the pharmacy literature that arrives in the daily mail and articles that appear in professional magazines and related newsletters one can learn much. **Continuing education** classes, seminars, and workshops are available to enhance the professional's knowledge of pharmacy and pharmacy affairs. Continuing education units (CEUs) are required to maintain certification as a pharmacy technician. A variety of apps can now be downloaded onto smartphones and tablets that also aid in staying up to date with the latest in research and drug information. One such app is Medscape; for more information, go to www.medscape.com.

POINTS TO REMEMBER

To become eligible for recertification every two years, certified pharmacy technicians must meet the requirements of obtaining 20 contact hours of pharmacy-related continuing education. At least 1 contact hour must be in pharmacy law, which can be accomplished through various means, such as an educational meeting.

Continuing education credits can be obtained through many sources, as long as they are pharmacy related and in the scope of practice for pharmacy technicians. Continuing education work can be found at the American Association of Pharmacy Technicians (AAPTs) and various other agencies, educational institutions, and online resources. CEUs are often awarded for participation in professional seminars and workshops.

WHAT WOULD YOU DO?

You became a certified pharmacy technician nearly two years ago. The certification period is close to expiring, and you must receive continuing education as part of your recertification process. What are your options for meeting the continuing education requirement?

The Role of the Pharmacy

The pharmacy has a role and responsibility within the communities served. The public trusts that the counseling and medications they receive from the pharmacy is sound and safe. The pharmacy, pharmacists, and staff need to live up to the standards and maintain that trust. There is a huge difference of opinion regarding how many roles the pharmacies and pharmacists should allow pharmacy technicians to play. Some states limit the roles of pharmacy technicians to only clerical duties. Certification is becoming more of a requirement, in more states, every year. Every pharmacy technician, as well as every pharmacist, must be extremely up to date on the pharmacy laws in his or her state and receive continuing education. With more knowledge, skills, and education, job duties for pharmacy technicians sometimes expand; this also means that salaries may increase.

Some pharmacies allow pharmacy technicians to regularly enter prescription orders into computers, which was formerly done only by pharmacists. Pharmacists are becoming more clinical, focusing on patient counseling and education, and interfacing with medical staff members. Many pharmacy technicians perform roles that were traditionally associated only with pharmacists. These include transcribing orders, retrieving medications from storage, and filling prescriptions. When a pharmacy technician is skilled at an advanced level and has received additional education, tasks assigned to him or her may be much more complex. More and more colleges now offer specialized pharmacy technician training. Specialty roles now being offered to technicians include education in compounding, immunizations, informatics, pharmacy industry changes, medication therapy management, and quality improvement.

PROVIDING SERVICES TO THE COMMUNITY

A pharmacy practice should maintain high standards of medication dispensing in serving the needs of its customers. Giving out proper information and offering fair prices are also important parts of the daily business in a pharmacy. To a lesser degree today than previously, because of the availability of prepackaged medications, specialized compounding (inside the pharmacy) is occasionally required. Accessible, quality pharmaceutical care, given with compassion and concern for patients, is essential to the success of the pharmacy. The pharmacy staff should continually strive to improve, regularly treating all customers with the dignity and respect they deserve. Other activities that are extensions of regular pharmacy practice include health fairs and fundraisers. These activities serve to heighten community awareness of support groups and available assistance for specific diseases and conditions.

RESPONSIBILITY TO THOSE BEING SERVED

Developing methods for standardization and control of medicinal agents is vital. In manufacturing laboratories, pharmacists often perform physical and chemical analyses either in the course of developing dosage forms of new products or in the control of standard products. In small laboratories, the responsibility for performing analyses may be delegated entirely to pharmacy staff members. However, even if pharmacists are not conducting analyses, they should at a minimum understand the basic principles involved in the standardization and control of the medicinal agents dispensed. The use of an analytical method is justified only after it has been proved to be valid, accurate, and selective. **Drug control** is the most important goal for a medication that may be taken by patients. Control is a method used to eliminate or reduce the potential harm of the drug distributed. Drug control is a means for providing knowledge, understanding, judgments, procedures, skills, and ethical standards that ensure optimal safety in distribution and use of medication.

Control of the Drug-Use Process

When multiple institutions such as hospitals, clinics, nursing homes, and drugstores (community pharmacies) are involved jointly in manufacturing, repackaging, and relabeling of drugs, they fall under the jurisdiction of the federal Food, Drug, and Cosmetic Act and, thus, government regulation. Control of quality is essential in the formulation, manufacture, and distribution of pharmaceutical products. This control serves to provide and maintain the desired features of purity, potency, and stability. These must fall within established levels so that all merchandise meets professional requirements, legal standards, and also additional standards that the management of a firm may adopt. The control of quality is the principle adopted by the Pharmaceutical Manufacturers Association, which applies equally to any institution whether a drug manufacturer or a pharmacy. Whatever control system is devised, it must be adequate and effective in attaining its purposes.

Pharmaceutical production presents many problems and conditions that make it a complicated operation, especially when the quantity prepared is large. **Quality control** must be built into the manufacturing process itself; it is not something that can be added after the product is made. Quality control is an organized effort of all individuals directly or indirectly involved in the production, packaging, and distribution of quality medications that are safe, effective, and acceptable. Its ultimate success depends upon the cooperation of all individuals. In hospital or community pharmacies, quality control not only should encompass formulation, compounding, and dispensing, but also must include packaging, purchasing, storage, and distribution of medication to the ultimate user, the patient. The total control of quality for drugs is a pharmacy department responsibility, but the responsibility for auditing the control system and evaluating product quality is that of a **quality control unit**, sometimes referred to as an **assay and control unit**. This unit is independent and reports to the director of pharmacy services. The assay and control, or quality control, unit may consist of a **registered** pharmacist supervisor and technicians, depending upon the scope of service. The supervisor of the quality control unit should have the authority to approve, reject, or order the reprocessing of products or procedures.

Today in the Pharmacy

Most states now require new pharmacists to earn a PharmD degree. After completing two to four years of undergraduate coursework, and then passing the Pharmacy College Admissions Test (PCAT), students can begin a four-year pharmacy program. Courses in this program include anatomy, biology, chemistry, and physics. PharmD students also complete rotations in many clinical and pharmaceutical facilities. Pharmacists previously working in pharmacies with

Bachelor of Science degrees in pharmacy are still able to practice without a PharmD degree. To become licensed, a pharmacist must pass the examination offered by the NABP, and any additional examination required by the laws of his or her state. The pharmacist of today must have excellent communication skills in order to communicate well with physicians, patients, and a large variety of health care professionals.

The pharmacy technicians of today must be skilled in many different areas. Some states require them to receive additional education and be trained on the job. There are still no nationally standardized requirements for them. In community pharmacies, technicians enter and maintain patient medications and histories. They prepare prescriptions, compound specialize medications, and manage inventory while assisting with third-party billing. In hospitals and other *inpatient pharmacies*, technicians prepare parenteral medications, supply floor stock, manage inventory needed for automated dispensing machinery, and transcribe physician orders. Other areas of work include long-term care, nuclear pharmacies, insurance companies, and call centers. These usually require specialized training for technicians. Regardless of where they work, pharmacy technicians must have excellent communication and organizational abilities.

The entry-level technician must be very familiar with pharmacy laws and regulations, pharmacology, compounding, inventory, billing, medication safety, and multiple technologies. Specialty certifications are available that will allow them to provide specialty services. Often, certification organizations, professional licensing boards, and state laws govern what pharmacy technicians are able to perform. Some pharmacy technicians work under pharmacist's supervision and assist in anticoagulation services, pharmacokinetics, review of laboratory results, determination of drug concentrations, and comparison of patient therapeutic responses. This helps pharmacists to make required changes in medication strength. Other pharmacy technician specialization areas include compounding, geriatrics, oncology, and pediatrics. Additional highly specialized training is available in hazardous drug compounding, sterile products, chemotherapy, and medication reconciliation.

Professional Organizations

Professional people in the field of pharmacy, like those in other fields, have created organizations or associations to advance the purposes of their professions. The most important organizations in the pharmacy profession are discussed in the following sections.

AMERICAN ASSOCIATION OF COLLEGES OF PHARMACY

The American Association of Colleges of Pharmacy (AACP), established in 1900, represents all 129 pharmacy colleges and schools in the United States and is the national organization representing the interests of pharmaceutical education and educators. The AACP publishes the *American Journal of Pharmaceutical Education* and a monthly newsletter, as well as other publications.

AMERICAN ASSOCIATION OF PHARMACEUTICAL SCIENTISTS

The American Association of Pharmaceutical Scientists (AAPSs), formerly an academy of the American Pharmacists Association, represents pharmaceutical scientists employed in academia, industry, government, and other research institutions. The AAPS publishes the journals *Pharmaceutical Research, AAPS PharmSciTech*, and *The AAPS Journal*, as well as a newsletter.

AMERICAN ASSOCIATION OF PHARMACY TECHNICIANS

The American Association of Pharmacy Technicians (AAPTs), formerly called the APT, was founded in 1979. It is a national organization and has chapters in many states. It represents pharmacy technicians and promotes certification of technicians. The association has established a Code of Ethics for Pharmacy Technicians.

AMERICAN COLLEGE OF CLINICAL PHARMACY

The American College of Clinical Pharmacy (ACCP) is a professional and scientific society that provides leadership, education, advocacy, and resources for clinical pharmacists.

ACCREDITATION COUNCIL FOR PHARMACY EDUCATION

Founded in 1932, the Accreditation Council for Pharmacy Education (ACPE) is the national accrediting agency for pharmacy education programs recognized by the U.S. Secretary of Education.

AMERICAN PHARMACISTS ASSOCIATION

The largest of the national pharmacy organizations, the *American Pharmacists Association (APhA)* consists of three academies: the Academy of Pharmacy Practice and Management (APhA-APPM), the Academy of Pharmaceutical Research and Science (APhA-APRS), and the Academy of Student Pharmacists (APhA-ASP). The APhA publishes the bimonthly *Journal of the American Pharmacists Association*, the monthly magazine *Pharmacy Today*, and the monthly *Journal of Pharmaceutical Sciences*. The APhA also operates a political action committee, or PAC. According to the APhA, its mission is "to advocate the interests of pharmacists; influence the profession, government, and others in addressing essential pharmaceutical care issues; promote the highest professional and ethical standards; and foster science and research in support of the practice of pharmacy."

AMERICAN SOCIETY OF HEALTH-SYSTEM PHARMACISTS

The American Society of Health-System Pharmacists (ASHPs) is a large organization that represents pharmacists who practice in hospitals, HMOs, long-term care facilities, home care agencies, and other institutions. The ASHP is a national accrediting organization for pharmacy residency and pharmacy technician training programs. The ASHP publishes the *American Journal of Health-System Pharmacy*.

The ASHP has established a model curriculum for pharmacy technician training that includes the following categories of goals: personal and interpersonal knowledge and skills, foundational professional knowledge and skills, processing and handling of medications and medication orders, sterile and nonsterile compounding, procurement, billing, reimbursement, inventory management, patient safety, medication safety, technology, informatics, regulatory issues, and quality assurance.

NATIONAL PHARMACY TECHNICIAN ASSOCIATION

The National Pharmacy Technician Association (NPTA) is the world's largest professional pharmacy technician organization. It is composed of pharmacy technicians from all types of pharmacy settings. The NPTA was designed to help pharmacy technicians realize their full potential by offering support services that encourage professional and personal growth. The NPTA was founded in 1999 in Houston, Texas, and releases publications and videos focused on the needs of pharmacy technicians.

PHARMACY TECHNICIAN CERTIFICATION BOARD

The Pharmacy Technician Certification Board (PTCB) publishes the PTCE, described earlier. Any pharmacy technician who wishes to be certified in the United States takes the computerized PTCE voluntarily. This organization also oversees a recertification program for technicians.

PHARMACY TECHNICIAN EDUCATORS COUNCIL

The Pharmacy Technician Educators Council (PTEC) is an association of educators who prepare people for careers as pharmacy technicians. Membership includes a discounted subscription to the *Journal of Pharmacy Technology*, which is published in conjunction with Sage Publications.

UNITED STATES PHARMACOPEIA

The **United States Pharmacopeia (USP)** is a nonprofit organization that sets standards for the identity, strength, quality, purity, packaging, and labeling of drug products. The USP provides drug information online. It is also referred to as the United States Pharmacopeial Convention.

Code of Ethics

A code of ethics serves to encourage respect and fair treatment for all patients. The following are basic principles that make up a code of ethics in the field of pharmacy:

1. Hold the health and safety of each patient to be of primary consideration.
2. Form a professional relationship with each patient.
3. Honor the autonomy, values, and dignity of each patient.
4. Respect and protect the patient's right of **confidentiality**.
5. Respect the rights of patients to receive pharmacy products and services, and ensure that these rights are met.
6. Observe the law, preserve high professional standards, and uphold the dignity and honor of the profession.
7. Continuously improve levels of professional knowledge and skills.
8. Cooperate with colleagues and other health care professionals so that maximum benefits to patients can be realized.
9. Contribute to the health care system and to the health needs of society.
10. Never condone dispensing, promoting, or distributing of drugs or medical devices that do not meet the standards of law or that lack therapeutic value for the patient.
11. Be fair and reasonable when it comes to the amount charged for medications and services.

The American Pharmacists Association published a *Code of Ethics for Pharmacists*. This code of ethics was adopted in 1994. The American Association of Pharmacy Technicians published a *Code of Ethics for Pharmacy Technicians*. It was originally published in the *American Journal of Health-Systems Pharmacists* in 2003. Chapter 3 provides more depth of discussion on ethical principles impacting the field of pharmacy.

WHAT WOULD YOU DO?

Greg was dispensing a prescription for a patient. Accidentally, he dropped a few capsules on the floor. He immediately picked them up and put them into the prescription container. If you were Greg, what would you have done in this situation?

Job Opportunities

Good job opportunities are expected for full-time and part-time work in the future, especially for pharmacy technicians with formal training or previous experience. Job openings for pharmacy technicians will result from the expansion of retail pharmacies and other employment settings, and from the need to replace workers who leave the field. Employment of pharmacy technicians is expected to grow much faster than the average for all occupations through 2022 as a result of the increased pharmaceutical needs of a larger and older population. The increased numbers of middle-aged and elderly people, who, on average, use more prescription drugs than do younger people, will spur demand for pharmacy technicians in all practice settings. With advances in science, newer medications are becoming available to treat more conditions. Cost-conscious insurers, pharmacies, and health systems will continue to emphasize the role of pharmacy technicians. As a result, pharmacy technicians will assume responsibility for more routine tasks previously performed by pharmacists. Pharmacy technicians also will need to learn and master new pharmacy technology as it surfaces. For example, robotic machines are used to dispense medicine into containers, and pharmacy technicians must oversee the machines, stock the bins, and label the containers. Although automation is increasingly being incorporated into the job, it will not necessarily reduce the need for pharmacy technicians. Continuing changes in health care legislation will give more people access to health services including prescription services placing more demand on pharmacies and pharmaceutical care practices.

Summary

The foundation of pharmaceutical care has come a long way in a little more than a century. All of the following have been seen: the continued specialization of pharmacists in specific disease conditions, the growing trend for certification of pharmacy technicians, the rapid spread of technology to facilitate the provision of care, and a shift in the composition of its workforce.

The two examinations used today for pharmacy technician certification include the Pharmacy Technician Certification Board's PTCE and the National Healthcareer Association's ExCPT exam. Both are accredited by the National Commission for Certifying Agencies (NCCA), and are computerized tests with multiple-choice questions. Pharmacy technicians must also complete 20 continuing education credits within two years in order to remain certified. One unit of this continuing education must be in related law topics.

Pharmacy will remain an integral part of our health care delivery system and an exciting career choice for its practitioners. Good job opportunities are expected for pharmacy technicians in the future as the various types of pharmacy settings expand and grow. The increased pharmaceutical needs of a larger and older population guarantee that the pharmacy technician field will grow faster than many other occupations.

REVIEW QUESTIONS

1. The national testing of a pharmacy technician is administered by the:

    A. Illinois Council of Health-System Pharmacists.

    B. American Society of Health-System Pharmacists.

    C. Pharmacy Technician Certification Board.

    D. National American Pharmacy Technicians.

2. A pharmacy technician is recertified by:

    A. completing 10 hours of credit every two years in pharmacy-related study.

    B. completing 10 contact hours of credit that must be in pharmacy law.

    C. completing 20 hours of credit every two years in pharmacy-related study, which includes one unit of pharmacy law.

    D. completing 40 hours of credit every year in pharmacy-related study.

3. Pharmacists are those who are educated and licensed to:

    A. dispense drugs and provide drug information.

    B. dispense information but not drugs.

    C. dispense alternate remedies rather than the drugs prescribed.

    D. test pharmacy technicians and provide their certification.

4. The most important goal for the pharmacy technician is:

    A. speed of filling a prescription.

    B. patient safety.

    C. data entry.

    D. professionalism.

5. Pharmacy technicians perform some routine tasks, such as:

    A. prescribing medications.

    B. counting tablets and labeling bottles.

    C. referring questions to medical assistants.

    D. counseling patients and giving out free samples.

6. Of the questions on the Pharmacy Technician Certification Exam, 13.75% concern:

   A. pharmacy quality assurance.
   B. pharmacology for technicians.
   C. pharmacy inventory management.
   D. medication safety.

7. AAPT stands for:

   A. American Association of Pharmaceutical Terminology.
   B. Automatic Accreditation of Pharmacy Technicians.
   C. American Association of Pharmacy Technicians.
   D. American Association of Pharmaceutical Torts.

8. Which of the following organizations gives national accreditation for pharmacy technician training programs?

   A. PTCB
   B. ASHP
   C. PTEC
   D. APhA

9. To pass the Pharmacy Technician Certification Exam, one must have a score of at least:

   A. 350.
   B. 450.
   C. 650.
   D. 900.

10. All of the following are the basic principles of a code of ethics for pharmacy technicians, except:

    A. honor the autonomy, values, and dignity of each patient.
    B. contribute to the health care system and social health needs.
    C. condone the dispensing, promoting, or distributing of drugs that lack therapeutic value.
    D. respect the rights of patients to receive pharmacy products and services.

11. An activity that requires specialized education and intellectual knowledge is referred to as:

    A. a hobby.
    B. a profession.
    C. quality control.
    D. a religion.

12. The *Journal of Pharmacy Technology* is affiliated with which of the following agencies?

    A. American Society of Health System Pharmacists
    B. American Council on Pharmaceutical Education
    C. American College of Clinical Pharmacy
    D. Pharmacy Technician Educators Council

13. The *American Journal of Pharmaceutical Education* is published by which of the following?

    A. American Association of Colleges of Pharmacy
    B. American Association of Pharmaceutical Scientists
    C. American Association of Pharmacy Technicians
    D. American Pharmacists Association

14. How many questions on the Pharmacy Technician Certification Exam are actually scored?

    A. 60
    B. 80
    C. 140
    D. 180

15. Which of the following factors is essential in the formulation, manufacture, and distribution of pharmaceutical products?

    A.   Cost

    B.   Quality of life

    C.   Drug quality control

    D.   Crossover study

CRITICAL THINKING

    1.   Describe the factors that make an occupation a profession.

    2.   Discuss the value of professional organizations and the role they play within a profession.

    3.   Explain the importance of a code of ethics. How does this relate to the profession of pharmacy practice?

    4.   Which organization sets standards for drug product identity, strength, quality, purity, packaging, and labeling? How does this organization provide its information?

    5.   Who does the ASHP represent? What is contained in their model curriculum?

    6.   Which types of training improve job outlooks for pharmacy technicians? What is a major factor in the increasing need for pharmacy technicians?

WEB LINKS

Accreditation Council for Pharmacy Education: www.acpe-accredit.org

American Association of Colleges of Pharmacy: www.aacp.org

American Association of Pharmacy Technicians: www.pharmacytechnician.com

American Pharmacists Association: www.pharmacist.com

American Society of Consultant Pharmacists Foundation: www.ascp.com

American Association of Pharmaceutical Scientists: www.aaps.org

American College of Clinical Pharmacology: www.accp1.org

American Society of Health-System Pharmacists: www.ashp.org

JobPharm.com: www.jobpharm.com

National Association of Boards of Pharmacy: www.nabp.net

National Healthcareer Association®: www.nhanow.com/pharmacy-technician.aspx

National Pharmacy Technician Association: www.pharmacytechnician.org

Pharmacy Technician Certification Board: www.ptcb.org

Pharmacy Technician Educators Council: www.pharmacytecheducators.com

U.S. Pharmacopeial Convention: www.usp.org

Virtual Library Pharmacy: www.pharmacy.org

READING LIST

Holdford, D. A. (2017). *Introduction to Acute & Ambulatory Care Pharmacy Practice,* 2nd ed. Bethesda, MD: American Society of Health System Pharmacists.

Lauster, C. D., and Srivastava, S. B. (2013). *Fundamental Skills for Patient Care in Pharmacy Practice.* Burlington, NJ: Jones & Bartlett Learning.

Muench, J. (2016). *A Pharmacist's Guide to Inpatient Medical Emergencies: How to Respond to Code Blue, Rapid Response Calls, and Other Medical Emergencies.* Seattle, WA: CreateSpace Independent Publishing Platform.

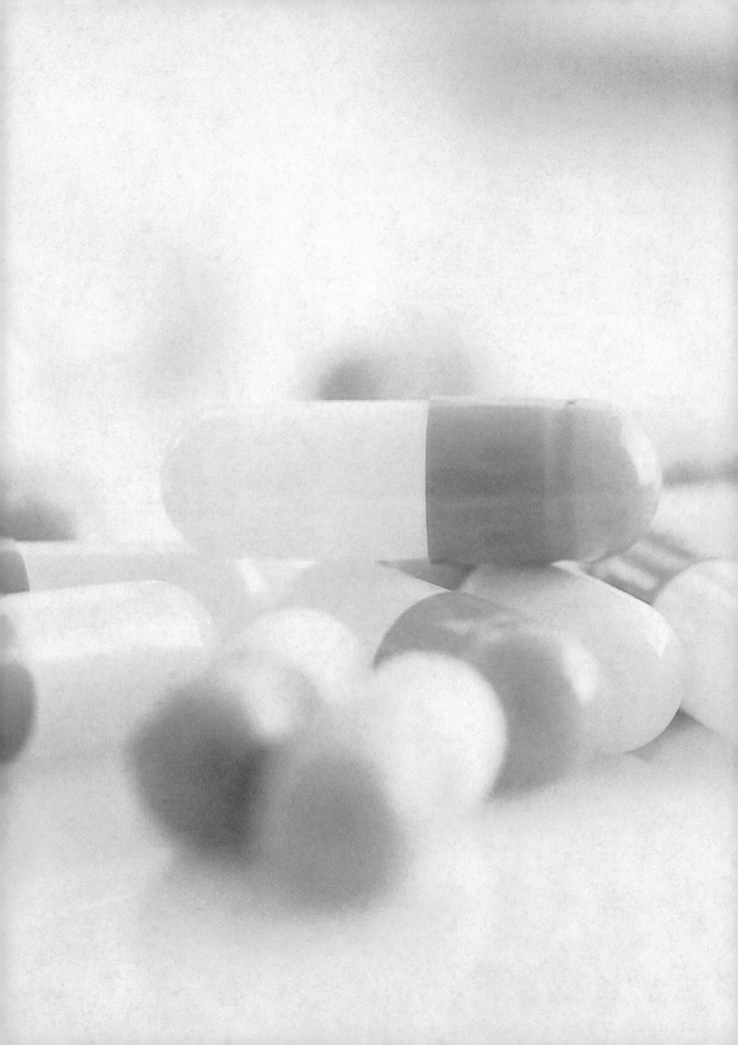

Pharmacy Law, Ethics, and Regulatory Agencies

OBJECTIVES

Upon completion of this chapter, the reader should be able to:

1. Explain the various types of law.
2. Discuss violations of the law related to the field of pharmacy.
3. Differentiate between state and federal pharmacy laws.
4. Explain the Controlled Substances Act and Schedule drugs.
5. Discuss the Drug Listing Act of 1972.
6. List various DEA forms used for controlled substances.
7. Discuss the Orphan Drug Act of 1983.
8. Explain the Occupational Safety and Health Administration (OSHA).
9. State the regulations of the Health Insurance Portability and Accountability Act (HIPAA).
10. Explain the roles of pharmacy technicians in working with controlled substances.

KEY TERMS

accessory	criminal	law	negligence
administrative law	criminal law	malpractice	orphan drug
adulterated	Drug Enforcement	medical ethics	regulatory law
barbiturates	Administration (DEA)	misbranding	standard code sets
bioethics	felony	misdemeanor	standards
civil law	Food and Drug	National Drug Code (NDC)	statutes
crime	Administration (FDA)	National Formulary (NF)	tort

Overview

Pharmacy technicians must be familiar with the legal requirements that relate to their daily professional activities. The laws relevant to the practice of pharmacy may come from different sources, such as the U.S. Food and Drug Administration (FDA), the state board of pharmacy, and the **Drug Enforcement Administration (DEA)**. Moreover, laws may appear in different forms, such as statutes, regulations, or court decisions.

There are several types of law. Each type of law is applicable to pharmacists and pharmacy practice. Federal laws primarily relate to the drug products, whereas state laws and regulations primarily relate to the people who practice pharmacy and the sites where they perform their professional duties.

In this chapter, laws, ethics, and different terms that are essential knowledge for pharmacy technicians are discussed. Pharmacy technicians should be familiar with the legal system and understand the legal terminology that relates to their profession.

Law and Ethics in Pharmacy

Laws, standards, and ethics can exercise controls on pharmacy and drugs. A **law** is a rule or regulation established by a governing body. Laws are enacted both to protect society and to maintain order and standards of living. Violation of a law can result in criminal penalties. **Standards** are guidelines for practice established by professional organizations. Professionals in a particular area of practice share a common philosophy (a basic viewpoint or shared beliefs, concepts, attitudes, and values). This common philosophy dictates the etiquette or standards of behavior considered appropriate for that profession. The philosophy and etiquette established within a profession drive the standards that are established for the profession. Pharmacists and pharmacy technicians are responsible for upholding legal and ethical standards in their profession.

Ethics is the study of values or principles governing personal relationships. These values and principles are used to determine whether actions are right or wrong. Ethics is based on morals, particular behaviors, or rules of conduct that are formed through the influences of family, culture, and society. **Medical ethics** is the term used to describe the discipline of evaluating merits, risks, and social concerns about medical activities.

CODE OF ETHICS IN PHARMACY

As noted in Chapter 2, the American Pharmacists Association developed a Code of Ethics for Pharmacists. The code addresses five overarching principles:

1. *Beneficence* concerns actions designed to positively benefit patients and pharmacy customers. Actions should be performed without prejudice.
2. *Fidelity* means that promises are kept so that patient needs are fulfilled correctly and on time. This also encompasses the maintenance of patient confidentiality.
3. *Veracity* concerns telling the truth, both for the benefit of patients in their care and in the effort to stop drug diversion or to ensure correct reporting of medication errors.
4. *Justice* is based on lawful actions that are fair and equal to all.
5. *Autonomy* involves self-reliance, wherein pharmacy technicians work to support the pharmacist, but also with initiative, reliability, and dependability. Pharmacy staff must also acknowledge and encourage patients to participate in their health care decisions.

The purpose of all actions in the pharmacy should be to benefit patients to the greatest degree, with uniformity. All actions have a consequence, and acting without consideration to the outcome of the action is not in the best interest of the pharmacy or the patient. Further, there should be consistency to the actions; all patients should be treated in the same manner. Expectations exist between pharmacists, pharmacy technicians, and patients. It is expected that the pharmacist and pharmacy technician interact with patients with sensitivity, kindness, patience, reliability, and tact.

Legal Language

It is very common for various professions to develop a language or vocabulary specific to the profession. Similar to the way the medical and pharmacy professions communicate using medical terminology, the legal profession has legal terminology. It is in the best interest of the pharmacy technician to have a working knowledge of basic legal terminology. Table 3-1 lists common legal terms with their definitions.

Table 3-1 Legal Terms to Know	
Assumption of risk	This refers to a patient who does not follow medical advice, and, therefore, becomes responsible for any problems that occur as a result of his or her decision.
Defendant	The person or group against whom charges are brought in a court action.
Deposition	An oral testimony taken by a court reporter at a location outside the courtroom, subject to the same requirements for truth as court testimony.
Interrogatory	A written set of questions that must be answered under oath as if in a court, within a specific period.
Jurisdiction	The power, right, and authority given to a court to hear a case and to make a judgment.
Litigant	A party to a lawsuit.
Litigation	A lawsuit or a contest in court.
Plaintiff	The person who files a lawsuit initiating a civil legal action. In criminal actions, the prosecution (government) is the plaintiff, acting on behalf of the people.
Statute of limitations	The law that limits the period during which a person can sue. The period varies from one to three years.
Subpoena	A court order that requires an individual to appear as a witness in court or to make himself or herself available to be deposed.

Governing Bodies

Laws are created and upheld by federal, state, and local government. In the United States, the federal government is divided into three branches:

1. *Legislative branch*: consists of the Congress (i.e., the House of Representatives and the Senate). This branch is responsible for creating laws.
2. *Executive branch*: consists of the president and vice president, cabinets, and various smaller organizations. This branch of government enforces law.
3. *Judicial branch*: consists of the Supreme Court and lower federal courts. This branch interprets laws.

The federal government creates, enforces, and interprets laws for the general population. State and local governments are responsible for determining the specifics of certain laws within their jurisdictions.

Regulatory agencies are government-based departments that create specific rules about what is and is not legal within a specific field or area of expertise. The regulatory agency for the field of pharmacy is the U.S. **Food and Drug Administration (FDA)**, which is a branch of the U.S. Department of Health and Human Services. Among other things, the FDA regulates all drugs with the exception of illegal drugs. All legislation pertaining to drug administration is initiated, implemented, and enforced by the FDA. The FDA is responsible for the approval of drugs, over-the-counter (OTC) and prescription drug labeling, and standards for drug manufacturing.

The core mission of the FDA is to provide consumers with assurance that medical drugs and devices that reach the marketplace have proven safety and efficacy in the roles for which they have been tested and approved. The path from initial demonstration that a molecule may have therapeutic potential to the production of an approved drug involves preclinical testing, complex clinical trials in humans, and posttrial regulatory approval by the FDA. For drugs, this process can take 10 to 15 years and cost millions of dollars. About 1 of every 1000 potential drugs will reach human clinical trials after preclinical testing. About 9 of every 10 drugs then fail in the human testing phase. All drugs must go through review by a committee, or *new drug division*, specializing in the class of drug in question, on the basis of the anticipated purpose of the drug.

Clinical trials establish safety, efficacy, and effectiveness of new drugs, and they are divided into Phase 0, II, III trials, and I. Phase 0 is *exploratory*, with the drug tested in 10 to 15 healthy volunteers. Phase I tests the drug in 20 to 80 healthy volunteers to determine toxicity and safety. Phase II tests it in 100 to 300 volunteers who have the targeted medical condition to explore efficacy and less-common side effects. Phase III tests the drug in 1000 to 3000 subjects with the targeted medical condition to test clinical efficacy. There may also be a Phase IV with the number of subjects depending on trial end points. However, after Phase III is completed, the drug sponsor can file a New Drug Application with the FDA, which is basically a request to manufacture and sell the drug in the United States. The FDA review of the application occurs within 180 days of receiving it. Arguably, the United States has the most stringent regulations regarding approval of medical drugs and devices in the world.

Types of Law

As society grows and changes, laws change to conform to current realities and to try to govern future realities. The main types of law are constitutional, statutory, administrative, common, and international. *Constitutional law* is derived from both federal and state constitutions. *Statutory law* is established by legislation; the results are **statutes**, which are the rules and regulations established by legislative decisions. *Administrative law* is derived from governmental administrative agencies. *Judges, based upon previous court decisions, create common law. International law* is based on treaties and other agreements between two or more countries. The term *criminal law* relates to offenses against the general public or society. *Civil law* focuses on rights of private citizens and is also referred to as *case law*. *Tort law* and *contract law* are derived from civil law.

CRIMINAL LAW

Criminal law governs the relationship of the individual to society as a whole. Violations against the government or the state are governed by criminal law. For example, if a pharmacist is practicing pharmacy without a license, then he or she is criminally liable and may be prosecuted by the government. These offenses are described as "harming the general public." Offenses under criminal law include misdemeanors, felonies, and treason. When a person is accused of a criminal violation, he or she has the right to *due process*, meaning that the accused will be allowed the opportunity to defend himself or herself against all charges. Criminal law governs intent to defraud pharmacy customers by cheating the customer with regard to drug quality or pricing or misleading a customer as to the facts about his or her prescriptions.

Misdemeanors

Misdemeanors are usually punishable by fines and may include imprisonment up to one year, usually in a city or county jail. Lesser misdemeanors are called *infractions* (which include minor offenses such as traffic violations), punishable by fines without imprisonment. Each state lists its own unique classes and subclasses of misdemeanors. These are usually grouped as Class A, Class B, and so on.

Felonies

Felonies are serious crimes punishable by larger fines than misdemeanors, or imprisonment for more than one year in a state penitentiary, or both. Felonies include murder and rape. First-degree felonies are considered the most serious type, and they evoke the most severe penalties of all the degrees of felonies. Convicted felons commonly lose many of their rights as private citizens, including the right to possess guns, run for public office, and vote. Voting rights are reinstated in most states after completion of the sentence being served.

Treason

Treason is considered the most serious type of crime, as it consists of attempts to overthrow the government of the country. Attempts to assassinate the president or other high-ranking government individuals may be considered treasonous acts. Attempts to destroy government buildings are other examples of treason. Treasonous acts differ from acts against the United States (such as the attacks of September 11, 2001) that may be deemed by the president to be acts of war.

CIVIL LAW

Civil law governs the relationship between individuals within society. Civil law is focused on noncriminal acts involving private individuals against other individuals, government agencies, or organizations. For example, a person or a patient can sue the pharmacy or the pharmacist. Civil law governs pharmacists who do not act in a professional manner with their customers, including areas such as libel, slander, violation of privacy, or unintentional (personal) bodily injury. Civil law is commonly referred to as *case law*. Civil law cases are decided by judges or by juries over which judges preside. There are many different types of civil law, with tort law and contract law most directly involved with the practice of pharmacy. Administrative law also plays an important role in pharmacy regulation.

Tort Law

Tort law allows for a person who has suffered harm from the wrongful acts of another to seek a remedy (which is usually monetary). A **tort** is a private wrong against another person or his or her property. Medical malpractice is regulated under tort law. In this type of law, the person bringing the tort (the plaintiff) is required to prove that the respondent (defendant) was legally obligated to act in a certain way, which he or she did not do. Injury or damage resulting from this action or lack of action by the defendant must also be proven, with the amount or seriousness of the damage demonstrated.

Examples of tort law include libel and slander. *Intentional torts* are committed when a person's rights are infringed upon intentionally. Examples of intentional torts include assault and battery. Assault is defined as attempting or threatening to touch or harm another person. Battery is defined as carrying out the intended assault. *Unintentional torts* are those committed against a person inadvertently, without intent to harm. They also describe a lack of action when that action is required for a positive patient outcome. Examples of unintentional torts include **negligence** and **malpractice**. Negligence involves not doing something that a reasonable person would do in a given situation or doing something that a reasonable person would not do in a similar situation. Malpractice is defined as negligence that occurs within a profession. Malpractice may also be referred to as *professional negligence* because a failure to act in a specific manner may result in patient harm. Medical malpractice involves an action or lack of action that may be considered improper within the confines of normal medical practice. An example of medical malpractice in the pharmacy would be a pharmacist who does not counsel a Medicare patient about a new medication, resulting in harm to the patient because of misunderstanding about how to take the medication properly.

POINTS TO REMEMBER

The elements that must be proven by a plaintiff in a negligence case include:

- That the defendant owed a duty of care to the plaintiff
- That the defendant breached this duty of care
- That the injury to the plaintiff was the result of the defendant's negligence
- That the plaintiff suffered injury and that the injury may be compensated for under the law

WHAT WOULD YOU DO?

David was working in the retail pharmacy and was upset at a co-worker for taking a longer-than-allowed break, especially since the pharmacy was very busy at that time. When the co-worker returned, they got into a verbal argument, and then the co-worker pushed David into a wall, threatening him never to talk to him that way again. If you were David, what would you do in this situation?

Contract Law

Contract law involves agreements that create obligations between several parties. These obligations may be created, eliminated, or changed by an agreement (contract). Written and oral contracts both provide for legal recourse, with both types binding parties to act in a predetermined manner. Contract law is directly affected by the *Uniform Commercial Code*, which was established to provide uniformity to sales and transactions throughout the United States. Individuals, who are not allowed to enter into a contract, include minors, the mentally ill, and individuals who are intoxicated by drugs or alcohol.

ADMINISTRATIVE LAW

Administrative law consists of rules and regulations established by agencies of the federal government. This type of law is also called **regulatory law**. Laws enacted by the legislature are referred to as *statutory law*. Administrative law agencies are given authority by Congress. Examples of administrative law include codes and regulations instituted by the Occupational Safety and Health Administration (OSHA), the Internal Revenue Service (IRS), the FDA, the Social Security Administration (SSA), and the Centers for Medicare and Medicaid Services (CMS).

Violations of the Law

A violation of the law is a **crime**. A crime can be classified as either a misdemeanor or a felony. An example of a misdemeanor in a pharmacy setting would be theft, such as by shoplifting. An example of a felony in the pharmacy setting would be illegal selling of drugs, burglary of the pharmacy, or arson.

The individual in violation of the law is called a **criminal**. An individual who helps someone commit a crime is called an **accessory**. An accessory can aid the perpetrator of a crime either directly or indirectly.

Violations of pharmacy laws are punishable by fines or by the revocation or suspension of a license to practice. Some state laws specify that violations of the pharmacy act are punishable as misdemeanors. Boards of pharmacy are authorized to make rules and regulations for the enforcement and administration of the pharmacy law. The board is an administrative agency, not a legislative one. It is important to understand various violations of the law, which are defined in Table 3-2.

Pharmacy Law and Regulation at the State Level

Regulation of pharmacy practice is primarily a function of the state and not of the federal government. Its basis is found in the power of the state to protect the health, safety, and welfare of its citizens. Pharmacy laws of individual states differ, but they are based on the same principles, objectives, and goals of pharmaceutical practice. State pharmacy law requires minimal qualifications for a class of individuals who are involved with pharmacy practice. No one may practice pharmacy without a license, except those exempted by the state legislation that creates the license requirement. Any individuals who are qualified to be licensed must successfully complete the requirements of the board of pharmacy. The pharmacy board is a subagency of the licensing division of the health department. Once licensure is gained, it is not revoked easily. The state can suspend, revoke, or terminate an individual's license but

Table 3-2 Violations of Pharmacy Laws

Violation	Definition	Example
Fraud	Dishonest and deceitful practices undertaken to induce someone to part with something of value or legal right.	A pharmacist or a technician promises patients "miracle cures" or accepts fees from patients for spiritual powers to heal.
Libel	Defamatory writing, such as published material, or pictures that injure the reputation of another.	A pharmacy advertises that a competing pharmacy does not stock medications of the same quality.
Slander	Spoken words that jeopardize someone's reputation or means of livelihood.	A pharmacy worker tells a customer that another pharmacy's staff is not qualified.
Negligence	Failure to use a reasonable amount of care to prevent injury or damage to another.	A pharmacist or technician fails to exercise ordinary care, and a patient is harmed.
Abuse	The improper use of equipment, a substance (such as a drug), or a service (such as a program).	A patient is harmed because a pharmacy worker gives him or her the wrong substance, strength, amount, or type of medication.

only after due process and for just cause as set out in the appropriate legislation. Licensed pharmacists have gained a profession, the practice of which is safeguarded by the federal and state constitutions as a property right. In most states, certificates of registration are granted for one or two years. Evidence of continuing education training is a requirement for maintaining certification and licensure. Under special circumstances, certificates of registration or pharmacy licenses may be canceled or revoked. The National Association of Boards of Pharmacy (NABP) has developed a Model State Pharmacy Practice Act (MSPPA). This act provides a greater degree of uniformity between states but still offers flexibility to the states that adopt it. Articles that deal with various aspects of regulating pharmacy practice organize the MSPPA.

POINTS TO REMEMBER

- Most states have their own unique regulations regarding state law.
- State laws are frequently more stringent than federal law. When there are differences between federal and state laws, the state law must be followed in these circumstances.

WHAT WOULD YOU DO?

Cheyenne, a pharmacy technician, passed her board certification exam and was working in a local pharmacy. Her state required her to be registered in order to practice, but she and her employer ignored this because they were related by marriage. If you were Cheyenne, what would you do? What can happen to the pharmacist and the business if the state discovered Cheyenne was working without being registered?

Pharmacy Law and Regulation at the Federal Level

Pharmacy practice is regulated by a series of rules, regulations, and laws that are enforced by local, state, and federal governments. Laws are continually reviewed and may be amended or changed as societal and industry needs evolve and change. New laws are also put into place as deemed necessary by government and regulatory agencies.

THE PURE FOOD AND DRUG ACT OF 1906

In 1906, the U.S. Congress passed the first important law to regulate the development, compounding, distribution, storage, and dispensing of drugs. The Pure Food and Drug Act of 1906 prohibited interstate distribution or sale of **adulterated** and misbranded food and drugs. The 1906 act was believed to be inadequate for the following reasons:

- It did not include cosmetics.
- It did not provide authority to ban unsafe drugs.
- A manufacturer could make false statements about a drug.
- Labels were not required to identify contents of medications.

In 1912, Congress addressed the false statement problem and included within the definition of **misbranding** false or fraudulent claims for the curative powers of drugs. The Sherley Amendment to the act, which Congress enacted during 1912, first regulated labeling. A deficiency in this revision was that the enforcement agency was required to show deliberate fraud to establish a violation. Under the FDA labeling regulations, since most drug containers do not allow enough space for thorough drug information, package inserts (*monographs*) must be supplied along with them. Information found in package inserts includes accurate summaries of essential scientific information for safe and effective use; wording that is not false, misleading, or promotional; and data based on human experience. Package inserts cannot make claims or suggest uses for drugs if there is insufficient evidence of safety and unproven evidence of effectiveness. Information in a package insert may also be referred to as prescribing information or professional labeling.

POINTS TO REMEMBER

Monographs (package inserts) must include all of the following information about the referenced medication: indications and usage, dosage and administration, dosage forms and strengths, contraindications, warnings and precautions, adverse reactions, drug interactions, use in specific populations, drug abuse and dependence, overdosage, description of chemical agents and ingredients, clinical pharmacology, nonclinical toxicology, clinical studies, references, how supplied, storage and handling, and patient counseling information.

POINTS TO REMEMBER

On a manufacturer's insert, a boxed warning may appear, which is encased in a bold border. Health care professionals as black box warnings commonly refer to boxed *warnings*. They are required for medications and other products that carry a high level of potential risk to the consumer. They indicate the necessary proper use of the drug, to avoid or decrease possibility of serious or life-threatening adverse effects.

POINTS TO REMEMBER

There are five *pregnancy categories* established by the FDA concerning the potential of a drug to cause fetal abnormalities if taken by pregnant women. Category A signifies no risk in thorough studies. Category B signifies that animal studies have shown no risk, but there have been no adequate studies in pregnant women. Category C signifies that animal studies have shown adverse effects, there have been no adequate human studies, and potential benefits may outweigh risks. Category D signifies there is positive fetal risk from human studies, yet potential benefits may still outweigh risks. Category X signifies that the drug should be avoided in pregnant women at all costs, due to proven fetal abnormalities with insufficient benefits.

THE HARRISON NARCOTICS ACT OF 1914

The Harrison Narcotics Act of 1914 was passed based upon international treaties intended to stop the recreational use of opium. As a result of this act, opium could no longer be purchased without a prescription, making the drug more difficult to obtain for nonmedical purposes. This act required registration of practitioners, documentation of prescriptions and their dispensing, and new restrictions surrounding the importation, sale, and distribution of opium, as well as coca leaves and any derivative products.

THE FOOD, DRUG, AND COSMETIC ACT OF 1938

In 1938, further amendments were made to the Pure Food and Drug Act. The Food, Drug, and Cosmetic Act of 1938 created the FDA and required pharmaceutical manufacturers to file New Drug Applications with the FDA. Under this act, manufacturers must be concerned with the purity, strength, effectiveness, safety, and packaging of drugs. Foods and cosmetics are also regulated. By this act, the FDA has the power to approve or deny new drug applications and even to conduct inspections to ensure compliance. The FDA approves the investigational use of drugs on humans and ensures that all approved drugs are safe and effective.

THE DURHAM–HUMPHREY AMENDMENT OF 1951

During the 1940s, the FDA began to use internal regulations to create classifications of prescription (legend drugs) and nonprescription (OTC) drugs. This process did not work very well. Therefore, in 1951, Senator Hubert Humphrey, a pharmacist from Minnesota, and Congressman Carl Durham, a pharmacist from North Carolina, supported legislation to establish clear criteria for such decisions. The Durham–Humphrey Amendment of 1951 prohibits dispensing of legend drugs without a prescription. Nonlegend, OTC drugs were not restricted for sale and use under medical supervision.

THE KEFAUVER–HARRIS AMENDMENTS OF 1962

The federal Food, Drug, and Cosmetic Act was amended again with the Kefauver–Harris Amendments of 1962 to require that drug products, both prescription and nonprescription, must be effective and safe. Prescription drug advertising was placed under supervision of the FDA and qualifications of drug investigators were subjected to review. These amendments provided for registration of manufacturers and inspection of manufacturing sites, and they required an unprecedented program of accountability from manufacturers.

THE COMPREHENSIVE DRUG ABUSE PREVENTION AND CONTROL ACT OF 1970

This act, also called the Controlled Substances Act (CSA), directs the manufacture, distribution, and dispensing of controlled substances that have the potential for addiction and abuse. This law replaced most previous narcotic and drug abuse control laws. It is enforced by the DEA, which is part of the U.S. Department of Justice. Under the jurisdiction of the CSA, drugs with potential for abuse are classified into five schedules: I, II, III, IV, and V. Drugs in Schedule I have the highest potential for abuse and addiction, and those in Schedule V have the least potential.

Schedule I

Schedule I agents have a high potential for abuse, and they are not accepted for medical use in the United States. Properly registered individuals may use Schedule I substances for research purposes.

Schedule II

Schedule II agents also have a high potential for abuse, but they are currently accepted for medical use in the United States. The abuse of these drugs may result in severe psychological or physical dependence. The broad categories of Schedule II drugs include opiates and opium derivatives, derivatives of cocoa leaves, and certain central nervous system stimulants and depressants. The quantity of the substance in a drug product often determines the schedule that will control it. For example, amphetamines and codeine usually are classified in Schedule II; however, Schedules III and IV control specific products containing smaller quantities of Schedule II substances, most often in combination with a noncontrolled substance.

A practitioner must issue a prescription for a controlled substance for a valid medical purpose. Prescriptions for Schedule II drugs must be written and not faxed or called in unless an absolute emergency exists that requires a faxed or phone order. Exceptions are made for hospices and nursing homes, however. No prescription for Schedule II controlled substances may be refilled.

Schedule III

Schedule III agents have a moderate potential for abuse and are accepted for medical uses in the United States. They have a lower potential for abuse than Schedule I and II drugs. Schedule III drugs contain limited quantities of certain narcotic and non-narcotic drugs.

Prescriptions for Schedule III or IV controlled substances may be refilled if authorized by a practitioner. These prescriptions may not be filled or refilled more than six months after the date issued. They also cannot be refilled more than five times after the date they were issued. After six months, or five refills, the practitioner may renew the prescription.

Schedule IV

Schedule IV agents have a low potential for abuse relative to those in Schedule III. Schedule IV drugs are generally long-acting **barbiturates** (central nervous system depressants), certain hypnotics, and minor tranquilizers.

Schedule V

Schedule V agents have the lowest abuse potential of the controlled substances and consist of preparations containing limited quantities of certain narcotic drugs, generally used for antitussive and antidiarrheal purposes. Schedule V drugs are still considered to be legend drugs that require a prescription. The combination of diphenoxylate hydrochloride and atropine sulfate (Lomotil®) is an example of one of these medications.

In some states, adults older than age 18 can request Schedule V drugs from the pharmacy counter. These are called behind-the-counter drugs. Antidiarrheals and antitussives with low doses of narcotics that are purchased in this way are referred to as "exempt" narcotics. When individuals purchase drugs in this manner, they are required to show their identification and sign a register. There are limits to the amount of Schedule V drugs that can be purchased in

Table 3-3 Drug Schedules

Schedule	Abuse Potential	Prescription Requirement	Examples
I	High abuse potential; no accepted medical use	No prescription permitted	Heroin, LSD, marijuana (except in certain states), mescaline, and peyote
II	High abuse potential; accepted medical use	Prescription required; no refills permitted without a new written prescription	Cocaine, codeine, methamphetamine (Desoxyn®), methadone hydrochloride (Methadose®), morphine (Astramorph®), opium (deodorized), methylphenidate (Ritalin®), and secobarbital (Seconal®)
III	Moderate abuse potential; accepted medical use	Prescription required; five refills permitted in six months	Certain drugs compounded with small quantities of narcotics; also other drugs with high potential for abuse (Tylenol® with Codeine tablets), and certain barbiturates
IV	Low abuse potential; accepted medical use	Prescription required; five refills permitted in six months	Barbital, chloral hydrate (Noctec®), diazepam, (Valium®), chlordiazepoxide (Librium®), and pentazocine hydrochloride (Talwin®)
V	Low abuse potential; accepted medical use	Prescription required for some, while others may be requested at the pharmacy counter in some states by individuals older than age 18	Cough syrups with codeine, diphenoxylate hydrochloride with atropine sulfate (Lomotil®), and pregabalin (Lyrica®)

a specific amount of time. In some states, pseudoephedrine is an example of a common Schedule V medication that can be purchased from the pharmacy counter without a prescription. Paregoric is a medication that treats diarrhea; although once available for purchase in this manner, it is now restricted to prescription sales, only, and is included in Schedule III. Table 3-3 shows drug schedules and some examples.

Registration

Individuals who manufacture, dispense, or distribute any controlled substance are obligated to register with the DEA unless they are exempt. Registrations vary in length from one to three years. Most pharmacy registrations are issued for three years. A DEA number must be assigned to those who are registered under the law as manufacturers, distributors, wholesalers, pharmacies, hospitals, and practitioners such as physicians, dentists, veterinarians, and scientists. Pharmacies must register with the DEA to dispense controlled substances, but pharmacists do not have to register. The one exception is that a pharmacist who owns a pharmacy as a sole proprietor must be registered. The DEA's "New Application for Registration" is also known as Form 224. This form can be viewed online at: www .reginfo.gov/public/do/PRAViewIC?ref_nbr=200811-1117-001&icID=12313.

Applications for re-registration are mailed by the DEA to each registered person approximately 60 days before the expiration date of the registration. The DEA can suspend or revoke a registration if the registrant has falsified his or her application or has been convicted of a felony under the federal CSA. A DEA number consists of a two-letter prefix, followed by seven digits. The first letter determines the type of practitioner, while the second letter signifies the first letter of the practitioner's last name. Pharmacy technicians may have to determine if the DEA number is valid on prescriptions. This is done by adding the second, fourth, and sixth digits together and multiplying this answer by two. Next, add the sum of the first, third, and fifth digits to this answer. If the last digit of the answer matches the seventh digit of the DEA number, the number is valid.

Ordering Controlled Substances

DEA Form 222 is used to order controlled substances from Schedules I or II. This form, which is filled out in triplicate, may be ordered from the DEA by phone, mail, or online and is free of charge. Anyone attempting to order controlled substances must have a DEA license. DEA Form 222 is not required when ordering Schedule III, IV, or V substances, which can be ordered directly from manufacturers or drug wholesalers. Form 222 requires the person ordering the substances to supply the following information: company name and address, ordering date, number of packages of each item, size of package of each item, name of each item, signature of purchaser or their attorney or agent, and DEA registration number.

POINTS TO REMEMBER

Only a maximum of 10 different items may be ordered on one DEA Form 222.

When the supplier receives each form and processes the order, the supplier must add the following information to the form: their DEA registration number, the national drug code (NDC) of each item, an indication of the packaging being shipped, and the date of each shipment. The supplier must have a copy of the purchasing company or individual's DEA certificate on file prior to shipping any order. The supplier can ship only to the purchaser's address that is listed on both the Form 222 and the corresponding DEA certificate. Form 222 is shown in Figure 3-1.

BLANK DEA FORM - 222
U.S. OFFICIAL ORDER FORM—SCHEDULES I & II

See Reverse of PURCHASER'S Copy for Instructions	No order form may be issued for Schedules I and II substances unless a completed application form has been received, (21 CFR 1305.04).	OMB APPROVAL NO. 1117-0010

TO: *(Name of Supplier)* | STREET ADDRESS

CITY and STATE | DATE | TO BE FILLED IN BY SUPPLIER — SUPPLIERS DEA REGISTRATION No.

LINE No.	No. of Packages	Size of Packages	Name of Item	National Drug Code	Packages Shipped	Date Shipped
1						
2						
3						
4						
5						
6						
7						
8						
9						
10						

TO BE FILLED IN BY PURCHASER

NO. OF LINES COMPLETED | SIGNATURE OF PURCHASER OR HIS ATTORNEY OR AGENT

Date Issued | DEA Registration No. | Name and Address of Registrant

Schedules 2, 2N, 3, 3N, 4, 5

Registered as a PHARMACY | No. of this Order Form

DEA Form-222 **U.S. OFFICIAL ORDER FORMS—SCHEDULES I & II**
DRUG ENFORCEMENT ADMINISTRATION
SUPPLIER'S COPY 1

SAMPLE

Figure 3-1 DEA Form 222.

Theft of Controlled Substances

If a controlled substance is stolen or lost from a pharmacy, the nearest DEA office must be notified, using DEA Form 106 (see Figure 3-2). Reports to the DEA in these situations must include the company's name and address, DEA number, the date the theft or loss occurred, the type of loss or theft, a complete list of missing controlled substances, the local police department's information, explanation of the pharmacy's container marking system, and related costs. The pharmacy should keep the original copy of the report, send two copies to the DEA, and in most states, send one copy to the board of pharmacy. Additionally, a copy may be required to be sent to the local police (this is per local ordinances).

POINTS TO REMEMBER

If a controlled substance is lost at any pharmacy, the nearest DEA office must be notified of the theft or significant loss upon discovery by submission of a DEA Form 106.

U.S. Department of Justice
Drug Enforcement Administration

REPORT OF THEFT OR LOSS OF CONTROLLED SUBSTANCES

Federal Regulations require registrants to submit a detailed report of any theft or loss of Controlled Substances to the Drug Enforcement Administration.

Complete the front and back of this form in triplicate. Forward the original and duplicate copies to the nearest DEA Office. Retain the triplicate copy for your records. Some states may also require a copy of this report.

OMB APPROVAL No. 1117-0001

1. Name and Address of Registrant (include ZIP Code) ZIP CODE
2. Phone No. (Include Area Code)
3. DEA Registration Number 2 ltr. prefix 7 digit suffix
4. Date of Theft or Loss
5. Principal Business of Registrant (Check one)
   1 ☐ Pharmacy 2 ☐ Practitioner 3 ☐ Manufacturer 4 ☐ Hospital/Clinic 5 ☐ Distributor 6 ☐ Methadone Program 7 ☐ Other (Specify) ________
6. County in which Registrant is located
7. Was Theft reported to Police? ☐ Yes ☐ No
8. Name and Telephone Number of Police Department (Include Area Code)
9. Number of Thefts or Losses Registrant has experienced in the past 24 months
10. Type of Theft or Loss (Check one and complete items below as appropriate)
   1 ☐ Night break-in 2 ☐ Armed robbery 3 ☐ Employee pilferage 4 ☐ Customer theft 5 ☐ Other (Explain) 6 ☐ Lost in transit (Complete Item 14)
11. If Armed Robbery, was anyone:
   Killed? ☐ No ☐ Yes (How many) ________
   Injured? ☐ No ☐ Yes (How many) ________
12. Purchase value to registrant of Controlled Substances taken? $
13. Were any pharmaceuticals or merchandise taken? ☐ No ☐ Yes (Est. Value) $
14. IF LOST IN TRANSIT, COMPLETE THE FOLLOWING:
   A. Name of Common Carrier
   B. Name of Consignee
   C. Consignee's DEA Registration Number
   D. Was the carton received by the customer? ☐ Yes ☐ No
   E. If received, did it appear to be tampered with? ☐ Yes ☐ No
   F. Have you experienced losses in transit from this same carrier in the past? ☐ No ☐ Yes (How Many) ________
15. What identifying marks, symbols, or price codes were on the labels of these containers that would assist in identifying t he products?
16. If Official Controlled Substance Order Forms (DEA-222) were stolen, give numbers.
17. What security measures have been taken to prevent future thefts or losses?

PRIVACY ACT INFORMATION

AUTHORITY: Section 301 of the Controlled Substances Act of 1970 (PL 91-513).
PURPOSE: Report theft or loss of Controlled Substances.
ROUTINE USES: The Controlled Substances Act authorizes the production of special reports required for statistical and analytical purposes. Disclosures of information from this system are made to the following categories of users for the purposes stated:
A. Other Federal law enforcement and regulatory agencies for law enforcement and regulatory purposes.
B. State and local law enforcement and regulatory agencies for law enforcement and regulatory purposes.
EFFECT: Failure to report theft or loss of controlled substances may result in penalties under Section 402 and 403 of the Controlled Substances Act.

Under the Paperwork Reduction Act, a person is not required to respond to a collection of information unless it displays a currently valid OMB control number. Public reporting burden for this collection of information is estimated to average 30 minutes per response, including the time for reviewing instructions, searching existing data sources, gathering and maintaining the data needed, and completing and reviewing the collection of information. Send comments regarding this burden estimate or any other aspect of this collection of information, including suggestions for reducing this burden, to the Records Management Section, Drug Enforcement Administration, Washington, D.C. 20537; and to the Office of Information and Regulatory Affairs, Office of Management and Budget, W ashington, D.C. 20503.

DEA Form - 106 (Dec. 1985) Previous edition dated 03/83 is OBSOLETE CONTINUE ON REVERSE

Figure 3-2 DEA Form 106.

Dealing with Outdated or Damaged Controlled Substances

When controlled substances become out of date, DEA Form 41, which can be obtained from the closest DEA office, must be used. The pharmacist must write a cover letter explaining the situation and requesting DEA permission to destroy these substances. The cover letter must be attached to the completed Form 41. Retail pharmacies may request DEA permission to destroy these substances once per year. The request must be sent to the DEA two weeks prior to the intended date of destruction. The DEA must approve the destruction of the substances before they may be destroyed. Two witnesses (either physicians, pharmacists, mid-level practitioners, nurses, or law enforcement officers) must witness the destruction of the substances. After the substances are destroyed, signed copies of Form 41 must be sent to the DEA (Figures 3-3A and 3-3B).

As of 2014, hospitals or clinics with on-site pharmacies, authorized manufacturers, distributors, reverse distributors, narcotic treatment programs, and retail pharmacies are allowed to collect pharmaceutical controlled substances from ultimate users by voluntarily administering mail-back programs and maintaining collection receptacles. Hospitals, clinics, and retail pharmacies are also allowed to voluntarily maintain collection receptacles at long-term care facilities.

| | OMB Approval No. 1117 - 0007 | U. S. Department of Justice / Drug Enforcement Administration **REGISTRANTS INVENTORY OF DRUGS SURRENDERED** | PACKAGE NO. |

The following schedule is an inventory of controlled substances which is hereby surrendered to you for proper disposition.

FROM: *(Include Name, Street, City, State and ZIP Code in space provided below.)*

Signature of applicant or authorized agent

Registrant's DEA Number

Registrant's Telephone Number

NOTE: CERTIFIED MAIL (Return Receipt Requested) IS REQUIRED FOR SHIPMENTS OF DRUGS VIA U.S. POSTAL SERVICE. See instructions on reverse (page 2) of form.

NAME OF DRUG OR PREPARATION	Number of Containers	CONTENTS (Number of grams, tablets, ounces or other units per container)	Controlled Substance Content, (Each Unit)	FOR DEA USE ONLY		
				DISPOSITION	QUANTITY	
Registrants will fill in Columns 1,2,3, and 4 ONLY.					GMS.	MGS.
1	2	3	4	5	6	7
1						
2						
3						
4						
5						
6						
7						
8						
9						
10						
11						
12						
13						
14						
15						
16						

FORM DEA-41 (9-01)   Previous edition dated **6-86** is usable.   *See instructions on reverse (page 2) of form.*

© U.S. Drug Enforcement Agency

Figure 3-3A DEA Form 41.

NAME OF DRUG OR PREPARATION	Number of Containers	CONTENTS (Number of grams, tablets, ounces or other units per container)	Controlled Substance Content, (Each Unit)	FOR DEA USE ONLY		
				DISPOSITION	QUANTITY	
					GMS.	MGS.
Registrants will fill in Columns 1,2,3, and 4 ONLY.						
1	*2*	*3*	*4*	*5*	*6*	*7*
17						
18						
19						
20						
21						
22						
23						
24						

The controlled substances surrendered in accordance with Title 21 of the Code of Federal Regulations, Section 1307.21, have been received in _____packages purporting to contain the drugs listed on this inventory and have been: ** (1) Forwarded tape-sealed without opening; (2) Destroyed as indicated and the remainder forwarded tape-sealed after verifying contents; (3) Forwarded tape-sealed after verifying contents.

DATE _____   DESTROYED BY: _____

** *Strike out lines not applicable.*   WITNESSED BY: _____

INSTRUCTIONS

1. List the name of the drug in column 1, the number of containers in column 2, the size of each container in column 3, and in column 4 the controlled substance content of each unit described in column 3; e.g., morphine sulfate tabs., 3 pkgs., 100 tabs., 1/4 gr. (16 mg.) or morphine sulfate tabs., 1 pkg., 83 tabs., 1/2 gr. (32mg.), etc.

2. All packages included on a single line should be identical in name, content and controlled substance strength.

3. Prepare this form in quadruplicate. Mail two (2) copies of this form to the Special Agent in Charge, under separate cover. Enclose one additional copy in the shipment with the drugs. Retain one copy for your records. One copy will be returned to you as a receipt. No further receipt will be furnished to you unless specifically requested. Any further inquiries concerning these drugs should be addressed to the DEA District Office which serves your area.

4. There is no provision for payment for drugs surrendered. This is merely a service rendered to registrants enabling them to clear their stocks and records of unwanted items.

5. Drugs should be shipped tape-sealed via prepaid express or certified mail (**return receipt requested**) to Special Agent in Charge, Drug Enforcement Administration, of the DEA District Office which serves your area.

PRIVACY ACT INFORMATION

AUTHORITY: Section 307 of the Controlled Substances Act of 1970 (PL 91-513).
PURPOSE: To document the surrender of controlled substances which have been forwarded by registrants to DEA for disposal.
ROUTINE USES: This form is required by Federal Regulations for the surrender of unwanted Controlled Substances. Disclosures of information from this system are made to the following categories of users for the purposes stated.
    A. Other Federal law enforcement and regulatory agencies for law enforcement and regulatory purposes.
    B. State and local law enforcement and regulatory agencies for law enforcement and regulatory purposes.
EFFECT: Failure to document the surrender of unwanted Controlled Substances may result in prosecution for violation of the Controlled Substances Act.

Under the Paperwork Reduction Act, a person is not required to respond to a collection of information unless it displays a currently valid OMB control number. Public reporting burden for this collection of information is estimated to average 30 minutes per response, including the time for reviewing instructions, searching existing data sources, gathering and maintaining the data needed, and completing and reviewing the collection of information. Send comments regarding this burden estimate or any other aspect of this collection of information, including suggestions for reducing this burden, to the Drug Enforcement Administration, FOI and Records Management Section, Washington, D.C. 20537; and to the Office of Management and Budget, Paperwork Reduction Project no. 1117-0007, Washington, D.C. 20503.

Figure 3-3B DEA Form 41.

These entities, when desiring to be "collectors" of these drugs must modify their registration obtain authorization to be a collector. This can be done online at www.deadiversion.usdoj.gov. Once authorized, these entities are called "authorized collectors."

Returning Controlled Substances

When controlled substances from Schedule II are returned, DEA Form 222 must be used. These substances may be returned from only one DEA registrant to another. Any facility that does not have a DEA number cannot return controlled substances. All returned controlled substances must be properly labeled with product descriptions, quantities, product names, product sizes, strengths, NDC numbers, and manufacturer names.

Record Keeping

Any pharmacy that handles controlled substances must keep complete and accurate records of all drugs received and dispensed. The records must be kept for two years. Some states require that the records be kept for at least five years. Schedule II drug records must be kept separately from all other records. DEA officials must make any record that includes controlled substances available for inspection.

Inventory

Pharmacies must keep Schedule II drugs in a locked cabinet, but Schedule III, IV, and V drugs may be stored in various locations throughout the pharmacy. The CSA requires each registrant to make a complete and accurate record of all stocks of controlled substances on hand every two years. When the inventory of Schedule II controlled substances is performed, an exact count or measure must be made.

WHAT WOULD YOU DO?

Samantha is a highly regarded pharmacy technician in a retail pharmacy. She has worked there for 10 years. Her brother recently was diagnosed with a herniated disc but is afraid of having back surgery. His life is one of constant pain. His physician has prescribed only the minimum dosage of oxycodone to prevent the possibility of addiction and recommends back surgery. One day, Samantha's brother asks if she can obtain additional tablets of oxycodone for him. If you were Samantha, what would you do?

Prescriptions

A practitioner must issue a prescription for a controlled substance for a valid medical purpose. If a practitioner attempts to resupply office stock by writing prescriptions for such a purpose but in fact is using the substance to maintain drug-dependent individuals who do not have legitimate prescriptions, then this is a violation of the law. As noted earlier, prescriptions for a Schedule II drug may not be refilled. Prescriptions for Schedule III, IV, and V drugs may be refilled if a practitioner gives authorization. Physicians may write three consecutive prescriptions for 30-day supplies. However, these prescriptions may not be filled or refilled more than six months after the date issued, nor can they be refilled more than five times after the date issued. After six months or after five refills, the practitioner may renew the prescription. Most states prohibit pharmacy technicians from taking phone orders for prescription (legend) drugs, and all states require pharmacists to authorize phoned-in prescriptions for controlled substances per DEA regulations. Prescriptions may be entered into an electronic medical record system and electronically transmitted to a pharmacy. This is referred to as *electronic prescribing* or *e-prescribing* and is permitted in many states. Prescriptions may also be handwritten on preprinted prescription forms, or printed onto similar forms via a computer printer, or even upon plain paper in certain circumstances. They may be, in certain jurisdictions, transmitted orally by telephone, but this can increase chances for errors.

THE POISON PREVENTION PACKAGING ACT OF 1970

The Poison Prevention Packaging Act authorized the Consumer Product Safety Commission to create standards for child-resistant packaging. This act requires that most OTC and legend drugs be packaged in child-resistant containers. These containers cannot be opened by 80% of children younger than 5 years but can be opened by 90% of adults (Figure 3-4). There are only instances in which prescriptions may leave the pharmacy without a child-resistant container: (1) if the prescriber writes "no child-resistant caps" on the prescription, (2) if the prescription is being dispensed for patients in a hospital or nursing home, or (3) if the patient requests this and has signed the appropriate release. Elderly patients may have difficulty opening child-resistant containers and may request that their medications be dispensed in containers that are not child-resistant. One type of medication that may be approved for dispensing without a child-resistant container is nitroglycerin; patients on this drug need to access the medication as quickly as possible. Examples of substances that do not, in most states, require child-resistant packaging include stool softeners, dietary supplements, including most vitamins, inhalers, and unit-dose medications.

THE OCCUPATIONAL SAFETY AND HEALTH ACT OF 1970

President Nixon signed the Occupational Safety and Health Act in 1970. The OSHA administers the act, which is a part of the U.S. Department of Labor. OSHA's mission is to ensure workplace safety and a healthy environment within the workplace. The medical industry became involved in OSHA-related publicity in the late 1980s, when the threat of human immunodeficiency virus (HIV) infection extended to health care workers. Viral hepatitis and other

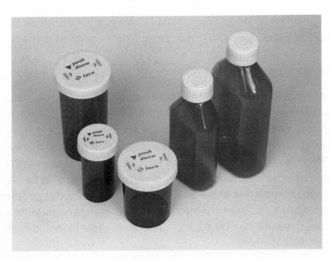

Figure 3-4 Drugs must be packaged in child-resistant containers.

pathogens already were concerns of health care workers, but when HIV, the virus that causes acquired immunodeficiency syndrome (AIDS), was identified, action was needed to better protect individuals who cared for patients with these infectious diseases. OSHA's final ruling on blood-borne pathogens became fully effective in July 1992. The act requires medical facilities to comply with the Blood-borne Pathogens Standard and to be able to prove that compliance to OSHA inspectors if necessary.

Common OSHA violations include the following: no eyewash facilities available, no labeling or improper labeling of hazardous chemicals, no documentation of initial employee training, no documentation of annual employee training, no annual hazard assessment performed, no proof of destruction of hazardous waste, no Emergency Action Plan in the facility, no Written Exposure Control Plan, OSHA Form 300A (Log of Work-Related Injuries and Illnesses) not posted during the required period, and no records of hepatitis B vaccinations on declaration forms.

Nuclear pharmacy is another area in which OSHA regulations apply. Nuclear pharmacy is probably the first specialty area in the pharmacy profession for which a special regulation at the state level has been established. Most regulations make it unlawful for any person to provide nuclear pharmaceutical services unless under the supervision of a qualified nuclear pharmacist. In nuclear medicine, exposure to chemotherapy requires special precautions and safety procedures.

Beginning in 1986, OSHA began requiring a *material safety data sheet (MSDS)* for every potentially dangerous chemical used in the workplace, including pharmacies. An MSDS must be kept on file in a designated, easily accessible binder, or be available in an electronic database. Each MSDS contains requirements for storage, procedures for handling, and steps to take if the chemical is splashed or sprayed into the eyes, or if it contacts the skin. Binders must be located in an easily accessible location. Commonly, licensed cleanup specialists are called in when a spill or exposure occurs. Law requires the use of the MSDS and there are penalties if not used correctly.

WHAT WOULD YOU DO?

Jeffrey was working in a hospital pharmacy and was splashed in the face by a disinfectant. His eyes were burning from the substance. He was not wearing protective goggles when the accident occurred. If you were Jeffrey, what is the first thing you would do?

THE DRUG LISTING ACT OF 1972

Under this act, each new drug is assigned a unique and permanent product code, known as a **National Drug Code (NDC)**, that identifies the manufacturer or distributor, the drug formulation, and the size and type of its packaging. Using this code, the FDA is able to maintain a database of drugs by use, manufacturer, and active ingredients and of newly marketed, discontinued, and remarketed drugs. The NDC for one product may not be used for another if any changes occur in product characteristics. A new NDC number must be assigned to the new product version.

THE MEDICAL DEVICE AMENDMENTS OF 1976

In 1976, the Medical Device Amendments were enacted. These amendments required manufacturers to register and list their products, follow good manufacturing practices during the making of these products, and report device failures. The amendments specify that before new devices are marketed, a panel of scientists to ensure their accuracy and preciseness to deliver the intended results must review them. A medical device is a machine or instrument recognized by the National Formulary or the United States Pharmacopeial Convention. Medical devices are used for the diagnosis, cure, mitigation, treatment, or prevention of disease. They may also be used to affect body structures as a part of treatment. There are three classes of medical devices. Class I includes needles, scissors, and others with a low potential to cause harm. Class II includes thermometers, catheters, and hearing aids, which all have performance standards that have been established by a panel of experts. Class III includes life-supporting systems that could cause serious injury or death if they fail.

THE ORPHAN DRUG ACT OF 1983

Before a new drug can be marketed, substantial evidence of both safety and effectiveness is required. The procedure is difficult, lengthy, and extremely expensive. Valuable new drugs with efficacy against diseases affecting only a small number of persons may not be developed because drug companies do not want to invest the millions of dollars and years of research necessary to secure approval for drugs that may not recoup their development costs. A drug that falls into this category is called an **orphan drug**. Orphan drugs are used to treat diseases that affect fewer than 200,000 people in the United States. The Orphan Drug Act of 1983 offers federal financial incentives to commercial and nonprofit organizations to undertake the development and marketing of such drugs. These incentives include tax breaks and a seven-year monopoly on drug sales. Since the act went into effect in 1983, more than 100 orphan drugs have been approved, including those for the treatment of conditions such as AIDS, cystic fibrosis, blepharospasm (uncontrolled rapid blinking), and snakebites.

THE DRUG PRICE COMPETITION AND PATENT-TERM RESTORATION ACT OF 1984

The Drug Price Competition and Patent-Term Restoration Act of 1984 was largely consumer-oriented and designed to lower drug prices by providing a mechanism to increase competition in the drug industry. This law provides abbreviated applications for new drugs and an accelerated procedure for approval of generic versions (pertaining to a substance, product, or drug that is not protected by trademark) of approved drugs whose safeguard protection is about to expire. An abbreviated new drug application (ANDA) is an application for a U.S. generic drug approval, for an existing licensed medication or approved drug. This application is submitted to the FDA's Center for Drug Evaluation and Research, Office of Generic Drugs, which provides for the review and ultimate approval of a generic drug product. Generic drug applications are termed "abbreviated" because they are generally not required to include preclinical (animal and in vitro) and clinical (human) trail data to establish an effectiveness. Applicants, instead, must scientifically demonstrate that their product is *bioequivalent*, meaning that it performs in the same manner as the innovator drug.

THE PRESCRIPTION DRUG MARKETING ACT OF 1987

The Prescription Drug Marketing Act of 1987 deals with safety and competition issues raised by secondary markets for drugs, and it prohibits the reimportation of a drug into the United States by anyone but the manufacturer. This act also prohibits the sale or trading of drug samples, the distribution of samples to persons other than those licensed to prescribe them, and the distribution of samples except by mail or by common carrier.

THE ANABOLIC STEROIDS CONTROL ACT OF 1990

The Anabolic Steroids Control Act of 1990 became effective in February 1991 and placed anabolic steroids under the regulatory provisions of the CSA. Anabolic steroids are hormonal substances that are related to testosterone, estrogen, progestins, and corticosteroids, which promote muscle growth. Athletes to increase physical performance use these agents occasionally. This act is significant because some observers believe that it reflects an essential change of direction for drug abuse control.

THE OMNIBUS BUDGET RECONCILIATION ACT OF 1990

The Omnibus Budget Reconciliation Act of 1990 (OBRA '90) requires pharmacists to offer to discuss information about new and refill prescriptions with Medicaid recipients (patients). However, as a result of this act, pharmacists now usually counsel all patients about their prescribed medications, not only those who have Medicaid. OBRA '90 requires states that seek reimbursement from the federal government for the cost of drugs provided to Medicaid patients to adopt programs that directly affect the pharmacy profession. With few exceptions, only costs for drugs approved as "safe and effective" are reimbursed. States must require pharmacists who provide services under the program to give consulting services. Drug utilization evaluation (DUE) must be conducted to ensure that all prescribed medications are reviewed for appropriateness. Matters that may be discussed in counseling should include the following information:

- Name and description of medication
- Dosage form, dosage, route of administration, and duration of drug therapy
- Common severe side effects or adverse effects
- Interactions (with other drugs or food) and therapeutic contraindications
- Self-monitoring of the medication therapy
- Proper storage
- Action in the event of a missed dose
- Special directions for and precautions to be taken by the patient

THE DIETARY SUPPLEMENT HEALTH AND EDUCATION ACT OF 1994

In 1994, Congress passed the Dietary Supplement Health and Education Act to clarify the regulatory framework applicable to nutritional supplements and to create specific labeling requirements. The products covered by this act are vitamins, minerals, herbs, botanicals, amino acids, other dietary supplements intended to increase total dietary intake, concentrates, metabolites, constituents, extracts, or any combination of these products. These supplements come in different forms, including capsules, powders, softgels, gelcaps, tablets, and liquids. This act placed the burden of proof squarely on the FDA, meaning that supplements whose safeness was questioned had to be proved harmful by the FDA.

THE HEALTH INSURANCE PORTABILITY AND ACCOUNTABILITY ACT OF 1996

The Health Insurance Portability and Accountability Act (HIPAA) was signed into law in August 1996. It amended the IRS Code of 1986, also known as the Kassebaum–Kennedy Act. HIPAA was one of the last acts of the Clinton Administration. Its Administrative Simplification provision contained four parts, each of which has generated various rules and standards as follows:

1. Electronic Health Transaction Standards: Under this provision, health organizations were required to adopt **standard code sets** to be used in all health transactions. For example, coding systems that describe diseases, injuries, and other health problems, as well as their causes, symptoms, and actions taken, had to be made uniform. All parties to any transaction were also required to use and accept the same coding. Although the code sets proposed as HIPAA standards were already being used by many health plans, clearinghouses, and providers, this standardization was intended to reduce mistakes, duplication of effort, and costs. Compliance was required by 2005.

2. Unique Identifiers: Previously, the use of multiple identification numbers was allowed when organizations dealt with each other. This was confusing, conducive to error, and costly. The goal of the HIPAA standard identifiers was to reduce such problems.

3. Security and Electronic Signature Standards: The Security Standard mandated safeguards for physical storage and maintenance, transmission, and access to individual health information. It applies not only to the transactions adopted under HIPAA but also to all individual health information that is maintained or transmitted; however, the Electronic Signature standard applies only to the transactions adopted under HIPAA. These standards were implemented in 2004.

4. Privacy and Confidentiality Standards: Implemented in 2003, the Privacy Standards limited the nonconsensual use and release of private health information, now termed *protected health information*; gave patients new rights to access their medical records and to know who else had accessed them; restricted most disclosure of health information to the minimum needed for the intended purpose; established new criminal and civil sanctions for improper use or disclosure of health information; and established new requirements for access to records by researchers and others.

POINTS TO REMEMBER

Patient confidentiality may be breached if protected health information is discussed in an area where the conversation may be overheard by someone not authorized to hear it, if computer screens or printed materials may be accidentally viewed by those not authorized to view them, if contact information is given out to people not authorized to receive it, if information is accessed by a health care worker who does not have permission to view it, and if information is given over the phone to an individual whose identity has not been not substantiated.

THE DRUG ADDICTION TREATMENT ACT OF 2000

This act allows physicians to prescribe DEA-preapproved controlled substances from Schedules III, IV, or V to people who are addicted to opioids, as part of maintenance or detoxification treatments. It differs from regulations controlling treatment for opioid addiction that uses methadone. Under this act, the patient must be in a treatment program that includes additional support services. The attending physicians must receive special training and be registered or certified with the DEA. Initially, private practice physicians can only treat 30 or fewer patients at one time; however, after one year, they may apply to treat as many as 100 patients simultaneously.

THE MEDICARE PRESCRIPTION DRUG, IMPROVEMENT, AND MODERNIZATION ACT OF 2003

This act was designed to provide senior citizens and disabled individuals with a prescription drug benefit, additional choices (via its Medicare Advantage plans), and more Medicare benefits. It established Medicare Part D, which is a voluntary prescription drug benefit program. This act is also referred to as the Medicare Modernization Act (MMA). It also offered tax breaks for prescription drugs, and partially privatized the Medicare system by establishing pretax medical savings accounts. However, certain fees for wealthier senior citizens were raised, leading to controversy. Overall, most senior citizens have benefited from this act because it helped them to better afford the increased price of many drugs vital to their health. It also enabled employers to offer employee drug benefits through drug subsidies.

THE COMBAT METHAMPHETAMINE EPIDEMIC ACT OF 2005

This act was designed to stop illegal use of drugs such as methamphetamine, crack cocaine, and others. It is an extension of the Patriot Act, initially passed in October 2001 in response to the September 11, 2001, terrorist acts, for the purpose of intercepting and obstructing terrorist acts. This act regulates drug trafficking that is used to financially support terrorism, greatly increasing the government's ability to prosecute and penalize individuals involved in these crimes. Legal drugs that can be utilized in the manufacture of the named illegal drugs under this act must be kept behind counters or in locked cases. These legal drugs include ephedrine and pseudoephedrine, and customers providing identification and their signature must track their purchase. Only *9 g per month per person* are allowed to be sold. There is also a daily limit of 3.6 g per day. As an example of a daily sales limit, regulated sellers may sell no more than 146 tablets of a 30 mg pseudoephedrine (as hydrochloride) product per day. This act also sets monthly sales limits for mobile retail vendors—those who sell products from movable or temporary stands or locations—and mail order distributors. Everyone selling these legal drugs must be registered with the U.S. Attorney General and receive training about this act.

ACCUTANE iPLEDGE PROGRAM OF 2006

This program was designed to mandate distribution in the United States for the drug known as isotretinoin (commonly sold under the trade name Accutane). This drug is used to treat severe cystic acne when other methods have not been successful. The program was intended to prevent use of the drug during pregnancy (or potential pregnancy) due to the high risk of birth defects. Physicians and pharmacists are now required by the FDA to register and use a specific website in order to receive this medication. The physician prescribing the drug enters patient information on the iPLEDGE website and pharmacists must review this information prior to filling the prescription. Mandatory patient counseling and reporting in the online system is still required for all patients. Since December 31, 2005, all patients receiving Accutane are required to be registered in the iPLEDGE Program.

RYAN HAIGHT ONLINE PHARMACY CONSUMER PROTECTION ACT OF 2008

This act amended the CSA to prohibit the delivery, distribution, or dispensing of a controlled substance that is a prescription drug over the Internet without a valid prescription but exempted telemedicine practitioners. It also defined the terms "valid prescription" and "online pharmacy," and imposes registration and reporting requirements on online pharmacies that dispense 100 or more prescriptions, or 5000 or more dosage units, of all controlled substances combined in one month. The act also increased criminal penalties involving controlled substances in Schedules III, IV, and V; authorized state actions against online pharmacies deemed to be threats to their citizens; and required the DEA to report to Congress on foreign suppliers of controlled substances over the Internet.

PATIENT PROTECTION AND AFFORDABLE CARE ACT OF 2010

This highly contested act represents the most significant overhaul of the U.S. health care system since the passage of Medicare and Medicaid. Its goal is to increase the quality and affordability of health insurance, lower the uninsured rate by expanding public and private insurance coverage, and reduce costs of health care for individuals and the government. It also requires insurance companies to cover all applicants within new minimum standards and to offer the same rates regardless of preexisting conditions or gender. Implementation began in 2013, amid intensive scrutiny, and various provisions and exemptions continue to evolve.

SYNTHETIC DRUG ABUSE PREVENTION ACT OF 2012

This act banned compounds commonly found in synthetic marijuana sold as "K2" or "Spice," synthetic stimulants such as bath salts, and hallucinogens by placing them under Schedule I of the CSA. This act was a part of the FDA Administration Safety and Innovation Act of 2012, which gave the FDA authority to collect user fees from the medical industry to fund reviews of innovator drugs, medical devices, generic drugs, and biologically similar biologics.

DRUG QUALITY AND SECURITY ACT OF 2013

This act created FDA oversight for large-volume compounding operations, allowed pharmacists to provide traditional compounding services to individual patients, and created track-and-trace requirements for drug products that will take effect over the next 10 years. Technology is being incorporated into packaging so that manufacturers can track unit-level drug products while they move through the nation's supply chain. This act helps to clarify current federal law regarding pharmacy compounding.

COMPREHENSIVE ADDICTION AND RECOVERY ACT OF 2016

This act addressed the full continuum of care—from primary prevention to recovery support—including significant changes to expand access to addiction treatment services and overdose reversal medications. It also included criminal justice and law enforcement-related provisions. This act improved access to overdose treatment; authorized grants to states to implement strategies for pharmacists to dispense naloxone; awarded grants to state substance abuse agencies, local government, and nonprofit organizations in areas with high rates of, or rapid increases in, heroin or other opioid use to expand availability of medication-assisted treatment; changed the law regarding office-based opioid addiction treatment with buprenorphine; improved treatment for pregnant and postpartum women; and gave grants to states to establish a response plan to the opioid epidemic.

Federal Regulatory Agencies

Three federal agencies that play a role in securing the health of Americans when it comes to diseases and drugs are the FDA, Centers for Disease Control and Prevention (CDC), and DEA.

FOOD AND DRUG ADMINISTRATION

The FDA is a branch of the U.S. Department of Health and Human Services. The agency oversees all domestic and imported food, bottled water, and wine beverages with less than 7% alcohol. It is also responsible for cosmetics, medicines, medical devices, radiation-emitting products, and even the feed and drugs used for farm animals. Thus it controls all drugs for legal use. All laws pertaining to drug administration are initiated, implemented, and enforced by the FDA.

CENTERS FOR DISEASE CONTROL AND PREVENTION

The CDC is a federal agency that provides facilities and services for the investigation, identification, prevention, and control of disease. In this context, it also oversees all foods and food-borne diseases. It provides statistics and information to health professions about the treatment of common and rare diseases worldwide. Its primary function is to issue regulations for infection control. It was established in 1946 as the Communicable Disease Center and became the Centers for Disease Control in 1970; the words "and Prevention" were added in 1992, but Congress requested that "CDC" remain the agency's initials. This agency also has been deeply involved in the war against HIV infection and AIDS.

DRUG ENFORCEMENT ADMINISTRATION

The DEA oversees controlled substances, including the investigation and prosecution of individuals who grow or manufacture substances for illegal distribution. The mission of the DEA is to enforce controlled substance laws and regulations and to prosecute both individuals and organizations who grow, manufacture, or distribute illegal substances. The DEA also targets people who use violence to coerce others to help them in their illegal activities and disseminates information about illegal substances to educate and inform the populace, who can then, in turn, help the DEA in its efforts. The DEA also interfaces with other governments to assist in the global enforcement of laws that regulate those who traffic drug and drug-related items.

Drug Recalls

The medical staff of the FDA determines the health hazard potential of a product and assigns a drug recall classification. Drug recalls are divided into three classes:

1. Class I: The use or exposure to the product will cause severe adverse reactions or death.
2. Class II: The use or exposure to the product may cause temporary or medically reversible adverse health hazards.
3. Class III: The use or exposure to the product is not likely to cause adverse health hazards.

Drug Standards

Drug standards are the set of requirements for the formulation of drug substances, ingredients, and dosage forms. Drugs stocked in the pharmacy must be compendia (listed) drugs, and a drug formulary or list of drugs stocked by the pharmacy must be maintained. These drug standards are contained in the United States Pharmacopeia (USP) and the **National Formulary (NF)**, published by the U.S. Pharmacopeial Convention, Inc. Pharmaceutical services must be under the general supervision of a licensed pharmacist. The pharmacist working within an institutional setting, such as a nursing home, must schedule regular visits to the facility to supervise the drug handling and administration procedures. At least monthly, he or she must review the drug regimen of each patient and report any discrepancies or irregularities to the administrator and the medical director. This is a significant requirement in terms of patient safety and professional integrity.

The Ethical Foundation of Pharmacy

As previously noted, in this chapter and in Chapter 2, ethics is a branch of moral philosophy that is concerned with the thoughts, judgments, and actions about issues that have greater implications of moral right and wrong. A pharmacy technician is an integral member of the health care team, in general, and the pharmacy team, specifically. Providing information about the risks and side effects of drug regimens is an ethical responsibility of physicians, pharmacists, and nurses. It is grounded in the principle of respect for the distinctive capacity of humans to make their own choices about their own lives. Patients must be aware of the benefits and risks of drugs that they may be taking.

Bioethics is a discipline that deals with the ethical and moral implications of biological research and applications, especially as they relate to life and death. It has relevance in the fields of pharmacology, anatomy, physiology, pathology, and biochemistry. This area of ethics also attempts to address the ethical questions raised by genetic research in the current era.

Summary

Laws, regulations, standards, and ethics govern the control of drugs in the practice of pharmacy. There are several types of law: civil, criminal, and statutory. Pharmacy technicians should understand the different terminologies used in law and which punishments may be given for which violations. The regulation of pharmacy practice is primarily a function of the state and not of the federal government. There may be some differences in pharmacy law among the different states.

Medical ethics is the term used to describe the discipline of evaluating merits, risks, and social concerns about medical activities. The five principles of the pharmacy code of ethics are beneficence, fidelity, veracity, justice, and autonomy. The purpose of all actions in the pharmacy should be to benefit clients to the greatest degree, with uniformity.

The U.S. Congress passed the first important federal law governing pharmacy, the Pure Food and Drug Act, in 1906. The Controlled Substances Act (CSA) governs the manufacture, distribution, and dispensing of substances that have the potential for addiction and abuse. Under this act, drugs are classified into five schedules. Since 1970, Congress has passed several important laws relating to drug research, manufacture, safety, or marketing. Among these are the Poison Prevention Packaging Act to prevent and protect children from accidental poisoning (child-resistant packaging), the Orphan Drug Act to provide research for new drugs needed by fewer people, the Occupational Safety and Health Act, and the Health Insurance Portability and Accountability Act (HIPAA). Beginning in 1986, OSHA began requiring a safety data sheet for every potentially dangerous chemical used in the workplace, including pharmacies.

REVIEW QUESTIONS

1. Standards of behavior considered appropriate within a profession are called:

   A. etiquette.
   B. ethics.
   C. philosophy.
   D. morals.

2. The drugs with the highest potential for abuse and addiction are classified as which one of the following schedules?

   A. I
   B. II
   C. IV
   D. V

3. Which of the following agencies oversees controlled substances and prosecutes individuals who illegally distribute them?

    A.   FDA
    B.   CDC
    C.   HIPAA
    D.   DEA

4. Which of the following laws offers federal financial incentives to commercial and nonprofit organizations to develop and market drugs that were previously unavailable in the United States?

    A.   Drug Listing Act
    B.   Orphan Drug Act
    C.   Poison Prevention Packaging Act
    D.   Controlled Substances Act

5. The FDA is a branch of which department that controls all drugs for legal use?

    A.   U.S. Department of Health
    B.   U.S. Department of Health and Human Services
    C.   U.S. Department of Agriculture
    D.   U.S. Department of Labor

6. A less serious crime, punishable by a fine or imprisonment for less than one year, is called a(an):

    A.   felony.
    B.   assault.
    C.   misdemeanor.
    D.   slander.

7. Pharmacy practice regulation is primarily a function of the:

    A.   DEA.
    B.   federal government.
    C.   state board of pharmacy.
    D.   U.S. Department of Health and Human Services.

8. A list of officially recognized drug names is known as the:

    A.   National Pharmacopeia.
    B.   U.S. Drug Code.
    C.   National Formulary.
    D.   International Pharmacopeia.

9. An example of a criminal law being broken would be which of the following?

    A.   A pharmacy technician packaging drug products
    B.   A patient suing the pharmacist
    C.   A pharmacist giving out free information
    D.   A pharmacist practicing without a license

10. The three branches of the federal government include all of the following, except:

    A.   regulatory.
    B.   judicial.
    C.   executive.
    D.   legislative.

11. Assumption of risk refers to a patient who:

    A. continues to drink alcohol when it interacts with his or her prescription medication.
    B. smokes cigarettes while pregnant against her physician's advice.
    C. is a diabetic and does not monitor his or her diet carefully.
    D. does all of the above.

12. In the pharmacy setting, an example of a crime that would be considered a misdemeanor is:

    A. shoplifting.
    B. arson.
    C. burglary.
    D. selling legend drugs without a prescription.

13. Failure to use a reasonable amount of care to prevent injury or damage to a pharmacy's customers would result in a charge of:

    A. libel.
    B. slander.
    C. negligence.
    D. abuse.

14. In most states, pharmacists are usually given certificates of registration, which are granted for a period of:

    A. 10 to 12 years.
    B. 6 months.
    C. 1 to 2 years.
    D. up to 5 years.

15. Which type of scheduled drugs has a high potential for abuse but is currently accepted for medical treatment in the United States?

    A. Schedule I
    B. Schedule II
    C. Schedule III
    D. Schedule IV

CRITICAL THINKING

1. Explain why it is necessary to uphold laws and ethical standards in the field of pharmacy. What do these laws prevent? What could be the result if these laws did not exist?

2. Research a legal case in your area involving violation of the laws regulating pharmacy. What was the violation? What were the arguments in the case? What was the outcome of the case?

3. Why is privacy such an important issue in health care and the field of pharmacy? Explain how the latest HIPAA regulations help protect a patient's privacy.

4. What were the key points of the Drug Listing Act of 1972?

5. What DEA forms are used for controlled substances?

6. What are the duties of the OSHA?

7. What are pharmacy technicians allowed to do when working with controlled substances?

8. What are the three classes of drug recalls and their descriptions?

WEB LINKS

American Bar Association: www.americanbar.org

American Society of International Law: www.asil.org

Centers for Disease Control and Prevention: www.cdc.gov

Drug Recalls: www.recalls.gov

Drug Topics: www.drugtopics.com

Mobile Sales under the Combat Methamphetamine Epidemic Act: www.deadiversion.usdoj.gov/meth/trg_mobile_081106.pdf

National Institutes of Health (NIH): www.nih.gov

U.S. Department of Health and Human Services (USDHHS): www.hhs.gov

U.S. Department of Justice DEA Office of Diversion Control: www.deadiversion.usdoj.gov

U.S. Drug Enforcement Administration: www.dea.gov

U.S. Food and Drug Administration: www.fda.gov

U.S. Pharmacopeial Convention: www.usp.org

READING LIST

Abood, R. R., and Burns, K. A. (2015). *Pharmacy Practice and the Law*, 8th ed. Burlington, NJ: Jones & Bartlett Learning.

Moini, J. (2020). *Law & Ethics for Pharmacy Technicians*, 3rd ed. Boston, MA: Cengage Learning.

Reiss, B. S., and Hall, G. D. (2016). *Guide to Federal Pharmacy Law*, 9th ed. Boynton Beach, FL: Apothecary Press.

Veatch, R. M., Haddad, A., and Last, E. J. (2017). *Case Studies in Pharmacy Ethics*, 3rd ed. Oxford, UK: Oxford University Press.

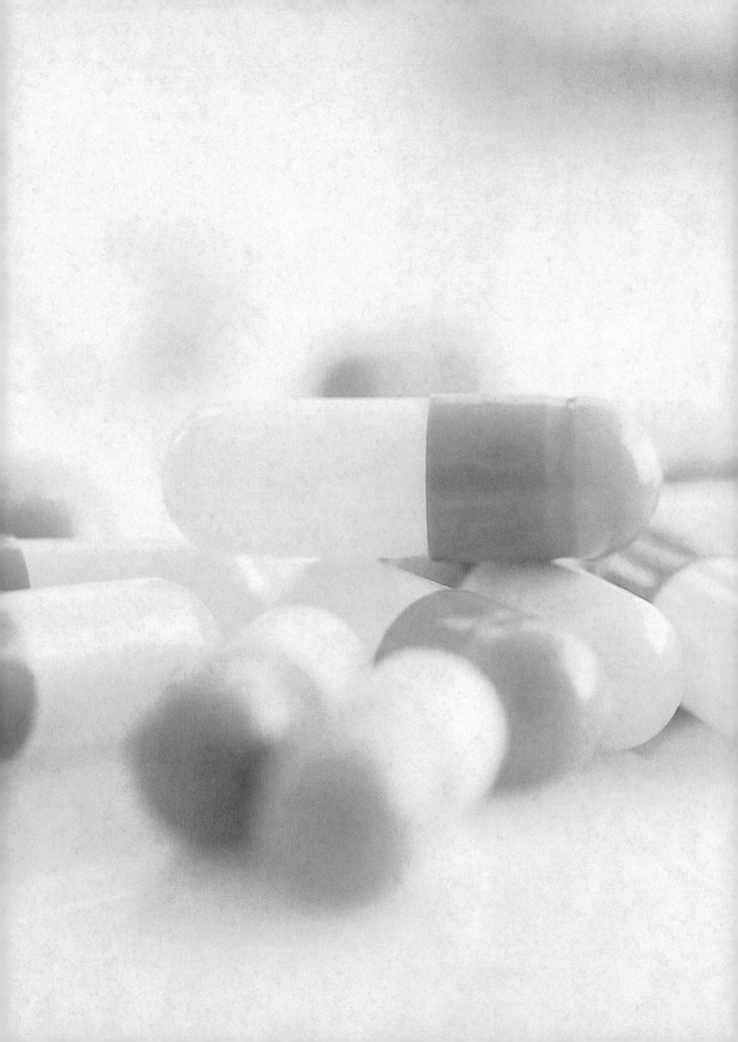

Communication with Patients and Customers

Professionalism
Autonomy
Honesty
Attitude
Confidentiality
Faithfulness
Appearance
Sexual Harassment
Grief

Barriers to Communication
Environmental (Physical Impairment)
Patients with Special Needs
Non–English-Speaking People
Hearing Impairment
Prejudice

Negative Communication

Defense Mechanisms
Regression
Projection
Repression
Rationalization
Compensation
Sublimation
Displacement
Apathy
Sarcasm
Denial

Dealing with Conflict

Eliminating Barriers to Communication
Time

OBJECTIVES

Upon completion of this chapter, the reader should be able to:

1. Explain the communication process and the communication cycle.
2. Describe the positive or "open" style of receiving feedback.
3. Differentiate between verbal and nonverbal communication.
4. State the various methods of communication.
5. Discuss the principles of autonomy and confidentiality.
6. Describe sexual harassment.
7. Explain some of the barriers to effective communication.
8. Discuss techniques for dealing with patients who have special needs.
9. Define negative communication.
10. Describe defense mechanisms and give examples.

KEY TERMS

apathy	decode	internal noise	repression
autonomy	defense mechanisms	prejudice	sarcasm
channels	denial	projection	sexual harassment
communication	displacement	rationalization	sublimation
compensation	expressive aphasia	receptive aphasia	
consumer	external noise	regression	

Overview

The pharmacy technician may work in very diverse practice settings such as hospitals, community pharmacies, clinics, health maintenance organizations, home health care organizations, retirement centers, and nursing homes. It is essential that pharmacy technicians are able to communicate effectively with patients, their caregivers, and other health care providers. An individual's success as a pharmacy technician begins and ends with the ability to communicate both professionally and courteously. It starts at the time of first contact with a potential employer and influences every aspect of the technician's career. Maintaining good relationships with co-workers and successfully developing rapport with clients depend on the pharmacy technician's ability to present himself or herself as competent, caring, knowledgeable, and presentable. It encompasses appearance as well as verbal and nonverbal communication. It takes place face to face, via telephone or fax, on the Internet, or through written documentation. First impressions have an enormous impact on those we meet and generally influence the course of any relationship, personal or professional. One would not feel comfortable trusting a dentist with poor oral hygiene or an ophthalmologist with dirty, broken glasses, or a surgeon with dirty hands and would doubt the teachings of an English professor who mispronounced even the simplest of words. Similarly, a patient meeting the pharmacy technician for the first time has certain expectations. An individual's presentation ultimately reflects back on his or her employer.

Communication Process

The communication process consists of the communication cycle, which involves two or more individuals participating in an exchange of information. The cycle involves the sender, or source, communicating a message to the receiver through a chosen channel of communication, to which the receiver responds with feedback (see Figure 4-1).

The communication cycle includes five basic elements:

- The sender or source
- The message
- The channel or mode of communication
- The receiver
- Feedback

SENDER

The sender is the person who sends a message through a variety of different **channels**. Channels can be spoken words, written messages, or body language. The sender encodes the message, which simply means that he or she chooses a specific way of expression using words or other channels.

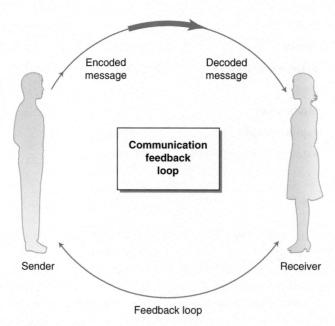

Figure 4-1 The communication loop.

MESSAGE

The message must contain all necessary information (complete). The message must not contain any unnecessary information (concise). It must be free from obscurity and ambiguity (clear). The message must be organized and logical (cohesive), and the message must be respectful and considerate of others (courteous).

CHANNEL

A channel is a path that a message takes from the sender to the receiver. It may be downward (from superiors to employees), upward (from employees to superiors), or horizontal (used between people on similar levels of responsibility).

RECEIVER

The receiver **decodes** the message according to his or her understanding of what is being communicated. However, there are times that the receiver understands the message incorrectly. This is often because of noise, which is anything that interferes with the message being sent. There are two kinds of noise: external and internal. **External noise** is literal noise, such as a radio or a jackhammer on the street outside. **Internal noise** includes the receiver's own thoughts, prejudices, and opinions.

POINTS TO REMEMBER

When a person wishes to share information with another, the sender must choose how to transmit that message.

FEEDBACK

Feedback can be verbal expressions or body language, expressing the fact that the receiver understood the message he or she received. When you communicate information to a patient or ask customers a question, always look for feedback. For example, when a technician dispenses a prescription and the patient needs consultation, the technician can ask the patient if he or she can wait until the pharmacist finishes a phone call so that he or she can answer the patient's questions. The technician should look for a response. If the patient responds positively, the pharmacy technician then knows that the patient will wait for the pharmacist to be able to talk with him or her directly.

The basic guidelines for giving feedback are as follows:

- Be clear.
- Have a positive emphasis—feedback is intended to help, not hurt.
- Be specific—avoid generalized comments. Notice when the person uses terms such as "always" or "never" and ask him or her to be more specific.
- Focus—highlight the person's behavior.
- Refer—to behavior that might be changed.
- Be descriptive—avoid evaluations.
- Own your feedback—use "I" statements.
- Be very careful with your advice—the person usually needs to understand how his or her actions can be improved in the future.

Feedback is sometimes called *criticism*, but this term negatively affects the perceptions of what feedback really is. Feedback is a way to let people know whether they are effectively communicating their message to you. It helps everyone to become more effective communicators. Feedback is not designed to harm the person who is receiving it, only to help him or her to become a better communicator and also to become more effective in actions on a daily basis. The following types of negative or "closed" styles of receiving feedback should be avoided:

- Defensive—defends personal actions and objects to the feedback that is being given
- Attacking—verbally attacks the person giving feedback
- Denial—refutes the accuracy or fairness of the feedback
- Disrespectful—devalues the speaker and the feedback provided
- Closed—ignores the feedback and is not interested in it
- Inactive listening—makes no attempt to understand the feedback
- Rationalizing—finds explanations that remove personal responsibility
- Patronizing—listens, but shows little interest
- Superficial—listens and agrees without intending to use the feedback to make any changes

The positive or "open" style of receiving feedback includes the following:

- Open—listens without interruptions or objections
- Responsive—listens without "turning the tables"
- Accepting—accepts the feedback without denying it
- Respectful—recognizes the feedback's value as well as the value of the giver of the feedback
- Engaged—interacts well with the speaker and asks for clarifications
- Active listening—listens carefully and tries to understand
- Thoughtful—tries to understand the personal behaviors that influenced the feedback being given
- Interested—shows genuine interest in getting feedback
- Sincere—really wants to make personal changes if they are appropriate

It is a good idea for the receiver to take notes about feedback received, especially in a group situation. One will not be able to remember everything spoken about, especially if there are numerous points. It is wise to have a written record to review to be able to act on every point covered.

To give feedback well, one should strive to be supportive, direct, sensitive, considerate, descriptive, specific, thoughtful, and helpful and try to give the feedback at a healthy time. For example, after the patient received and understood the message, you should ask him or her a question as feedback. One should avoid attacks; giving indirect feedback; being insensitive, disrespectful, or judgmental; giving feedback that is too generalized; and completely avoid being impulsive or selfish so that the receiver does not feel that the feedback was initiated only for personal reasons. Also, avoid poor timing because the receiver at such times may be ill-prepared to receive the feedback from the outset. For example, if you make an effort to develop good interpersonal skills, it will not be difficult to communicate with most individuals. You will, however, encounter patients in special circumstances that may cause them to be anxious or angry, and this will affect your interactions with them. Start with the most important things first. Be as brief as possible, and do not overly focus on small points because the receiver may then feel that the feedback is "nitpicking" or unfair.

Giving feedback about feedback is also a good practice. The receiver of the feedback should be given a chance to express his or her views about what was said and to discuss what he or she thought about the feedback (e.g., it was embarrassing, too general, repetitive, shallow, or too critical). This interaction can quickly show whether the receiver was disappointed with the quality of the feedback received and help to solve any existing difficulties that otherwise might go unaddressed.

In giving feedback, be honest but not brutal. In receiving feedback, try to use it to change what can be changed, and ask more questions about the rest—there is no reason to feel overwhelmed by a lot of feedback and then not act on it. Giving and receiving feedback is a continual learning process for both the speaker and receiver.

POINTS TO REMEMBER

A constructive pharmacy technician–patient relationship is essential to sound health care practice and the optimal well-being of the patient.

Verbal Communication

The goal of all communication is understanding. **Communication** is the sharing of information, ideas, thoughts, and feelings. It involves not just the spoken word, but also what is transported through inflection, vocal quality, facial expression, body posture, and other behavioral responses (see Figure 4-2). Whether or not a person complies with the medical regimen set down by his or her physician depends on a full understanding of the reasons behind the treatment prescribed. The communication between a client and the pharmacy technician may determine the treatment outcome. If a patient comprehends why it is important to take a medication in the exact manner in which it is prescribed, he or she is much more likely to comply. Many times individuals will alter the dose or duration of medications based on how they feel if they are unaware of the reasons behind the specific directions. If pharmacy technicians understand their role in treatment, they also understand the crucial position they hold and will gain and maintain knowledge through education and communication with all persons involved.

POINTS TO REMEMBER

To provide quality patient care, pharmacy technicians must have the desire and ability to communicate effectively with supervisors, co-workers, patients, and other health care providers.

Verbal communication consists of much more than just words. Tone, inflection, and level of pitch determine the meaning of the message we are sending even more than the words we choose. Phrasing, which refers to the style of speaking and the words we use to express ourselves, communicates to the receiver its own message. Choice of words is no more important than the way we pronounce them or the way we present them in determining how another person understands us. Proper diction and enunciation are required for speaking clearly and accurately. Quality communication requires much more than the giving of information. It includes the full scope of skills of listening, comprehending, imparting that information to others, obtaining feedback to validate that the information was received accurately and fully, and documenting the fact that each step in the process of communication was followed.

There are a variety of ways that help to improve verbal skills. These include increasing your vocabulary by reading, using communication aids such as the Internet, compact discs (CDs), and digital video discs (DVDs). There are

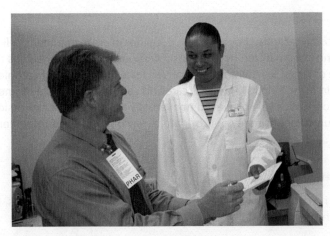

Figure 4-2 Communication is not just words. Facial expression, posture, and behavior all play a role in the message that is sent.

communication courses available from many different universities and colleges. When communicating with customers, it is important to think how they might feel about a situation. Often, a customer is in pain or feeling poorly, and it may be hard for him or her to control emotions. As a pharmacy technician, you should always be in control of your emotions, however. When a customer attempts to argue, you must not engage in the argument and try to remain positive at all times. Pharmacy technicians, however, should not deal with any customer who is abusive—the supervision pharmacist should be alerted to the situation, which may require help from a security person.

Written Communication

Excellent written communication skills are also important in the pharmacy setting. The pharmacy technician should be concerned about his or her writing. Inaccurate or confusing writing in the pharmacy setting not only irritates others but also leads to harmful patient care. The pharmacy technician will often be responsible for many kinds of writing, including memos, e-mail messages, ordering supplies, and record keeping. Written communication can reinforce or back up oral instructions or explanations of possible side effects of medications and can clarify misunderstandings to others.

Nonverbal Communication

By far, most of our communicative transmissions are nonverbal. We express ourselves both consciously and unconsciously through what is known as body language. Body language involves eye contact, facial expressions, hand gestures, grooming, dress, space, tone of voice, posture, touch, and much more.

EYE CONTACT

Certain aspects of body language are universal, such as smiles or frowns, and others are culture specific. Maintaining good eye contact is the most important nonverbal communication skill. It imparts to the receiver the impression that one is indeed interested in and paying attention to him or her. Anyone coming to a pharmacy rightly believes that he or she automatically deserves the undivided attention of the pharmacy technician for the duration of the transaction. With direct eye contact, the pharmacy technician is conveying to the client that he or she is indeed receiving undivided attention. Conversely, the pharmacy technician needs to be aware of the possible adverse effect that eye contact can create when interacting with individuals coming from different cultures who believe that looking directly at someone's face is rude and invasive. By being sensitive and attentive, the pharmacy technician should be able to modify his or her approach accordingly. Eye contact is not comparable to staring, which is impolite and invasive. Staring is rarely, if ever, eye-to-eye contact, and it is often perceived as communicating a judgmental and negative message, if not an openly aggressive one.

FACIAL EXPRESSIONS

Often, when individuals become patients, they experience feelings of embarrassment, self-consciousness, decreased self-esteem, and fear of being dehumanized by medical professionals. Facial expressions that accompany direct eye contact can either reinforce or dispel a patient's preconceived fears. The pharmacy technician can and must demonstrate professional interest in the individual as well as care and concern. Shocked, judgmental, disapproving, or disbelieving attitudes are almost exclusively conveyed nonverbally through facial expressions and body language in general, and under no circumstance are they appropriate behavioral attitudes to be demonstrated in the professional setting.

POINTS TO REMEMBER

A great deal of information is communicated through head and facial movements, but the movements of a person's eyes may provide more information than any other facial structure.

HAND GESTURES

The way one holds or moves the arms and hands (and the rest of the body) can project strong nonverbal messages. Primarily, the hands are used to emphasize important aspects of the words being said by the speaker.

GROOMING AND DRESS

Appearance is an integral part of nonverbal communication. It influences the way others view us and can present a conflicting message or even a totally incorrect message. When we see someone who is dressed or groomed in a way that is very different from our own style, we assume that our personalities are the opposite. This is not always true. Although we should not judge people by the way they dress or how they are groomed, it is difficult not to form opinions based on what is seen.

SPATIAL AWARENESS

Another aspect of nonverbal communication that requires cultural awareness is perceived territory. Generally speaking, Anglo-Saxon Americans tend to require more personal space than persons of other cultures and feel most comfortable at arm's length in all but intimate relations. In some other cultures, too much separation between interacting individuals is viewed as insulting or dismissive. As with direct eye contact, an awareness of the client's response to the approach taken will assist in modifying and improving interactions.

TONE OF VOICE

Use of the correct tone of voice in all situations with patients and customers cannot be emphasized enough. All people respond more favorably when spoken to in a tone that makes them feel respected, cared for, and understood. Your voice should convey an attitude of helpfulness and respect. You should reflect positive feelings about your job, patients, and skills. The sound of your voice should always remain calm, confident, and respectful. Pharmacy technicians should be aware of their vocal tone and never sound sarcastic, impatient, bored, parental, bullying, weak, or hesitant.

POSTURE

Posture is the position of the body with respect to the surrounding space. A posture is determined and maintained by coordination of the various muscles that move the limbs by the sense of balance. During communication, posture can usually be described as open or closed.

Open Posture

Open posture signifies a feeling of receptiveness and friendliness. An open posture position consists of the arms lying comfortably at the sides or in the lap. One should face the person to whom one is speaking and lean forward to indicate interest in what is being said. All these actions signify that one is listening and demonstrate positive forms of communication.

Closed Posture

A closed posture conveys the opposite—a feeling of not being totally receptive to what is being said. It can also signal that someone is angry or upset. A person in a closed posture may hold the arms rigidly or fold them across the chest. This person may lean back in a chair, away from the other person or may turn away to avoid eye contact. Slouching is a kind of closed posture that can convey fatigue or lack of caring.

PHYSICAL CONTACT

Touching can be an extremely powerful tool for the medical professional when utilized appropriately and therapeutically. The boundary between appropriate and inappropriate touching is well defined and inviolable without grave repercussions. On the other hand, one must also be aware of the proper use of appropriate touching in the workplace. Touching another person without his or her permission is never acceptable, and it is essential that the pharmacy technician understand the different forms of consent that may be offered or denied other than verbally. Occasionally, the technician might be required to demonstrate the proper use or application of a prescribed treatment. It is, however, important to ask permission or explain the necessity of any procedure that requires a hands-on approach before acting. The mere act of asking permission imparts respect and facilitates cooperation. It also creates an atmosphere of safety and comfort.

Communication with Others

The first priority when communicating with another is to have one's message received accurately. One way of accomplishing this is to show consistency between verbal and nonverbal communication. Do nonverbal characteristics emphasize the words spoken or misrepresent them? If a person is smiling or, worse, happy when offering condolences, the communication sent is inconsistent. Rarely is the verbal message received over the more believable nonverbal message. Another method used to determine whether or not your message has been received accurately is to ask the other individual to provide feedback. Ask questions that encourage specific details relating to the information given. The answers received will determine whether or not further explanation is required. The second and equally important concern is to ensure that one has accurately received the message sent. Provide feedback by restating the message heard, thereby providing opportunity for clarification or validation. A pharmacy technician will be instructing the client about the prescribed use of medications. This includes many details such as dose, amount, route of administration, frequency, and duration of use. It is essential that the client understand accurately because misunderstandings could have lethal consequences. Providing accurate written instructions is an added reinforcement of the verbal instructions, not a substitute for them.

Methods of Communication

One-on-one, face-to-face communication will be the method the pharmacy technician will be engaged in the most, although there are numerous other modes he or she will be required to use during the course of a workday. In the pharmacy, these might include telephones, computers, e-mails, networking through the Internet, telecommunication conferences, pagers, and voice mails. The pharmacy technician will also be required to provide written documentation. Each method of communication has its own specific characteristics; however, it is important to remember that all require courtesy, clarity, and accuracy of information both given and received.

TELEPHONES AND TELEPHONE SKILLS

The pharmacy technician will be required to conduct much of the pharmacy's daily business over the telephone. The manner in which he or she answers the phone sets the tone for the rest of the conversation (see Figure 4-3). The tone of voice should be pleasant yet professional. Properly identify the place of business and yourself by name followed by an offer of assistance. Remember that only half of the introductions have been made. Allow the caller time to complete the introductory phase of the communication including the purpose of the call before placing him or her on hold. This will reflect positively on you, your employer, and your place of business. When placing a telephone call, introduce yourself and your place of employment followed by a short statement of the purpose of the call. Be prepared before initiating the telephone call to ensure that you communicate precisely, accurately, and cohesively.

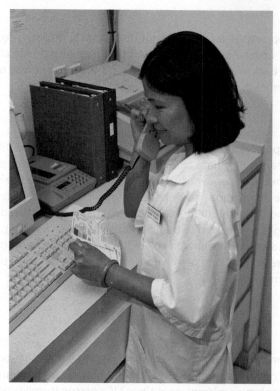

Figure 4-3 Telephone skills are important and should demonstrate professionalism.

Proper Taking of Telephone Messages

Proper written message taking is essential when the technician answers the telephone. Several calls may be answered before there is an opportunity to relay a message or carry out a promise of action. Numerous types of message pads are available today to facilitate proper message taking (see Figure 4-4). Never use small scraps of paper for messages; they are too easily lost. Bear in mind that the message book should be kept indefinitely in the pharmacy, because it could be used as evidence in a court of law.

At least seven items are needed to take a telephone message correctly:

- The name of the person to whom the call is directed
- The name of the person calling
- The caller's daytime or evening telephone number, or both
- The reason for the call
- The action to be taken
- The date and time of the call
- The initials of the person taking the call

The nature of the message will determine whether it should be reported immediately. The person who completes the call must sign and date the message. The message procedure is not complete until the necessary action has been taken.

CELL PHONES

Cellular phones have become a part of most people's daily lives. More than 92% of adults in the United States have some type of cell phone and more than 61% have some type of smartphone. Pharmacy technicians must avoid use of their personal cell phones in the workplace. Personal cell phones should be used only when on a break and not when actually working. If you receive an urgent call or text message, you must get permission with your supervisor to reply. The most important duty of pharmacy technicians is to focus on excellent patient care and avoid distractions.

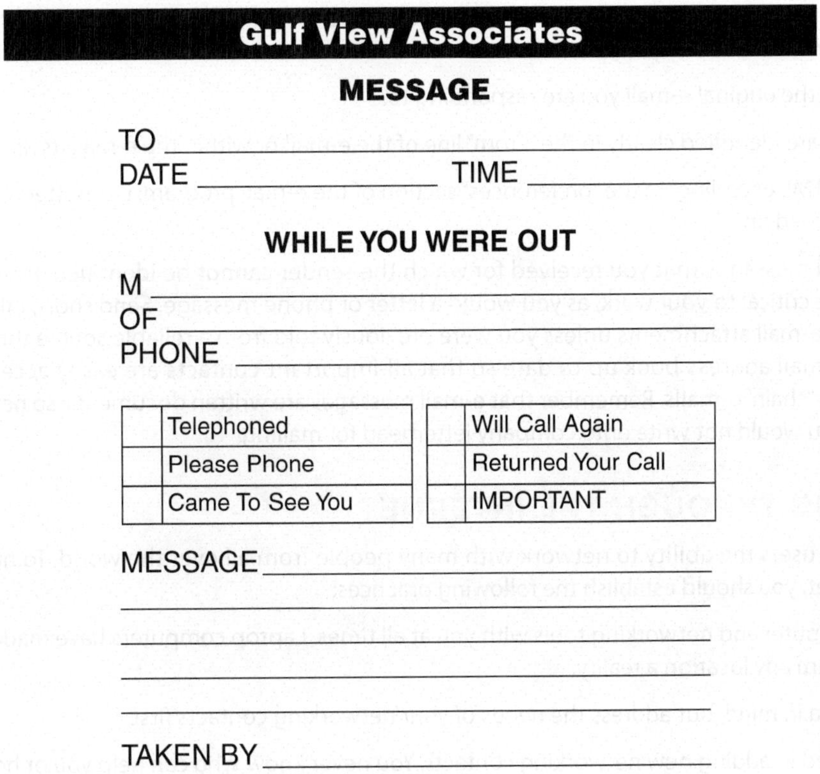

Gulf View Associates

MESSAGE

TO _____

DATE _____ TIME _____

WHILE YOU WERE OUT

M _____

OF _____

PHONE _____

Telephoned		Will Call Again	
Please Phone		Returned Your Call	
Came To See You		IMPORTANT	

MESSAGE _____

_____

_____

_____

TAKEN BY _____

Figure 4-4 A message pad used to facilitate proper message taking.

FAX MACHINES

The use of fax machines has greatly increased the efficiency of day-to-day operations in the pharmacy. Connected to a normal phone line, a fax machine allows transmittal of documents to the fax machines of other people instantly. Advances in technology have created systems wherein fax machines can correspond with computer programs as well as other fax machines. Doctors regularly fax written information to pharmacies, helping to avoid errors in communication caused by not hearing or not understanding information spoken over the phone or phone calls that are interrupted by static and other noise. One key to reducing medication errors is to provide real-time decision support and timely notification of inappropriate medication orders to the health care providers responsible for patient care. Pharmacy technicians should be very familiar with the use of fax machines, because they are used every day in the pharmacy.

COMPUTERS

Computers are another tool for communication. The pharmacy technician should learn how to use the available technology with accuracy and efficiency. Today, the Internet affects all types of business communications. It is used to do research, work with customers, handle voice and video conferences, and communicate using e-mail.

E-MAIL

Electronic mail has become a very popular method of communication in the medical community, as in every sphere of society. The inexpensiveness and ease-of-use of e-mail makes it the preferred method of communication compared with regular mail delivery. Some important factors to consider when using e-mail are the following:

- Use normal uppercase and lowercase letters. Avoid using all capital letters because this is used for emphasizing certain words; using all capitals is considered "shouting."

- Do not assume your intentions will be understood, because people cannot see your face or body language.

- Do not send insulting remarks by e-mail; this is referred to as "flaming."

- Double check e-mails by rereading them, and never send an e-mail in anger.

- Remember that e-mail can be easily forwarded without the sender's knowledge and is not necessarily a private communication between two people.

- Include part of the original e-mail you are responding to.

- Make sure you are identified clearly in the "From" line of the e-mail or within the e-mail itself.

- Turn off the "HTML encoding" in the "preferences" section of the e-mail program; it is better to have the "Plain text" option turned on.

Delete all e-mail messages that you received for which the sender cannot be identified. It is all right to ignore e-mails that are not critical to your work, as you would a letter or phone message. Send short, informal e-mail messages. Never open e-mail attachments unless you were previously told from a reliable source that they were being sent. Keep your e-mail address book up to date so that all-important contacts are easily accessible. Do not get involved in sending "chain" e-mails. Remember that e-mail messages are written documents, so never put something in an e-mail that you would not write onto company letterhead for mailing!

NETWORKING THROUGH THE INTERNET

The Internet offers users the ability to network with many people from all over the world. To network effectively through the Internet, you should establish the following practices:

- Have your computer and networking tools with you at all times. Laptop computers have made quick accessibility from any location a reality.

- Have an agenda in mind, but address the needs of your networking contacts first.

- Be open-minded in adding new networking contacts. You never know who can help you or how one can help you in the future.

- Manage your time effectively.

- Ask for referrals.

- Make notes about each conversation and place these notes in an easily accessible computer location.

- Follow-up on all leads you are given, and stay in touch with the contacts who referred you.

- Ask for information and advice.

- Stay positive and upbeat at all times.

TELECOMMUNICATION CONFERENCES

The use of teleconferences over the phone or via computers has grown greatly in the past few years. For example, a pharmacist in Florida may converse with medical centers, hospitals, or other pharmacies out of state to discuss problems, solutions, costs, or medications in a group setting. This allows many different people to share differing knowledge of important and complicated subjects in a forum that is easy to use and offers very efficient use of time to accomplish tasks and goals. Occasionally pharmacy technicians will be included in teleconferences, and it is important for them to be aware of the basic etiquette and manner of utilizing these new technologies to their best potential.

PAGER AND VOICE MAIL

A new phenomenon in the pharmacy setting is the use of customer paging systems. After customers put in their prescription orders at the pharmacy, they are given a paging device and are allowed to move around the store while their order is being prepared. When their order is ready, their pager signals them to return to the pharmacy counter, where they can then pick up their prescription. Another popular type of technology used in pharmacies is the voice mail message system. Refills may be called in by leaving a voice mail message for what is needed from the pharmacy. This system utilizes touch-tone phones to make selections and enter data through a computer that controls the message system. Patients can enter their prescription number, name, Social Security number, name of the prescription medication they need to be refilled, and any other required information. Most of their refills are then processed and ready for pickup within 24 hours.

WRITTEN DOCUMENTATION

State boards of pharmacy require pharmacy records to be kept for two years. It is important to keep track of all dispensed medications, manufacturer data, lot numbers, and patient records to ensure proper management and business practices. A competent plan for records management on a day-to-day basis can save a pharmacy a lot of time and trouble in the future. This is especially true if legal issues arise. The pharmacy can protect itself greatly by having a good record of activities to prove proper business management and good patient service.

Types of Customers

In a pharmacy, customers are not only clients with a prescription. Customers are also the physicians who write the prescriptions, the nurses who call in the prescriptions, and others such as pharmaceutical representatives.

CONSUMERS

In the community pharmacy setting, the **consumer** is the person coming to the pharmacy for the filling of prescriptions or the purchase of over-the-counter remedies for a wide variety of situations. Above all, the consumer is seeking information. The pharmacy technician will be called upon to answer many questions. It is important for the technician to remember that he or she cannot be expected to know all things, and the most valuable technician will know when to refer questions or concerns directly to the pharmacist.

PHYSICIANS

Physicians are the pharmacist's livelihood. Most contact with them will be via the telephone. It is important for the pharmacy technician to be respectful, pleasant, and courteous when taking their calls.

POINTS TO REMEMBER

Using the first name of anyone other than a friend is considered inappropriate or discourteous in most cultures.

NURSES

Often the nurse working with a physician will be the person calling in a prescription. He or she should be treated with respect.

PHARMACEUTICAL REPRESENTATIVES

Pharmaceutical sales have enormous implications for the business of pharmacy. The development of new drugs is time-consuming and expensive, and the marketing of approved drugs is extremely competitive. Pharmaceutical representatives from leading manufacturers regularly contact physicians in their coverage area to promote the use of their products and the companies they represent. These individuals must have current information on new medicines, research, and technologies that relate to drugs and usage of drug products.

Professionalism

Professionalism is behavior based on a body of knowledge and ethical standards to serve the public. Pharmacy technicians must maintain professional behavior, show respect, and exhibit a positive attitude in all of their dealings with customers and other medical personnel.

The most important characteristics a good pharmacy technician can display are honesty, reliability, dependability, integrity, and organization. The pharmacist and other personnel must be able to rely on the technician to maintain professional behavior at all times. They must be able to trust that the technician will behave ethically and maintain confidentiality regardless of the presence or absence of direct supervision.

AUTONOMY

The principle of **autonomy** establishes a patient's right to self-determination. He or she can choose what will be done to his or her body. This right is considered paramount even if a health professional may judge a patient's decision as being damaging to his or her health. One area of importance is patient respect in situations involving death with dignity and euthanasia. Health professionals should respect the wishes of all patients uncritically, enhancing their sense of self-worth and focusing on the active involvement of competent patients. Informed consent must be given to the health professional by the patient before any procedure is undertaken.

HONESTY

The honesty principle states that patients have the right to tell the truth about their medical condition, the course of their disease, treatments recommended, and alternative treatments available.

ATTITUDE

Pharmacy technicians must be warm and caring and display a genuine interest in helping people. They must be able to perform their duties effectively and efficiently while keeping in mind that their first priority is to the patient met in the hospital or the client coming to the neighborhood pharmacy.

CONFIDENTIALITY

Confidentiality assures patients that information about their medical conditions and treatment will not be given to third parties without permission. Confidentiality is essential for preserving the human dignity of the patient. Patients are expected to reveal the most personal details of their existence to virtual strangers. They must be able to trust that this information will not be shared with others not involved in their medical care.

Unnecessary conversation that is often negative is referred to as *gossip*. It should always be avoided. Gossip can result in legal outcomes. It is a totally unprofessional breach of another person's trust and confidentiality. You must always avoid others who try to engage you in gossip, stating that it is unfair, inappropriate, and wastes valuable time. Gossip that is focused on a patient is a strict breach of confidentiality. Patients' names should never be used in conjunction with the description of their conditions, since people who are not authorized to be made aware of such information may overhear these.

Also, all written materials that contain patient information must be secured from unauthorized people coming into contact with them. Anything with a visible patient name must be considered confidential. Such written paperwork should never be left where unauthorized individuals, who include other patients, visitors to the facility, and even vendors of supplies and equipment, may see it.

FAITHFULNESS

The right of patients to have health professionals provide services that promote the patient's interest rather than those that serve a competing or conflicting interest is faithfulness. A pharmacist or technician who encourages the use of vitamins the patient does not need may be promoting his or her financial well-being at the expense of the patient. Ethically, the responsibility of a health professional is, first and foremost, the welfare of the patient.

APPEARANCE

Pharmacy technicians are professionals and should not only act professionally but also dress professionally. Cleanliness and neatness say more about an individual than dressing in the latest fad and instill good impressions in others.

SEXUAL HARASSMENT

Sexual harassment occurs whenever any person makes intentional, clearly understood statements or takes intentional, clearly understood action that causes another to feel that his or her job is at risk if the sexual advances are rejected. Harassment may be physical or verbal, expressed in gestures or images, or written or spoken. It can occur at any level within the hierarchy of the work environment and can result in personal distress. The legal implications can be extremely distressing and debilitating for all concerned.

WHAT WOULD YOU DO?

You are helping a customer in your pharmacy when you notice that a regular male customer has entered and gets in line. Your co-worker is an attractive female pharmacy technician. She takes care of the man's prescription, remaining professional while he obviously flirts with her. He returns several times in the next few weeks, each time becoming more "pushy" with his flirting, until he asks her to go out with him. She declines, professionally and quietly so as not to embarrass him. The next night, he returns close to the end of her shift and stands off to one side, watching her as she prepares to go home. You are worried that he will continue to bother her once she leaves the building. What would you do?

GRIEF

Grief is a term that refers to a variety of intense physical and psychological responses occurring after some type of loss. It is a natural adaptive response to loss. There are two primary adaptive processes of grief. These include *mourning* and *bereavement*. Mourning is when grief is expressed, and the loss is integrated as well as resolved. Bereavement is the period after the death of a loved one. Stages of grief include *shock*, *reality*, and *recovery*. The various types of grief include *anticipatory*, *disenfranchised*, *dysfunctional*, and *uncomplicated* grief.

Barriers to Communication

The number of barriers to good communication in any situation is great, but they present especially challenging dilemmas in the pharmaceutical setting. The potential for life-threatening mistakes make it essential that communication be accurate and timely. Work conditions may be crowded and noisy. The physical environment may not allow for privacy and ease of confidentiality. Personal characteristics and concerns of clients and co-workers alike can interfere with the smooth communication in the workplace. Time constraints add pressure and may increase stress. The general administrative philosophy also plays a part in setting the tone of working relationships.

ENVIRONMENTAL (PHYSICAL IMPAIRMENT)

A pleasant environment is one in which, among other things, acoustics are sufficient to carry on a conversation without having to raise one's voice. Also, an environment in which good rapport can be established and confidentiality assured is essential for any pharmacy. If a patient does not feel that all communication is treated with care, concern, courtesy, and, above all else, confidentiality, that patient will, at best, be less than direct and honest. This not only prolongs the time needed to properly understand and accurately meet the needs of the individual, but it also could easily lead to misinformation and inaccurate treatment. At worst, the patient's health and, in fact, life are placed in jeopardy. Another result of an uncomfortable or unpleasant atmosphere could be the loss of that patient's continuing his or her relationship with the pharmacy. The client loses good continuity of care, the pharmacist loses business, and eventually his or her reputation suffers. The pharmacy technician who is aware of the relationship between excellent medical care and an environment conducive to good communication will be seen as a valuable asset.

PATIENTS WITH SPECIAL NEEDS

There are a variety of special situations that may affect patients in regard to effective communication with pharmacy staff. Patients who are terminally ill may have great difficulty communicating and in many cases require others to assist them. It is difficult for all people, including those in various medical professions, to communicate effectively with patients who are terminally ill. However, it is essential that professionalism be maintained in all such communications. In some cases, medical professionals are the primary remaining connections that these patients have with life. To help terminally ill patients with goals they may have to complete various tasks in their lives, medical professionals should seek out opportunities for better communication. Empathetic listening is an essential skill in communicating with terminally ill patients.

Communications may also be more difficult with patients who are experiencing pain, are under the influence of strong medications, or are confused or disoriented. Though pharmacy technicians may be in contact with these types of patients less frequently than other medical professionals, they should still understand the guidelines for behavior when communicating with them. With these patients, it is essential to identify yourself and maintain eye contact. You should state the patient's name, and always speak slowly and clearly, using simple language. You should attempt to keep your messages brief and focused on important information, allowing the patient time to respond. Touching the patient is acceptable if he or she feels comfortable with this. For patients in significant pain, you should only attempt to communicate when medications have been given to lessen the pain significantly. However, medications may make patients unable to easily communicate, so keep your messages clear and simple, repeating them if needed. You should review what was communicated with the patient to verify understanding, and that the information is remembered. If appropriate, written information should be left with the patient to review later.

NON-ENGLISH-SPEAKING PEOPLE

Language barriers occur when an individual neither speaks nor comprehends an adequate amount of English. This presents unique challenges for the pharmacy technician. Communication can often be facilitated by the use of proper English and elimination of complex words or phrases. Use of demonstrative gestures may also help. The availability of preprinted instructions in a variety of languages is a valuable aid.

HEARING IMPAIRMENT

The client's role in the communication process is multifaceted. Barriers to good communication on the client's part can be of a physical or psychological nature. The important role of the pharmacy technician is to observe early on whether or not the client has any limitations that might interfere with good communication. There are a number of physical abnormalities that could limit the client's ability to participate fully or accurately in the communication process. Is the person hearing correctly under all circumstances? A client may hear perfectly well in a small room with only one other person communicating but may be unable to hear accurately in a room full of background noise. Is the client capable of hearing lower tones well but cannot follow the conversation of someone with a high, soft voice? A client might be deaf and communicate only through sign language, an interpreter, or by reading lips. Pharmacy technicians may also interact with clients whose hearing is unimpaired but who have other forms of physical impairment that make communication challenging. **Receptive aphasia** is a physical limitation that occurs after certain neurological injuries and leaves the person incapable of understanding all that is said. Another client might exhibit **expressive aphasia**, a condition in which he or she cannot form language and express his or her thoughts accurately even though thought processes are intact.

PREJUDICE

Personal and social bias, which brings about discrimination, is called **prejudice**. The word *discrimination* is used to describe unfair treatment of a person because of race, gender, religious affiliation, handicap, or any other reason. Discrimination is unethical, immoral, and socially wrong. Sometimes it is even illegal, and it also prevents effective communication.

Negative Communication

The pharmacy technician should be aware of the negative impression he or she can have on others. Some examples of negative communication include the following:

WHAT WOULD YOU DO?

One of your co-workers in the pharmacy regularly complains about his hours, the customers, having to handle shipping and receiving, and generally anything that the other staff members tolerate well. You ask him if he wants to talk about anything because he seems unhappy. He tells you to mind your own business. His actions regularly distract you from your work, and you are concerned that you might be more likely to make an error because of this. What would you do?

- Speaking too softly or indistinctly

- Appearing bored or disinterested

- Appearing impatient (e.g., drumming fingers or clicking a pen)

- Interrupting

- Ignoring common courtesies such as saying "please" and "thank you"

- Speaking too quickly or sharply

- Confronting or being loud and aggressive

- Using negative body language (e.g., chomping gum or slouching)

- Appearing judgmental (e.g., frowning or crossing one's arms)

- Avoiding eye contact or staring

Defense Mechanisms

The human body may react to anxiety or stress in many different ways. **Defense mechanisms** are tools an individual uses when required to deal with uncomfortable or threatening situations. These are often subconscious reactions designed for emotional protection. They help us to deal with whatever difficult event has triggered such a response. There are many types of defense mechanisms, and pharmacy technicians should be familiar with them to better communicate with patients and others they come into contact with in the course of their duties. Commonly employed defense mechanisms include the following.

REGRESSION

Responding to a perceived threat or conflict in an immature way is called **regression**. The individual calls upon coping skills learned early in life to avoid or escape conflict in the present. Examples include making excuses for not doing a certain thing or saying that it cannot be done, instead of the truth—that the person does not want to do it.

PROJECTION

Shifting one's own unacceptable feelings onto another person is called **projection**. An example is when a man who has competitive or hostile feelings about another says that the other person "does not like him."

REPRESSION

Repression is characterized by pushing uncomfortable thoughts or conflicts out of consciousness to avoid the discomfort of confrontation. Examples include blocking a problem out of the mind and changing the subject when it is mentioned.

RATIONALIZATION

Giving reasonable justification to explain unreasonable behavior is called **rationalization**. An example is when you buy something you want because you are convinced that a similar item you already own will not be of value much longer.

COMPENSATION

Exaggerating one acceptable characteristic to make up for an unacceptable one is called **compensation**. A person who compensates makes up for one behavior by stressing another. Compensation is not always a negative response, but it is often used as an excuse for not accomplishing what should be accomplished. An example is a person with a deficiency in one area who becomes extremely proficient in a different area.

SUBLIMATION

Sublimation is redirecting a socially unacceptable impulse into a socially acceptable act. An example is using work or hobbies to divert your thoughts from a problem you do not want to address.

DISPLACEMENT

Displacement is giving one's own negative feelings to someone or something else unrelated to the situation. When faced with situations that are uncomfortable and potentially volatile, the pharmacy technician should remain calm, observant, flexible, patient, and be willing to try different approaches. The technician should not hesitate to request assistance from a supervisor or employer if needed. An example of displacement behavior is when a person who has been angered at work goes home and punishes his or her child for a behavior that is usually tolerated.

APATHY

A lack of feeling, emotion, interest, or concern is called **apathy**. An apathetic person shows indifference to what is happening or a pretense of not caring about a situation. Apathy is sometimes a sign of depression. An example is when an individual does not do regular menial tasks that should be done because he or she has no interest in the outcome of being responsible for them.

SARCASM

In most cases, the use of **sarcasm** is hostile and cruel; however, some individuals use it constantly, thinking that it is quite witty. On the contrary, it often makes bitter enemies of its victims. An example is when an individual makes fun of a co-workers' behavior or mistakes to improve his or her standing in the office, even though it only causes him or her continuing embarrassment.

DENIAL

Denial is a psychological defense mechanism in which confrontation with a personal problem or with reality is avoided by denying the existence of the problem or reality. An example is a parent who reacts with hostility to some-one who discusses his or her child's affliction, saying that the person is overreacting or misinformed even though the child's condition is a medical certainty.

Dealing with Conflict

Conflict may develop in the pharmacy over many issues, including pricing, prescriptions, and the perceptions of patients or customers. Conflict can be dealt with in many ways. The first way to assure good communication is for pharmacy technicians to be open and willing to listen to the people they talk to about health problems and medi-cation requirements. Second, pharmacy technicians should avoid confrontational terms and keep the focus of their discussions on the good of the patient. They should never enter into any discussion that is beyond their scope of training and should always refer customers directly to the pharmacist or back to their physician if needed. The most important thing for pharmacy technicians to remember is to remain professional at all times. If a situation starts to get out of hand, it is best to alert the pharmacist so the proper decision can be made regarding the customer's com-plaint or problem.

Eliminating Barriers to Communication

The elimination of barriers to good communication requires the realization that they exist, the identification of the specific nature of the barriers, and the willingness to take appropriate action to eliminate them. This is the respon-sibility of every member of the working team. Good working relationships can compensate for any barrier created by the actual physical space occupied by the pharmacy. Working conditions will improve with recognition of the barriers present and with the staff working together as a team. This will result in increased quality of services and increased client satisfaction, which will be evidenced by increased revenues.

TIME

In the world we live in today, few of us have too much time on our hands. The pharmacist cannot and usually will not tolerate unnecessary delays in the routine workings of his or her place of business. The pharmacy technician must prioritize his or her time with extreme care to complete each task efficiently before the next is due to begin. Every worker must operate under similar time constraints. Most clients have only limited available time as well. For any facility to function within the designated time constraints of all, good communication is the essential key.

Summary

How you present yourself will determine the course your career will take. The pharmacy technician who pays attention to how others perceive him or her and who acts, speaks, and dresses accordingly will have greater job satisfaction and security. Verbal communication depends on words and sound, whereas nonverbal communication consists of messages that are conveyed to another without the use of words. Eye contact, facial expressions, and hand gestures are some of the many ways we use body language to communicate. Some of the barriers to communication include physical impairment, language differences, and prejudice. Defense mechanisms are psychological methods of dealing with stressful situations and include regression, projection, repression, rationalization, compensation, sublimation, displacement, and several others.

REVIEW QUESTIONS

1. An individual's success as a pharmacy technician begins and ends with the ability to:

   A. work in very diverse practice settings.
   B. communicate both professionally and courteously.
   C. become certified.
   D. explain the value of listening.

2. The communication cycle includes the sender, the message, the channel, the receiver, and the:

   A. documentation.
   B. first impressions.
   C. presentation.
   D. feedback.

3. The goal of all communication is:

   A. completeness.
   B. cohesiveness.
   C. body language.
   D. understanding.

4. Pharmacy technicians must have excellent oral, nonverbal, and _____ communication skills.

   A. phrasing
   B. written
   C. prescribing
   D. receiving

5. The pharmacy technician can and must demonstrate _____ to patients, as well as care and concern.

   A. professional interest
   B. body language
   C. hand gestures
   D. spatial awareness

6. The type of communication you, as a pharmacy technician, will be engaged in the most is:

   A. written.
   B. face-to-face.
   C. telephone.
   D. e-Mail.

7. When answering the pharmacy's phone, you should properly identify:

   A. the hours of operation.
   B. the place of business and yourself by name.
   C. the caller's name first.
   D. whether the pharmacy is having a sale on certain medications.

8. Which of the following is *not* one of the seven items you should write down when taking a telephone message properly?

   A. The name of the person to whom the call is directed
   B. The caller's daytime and/or evening telephone number
   C. The caller's Social Security number
   D. The date and time of the call

9. As a pharmacy technician, it is important to know when to:

   A. close the store for the day.
   B. take your breaks during the day.
   C. exhibit a positive attitude.
   D. refer questions or concerns directly to the pharmacist.

10. One of the most important characteristics a good pharmacy technician can display is:

   A. knowing the prices of over-the-counter medications.
   B. being at least an hour early into work.
   C. integrity.
   D. giving prescription advice and opinions to customers.

11. The principle of _____ establishes a patient's right to self-determination.

   A. ethics
   B. autonomy
   C. confidentiality
   D. faithfulness

12. Sexual harassment may be verbal, written, or:

   A. physical.
   B. intentional.
   C. legal.
   D. illegal.

13. Personal and social bias, which brings about discrimination, is called:

   A. prejudice.
   B. unfairness.
   C. negative.
   D. confrontational.

14. _____ are tools an individual uses when required to deal with uncomfortable or threatening situations.

    A. Social wrongs
    B. Negative communicators
    C. Defense mechanisms
    D. Conscious reactions

15. _____ is a psychological defense mechanism in which confrontation with a personal problem, or with reality, is avoided by not admitting the existence of the problem or reality.

    A. Sublimation
    B. Displacement
    C. Hostility
    D. Denial

CRITICAL THINKING

1. Think about a situation in which you have dealt with someone who left you feeling angry or disappointed. What was it about the encounter that made you feel this way? What could have improved the outcome of the encounter?

2. Now think about an encounter in which you have dealt with someone who left you feeling satisfied and happy. What was it about this encounter that made you feel this way?

WEB LINKS

National Communication Association: www.natcom.org

The People's Pharmacy: www.peoplespharmacy.com

Pharmacy Times: www.pharmacytimes.com

Resource Pharm: www.resourcepharm.com

CHAPTER 5

Pharmaceutical Information and References

OUTLINE

OBJECTIVES

Upon completion of this chapter, the reader should be able to:

1. Identify which primary drug information resource does not include all available drugs, and why.

2. Explain why the loose-leaf version of "Drug Facts and Comparisons" is extremely popular in pharmacies.

3. Identify the best source to use to determine whether a generic drug is equivalent to a brand name drug.

4. Discuss the reference that accesses all FDA official standards and lists new products being developed and approved.

5. Identify the reference source preferred by hospital pharmacies.

6. Explain the reference source that focuses on pharmacogenomics, drug transporting, pharmacokinetics, and pharmacodynamics.

7. Identify the reference source that discusses medical foods, nondrug and preventive measures for self-treatable disorders, nonprescription medications, and nutritional supplements.

8. Explain the databases that have been incorporated into many online drug resources, such as Clinical Pharmacology and Micromedex.

9. Identify three online sources of drug information provided by the U.S. government.

10. List the two most popular pharmacy journals.

Sources of Drug Information

In the pharmacy various sources of drug information are used. These sources must be current and up to date. Most of them give basic information, and a few are very technical. Sources of drug information are either computerized or printed. Many sources of drug information are available; the following discussion focuses on those most commonly seen in the pharmacy.

PHYSICIAN'S DESK REFERENCE

Most physician offices and many pharmacies utilize the *Physician's Desk Reference (PDR)*, which is updated each year. It contains six sections: Manufacturer Indexing, Generic and Trade Names, Product Category Index, Product Identification Guide, Product Information, and Diagnostic Product Information. Each drug listed has a complete monograph, including chemical structure and results of drug studies. There is also a miscellaneous information section. The PDR compiles official drug package inserts from manufacturers who pay a fee for their products to be listed; therefore, not all available drugs are included. The PDR lists only FDA-approved drugs, along with contact information of drug manufacturers. It is available as a hardback book, CD-ROM, and in an online version that is free for prescribers (www.pdr.net).

DRUG FACTS AND COMPARISONS

Drug Facts and Comparisons is one of the most popular sources of drug information used by pharmacists. It contains vital information and is easy to use. It is organized into five sections: Index, Keeping Up, Drug Monographs, Drug Identification, and Appendix. This publication includes indications, dosage strengths, dosage forms, sizes, and manufacturers. In most pharmacies, the loose-leaf version of this publication is used so that monthly updates to its pages may be easily made. It is also available in a standard, hardback, bound version, pocket-sized version or as an electronic subscription called *Facts and Comparison eAnswers* (www.wolterskluwercdi.com).

ORANGE BOOK (APPROVED DRUG PRODUCTS WITH THERAPEUTIC EQUIVALENCE EVALUATIONS)

Provided by the FDA, the *Orange Book* is an annually updated, comprehensive listing of approved drug products and therapeutic equivalence evaluations. It is the best source to use in determining whether a generic drug is equivalent to a brand name drug. Included are approval lists, discontinued drug products, and orphan product designations. Searches may be conducted in various ways, including by active ingredient, patient number, applicant holder, application number, or proprietary name. The *Orange Book* is now provided as a PDF file, which is updated annually and can be accessed for free (www.accessdata.fda.gov/scripts/cder/ob/index.cfm). Periodic updates are also available online.

DRUG TOPICS REDBOOK

Drug Topics Redbook is one of the oldest sources of drug information published, focusing on average and wholesale drug costs and prices. It is more commonly used in community pharmacies than in hospital pharmacies. The book has 10 sections: Emergency Information, Clinical Reference Guide, Practice Management and Professional Development, Pharmacy and Health Care Organizations, Drug Reimbursement Information, Manufacturer/Wholesaler Information, Product Identification, Prescription Product Listings, Over-the-Counter/Nondrug Products Listing, and Complementary/Herbal Product Referencing. It contains quick reference charts by drug type, including those that are excreted in breast milk, those that should not be crushed, and others that are either alcohol- or sugar-free. Pharmacy calculation examples and Spanish-language dosing instructions are also featured. This extensive book is rather difficult to reference unless the user is aware of the drug section abbreviations it contains. It also contains lists of all nontraditional PharmD programs, their requirements, and current enrollment information. The book is published in a softcover bound version, on CD-ROM, and in an online version (www.fda.gov/regulatory-information/search-fda-guidance-documents/guidance-industry-and-other-stakeholders-toxicological-principles-safety-assessment-food-ingredients-0).

UNITED STATES PHARMACOPEIA–NATIONAL FORMULARY (USP–NF)

This publication accesses FDA official standards and guides users in the tests, procedures, and acceptance criteria related to pharmaceutical manufacturing and quality control. It helps pharmacy personnel to comply with the official standards and lists new products being developed and approved. It is available in a hardback version, CD-ROM, and as an online subscription (www.uspnf.com/purchase-usp-nf).

UNITED STATES PHARMACISTS' PHARMACOPEIA

This comprehensive publication includes compounding products and ingredient information, safety information, and products used for specific conditions. It also includes recent sterile preparation guidelines for U.S. pharmacists, common nonformulary agents, dietary supplements, veterinary compounding, and related laws. It is available in a hardback version and as an online subscription (www.usp.org/).

AMERICAN HOSPITAL FORMULARY SERVICE DRUG INFORMATION

This publication is favored in hospital pharmacies and provides drug monographs that feature uses, dosages, administration information, interactions, adverse reactions, toxicities, compounding information, chemistry, stability, mechanisms of action, antibiotic spectrum and resistance, pharmacology, pharmacokinetics, and references for laboratories and testing. Contributors to this publication include medical, pharmacy, and management experts. It is available in hardback, electronic, and mobile application versions (www.ahfsdruginformation.com/).

MARTINDALE'S "THE COMPLETE DRUG REFERENCE"

This hardback book provides information on drugs in clinical use worldwide. It includes information on herbal and complementary medicines, vitamins, nutritional agents, vaccines, radiopharmaceuticals, toxic substances, drugs of abuse, recreational drugs, and many other topics (www.wolterskluwercdi.com/lexicomp-online/martindale/).

PEDIATRIC AND NEONATAL DOSAGE HANDBOOK

This hardback or CD-ROM handbook provides information on suggested current dosages for pediatric patients (webstore.lexi.com/Pediatric-Dosage-Handbook).

GERIATRIC DOSAGE HANDBOOK

This hardback or CD-ROM handbook provides information on suggested current dosages for geriatric patients (www.wolterskluwercdi.com/lexicomp-online/).

AMERICAN DRUG INDEX

The *American Drug Index* lists over 22,000 prescription and over-the-counter drugs. Information includes active ingredients, dosage forms, drugs that should not be chewed or crushed, look-alike and sound-alike drugs, manufacturers, normal laboratory values and related information, packaging and uses, pronunciations of drug names, storage requirements for USP drugs, strengths, and a trademark glossary. This book is available in electronic and hardback formats (www.worldcat.org/title/american-drug-index-2016/oclc/919342176).

GOODMAN & GILMAN'S "THE PHARMACOLOGICAL BASIS OF THERAPEUTICS"

Goodman & Gilman's *The Pharmacological Basis of Therapeutics* contains information such as drug metabolism pharmacogenomics, drug transport/drug transporters, pharmacokinetics, pharmacodynamics, and principles of therapeutics in all areas of the body system. It is available as online subscription and also in hardback format www.medicosrepublic.com/goodman-and-gilmans-the-pharmacological-basis-of-therapeutics-13th-edition-pdf-free-download/.

HANDBOOK OF NONPRESCRIPTION DRUGS

The *Handbook of Nonprescription Drugs* is published by the American Pharmacists Association (APhA). It provides self-care options for complementary and alternative medicine/therapies, FDA-approved dosing information, FDA-evidence-based research on efficacy and safety considerations of nonprescription, and herbal and homeopathic medications. It also discusses medical foods, nondrug and preventive measures for self-treatable disorders, nonprescription medications, and nutritional supplements. It is available as a downloadable e-book and in hardback format (pharmacylibrary.com/doi/book/10.21019/9781582122656).

REMINGTON'S "PHARMACEUTICAL SCIENCES: THE SCIENCE AND PRACTICE OF PHARMACY"

Remington's *Pharmaceutical Sciences: The Science and Practice of Pharmacy* covers all areas of pharmacy, including its history, ethics, and the specifics of pharmacy practice and industrial pharmacy. Specific areas include disease state management, immunology, pathophysiology and manifestations of diseases, professional communication, pharmacy practice specialization, and patient care. The book is available in hardback format and online (www.pharmacystudent.me/remington-the-science-and-practice-of-pharmacy/).

TRISSEL'S "HANDBOOK ON INJECTABLE DRUGS"

Lawrence Trissel's *Handbook on Injectable Drugs* is a popular reference book used primarily in the hospital setting. It contains significant information about parenteral medications. Its monographs discuss administration, drug products, stability, and compatibility with both other drugs and infusion solutions. While pharmacy technicians cannot pass information from this book to nurses or physicians, they can locate the information and present it to the pharmacist. Therefore, this allows for a rapid response from the pharmacy to the medical personnel involved. The book is available in electronic, hardback, mobile application, and online formats. Today, the Trissel databases have been incorporated into many online drug compendia, including *Clinical Pharmacology* and *Micromedex* (www.ahfsdruginformation.com/handbook-on-injectable-drugs/).

THE INTERNET

The Internet contains numerous sources of drug information but not all are accurate or up to date. Information posted online by colleges, universities, and publishers is usually a good place to start. Continuing education is also provided by many online sources. Good online sources of drug information include www.cdc.gov, www.cms.gov, www.drugs.com, www.drugtopics.com, www.fda.gov, www.nih.gov/health-information, www.mayoclinic.org, www.medicare.gov, medlineplus.gov, www.medscape.com, www.pdr.net, www.rxlist.com, www.webmd.com, and dailymed.nlm.nih.gov.

PHARMACY JOURNALS AND MAGAZINES

Various pharmacy journals and magazines are also available, in printed and digital formats. The most commonly perused pharmacy journals are the *American Journal of Health-System Pharmacy* (www.ashp.org) and *Journal of Pharmacy Technology* (journals.sagepub.com/home/pmt). The most commonly read pharmacy magazines include the *American Association of Pharmacy Technicians* (www.pharmacytechnician.com), *Computer Talk for the Pharmacist* (www.computertalk.com), *Hospital Pharmacy* (journals.sagepub.com/home/hpx), *Drug Topics* (www.drugtopics.com), *Today's Technician* (www.pharmacytechnician.org), *Pharmacy Times* (www.pharmacytimes.com), *Pharmacy Today [JAPhA]* (www.pharmacytoday.org), *The Script Newsletters* (www.pharmacy.ca.gov/publications), and *U.S. Pharmacist* (www.uspharmacist.com).

REVIEW QUESTIONS

1. Which of the following drug information resources does not include all available drugs?

   A. *Drug Facts and Comparisons*
   B. Goodman & Gilman's *The Pharmacological Basis of Therapeutics*
   C. Trissel's *Handbook on Injectable Drugs*
   D. *Physician's Desk Reference*

2. Which of the following drug information resources is extremely popular in pharmacies?

   A. *Physician's Desk Reference*
   B. *Drug Facts and Comparisons*
   C. *Handbook of Nonprescription Drugs*
   D. *United States Pharmacopeia–National Formulary*

3. Which of the following is the best source to use for determining whether a generic drug is equivalent to a brand name drug?

    A. *Orange Book*
    B. Goodman & Gilman's *The Pharmacological Basis of Therapeutics*
    C. Pharmacy journals and magazines
    D. *Physician's Desk Reference*

4. Which of the following reference sources is preferred by hospital pharmacies?

    A. *Drug Facts and Comparisons*
    B. *Handbook of Nonprescription Drugs*
    C. *American Hospital Formulary Service Drug Information*
    D. *The Pharmacological Basis of Therapeutics*

5. Which of the following drug information sources does the U.S. government provide?

    A. FDA.gov
    B. ClinicalPharmacology.com
    C. ASHP.org
    D. PDR.net

6. Which of the following drug information resources focuses on pharmacokinetics?

    A. *American Hospital Formulary Service Drug Information*
    B. *Physician's Desk Reference*
    C. The Internet
    D. Goodman & Gilman's *The Pharmacological Basis of Therapeutics*

7. Which of the following references sources discusses medical foods and preventive measures for self-treatable disorders?

    A. Trissel's *Handbook on Injectable Drugs*
    B. *Handbook of Nonprescription Drugs*
    C. Goodman & Gilman's *The Pharmacological Basis of Therapeutics*
    D. *United States Pharmacopeia–National Formulary*

8. Which of the following information has been incorporated into many online drug resources?

    A. Trissel's *Handbook on Injectable Drugs*
    B. *Handbook of Nonprescription Drugs*
    C. *American Hospital Formulary Service Drug Information*
    D. *Orange Book*

9. Which of the following lists new products being developed and approved and accesses FDA standards?

    A. Martindale's *The Complete Drug Reference*
    B. *Drug Facts and Comparisons*
    C. *Handbook of Nonprescription Drugs*
    D. *United States Pharmacopeia–National Formulary*

10. Which of the following is the most popular journal used in pharmacies?

    A. *Hospital Pharmacy*
    B. *Journal of Pharmacy Technology*
    C. *Pharmacy Today*
    D. *U.S. Pharmacist*

WEB LINKS

Clinical Pharmacology: clinicalpharmacology.com

Medical Office Pharmacology: www.mapharm.com

Micromedex Healthcare Series: www.ibm.com/watson-health/learn/micromedex

National Institutes of Health: www.nih.gov/health-information

CHAPTER 6

Prescriptions and Processing

OUTLINE

The Prescription
    Processing Prescriptions—Dispensing
    Receiving the Prescription
    Reading, Checking, and Computer Entry
    Numbering and Dating
    Labeling
    Preparing
    Packaging
    Rechecking
    Patient Counseling
    Recording and Filing
    Pricing
    Refilling

OBJECTIVES

Upon completion of this chapter, the reader should be able to:

1. Explain prescriptions, their uses, requirements, and components.
2. Differentiate between legend and over-the-counter (OTC) drugs.
3. List the component parts of a prescription.
4. Discuss how prescriptions are processed, received, and checked.
5. Describe the ways prescriptions are numbered, dated, and labeled.
6. Explain the differences between generic and trade names.
7. Differentiate between a control number and a National Drug Code.
8. Explain the importance of rechecking of prescriptions.
9. Identify methods for recording and filing prescriptions.
10. Explain requirements for refilling prescriptions.

KEY TERMS

inscription	over-the-counter (OTC)	signa	superscription
legend drug	pharmacy compounding	subscription	

OVERVIEW

Prescriptions are required for all drugs that are not sold over-the-counter (OTC). Pharmacy technicians must be able to interpret prescriptions and correctly discuss them with customers as well as pharmacists. They must be familiar with the handwriting of prescribers as well as the electronic prescription processing method used in the pharmacy. Technicians must be familiar with abbreviations used in prescriptions.

The Prescription

An order for medication issued by a physician, dentist, or other licensed medical practitioner is called a prescription. In certain states, nurse practitioners and even pharmacists can issue prescriptions with certain restrictions. The prescription order is a part of the professional relationship among the prescriber, the pharmacist, and the patient. It is the pharmacist's responsibility in this relationship to provide quality pharmaceutical care that meets the medication needs of the patient. The pharmacist or pharmacy technicians not only must be precise in the manual aspects of filling the prescription order but also must provide the patient with the necessary information and guidance to ensure the patient's compliance in taking the medication properly. There are two broad legal classifications of medications: those that can be obtained only by prescription and those that may be purchased without a prescription. The latter are termed *nonprescription drugs* or **over-the-counter (OTC)** drugs. A medication that may be dispensed legally only by prescription is referred to as a *prescription drug* or **legend drug**.

Prescriptions may be written by the prescriber and given to the patient for presentation at the pharmacy, telephoned or sent directly to the pharmacist by means of a fax machine, or sent electronically from a physician's computer to a pharmacist's computer. The component parts of a prescription include the following:

- Address of the prescriber's office
- Name and address of the patient
- Date
- Medication prescribed (**inscription**)
- Rx symbol (**superscription**)
- Dispensing directions to pharmacist (**subscription**)
- Directions for patient (**signa**)
- Refill and special labeling
- Prescriber's signature and license or Drug Enforcement Agency (DEA) number

An example of a physician's prescription is shown in Figure 6-1.

WHAT WOULD YOU DO?

You receive a prescription for a customer that reads "prednisone, 50 mg, five tablets per day." On hand there are 10 mg tablets of prednisone. Should you assume that the physician meant "five 10 mg tablets of prednisone per day," which would total 50 mg, or that he actually meant "five 50 mg tablets of prednisone per day," which would total 250 mg? If you were this pharmacy technician, what would you do?

PROCESSING PRESCRIPTIONS—DISPENSING

Proper procedures and correct steps for processing prescriptions and dispensing include receiving, reading and checking, numbering and dating, labeling, preparing, packaging, rechecking, delivering and patient counseling, recording and filing, pricing, and refilling.

Receiving the Prescription

The pharmacy technician receives the prescription order directly from the patient. This is a good opportunity to enhance the pharmacist–patient or the technician–patient relationship and facilitates the gathering of essential information from the patient, such as a history of diseases and other drugs being taken. This information is critical for the provision of quality pharmaceutical care. The technician can also obtain the patient's correct name, address, and other necessary information and determine whether the patient's medications are provided through insurance coverage. Pharmacy technicians should ask the patient whether he or she wishes to wait, call back, or have the medication delivered. Many pharmacists try to price prescriptions before dispensing, especially for unusually expensive medication, to avoid subsequent questions concerning the charge.

Reading, Checking, and Computer Entry

Pharmacy technicians should read the prescription completely and carefully to be sure the ingredients or quantities prescribed are clear. The pharmacy technician should take the time to update the patient's profile. From the computer, the technician should determine the compatibility of the newly prescribed medication with other drugs being taken by the patient. He or she must enter the prescription into the computer database, bill the patient's insurance company, and calculate the amount that the patient must pay. The pharmacist, who is required to compare it with the prescription and container label, must verify the pharmacy technician's computer entry for accuracy.

The technician should determine whether drug–food or drug–disease interactions are possible. If some part of the information is illegible or if it appears that an error has been made, the technician should notify the pharmacist. Then the pharmacist should consult another pharmacist or the prescriber. Unfamiliar or unclear abbreviations are a source of errors in interpreting and filling prescriptions. The pharmacist must take great care and use his or her broad knowledge of drug products to prevent dispensing errors. The amount and frequency of a dose must be noted carefully and checked. In determining the safety of the dose of a medicinal agent, the age, weight, and condition of the patient, dosage form prescribed, possible influence of other drugs being taken, and the frequency of administration all must be considered (see Figure 6-2).

COMMUNITY MEDICAL CLINIC
1700 South Tamiami Trail, Sarasota, FL 34239,   (813) 952-2577

Patient Name: _Mary Chase_ _____ Date: __12-10-xx__

Address: _____

R̥

Cephalexin 250 mg
28
Tqid

Private Pay
Private Insurance
Medicaid
CMC

Refill: __0__ Physician Signature: __J. Brown__ M.D.

Physician Name (printed): __J. Brown__

Physician DEA#: _____

Figure 6-1 Prescriptions.

MEDICATION ERROR ALERT

A typical community pharmacy that fills 2000 prescriptions per week may generate up to two clinically significant prescription errors. This is an important fact concerning the need for improved accuracy in community pharmacy, and pharmacy professionals continually work toward reducing the likelihood of errors by improving community pharmacy standards.

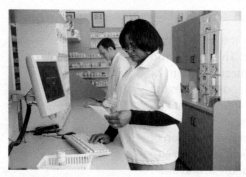

Figure 6-2 One of the primary duties of the pharmacy technician is to enter and update prescription and customer information into the computer database.

POINTS TO REMEMBER

Once the prescription has been read, reviewed, and compared with the information in the patient's computer profile, the pharmacy technician must enter the prescription information into the pharmacy computer system and print the prescription label.

Numbering and Dating

It is a legal requirement that the prescription order be numbered and that the same number be placed on the label. This numbering helps to identify the bottle or package. Consecutive numbers are assigned by prescription computers or manually by using numbering machines. Including the date the prescription is filled on the label is also a legal requirement. This information is important in determining the appropriate refill frequency and patient compliance and can be used as an alternate means of locating the prescription order if the prescription number is lost by the patient.

Labeling

Medication labels give information on the dose contained in the package. For the patient's safety, a pharmacy technician must be able to identify and interpret the information on a medication label. He or she must read the label carefully and understand essential information. The technician must recognize the generic name, trade name, dosage strength, form, supply dosage, total volume, route of administration, directions for mixing, and cautions.

Medication labels also contain information such as expiration date, which indicates the date after which a drug should not be used. Other information can be seen on the back or side of a label, such as storage information, lot numbers, the name of the drug manufacturer, and a National Drug Code (NDC) number. Figure 6-3 provides an example of a drug label (this is a fictitious product) for reference in this section. Please look at examples of actual drug products for comparisons and to become familiar with the styles and variations of information that appear on a drug label.

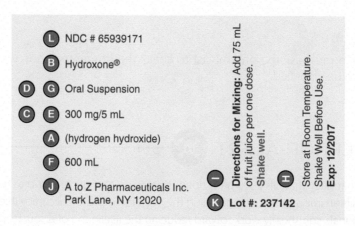

Figure 6-3 Drug label information includes: (A) generic name, (B) trade name, (C) dosage strength, (D) form, (E) supply dosage, (F) total volume, (G) administration route, (H) directions for mixing, (I) cautions, (J) manufacturer name and address, (K) control or lot number, and (L) NDC number.

Generic Names   The established generic (also called nonproprietary) name of a drug appears directly underneath its trade, brand, or proprietary name. Generic names are sometimes printed inside parentheses and must be identified on all drug labels by law. Prescribers as substitutes regularly order generic equivalents of many trade-name drugs. On these products, only the generic name appears. It is advisable for the pharmacy technician to always carefully cross-check names of all medications to avoid inaccurate dispensing to patients. On the label in Figure 6-3, hydrogen hydroxide is the generic name.

Trade Names   Manufacturers' names for their medications are called trade, brand, or proprietary names. These names are usually the most prominently printed names on drug labels and may appear in larger or bold type. They are often followed by the symbol "®," indicating that both the name of the drug and its formulation are registered. In Figure 6-3, the brand name is Hydroxone®.

POINTS TO REMEMBER

It is essential for the technician to cross-check the names of all medications, whether the label indicates only the generic name or both the trade and generic names, in order to accurately identify a drug.

Name of the Manufacturer   The manufacturer's name is present on all drug labels and usually contains the company's logo as well as its location (city, state, and zip code) (see Figure 6-3).

Control Numbers   Federal law must identify all medications identified with control numbers, sometimes called lot numbers (see Figure 6-3). For drug recalls, these numbers identify a particular group of medication packages that must be removed from store shelves. Using these numbers to remove groups of medications that may have been damaged or tampered with has helped to avoid the harming of large numbers of people.

National Drug Code   Every prescription medication must have a unique identifying number according to federal law. This number, with the letters "NDC" followed by three specific groups of numbers, is to appear on every manufacturer's label. For example, the NDC number for Procanbid® (procainamide) is NDC 61570-069-60.

The prescription label may be typewritten or prepared by computer, using the information entered by the pharmacist or pharmacy technician. Figure 6-4 shows a computer-prepared prescription, including the label.

A prescription should have a professional-appearing label. The size of the label used should be appropriate to the size of the prescription container. The name, address, and telephone number of the pharmacy are all legally required to appear on the label. The prescription number, prescriber's name, patient's name, directions for use, and date of dispensing also are legally required. The patient's name and address and strength of the medication are also commonly included. Some state laws require that the name or initials of the pharmacist dispensing the medication appear on the label. Auxiliary labels (also known as strip labels) are used to emphasize important aspects of the dispensed medication, including its proper use, handling, storage, refill status, and necessary warnings or precautions.

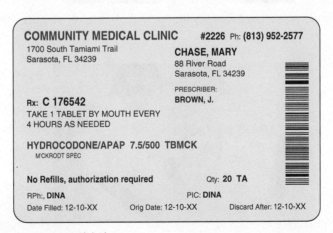

Figure 6-4 Computer-prepared prescription labels.

Certain medications must be taken with food, may make the patient sensitive to sunlight, or may change the color of urine. Auxiliary labels are available in various colors to give them special prominence. Figure 6-5 shows some examples of pharmacy auxiliary labels.

Preparing

Most prescriptions call for dispensing of medications already prefabricated into dosage forms by pharmaceutical manufacturers. In filling prescriptions with prefabricated products, the pharmacist should compare the manufacturer's label with the prescription to be certain it is the correct medication (see Figure 6-6). Medications that show signs of poor manufacture or deterioration or for which the stated expiration date on the label has passed should never be dispensed.

Tablets, capsules, and some other solid, prefabricated dosage forms usually are counted in the pharmacy using a device that is called the counting tray, which is shown in Figure 6-7. This device facilitates the rapid and sanitary counting and transferring of medication from the stock packages to the prescription container. To prevent

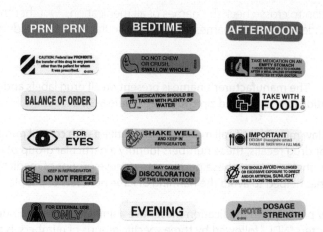

Figure 6-5 Auxiliary labels.

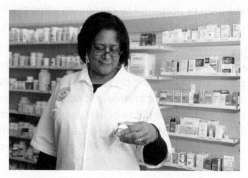

Figure 6-6 The pharmacy technician must carefully verify the contents of medication bottles when preparing to fill prescriptions.

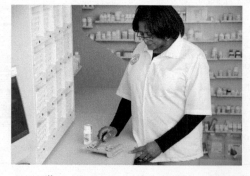

Figure 6-7 The pharmacy technician uses a pill counter to count the correct number of pills to fill a prescription.

contamination of capsules and tablets, the counting tray should be wiped clean after each use, because powder, especially from uncoated tablets, tends to remain on the tray.

Some prescriptions may require compounding, but these represent only a small percentage of the total. The pharmacist must have the knowledge and skills needed to prepare them accurately. **Pharmacy compounding** is defined as the preparation, mixing, assembling, packaging, or labeling of a drug or device. Extemporaneous compounding is essential in the course of professional practice to prepare drug formulations in dosage forms or strengths that are not otherwise commercially available. Extemporaneous compounding is discussed in Chapter 13.

POINTS TO REMEMBER

The dispensing of medications requires 100% accuracy. Pharmacy technicians must always be cautious and careful during the dispensing process.

Packaging

When the pharmacy technician is in the process of filling a prescription, he or she may select a container from various types with different shapes, sizes, mouth openings, colors, and compositions. Selection is based primarily on the type and quantity of medication to be dispensed and the method of its use. Figure 6-8 shows some types of medication containers.

All legend drugs intended for oral use must be dispensed to the patient in containers having child-resistant safety closures, unless the prescriber or the patient specifically requests otherwise. Drugs that are used by or given to patients in hospitals, nursing homes, and extended-care facilities need not be dispensed in containers with safety closures unless they are intended for patients who are leaving the confines of the institution. Examples of child-resistant containers are shown in Figure 6-9.

When pharmacy technicians place a medication into a container (see Figure 6-10), they must attach the printed label to the container immediately (see Figure 6-11).

Rechecking

The pharmacist must recheck every prescription that has been dispensed for verification. All details of the label should be rechecked against the prescription order to verify directions, patient's name, prescription number, date, and prescriber's name. Rechecking is especially important for those drug products available in multiple strengths (see Figure 6-12).

Patient Counseling

Either the pharmacist or the pharmacy technician may present the prescription medication to the patient or his or her family member. The pharmacy technician should always refer the patient to the pharmacist for counseling. Only a licensed pharmacist should counsel patients about their medications.

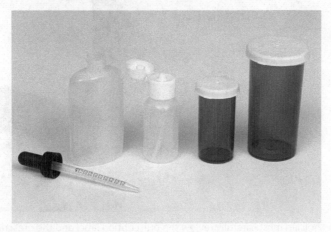

Figure 6-8 Various types of medication containers.

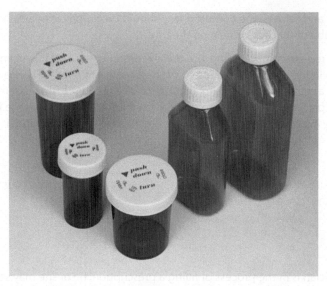

Figure 6-9 Various child-resistant caps.

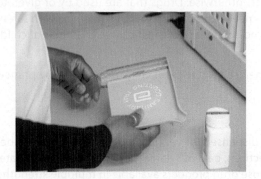

Figure 6-10 The pharmacy technician carefully fills the prescription bottle.

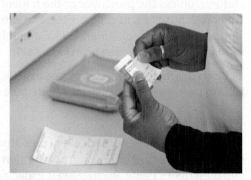

Figure 6-11 The pharmacy technician labels the prescription bottle.

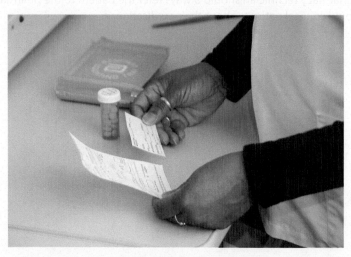

Figure 6-12 The pharmacy technician must carefully review the prescription label and the prescription to be sure they match.

There has been an increased awareness that labeling instructions are often inadequate to ensure the patient's understanding of his or her medication. The prescriber and the pharmacist share the responsibility for ensuring that the patient receives specific instructions, precautions, and warnings for safe and effective use of the prescribed drugs.

WHAT WOULD YOU DO?

A customer in your community pharmacy asks you, the pharmacy technician, about a prescription high blood pressure medication that he had just picked up about 5 hours earlier. He states that sometimes after taking the medication, he feels very dizzy. He asks you if he can take a smaller dosage each time but take it more times during the day to receive the prescribed amount. He tells you that his physician said he shouldn't do this, but asks for your opinion, "since you deal with prescriptions like this every day." What would you do?

Recording and Filing

A record of the prescriptions dispensed is maintained in the pharmacy through the use of computers and hard copy prescription files. Many chain drug stores have central computer systems today, which allow pharmacists from any place in the system to access a patient's record and refill a prescription previously dispensed at another store. There are various types of units available to keep original prescription orders. Metal or cardboard units, which conveniently store approximately 1000 prescriptions, are commonly used (see Figure 6-13). Partitioned drawers often are used for filing. The least common method of filing is microfilming of prescriptions.

Pricing

The pharmacy is a business practice. The pharmacy technician must assist in the financial aspects of this practice so that the business is maintained and makes a fair profit. A method of pricing prescriptions should be established to ensure the profitable operation of the prescription section. The charge applied to a prescription should cover the costs of the ingredients, which include the container and label, the time of the pharmacist or pharmacy technician

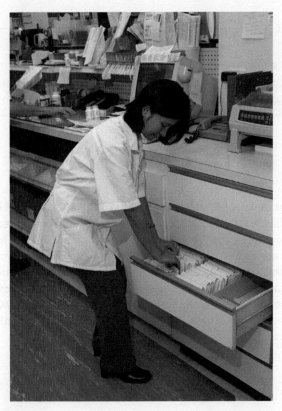

Figure 6-13 Prescription filing system.

and auxiliary personnel involved, the cost of inventory maintenance, and operational costs of the pharmacy. It is obvious that pricing the prescription must provide a reasonable margin of profit on investment.

Refilling

The prescriber must provide instruction for refilling a prescription by indicating on the original prescription the number of appropriate refills. Federal law does not limit the number of refills of prescriptions for noncontrolled medications. State laws may impose such limits. On the other hand, the refilling of prescriptions for controlled agents is strictly regulated. For Schedule II, no refills are permitted without a new written prescription. For Schedules III and IV, a maximum of five refills per prescription are permitted within six months. No prescription should be renewed indefinitely without the patient being reevaluated by the prescriber to ensure that the medication as originally prescribed remains the drug of choice. The maintenance of accurate records of refilling is important not only for complying with federal and state laws, but also for providing information on the patient's medication history.

POINTS TO REMEMBER

For most Schedule V drugs, no prescription is required for individuals age 18 or older, but these drugs may be sold only at pharmacies with a licensed pharmacist on premises.

WHAT WOULD YOU DO?

A customer returns to your pharmacy after eight days with a refill request for her pain medication. You remember talking to this woman the previous week about her chronic back pain and realize that her prescription should have lasted at least 20 days before needing to be refilled. What would you do?

MEDICATION ERROR ALERT

Nearly 250,000 senior citizens are hospitalized every year because of reactions between prescription and OTC medications. Another related danger is that many OTC products contain ingredients such as *acetaminophen* that may also be present in the prescription medications a patient is taking, leading to a potential overdose.

Summary

As the practice of pharmacy has developed, so have the roles of the pharmacy technician. Technicians regularly receive and review new and refill prescriptions and handle dispensing, labeling, record keeping, pricing, patient profiles, purchasing, billing, phone calls, cash registers, receiving, and inventory. The computer is a major part of their daily routines. Technicians are accountable for all of these tasks, trying to perform them with as few errors as possible, in addition to maintaining high ethical and professional standards, having strong communication skills, and being good team players who can handle the high pace and high stress of their jobs. The number of prescriptions dispensed in the United States has rapidly increased, as have the different settings in which the pharmacists practice. To keep up with the rising demand for pharmaceutical products and services, technicians will play a much greater role to support pharmaceutical care.

REVIEW QUESTIONS

1. A prescribed medication is also called a:

   A. superscription.
   B. subscription.
   C. inscription.
   D. legend drug.

2. Auxiliary labels are used to emphasize:

   A. important aspects of aseptic technique.
   B. important characteristics of the dispensed medication.
   C. that technicians should complete the dispensed medication.
   D. that technicians should satisfy the customers.

3. Child-resistant containers are used in which of the following conditions?

   A. Medications dispensed for patients in the hospital
   B. Medications dispensed for patients in nursing homes
   C. All dispensed legend drugs
   D. Drugs dispensed for extended-care facilities

4. Which of the following defines the "Rx" symbol?

   A. Superscription
   B. Subscription
   C. Inscription
   D. Signa

5. How many specific groups of numbers are contained in a National Drug Code?

   A. Two
   B. Three
   C. Five
   D. Seven

6. Refills for a prescription may be completed when the:

   A. prescription is lost.
   B. prescriber indicates that refills are allowed.
   C. refill blank is left blank.
   D. pharmacist tells the technician to refill the prescription.

7. Which of the following is correct in regard to a prescription?

   A. It must include the name and address of the patient.
   B. It must include the patient's Social Security number.
   C. It must include the pharmacy technician's signature.
   D. It must include the pharmacist's signature.

8. All of the following are common methods of filing original prescriptions in the pharmacy, *except*:

   A. computerized
   B. cardboard unit
   C. microfilming
   D. partitioned drawer

9. To prevent contamination of capsules and tablets, you should:

   A. wash your hands once a day before counting medications.
   B. use disinfecting spray on the counting tray.
   C. wipe the counting tray clean after each use.
   D. wipe the drug container with bleach prior to filling.

10. The component parts of a prescription include all of the following, *except*:

    A. date.
    B. medication prescribed (inscription).
    C. dispensing directions to the pharmacist (subscription).
    D. prescriber's signature and tax identification number.

11. How many refills are allowed for Schedule II drugs?

    A. 0
    B. 2
    C. 3
    D. 5

12. Tablets, capsules, and some other prefabricated dosage forms usually are counted in the pharmacy using a device called the counting:

    A. scanner.
    B. tray.
    C. counter.
    D. dispensary.

13. Unless the prescriber or the patient requests otherwise, all legend drugs intended for oral use must be dispensed by the pharmacy technician to the patient in containers having:

    A. tinted plastic to avoid sunlight damage.
    B. a chemical packet to keep contents dry.
    C. a device inside to remove the medication for use.
    D. a safety closure.

14. Which of the following is not a component of the pricing of a prescription?

    A. The cost of the ingredients
    B. The container and its labeling
    C. The operational costs involved
    D. The location of the pharmacy

15. Which of the following are responsible for ensuring that patients receive specific instructions, precautions, and warnings?

    A. Pharmacists and pharmacy technicians
    B. Physicians and pharmacists
    C. Nurses and pharmacy technicians
    D. Only physicians

CRITICAL THINKING

A pharmacy technician misread the handwriting on a prescription for 10 mg of Metadate ER and dispensed methadone 10 mg instead for a 7-year-old boy. Fortunately, the pharmacist read the information that accompanied the prescription and realized the error. It is the responsibility of the pharmacy technician to clarify any drug order that is doubtful in order to prevent medication errors.

1. If the handwriting on a prescription is not clear, what should a pharmacy technician do?

2. Do pharmacy computer systems normally alert the user to a medication that may be incorrect for a specific age of patient?

WEB LINKS

Compounding and the FDA: Questions and Answers: www.fda.gov/drugs/human-drug-compounding/compounding-and-fda-questions-and-answers

Frequently Asked Questions About Pharmaceutical Compounding: www.pharmacist.com/frequently-asked-questions-about-pharmaceutical-compounding

Prescription Process: prescriptionprocess.com/know-the-facts/how-prescriptions-are-processed-and-filled/

Processing Medication Orders and Prescriptions: basicmedicalkey.com/processing-medication-orders-and-prescriptions/

What Are Compounding Pharmacies? www.webmd.com/brain/news/20121010/what-are-compounding-pharmacies

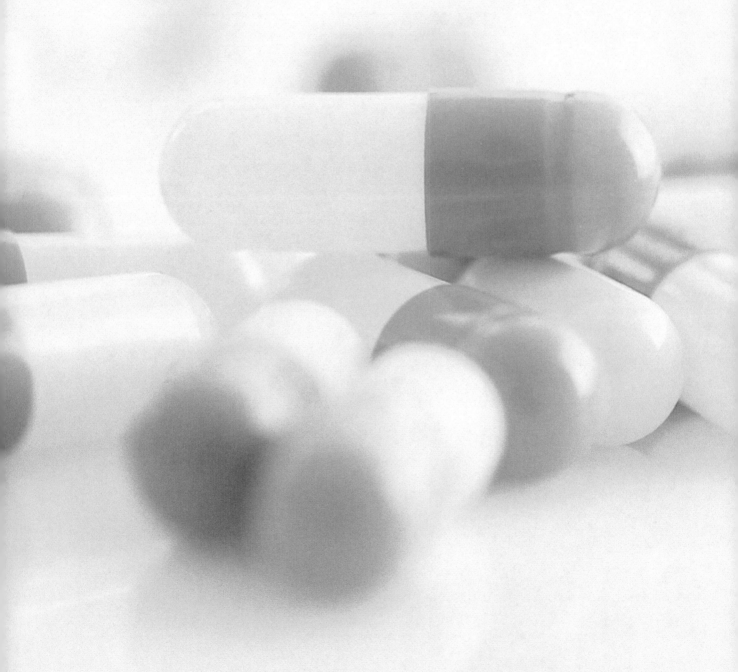

CHAPTER 7

Dosage Forms and Routes of Administration

OUTLINE

OBJECTIVES

Upon completion of this chapter, the reader should be able to:

1. Identify the five basic sources of drugs.
2. Explain the meaning of the term "dosage strength."
3. Identify the solid dosage forms of drugs.
4. Identify the semisolid dosage forms of drugs.
5. Identify the liquid forms of drugs.

6. Describe the oral route of drug administration and the equipment used.

7. Describe the parenteral route of administration and the basic equipment used.

8. Describe the topical route of administration and the basic equipment used.

9. Describe the inhalation route of administration.

10. Describe the basic equipment used for inhalation administration.

KEY TERMS

ampule	gavage	oral	sustained-release (SR)
aromatic water	gel	parenteral	syrup
buccal	gelcap	paste	tablet
buffered tablet	granule	pill	tincture
caplet	induration	plaster	topical
capsule	intradermal injection	powder	total volume
cream	intramuscular injection	solution	troche
dosage strength	intravenous injection	spirit	vial
elixir	liniment	subcutaneous injection	wheal
emulsion	lotion	sublingual	Z-track method
enteric-coated tablet	lozenge	supply dosage	
fluidextract	mixture	suppository	
form	ointment	suspension	

Overview

Any medication has the potential to cause serious harm to the patient. Therefore, the process of dispensing and administering medication orders must always be performed with great care. Each member of the health care team involved in medication administration must be constantly vigilant to prevent errors and deliver quality patient care. The pharmacy technician must be familiar with many different forms of medication as well as with their routes of administration, doses, and strengths. A medication should never be given until its purpose, possible side effects, precautions, and recommended dosages are known. Pharmacy technicians must learn many drug names and sources in order to be able to dispense medications.

Drug Sources

There are basically five sources of drugs: plant, animal (including humans), mineral or mineral products, synthetic (chemical substances), and engineered (investigational drugs). Today, chemicals and even human tissues such as those used in stem-cell therapy can be manipulated to create new drug sources.

PLANT SOURCES

Plant sources are grouped by their physical and chemical properties. Alkaloids are organic compounds that have been combined with acids to make a salt. Nicotine, morphine sulfate, and atropine sulfate are examples of these chemical compounds. An important cardiac glycoside is digoxin. Digoxin is made from digitalis, a derivative of the foxglove plant.

ANIMAL SOURCES

Animal sources, such as the body fluids and glands of animals, can act as drugs. The drugs obtained from animal sources include enzymes such as pancreatin and pepsin. Hormones such as thyroid and insulin are also derived from animal sources.

MINERAL SOURCES

Minerals from the earth and soil are used to provide inorganic materials unavailable from plants and animals. They are used as they occur in nature. Examples include iron, potassium, silver, and gold, which are used to prepare medications. Sodium chloride (table salt) is one of the best-known examples in this category. Gold is used to control severe rheumatoid arthritis, and coal tar is used to treat seborrheic dermatitis and psoriasis.

SYNTHETIC SOURCES

New drugs may be created from the application of chemistry, biology, and computer technology to previously identified substances from living organisms (organic substances) or nonliving materials (inorganic substances). These drugs are called synthetic or manufactured drugs because they are not found naturally in this state but rather are artificially created substances. Common examples of synthetic drugs include meperidine (Demerol®), sulfonamides, and oral contraceptives. Some drugs are both organic and inorganic, such as propylthiouracil, which is an antithyroid hormone.

POINTS TO REMEMBER

Certain organic drugs such as penicillin are semisynthetic and are made by altering their natural compounds or elements.

BIO OR GENETICALLY ENGINEERED SOURCES

The newest area of drug origin is gene splicing or genetic engineering. The newer forms of insulin for use in humans have been produced with this technique.

DOSAGE CONSIDERATIONS

Pharmacy technicians should understand the importance of dosages of drugs. Therefore, all of the following considerations are vital in providing excellent service to customers.

DOSAGE STRENGTH

The amount of the medication per unit of measure (the amount per tablet, capsule, milligram, or milliliter) is called the **dosage strength**. Dosage strength of a drug refers to its dosage weight, the amount of the drug provided in a specific unit of measurement. Milligrams are common dosage measurements. Some drugs have two different but equivalent dosage strengths, such as "milligrams per tablet" and "units per tablet." This allows either type of measurement to be used by prescribers.

Example

A bottle may contain 50 capsules; however, the dosage strength is the number of milligrams per capsule. On its label, a syrup shows 240 mL (the total volume), but the dosage strength is 15 mg/mL.

FORM

The **form** of a drug identifies its structure and composition. Solid dosage forms include tablets and capsules. Powders and granules can be directly combined with food and beverages. Some must be reconstituted (liquefied) and measured precisely, either in milliliters, drops, or ounces. These forms may be clear solutions (crystalloids) or suspensions (in which the liquid contains solid particles that separate from the solution in its container). Medicines to be injected may be available in a solution or in a dry powder form that is then reconstituted. After reconstitution, they are measured in cubic centimeters or milliliters. There are many other different forms of medications, including patches for transdermal administration, creams, and suppositories.

Labels may also use abbreviations or words that explain the form of the drug. Examples are LA (long-acting), SR (sustained release), CR (controlled release), DS (double strength), and XL (extra-long acting).

SUPPLY DOSAGE

Supply dosage is a term that refers to both dosage strength and form. For solid-form medications, supply dosage is read as "*X* measured units per tablet." For liquid medications, it is the same as the medication's concentration, such as "*X* measured units per milliliter."

Example

The medication may be read as 125 mg/2 mL (125 mg in 2 mL), whereas in tablets or capsules, the amount of medication may be stated as 25 mg/tablet (25 mg in 1 tablet) or 500 mg/capsule (500 mg in 1 capsule).

TOTAL VOLUME

Total volume refers to the *full quantity* contained in a vial, bottle, or package. For solid medications, it is the total number of individual items (e.g., capsules or tablets). For liquids, it is the total fluid volume. It is important to recognize the difference between the amount per milliliter and the total volume to avoid any errors.

ADMINISTRATION ROUTE

The administration route refers to the site of the body or the method of drug delivery intended, for example, oral (PO), intramuscular (IM), intravenous (IV), or topical. There are many different administration routes. Unless otherwise instructed, capsules, caplets, and tablets are intended for oral administration.

DIRECTIONS FOR MIXING AND RECONSTITUTING

Certain drugs are dispensed in powder form, which must be reconstituted before use. Often, an initial concentrate of a powdered drug is prepared by mixing it with sterile water or some specified agent, and then the solution is shaken vigorously until no large visible particles are seen. The reconstitution must be performed exactly as the label directs.

CAUTIONS

Often manufacturers print cautions or special alerts onto the packaging of medications. Some of these cautions or alerts are "refrigerate at all times," "protect from light," or "keep in a dry place." Suspensions that are reconstituted for the patient to use may be dispensed as ready-to-use medications, or there may be instructions to "shake well before using." All instructions given as cautions and alerts should be followed carefully.

Dosage Forms of Drugs

Pharmaceutical principles are the underlying physical and chemical properties of a substance that allow a drug to be incorporated in a pharmaceutical dosage form such as tablets and solutions. These principles apply whether the drug is extemporaneously compounded (prepared by the pharmacist) or manufactured for commercial distribution as a drug product. Drug dosage forms are classified according to their physical state and chemical composition. They may include gases, liquids, solids, and semisolids. Some substances can undergo a change of state or phase, from solid to liquid states (melting) or from liquid to gaseous states (vaporization).

POINTS TO REMEMBER

Certain drugs are soluble in water, some are soluble in alcohol, and others are soluble in a mixture of liquids.

SOLID DRUGS

The route for administering a medication depends on its form, its properties, and the effects desired. Intermolecular forces of attraction are stronger in solids than in liquids or in gases. Solid drugs include tablets, pills, plasters, capsules, caplets, gelcaps, powder, granules, troches, or lozenges (see Figure 7-1).

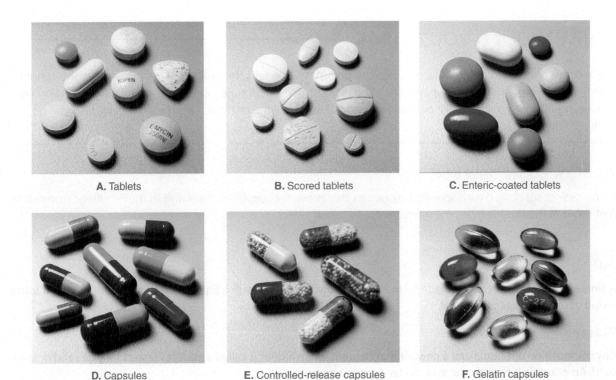

A. Tablets   **B.** Scored tablets   **C.** Enteric-coated tablets

D. Capsules   **E.** Controlled-release capsules   **F.** Gelatin capsules

Figure 7-1 Solid dosage forms.

MEDICAL TERMINOLOGY REVIEW

sublingual:

sub = *under*

lingual = *tongue*

under the tongue

buccal:

buc = *the cheek*

-al = *pertaining to*

pertaining to the check

Tablet

A **tablet** is a pharmaceutical preparation made by compressing the powered form of a drug and bulk filling material under high pressure (see Figure 7-1). Tablets are sometimes erroneously called pills, but that term more properly refers to a specific formulation, as explained later. Special forms of tablets include sublingual tablets and enteric-coated tablets. Most tablets are intended to be swallowed whole for dissolution and absorption from the gastrointestinal tract. Some are intended to be dissolved in the mouth, dissolved in water, or inserted as suppositories. Tablets come in various sizes, shapes, and colors, and they also vary in composition. The various forms of tablets include chewable, sublingual, buccal, enteric-coated, and buffered tablets. Chewable tablets must be chewed. They contain a flavored or sugar base. Chewable tablets are often recommended for children who cannot swallow other forms of medication. Antacids and antiflatulents commonly take this form. Sublingual tablets must be dissolved under the tongue for rapid absorption. An example is nitroglycerin for angina pectoris. Buccal tablets are placed between the cheek and the gum until they are dissolved and absorbed. An **enteric-coated tablet** has a special coating to protect against stomach acid, allowing the drug to dissolve in the alkaline environment of the intestines. A **buffered tablet** can prevent ulceration or severe irritation of the stomach wall. Antacids have been added to reduce irritation to the stomach by the active ingredients.

WHAT WOULD YOU DO?

A woman brings two different tablets into the pharmacy. She tells the pharmacy technician that she cannot remember which tablet is for hypertension. She explains that she put the tablets into an unlabeled bottle while traveling, after disposing of their original containers. If you were the pharmacy technician, what would you do to identify the two tablets?

POINTS TO REMEMBER

Some tablets are coated with specific substances that prevent them from dissolving in the mouth or stomach so that more of the drug reaches the intestine.

Pill

A single-dose unit of medicine made by mixing the powdered drug with a liquid such as syrup and rolling it into a round or oval shape is called a **pill**.

Plaster

Any composition of a liquid and a powder that hardens when it dries is called a **plaster**. Plasters may be solid or semi-solid. An example is the salicylic acid plaster used to remove corns.

Capsule

A **capsule** is a medication dosage form in which the drug is contained in an external shell (see Figure 7-1). Capsule shells are special containers that are usually made of gelatin and are sized for a single dose. They enclose or encapsulate powder, granules, liquids, or some combinations of these. They are used when medications have an unpleasant odor or taste. Capsules can be pulled apart, and the entire contents can be added as powder to food for individuals who have difficulty swallowing. Some forms of capsules provide a controlled-release dosage and are used over a defined period of time. These are called **sustained-release (SR)** or timed-release capsules. These drugs should never be crushed or dissolved, because this would negate their timed-release action. Capsules are available in various sizes, ranging from the number 000 to 5.

POINTS TO REMEMBER

The largest size of capsule is 000 and the smallest size is 5.

Caplet

A **caplet** is shaped like a capsule but has the form of a tablet. The shape and film-coated covering make swallowing easier.

Gelcap

A **gelcap** is an oil-based medication that is enclosed in a soft gelatin capsule (see Figure 7-1).

Powder

A drug that is dried and ground into fine particles is called a **powder**. Most antifungal foot medications are available in powdered forms to keep the area as dry as possible. Examples include nystatin powder and potassium chloride powder (Kato powder).

Granule

A small pill, usually accompanied by many others encased within a gelatin capsule is called a **granule**. In most cases, granules within capsules are specially coated to gradually release medication over a period of up to 12 hours (see Figure 7-1).

Troche or Lozenge

A hard or semisolid dosage form containing a medication intended for local application in the mouth or throat is called a **troche** or **lozenge**. These are flattened disks. Typically, a troche is placed on the tongue or between the cheek and gum and left in place until it dissolves. The medications most commonly administered by means of troches include cough suppressants and treatments for sore throat. An example of a medication available in troche form is clotrimazole, and an example of a medication available in lozenge form is cetylpyridinium chloride.

SEMISOLID DRUGS

Semisolid drugs are often used as **topical** (applied to the surface of the body) applications. These drugs are soft and pliable. Semisolid drugs include suppositories, ointments, creams, gels, lotions, and pastes. Semisolid drugs may be administered by means of a patch for transdermal absorption.

Suppository

A bullet-shaped dosage form intended to be inserted into a body orifice is called a **suppository**. Suppositories contain medication that is usually intended to provide a local effect at the site of insertion. Suppositories maintain their shape at room temperature but melt or dissolve when inserted. The most common sites of administration for suppositories are the rectum, vagina, and urethra.

Ointment

An **ointment** is a drug combined with an oil base, resulting in a semisolid medication that is intended for external application, usually by rubbing (see Figure 7-2). Medications that may be administered in ointment form include anti-inflammatory drugs, topical anesthetics, and antibiotics. Examples are erythromycin ophthalmic ointment and Ben-Gay® ointment.

WHAT WOULD YOU DO?

A pharmacist asks a pharmacy technician to compound an ointment for a patient. The technician notices that one of the ingredients has expired. If you were the pharmacy technician, what would you do?

MEDICAL TERMINOLOGY REVIEW

ophthalmic:

ophthalm = *eye*

-ic = *pertaining to*

pertaining to the eye

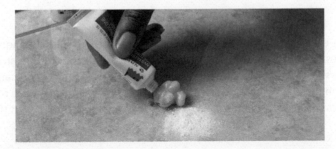

Figure 7-2 Semisolid dosage forms.

Cream

A **cream** is a semisolid preparation that is usually white and nongreasy and has a water base. It is applied externally to the skin or administered by means of an applicator intravaginally. Examples include hydrocortisone and betamethasone creams.

Gel

A **gel** is a jelly-like substance that may be used for topical medication. Some gels have a high alcohol content and can cause stinging if applied to broken skin. Examples include bullfrog gel and naftifine gel.

Lotion

A **lotion** is a semisolid preparation applied externally to protect the skin or to treat a dermatologic disorder. Examples include hydrocortisone and ammonium lactate lotions.

MEDICAL TERMINOLOGY REVIEW

transdermal:

trans = *across*

derm/o = *skin*

-al = *pertaining to*

pertaining to crossing the skin

Paste

A **paste** is a topical, semisolid formulation containing a pharmacologically active ingredient in a fatty base. An example is zinc oxide paste.

Patches

Transdermal patches (also called "skin patches") are medicated adhesive patches placed on the skin that deliver a medication into the bloodstream directly through the skin. Patches are advantageous in that they allow the medication to be released on a controlled basis into the skin. The first transdermal patch was used to administer the drug *scopolamine*, which is used to relieve the symptoms of motion sickness.

At one time, the nicotine transdermal patch was the most popular patch used in the United States. Patches are also commonly used to administer estrogen, fentanyl, lidocaine, nitroglycerin, antidepressants, hormonal contraceptives, and various drugs used to treat attention deficit hyperactivity disorder (ADHD).

POINTS TO REMEMBER

There are four basic types of transdermal patches: single-layer, multi-layer, reservoir (in which the drug layer is separated from the adhesive layer), and matrix (in which the adhesive surrounds the drug layer).

LIQUID DRUGS

Liquid preparations include drugs that have been dissolved or suspended. Examples of liquid drugs are syrups, solutions, spirits, elixirs, tinctures, fluidextracts, liniments, emulsions, mixtures, suspensions, aromatic waters, sprays, and aerosols. They are also classified by site or route of administration such as local (topical) on or through the skin, through the mouth, through the eye (ophthalmic), through the ear (otic), or through the rectum, urethra, or vagina. Liquid drugs may also be administered systemically by mouth or by injection throughout the body (see Figure 7-3).

Syrup

A drug dosage form that consists of a high concentration of a sugar in water is called a **syrup**. It may or may not have medicinal substances added. Examples include ipecac and metaproterenol syrups.

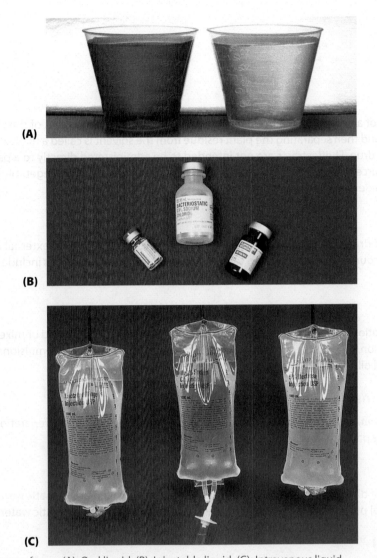

Figure 7-3 Liquid dosage forms. (A): Oral liquid. (B): Injectable liquid. (C): Intravenous liquid.

Solution

A **solution** is a drug or drugs dissolved in an appropriate solvent. An example of a solution is normal saline.

Spirit

An alcohol-containing liquid that may be used pharmaceutically as a solvent is called a **spirit**. It is also known as an essence. Examples include essence of peppermint and camphor spirits.

Elixir

A drug vehicle that consists of water, alcohol, and sugar is known as an **elixir**. It may or may not be aromatic and may or may not have active medicinal properties. The alcohol content of elixirs makes them convenient as liquid dosage forms for many drugs that are only slightly soluble in water. In these cases, the drug is first dissolved in alcohol, and then the other elixir components are added. All elixirs contain alcohol. They should be used with caution in patients with diabetes or a history of alcohol abuse. Some pediatric medications retain the name of elixir, although they no longer contain alcohol. Examples include theophylline and phenobarbital elixirs.

Tincture

A **tincture** is an alcoholic preparation of a soluble drug, usually from a plant source. In some cases, the solution may also contain water. Examples include iodine and digitalis tinctures.

Fluidextract

A concentrated solution of a drug removed from a plant source by mixing ground parts of the plant with a suitable solvent, usually alcohol, and then separating the plant residue from the solvent is called a **fluidextract**. Typically, 1 mL (1 cc) contains 1 g of the drug. Fluidextracts are not intended to be administered directly to a patient. Instead, they are used to provide a source of drug in the manufacture of final dosage forms. Only vegetable drugs are used. An example is glycyrrhiza fluidextract.

Liniment

A **liniment** is a mixture of drugs with oil, soap, water, or alcohol, which is intended for external application by rubbing. Most liniments are counterirritants intended to treat muscle or joint pain. Examples include camphor and chloroform liniments.

Emulsion

A pharmaceutical preparation containing two agents that cannot ordinarily be combined or mixed is called an **emulsion**. In the typical emulsion, oil is dispersed inside water. Most creams and lotions are emulsions. Examples include Petrogalar Plain® (mineral oil/emulsion) and cod liver oil.

Mixture and Suspension

In a **mixture** or a **suspension**, an agent is mixed with a liquid but not dissolved. These preparations must be shaken before being taken by the patient. An example is milk of magnesia (suspension).

Aromatic Water

In pharmacy, a mixture of distilled water with an aromatic volatile oil is called an **aromatic water**. Aromatic waters may be used for medicinal purposes. Examples include peppermint and camphor aromatic waters.

Spray and Aerosol

A liquid or fine powder that is sprayed in a fine mist is called an aerosol. The most commonly used aerosols are respiratory treatments for asthma and the various sprays used on the skin. Although most aerosolized medicines are liquids, some are powders whose particles are small enough to pass through the spray apparatus.

WHAT WOULD YOU DO?

A customer asked a pharmacy technician why he should shake the medication before giving it to his child. If you were the pharmacy technician, what would you do?

GASEOUS DRUGS

Pharmaceutical gases include the anesthetic gases such as nitrous oxide and halothane. Compressed gases include therapeutic oxygen (see Figure 7-4) and carbon dioxide.

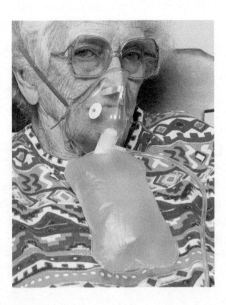

Figure 7-4 Gaseous dosage forms.

Principles of Drug Administration

The route of a drug refers to how it is administered to the patient. The chosen route of drug administration determines the rate and intensity of the drug's effect. A drug prepared for one route but administered by another route may not have any effect at all and is potentially dangerous. Each route requires different dosage forms.

Certain medications can be administered by more than one route, whereas a specific route must administer others. The route of administration is determined by a number of factors, including the following:

- The action of the medication on the body
- The physical and emotional state of the patient
- The characteristics of the drug

Other factors, such as age (pediatric and geriatric), the disease being treated, and the absorption, distribution, metabolism, and elimination of drugs, are also important. Three methods of administration are generally used: oral, parenteral, and topical. Each is described in detail in the sections that follow.

ORAL ROUTE

The **oral** route (taken by mouth) is the safest and most convenient route of administration for most medications. Medication taken by mouth is solid (tablet) or liquid (syrup). The presence or lack of food in the stomach affects absorption of many oral medications. Some drugs taken with food may have a slow absorption rate. Oral drugs may be swallowed or may be taken by the buccal or sublingual route. The oral route can also take many liquid forms of medications. These differ mainly in the type of substance used to dissolve the drug, such as water, oil, or alcohol, and were discussed earlier in this chapter. Generally, oral medications should be taken with enough water to send the drug to the stomach. Liquid medications are ideal for children. Oral syringes are an ideal way to administer liquid medications to children (see Figure 7-5). Liquid medications that may stain the teeth can be taken through a straw. If the patient has been vomiting or is nauseated, an alternative route of administration might be necessary.

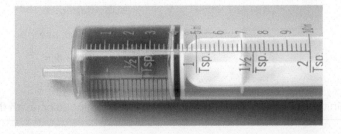

Figure 7-5 Liquid oral syringe.

WHAT WOULD YOU DO?

A child with a sore throat was prescribed amoxicillin powder by his or her pediatrician. The child's mother mixed the powder with water but did not refrigerate it. After one week, the mother called the pharmacy explaining that she had just read that she was supposed to refrigerate the mixture after each dosage but had not done so. If you were the pharmacy technician that took the call, what would you do?

Basic Equipment Needed for Oral Administration

Three measuring devices are used in the administration of oral medications (Figure 7-6):

- The medicine or water cup
- The medicine dropper/oral syringe
- The calibrated spoon

The medicine cup may be calibrated in fluid ounces, cubic centimeters (cc), milliliters (mL), teaspoons, or tablespoons. The medicine dropper may be calibrated in milliliters or drops. Calibrated spoons are usually marked up with 1/4 teaspoon and 1 cc measurements, up to two teaspoons (10 cc). Syringes are usually marked up with 1/2 cc increments.

Sublingual Route

Drugs given by the **sublingual** route are held under the tongue until they dissolve completely (see Figure 7-7). This method is used when rapid action is desired, for example, ergotamine tartrate (Ergostat®) for migraines and nitroglycerin for angina pectoris can be administered by the sublingual route.

Buccal Route

For administration of drugs via the **buccal** route, the medication is placed between the gum and cheek and left there until it is dissolved. The buccal route may administer oxytocin, used for inducing labor, but it is not often administered this way.

MEDICAL TERMINOLOGY REVIEW

intradermal:	**subcutaneous:**
intra = *within*	sub = *under, beneath*
derm/o = *skin*	cutane/o = *skin*
-al = *pertaining to*	-ous = *pertaining to*
pertaining to within the skin	pertaining to beneath the skin

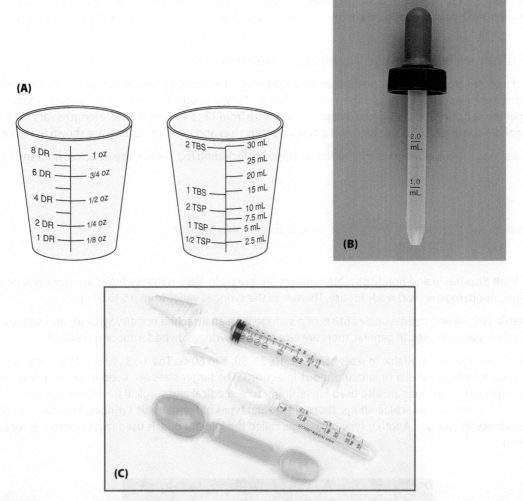

Figure 7-6 Tools to administer liquid dosages. (A): Medicine cup. (B): Medicine dropper. (C): Calibrated spoon and oral syringe.

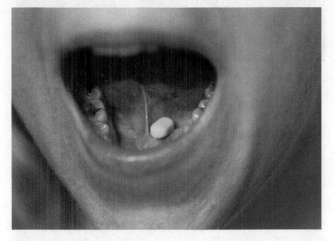

Figure 7-7 Sublingual medication administration.

PARENTERAL ROUTE

Administration of drugs other than through the digestive system is called **parenteral** administration. Thus, a parenteral medication, such as one given by injection, bypasses the gastrointestinal tract, such as with drugs given by injection. Medications are injected into the tissues of the body using a syringe and a needle for rapid effect and absorption. There are four main categories of parenteral administration, which are differentiated according to the site of the injection. Drugs may be injected into muscles, veins, skin (intradermal or subcutaneous), and the spinal column.

Basic Equipment Needed for Parenteral Administration

Two types of needles are available (disposable and nondisposable) for giving medications by the parenteral route. The most commonly used are the disposable needles. Gauge (G) of a needle is determined by the diameter of the lumen or opening at its beveled tip. Needle gauges range in size from 13 to 31 G, and needle lengths vary from 3/8 to 2 inches. A needle consists of a hub, a shaft, and a bevel. Various sizes and types of needles are shown in Figure 7-8.

Figure 7-9 shows the components of a hypodermic injection, including the needle, needle cover, hub, and syringe.

POINTS TO REMEMBER

The larger the gauge of a needle is, the smaller is the diameter of its lumen.

Syringes   Both disposable and nondisposable syringes are available. Disposable syringes are sterilized, prepackaged, nontoxic, nonpyrogenic, and ready for use. The size of the syringes varies from 0.5 to 60 cc.

A disposable syringe and needle unit consists of a syringe with an attached needle. Syringes are distinguished according to their sizes and uses. In general, there are two types of syringes: hypodermic and prefilled.

Hypodermic syringes are available in sizes of 1, 3, 5, 10, 20, 30, and 60 cc. The 1-, 3-, and 5-cc syringes are most commonly used for intramuscular or subcutaneous injections. The larger sizes are used to prepare intravenous admixtures. Hypodermic syringes are also used for venipuncture, medical and surgical treatment, aspiration, irrigations, and **gavage** (tube-to-stomach) feedings. There are several types of hypodermic syringes, including needleless, insulin, and tuberculin syringes. Another type of syringe, called the injector pen, is used most commonly for insulin administration.

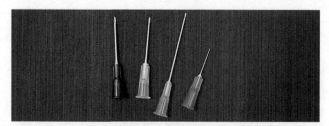

Figure 7-8 Various lengths and sizes of needles.

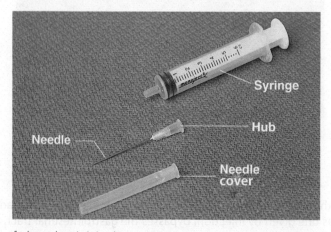

Figure 7-9 The components of a hypodermic injection.

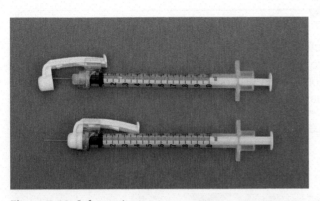
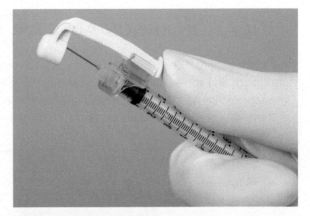

Figure 7-10 Safety syringe.

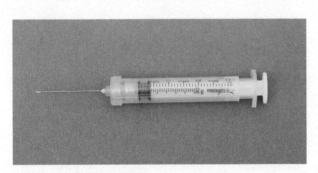
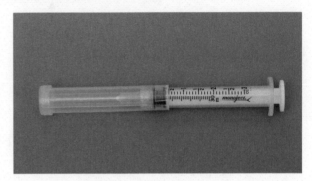

Figure 7-11 Safety syringe.

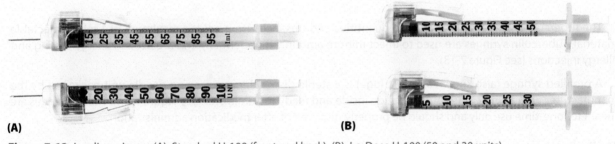

(A)   **(B)**

Figure 7-12 Insulin syringes. (A): Standard U-100 (front and back). (B): Lo-Dose U-100 (50 and 30 units).

Retractable needle cover syringes are used for prevention of needle sticks, as required by Occupational Safety and Health Administration (OSHA) standards. These syringes come with retractable needle covers to prevent needle sticks from contaminated syringes (see Figures 7-10 and 7-11).

POINTS TO REMEMBER

Never recap a needle—this will help to avoid needle sticks.

The insulin syringe is calibrated in units (U) specifically for use of diabetic patients. An international unit (IU) is an internationally accepted amount of a substance (e.g., vitamins or vaccines) used simply as a means of standardizing measures. An international unit does not have a specific, uniform definition of size. Insulin syringes are labeled as U-40 or U-100 (see Figure 7-12) and come in the following sizes: 0.3, 0.5, and 1.0 cc.

MEDICATION ERROR ALERT

The abbreviations "U" or "u," denoting units, and "IU" denoting international units are no longer accepted by most institutions and appear on the Joint Commission's "Do Not Use" list and the ISMP's "Error-Prone Abbreviations" list. The abbreviation "U" is often mistaken for the number "0" or "4," while "IU" is often mistaken for "IV" (intravenous). Use of these abbreviations increases the risk for medication errors. Thus, the Joint Commission recommends that the word "unit" always be written out.

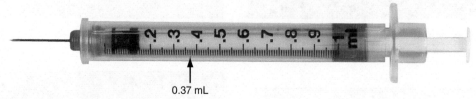

0.37 mL

Figure 7-13 Tuberculin syringe.

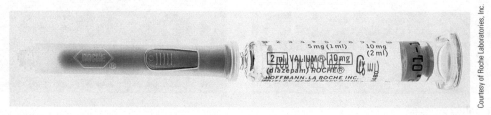

Courtesy of Roche Laboratories, Inc.

Figure 7-14 Prefilled, single-dose syringe.

The tuberculin syringe is used for small quantities of drugs, because it holds a maximum of 1 mL of injectable material. Tuberculin syringes are used to inject minute amounts intradermally and are used in allergy testing and allergy injections (see Figure 7-13).

A prefilled syringe (also known as a cartridge) is a sterile disposable syringe and needle unit packaged by the manufacturer with a single dose of medication inside and ready to administer (see Figure 7-14). These syringes are meant for one-time use only and should be properly disposed of after medication administration.

Medication Containers   Medications prescribed for injections are available in different containers such as ampules, vials, and sterile cartridges with premeasured medication.

An **ampule** is a small, hermetically sealed glass container that usually holds a single dose of medication (see Figure 7-15A). Ampules have a neck with a scored weak point that is broken just before use. A **vial** is a small bottle with a rubber stopper, through which a sterile needle is inserted to withdraw a dose of the medication inside. There are two types of vials: single and multiple doses. A multiple-dose vial may contain varying numbered doses of a drug. Vials vary in size from 2 to 100 mL (see Figure 7-15B). Because multidose vials are used more than once, extreme caution must be taken every time a needle is inserted into the medication to protect it from contamination, which could cause serious infections in future patients. If at any time the technician thinks that an error has been made or suspects possible contamination, the vial should be discarded. Unused medication should never be returned to the vial.

Parenteral Medication Forms

Parenteral forms of medication can be selected when a rapid response to a medication is desired or when a patient is not able to take a medication orally. Injectable drug forms may be available as a solution or a powder. A solution is a mixture of one or more substances dissolved in another substance, usually a fluid, to form a homogeneous mixture. A powder consists of dry particles of medications. The powder itself cannot be injected. It must be reconstituted to a liquid for injection. A diluent such as sterile water is added to the powder and mixed well.

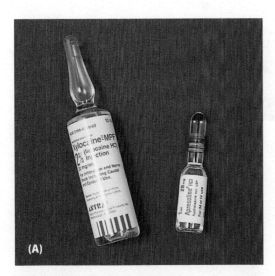

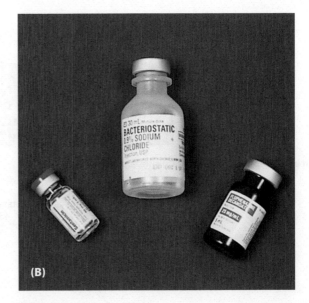

Figure 7-15 (A): Ampules. (B): Vials.

Parenteral Administration Routes

Parenteral medication can be administered through several routes, such as intradermal, subcutaneous, intramuscular, intravenous, epidural (into the subarachnoid space), and intra-articular. The most common of these are described in the following sections.

Intradermal Injection   An **intradermal injection** is given within the skin. If the injection is given correctly, a small **wheal** (a skin eruption that may follow injection of an antigen) occurs on the skin (see Figure 7-16). A 3/8-inch, 27- or 28-G needle is used for intradermal injections. The angle of insertion is 10 to 15 degrees, almost parallel to the skin surface (Figure 7-17). A common site of injection is the center of the forearm. Other sites that may be used are the upper chest and back areas. Skin tests for allergies and tuberculin tests are the most common uses for intradermal injections. One method of tuberculin screening is the tine test, which is administered using individually packaged disposable sterile stamps with four or six prongs on the end that have been treated with tuberculin solution. The tine test is not as accurate as the Mantoux (purified protein derivative [PPD]) intradermal screening test. With the Mantoux test, a 0.1-mL solution of PPD is injected into the intradermal layers. The site is then monitored for 48 to 72 hours. The result is considered positive if the resulting **induration** (hardening or firmness) is more than 15 mm in diameter. Allergy skin testing involves intradermally injecting a small amount of antigen and later examining the test site for a visible reaction. This test is more accurate than the scratch test. Extracts are injected into the intradermal layer of the skin, with the usual sterile technique, in a dose of 0.1 to 0.2 mL.

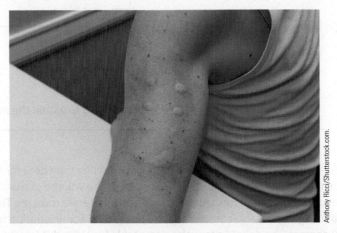

Figure 7-16 Formation of a wheal resulting from a positive reaction to allergen testing.

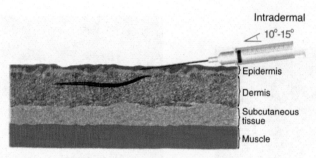

Figure 7-17 Intradermal injection sites and needle angle.

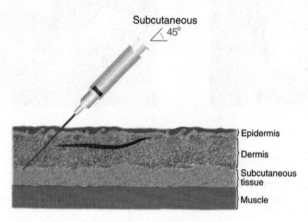

Figure 7-18 Subcutaneous injection sites and needle angle.

POINTS TO REMEMBER

When intradermal injections are used for allergy testing, 10 to 15 allergens may be tested at one time on each arm.

Subcutaneous Injection   A **subcutaneous injection** is given just below the skin and the layer of fatty tissue called adipose tissue. The most common sites for subcutaneous injections are the deltoid area, anterior thigh, abdomen, and upper back. The angle of insertion is 45 degrees for local anesthetics, allergy treatments, and epinephrine (see Figure 7-18); however, insulin and heparin are usually injected at a 90-degree angle. The amount of drug administered through the subcutaneous route should not be more than 2 mL.

MEDICAL TERMINOLOGY REVIEW

intramuscular:

intra = *within*   -ar = *pertaining to*

muscul/o = *muscle*   pertaining to within the muscle

Intramuscular Injection   A drug is injected into a muscle (**intramuscular injection**) for the following reasons: the drug will irritate the skin tissues, a more rapid absorption is desired, or the volume of the medication to be injected is large. In adults, the preferred sites are the gluteus, deltoid, and vastus lateralis muscles. The vastus lateralis is part of the quadriceps muscle in the thigh and is also considered the safest site of administration for infants (see Figure 7-19). The angle of insertion is 90 degrees. The deltoid site is also acceptable for older children. Muscles can absorb a greater amount of fluid than is usually given by subcutaneous administration. Dosage may vary from 0.5 to 5 mL. In adults,

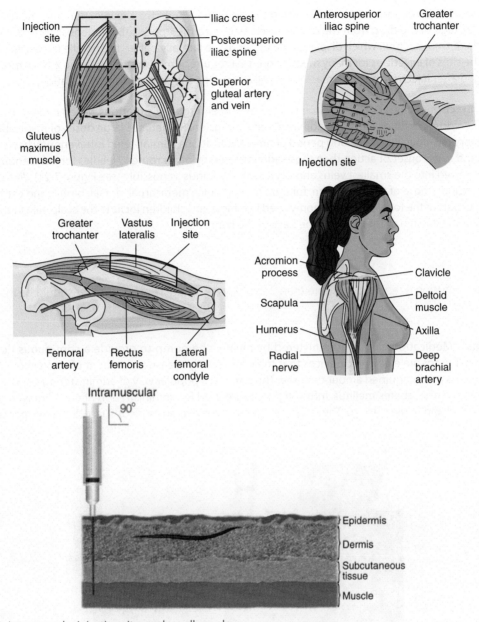

Figure 7-19 Intramuscular injection sites and needle angle.

up to 2 mL of medication can be injected into the deltoid muscle, whereas up to 5 mL can be injected into the vastus lateralis and gluteal sites. Infants and children should be given no more than 2 mL in the vastus lateralis or ventrogluteal sites. The needle is usually 1 to 3 inches in length, but longer needles are sometimes needed, especially for obese patients. The recommended gauge of the needle ranges from 20 to 23 G.

MEDICAL TERMINOLOGY REVIEW

intravenous:

intra = *within*

ven/o = *veins*

-ous = *pertaining to*

pertaining to within the veins

Some drugs injected intramuscularly are irritating to skin tissue. Therefore, the injection must be given in a way that prevents leakage of the drug from the deep muscle back into the upper subcutaneous layers. For these types of injections, the **Z-track method**, which displaces the upper tissue laterally before the needle is inserted, is used (see Figure 7-20). The sites of injections for many medications that require administration with the Z-track method should not be massaged after injection, because massaging will encourage the spread of the medication.

Intravenous Injection   **Intravenous injection** is used during emergency situations, when immediate effects are required, or when drugs or fluids are being administered by infusion. Sometimes large doses of medication must be given, either every few hours or over a long period of time. Medications administered intravenously have a faster rate of absorption and faster onset of action than those administered by other routes. Needles for intravenous injections are generally inserted into the smallest veins and as close to the hands as possible (see Figure 7-21). Veins commonly used in adults include those of the hand, arm, forearm (in particular, metacarpal, dorsal, basilic, and cephalic veins), and the dorsal plexus of the foot. Veins commonly used in infants and children include the scalp vein in the temporal area and veins in the dorsum of the foot and the back of the hand.

POINTS TO REMEMBER

If an intravenous infusion is required for more than 2 to 3 days, a central venous catheter should be inserted.

Pump Systems   Medication can be administered by means of a pump to provide a continuous flow into the patient's system. Pumps are electronic devices that force a precisely measured amount of intravenous fluid into a patient's vein over a predetermined amount of time. The pump is a popular way of administering a constant dose of insulin to a patient with diabetes mellitus. Infusion pumps are used for administration of most intravenous medications in institutional and home settings. These devices create a positive pressure of 10 to 25 pounds per square inch.

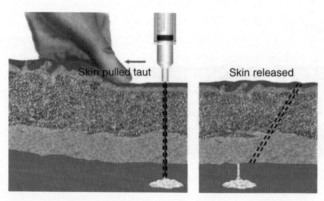

Figure 7-20 Z-track method of intramuscular injection.

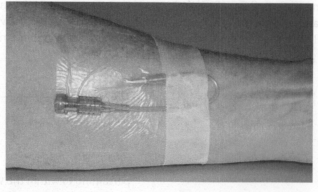

Figure 7-21 Intravenous injection.

They offer more accurate control over the rate of infusion than other devices. The infusion pumps flow at rates of up to 999 mL/hr and are able to provide a higher rate of infusion and higher pressure.

Urethral Route

This route involves application of a drug by insertion into the urethra. A solution can be instilled into the urinary bladder using a catheter. Other common dose forms include urethral suppositories. Urethral administration is commonly used to treat incontinence or impotence (in males). Disadvantages of this route are inconvenience and localized pain.

TOPICAL ROUTE

Topical medications are applied to the surface of the body (the skin or mucous membranes). The vast majority of drugs applied to the skin are designed to have local effects. For instance, topical anesthesia is the application to the skin of a drug that temporarily deadens nerve sensations. Other medications applied topically, such as the fentanyl patch, are designed to have systemic effects. Skin medication forms include lotions, liniments, ointments, and transdermal patches. Lotions are often used to control itching. Calamine lotion is an example. Some lotions are used to relieve congestion and pain in muscles and joints. After applying the lotion, the area may be covered with a thick dressing to retain heat. Liniments (emulsions) have a higher portion of oil than do lotions. They are often used to protect dried, cracked, or fissured skin. Ointments are applied to dry, scaly areas with little or no hair and can exert a prolonged effect.

Mucous membranes are useful sites of administration because of their ability to absorb medication designed to provide either a local or a systemic effect. The buccal, sublingual, rectal, and respiratory (inhalation) routes are most often chosen when a systemic effect of a topically applied drug is desired. Other routes, such as ophthalmic, otic, nasal, vaginal, or urethral, are most often used to administer drugs with local effects. Use of the sublingual, buccal, and urethral routes of drug administration was discussed earlier in this chapter.

Transdermal Patches

Certain medications can be absorbed slowly through the skin to create a constant, time-released systemic effect. Transdermal patches are dosage forms that release minute amounts of drug at a consistent rate (see Figure 7-22). As the drug is released from the patch, it is absorbed into the skin and carried off by the capillary blood supply. Examples of drugs administered transdermally include nitroglycerin, estrogen, testosterone, nicotine, and scopolamine.

Inhalation Administration

The act of drawing breath, vapor, or gas into the lungs is called inhalation. Inhalation therapy may involve the administration of medicines, water vapor, and gases such as oxygen, carbon dioxide, and helium. The medication is inhaled to achieve local effects within the respiratory tract through aerosols (see Figure 7-23), nebulizers, Spinhalers®, or metered-dose inhalers. Medications that are administered through inhalers include bronchodilators, mucolytic agents, and steroids.

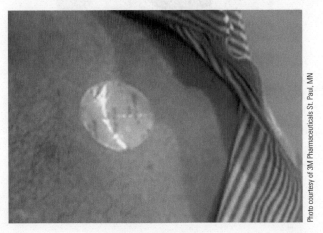

Photo courtesy of 3M Pharmaceuticals St. Paul, MN

Figure 7-22 Transdermal patch.

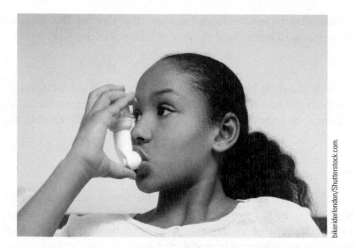

Figure 7-23 Inhaler.

When given therapeutically, oxygen is considered a medication. The dosage is based on individual needs, with the prescriber specifying the flow rate, concentration, method of delivery, and length of time for administration. Oxygen is ordered as liters per minute (LPM) and as percentage of oxygen concentration (%). Oxygen toxicity may develop when 100% oxygen is breathed for a prolonged period. A high concentration of inhaled oxygen causes alveolar collapse, intra-alveolar hemorrhage, hyaline membrane formation, and disturbance of the central nervous system and retrolental fibroplasias in newborns. Oxygen can be administered in several ways. The most commonly prescribed methods use nasal cannulas and masks.

Ophthalmic Administration

Drops and ointments instilled into the eye are generally absorbed slowly and affect only the area in contact. The medications are placed between the eyeball and the lower lid (see Figure 7-24). Ophthalmic preparations must be sterile to prevent eye infections and should be isotonic to minimize burning. Medications given as ophthalmic preparations include antibiotics, antivirals, decongestants, artificial tears, and topical anesthetics.

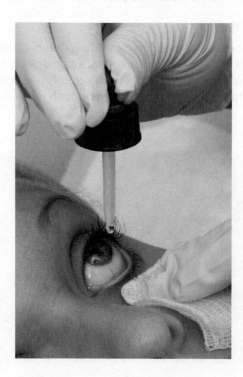

Figure 7-24 Ophthalmic route.

Otic Route

Dropping a small amount of a sterile medicated solution into the ear treats localized infection or inflammation of the ear. Very low dosages of medication are required, and the manufacturer must indicate that the medication is meant for otic usage. In children younger than 3 years of age, gently pull the earlobe down and back; in adults, gently pull the earlobe up and out (see Figure 7-25). The patient must remain with the head inclined to the opposite side for 5 minutes to allow the medication to coat the surface of the inner ear canal. The use of eardrops is usually contraindicated if the patient has a perforated eardrum.

Nasal Route

Nasal solutions act locally to treat minor congestion or infection. The medication should be drawn up in the dropper and held just over one nostril, and then the required number of nose drops should be administered (see Figure 7-26). If a nasal spray is used, the patient sits upright, one nostril is blocked, and the tip of the nasal spray is inserted into the nostril. As the patient takes a deep breath, a puff of spray is squeezed into the nostril.

Patients often misuse nasal decongestant sprays. Nasal medications are commonly used for blocked nasal passages (decongestants) and nosebleeds (hemostatics).

Vaginal Route

Vaginal suppositories, tablets, creams, and fluid solutions are used to treat local infections. Medications are deposited into the vagina. Douches may be used as anti-infectives. Local contraceptives are available as creams and foams. Vaginal instillation is most effective if the patient is lying down. Creams are instilled with applicators.

Rectal Route

Rectal medications are useful if the patient is nauseated, vomiting, or unconscious. Manufacturers supply rectal medications in the form of gelatin or cocoa butter-based suppositories, which melt in the warmth of the rectum and release the medication (see Figure 7-27), or in the form of enemas as a solution. Suppositories may be used to soften the stool or stimulate evacuation of the bowel. The best time to administer a rectal drug intended for a systemic effect is after a bowel movement or enema. An enema can be used to deliver a solution or medication into the rectum and colon. Enemas are most often used to cleanse the lower bowel in preparation for radiography, proctoscopy,

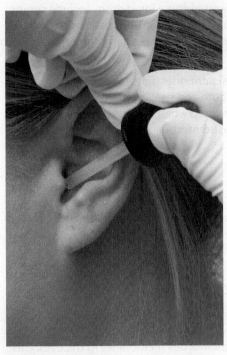

Figure 7-25 Otic route.

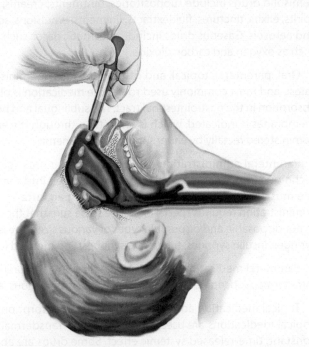

Figure 7-26 Nasal route.

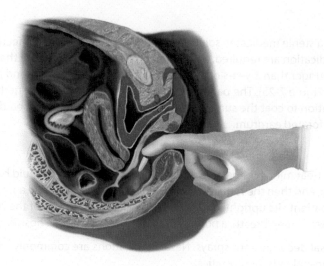

Figure 7-27 Rectal route.

sigmoidoscopy, and surgery. A Fleet® Enema is a ready-to-use device that promotes bowel evacuation by softening the feces and stimulating peristalsis. The Fleet ready-to-use enema does not cause burning, irritation, or dehydration and does not interfere with the absorption of vitamins or the actions of drugs.

Summary

Pharmacy technicians are required to have knowledge of many different drug names and sources. Drug names include chemical, generic (nonproprietary), and trade (proprietary, brand, or manufacturer) names. There are basically five sources of drugs: plant, animal (including humans), mineral or mineral products, synthetic (chemical substances), and engineered (investigational drugs). In addition, pharmacy technicians must learn many different types of dosage forms that are currently available in the market. These include gases, liquids, solids, and semisolids. Solid drug forms include tablets, pills, plasters, capsules, caplets, gelcaps, powders, granules, and troches (lozenges). Semisolid drugs include suppositories, ointments, creams, gels, lotions, and pastes. Liquid drugs include syrups, spirits, elixirs, tinctures, fluidextracts, liniments, emulsions, solutions, mixtures, suspensions, aromatic waters, sprays, and aerosols. Gaseous drugs include anesthetic gases such as nitrous oxide and halothane and compressed gases such as oxygen and carbon dioxide.

Oral, parenteral, topical, and other routes may administer drugs. Oral administration of drugs is the easiest, safest, and most commonly used route. The medication is placed in the mouth and swallowed into the stomach for absorption in the gastrointestinal tract. The sublingual and buccal routes are used when absorption through mucous membranes is indicated, which is faster than through the enteral (oral/gastrointestinal) route. Medication may be administered rectally by either suppository or enema.

Parenteral administration of medications requires special processes that must be carried out while sterile technique is maintained. Injections may be given into the dermis of the skin, into the subcutaneous tissue, into the muscles, or into the veins. Administering an intravenous injection is an advanced skill, and each route of administration requires special expertise to be sure that the medication reaches the desired location. Syringes come in nondisposable and disposable types of various sizes. These include hypodermic syringes, retractable needle cover syringes, insulin syringes, tuberculin syringes, and prefilled (cartridge) syringes.

Parenteral medications come in vials, ampules, and prefilled syringes. Parenteral administration routes include intradermal, subcutaneous, intramuscular, and intravenous, as well as the Z-track method.

Topical medication administration results in absorption of the drug through the skin or mucous membranes. Topical medications are used for local effects. Transdermal patches allow slow absorption through the skin for a constant, time-released systemic effect. Some drugs are absorbed through mucous membranes in the eyes, ears, nose, vagina, and respiratory tract. Inhalation administration is the act of drawing breath, vapor, or gas into the lungs.

REVIEW QUESTIONS

1. Which of the following determines needle gauges?

   A. The size of the shaft
   B. The diameter of the lumen
   C. The length of the hilt
   D. The size of the syringe

2. Which of the following is an example of a solution?

   A. Water and iodine
   B. Water and alcohol
   C. Water and sugar
   D. Normal saline

3. An agent mixed with a liquid but not dissolved is referred to as a(n):

   A. tincture.
   B. suspension.
   C. aromatic water.
   D. fluidextract.

4. Tablets are sometimes mistakenly called:

   A. pills.
   B. powders.
   C. buffered.
   D. gelcaps.

5. Which of the following is an example of semisolid drugs?

   A. Caplets
   B. Gelcaps
   C. Gels
   D. Granules

6. The best time to administer a rectal drug intended for a systemic effect is:

   A. early morning.
   B. after dinner.
   C. after a bowel movement.
   D. bedtime.

7. Any composition of a liquid and powder that hardens when it dries is called a:

   A. capsule.
   B. plaster.
   C. gelcap.
   D. lotion.

8. Nicotine and nitroglycerin are examples of drugs that may be administered:

   A. transdermally.
   B. nasally.
   C. vaginally.
   D. rectally.

9. Elixirs differ from tinctures in that they are:

   A. colorless.
   B. tasteless.
   C. sweetened.
   D. bitter.

10. Which of the following is an example of aromatic water?

    A. Milk of magnesia
    B. Peppermint
    C. Mineral oil
    D. Chloroform

11. Which of the following is the reason that you should never recap a needle?

    A. To avoid contamination
    B. To avoid infection
    C. To avoid needle sticks
    D. To prevent asepsis

12. Which of the following is not a method of parenteral administration?

    A. Intravenous
    B. Intradermal
    C. Intravaginal
    D. Epidural

13. An excessive hardening or firmness of any body site is called:

    A. induration.
    B. infarction.
    C. infection.
    D. infiltration.

14. Which of the following forms of liquid drugs consists of water, alcohol, and sugar?

    A. Syrup
    B. Elixir
    C. Spirit
    D. Tincture

15. Which of the following is the route of administration of a drug that is placed between the gums and the cheek?

    A. Transdermal
    B. Sublingual
    C. Buccal
    D. Topical

CRITICAL THINKING

1. Which are examples of synthetically created drugs, and what are the differences between organic and inorganic components of these?

2. How does the form of the drug affect the method through which it is administered? Choose a dosage form and explain why it is administered in a particular way.

3. What is the definition of the term "inhalation," and what types of substances may be administered in this way?

4. What are the types of equipment used to administer inhaled medications, and what are the most commonly prescribed methods used for oxygen administration?

WEB LINKS

DailyMed: dailymed.nlm.nih.gov

Drug Topics: www.drugtopics.com

Drugs.com: www.drugs.com

Mayo Clinic: www.mayoclinic.org

Medline Plus: medlineplus.gov

Merck & Co.: www.merckmanuals.com

Pharmacy Times: www.pharmacytimes.com

Pharmacy Today (JAPhA): www.pharmacytoday.org

RxList—The Internet Drug Index: www.rxlist.com

Today's Technician: www.pharmacytechnician.org

U.S. Pharmacist: www.uspharmacist.com

WebMD: www.webmd.com

Measurement Systems

OBJECTIVES

Upon completion of this chapter, the reader should be able to:

1. Explain the rules of the metric system and the basic units of weight, volume, and length.
2. Describe common equivalents in the metric system.
3. Discuss the apothecary system.
4. Explain the household system.
5. Convert metric measures to their equivalents in the other systems.
6. Name the metric equivalents that are used in the medical profession.
7. Define common prefixes used in the metric system.
8. Explain the rules concerning changing grams to milligrams and milliliters to liters.
9. Describe the international unit (IU).
10. Explain the use of milliequivalents (mEq) and units in dosage calculations.

KEY TERMS

apothecary system	household system	metric system	ounce
dram	international units	milliequivalent	unit
grain	liter	milliunit	
gram	meter	minim	

Overview

Administration of the medications prescribed for the patient must be accurate and the amounts must be correct. Pharmacy technicians must have a comprehensive knowledge of the weights and measures used in drug administration for prescribed amounts. Three systems are used for measuring medication and solutions: metric system, apothecary system, and household system. It is necessary for the pharmacy technician to know each system and be able to convert from one system to another. Most medications and measurements used in the health care field are calibrated and calculated using the metric system. Thus, knowledge of the metric system is very important, because dosage units are calculated in metric measurements. Although some medications are still prescribed in apothecary and household terms, health care workers will find that the majority of medication calculation and administration skills involve accurate use of the metric system.

Measurement of weight, volume, and length of the prescription and administration of drugs is done with three parameters in mind. Weight is the most utilized parameter. It is essential as a dosage unit. The metric weight units, such as milligrams and grams, are the most accurate. Measurement of volume is the next most important parameter. Volume is the parameter used for liquids. Volume also includes two additional parameters for dosage calculations: quantity and concentration. The most commonly used metric volume unit for dosage calculations is the milliliter. Today, household and apothecary measures such as teaspoons and ounces are used less commonly. Length is the least utilized parameter for dosage calculations.

The Metric System

The **metric system** of measure was introduced in 1799 in France. Its use in the United States was legalized in 1866. By an act of Congress in 1893, it became our legal standard of measure, and all other systems refer to it for official comparison. It is now the standard for scientific and industrial measurements and is used in approximately 90% of the world's developed countries. Today, the metric system is the system of choice when one deals with the weights and measures involved in the calculation of drug dosages. Its accuracy and simplicity are related to its utilization of the decimal system, which is based on units of 10. The use of decimals can eliminate errors in measuring medications. The three basic units of the metric system are the following:

1. **Gram:** the basic unit for weight
2. **Liter:** the basic unit for volume
3. **Meter:** the basic unit for length

Adding a prefix specifies parts of these basic units. Each prefix has a numerical value, which is shown in Table 8-1. It is essential for individuals who deal with measurement, calculation, and administration of drugs to be familiar with prefixes that are commonly used in the metric system.

It is also important that pharmacy technicians be familiar with common metric abbreviations, which are shown in Table 8-2.

International standardization of metric units was established throughout the world in 1960 with the introduction of the International System, or SI (from the French Système International). Table 8-3 shows SI standardized abbreviations.

Table 8-1 Metric Prefixes

Metric Prefix	Value
micro =	One millionth of a unit (0.000001) or $\frac{1}{1,000,000}$ of the base unit
milli =	One thousandth of a unit (0.001) or $\frac{1}{1000}$ of the base unit
centi =	One hundredth of a unit (0.01) or $\frac{1}{100}$ of the base unit
deci =	One tenth of a unit (0.1) or $\frac{1}{10}$ of the base unit
deka =	Ten units (10)
hecto =	One hundred units (100)
kilo =	One thousand units (1000)

Table 8-2 International Metric System Abbreviations

Weight	Volume	Length
gram (basic unit), g	liter (basic unit), L	meter (basic unit), m
milligram, mg	milliliter, mL	centimeter, cm
microgram, mcg	cubic centimeter, cc	millimeter, mm
kilogram, kg	deciliter, dL	kilometer, km

Table 8-3 The International System of Standardized Abbreviations

Metric System	Unit	Abbreviation	Equivalents
Weight	gram (basic unit)	g	1 g = 1000 mg
	milligram	mg	1 mg = 1000 mcg = 0.001 g
	microgram	mcg	1 mcg = 0.001 mg = 0.000001 g
	kilogram	kg	1 kg = 1000 g
Volume	liter (basic unit)	L or l	1 L = 1000 mL
	milliliter	mL	1 mL = 1 cc = 0.001 L
	cubic centimeter	cc	1 cc = 1 mL = 0.001 L
Length	meter (basic unit)	m	1 m = 100 cm = 1000 mm
	centimeter	cm	1 cm = 0.01 m = 10 mm
	millimeter	mm	1 mm = 0.001 m = 0.1 cm

POINTS TO REMEMBER

The metric system is the most accurate and popular system used today for drug prescriptions and drug administration.

GRAM

The gram is the basic unit of weight in the metric system. A gram equals approximately the weight of 1 cubic centimeter (cc) or 1 milliliter (mL) of water. One gram is equal to approximately 15 grains (gr), or 0.035 ounce (oz). Some medications are ordered as fractions of grams. A milligram (mg) is 1000 times smaller than a gram; medications may be ordered in milligrams. The kilogram is a very large unit that is not used for measuring medications. A kilogram is 1000 times larger than a gram. It is used to determine a patient's weight. Table 8-4 shows values equivalent to a gram.

Table 8-4 Value of the Gram

Gram	Equivalents
1 g	1,000,000 mcg
	1000 mg
	100 cg
	$^1/_{1000}$ kg

Example

How many milligrams are there in 0.65 g?

Solution:

Multiply 0.65 g by 1000 to determine that there are 650 mg in 0.65 g. The rule for converting between decimals and percentages can be expanded to include multiplying and dividing by 10, 100, or 1000 by moving the decimal point to the left or right for the same number of places as there are zeros. Multiplication by 1000 can be accomplished by simply moving the decimal point three places to the right, so 0.65 g equals 650 mg.

Conversion of weight in the metric system to the apothecary system was explained earlier, when we learned that 1 gr is equivalent to either 60 or 65 mg.

$$1 \text{ gr} = 60 \text{ mg or } 1 \text{ gr} = 65 \text{ mg}$$

The relationship between grains and milligrams or grams is more complex (see Table 8-5).

Example

How many kilograms does a 62-lb child weigh?

First fraction: 62 lb/X kg

Remember that 1 kg = 2.2 lb

Second fraction: 2.2 lb/1 kg

Table 8-5 Approximate Equivalent Measures for Weight

Metric	Apothecary
60 mg	1 gr
30 mg	½ gr
15 mg	¼ gr
1 mg	$^1/_{60}$ gr
1 g (1000 mg)	15 gr
0.5 g	7.5 gr
1 kg	2.2 lb

Write the proportion:

$$\frac{62\ lb}{X\ kg} = \frac{2.2\ lb}{1\ kg}$$

Cross-multiply to solve:

$$62 \times 1 = 2.2X$$
$$62 = 2.2X$$
$$X = \frac{62}{2.2} = 28.18$$

LITER

The liter is the basic unit of volume used to measure liquids in the metric system. It is equal to 1000 cc (cubic centimeters) of water. One cubic centimeter is considered equivalent to 1 mL (milliliter); thus, 1 L (liter) = 1000 mL or cc. The cubic centimeter is the amount of space that 1 mL of liquid occupies. One liter is equal to 1.056 qt (quarts), which is 0.26 of a gallon or 2.1 pt (pints). Table 8-6 summarizes metric volumes.

Example

How many liters are there in 350 mL?

Solution:

Divide 350 mL by 1000. The division by 1000 can be accomplished by simply moving the decimal point three places to the left, so 0.35 L equals 350 mL.

METER

The meter is used for linear (length) measurement. Linear measurements (e.g., meter and centimeter) are commonly used to measure the height of an individual and to determine growth patterns, not in the calculation of doses. Therefore, only the units of weight and volume are discussed in this chapter.

Household Measurements

Household measurements are not accurate enough for health care professionals to use in the calculation of drug dosages in the hospital or pharmacy. However, the **household system** is still in use for doses given primarily at home, as indicated by the name. It is perfectly safe to use for measurements in cooking but should be avoided for administration of medications. The household system is the least accurate of the three systems of measure. Capacities of utensils such as teaspoons, tablespoons, and cups vary from one house to another. The basic units of volume in the

Table 8-6 Metric Volumes	
Volume	**Liter**
1 kiloliter (kL)	1000.000 L
1 hectoliter (hL)	100.000 L
1 dekaliter (daL)	10.000 L
1 liter (L)	1.000 L
1 deciliter (dL)	0.100 L
1 centiliter (cL)	0.010 L
1 milliliter (mL)	0.001 L

Table 8-7 Approximate Equivalent Measures of Volume

Metric	Household	Apothecary
5 mL	1 tsp	—
15 mL	1 tbsp	—
30 mL	2 tbsp	1 oz
240 mL	1 cup	8 oz
480 mL	2 cups = 1 pt	16 oz
960 mL	2 pt = 1 qt	32 oz

household system, in increasing size, are the drop, teaspoon, tablespoon, ounce, cup, pint, quart, and gallon. Of these, the four smallest measures are most commonly used for medications.

When one discusses medications specifically, the word *ounce* generally implies volume, which is represented as *fluid ounces*. In other contexts, ounce may represent a unit of weight, as does the term *pound*. There are 3 tsp (teaspoons) in 1 tbsp (tablespoon). There are 2 tbsp in 1 oz, 6 oz are equal to an average teacup, and 8 oz are equal to an average cup or glass. Because spoons, cups, and glasses come in all sizes and shapes, one can understand why this system is not completely accurate. Table 8-7 shows a list of approximate equivalents among the metric, household, and apothecary measurement systems.

POINTS TO REMEMBER

Household measurements in the United States are also called customary measurements; the "household system" is the least accurate measurement system.

Apothecary System

The **apothecary system** is also called the wine measure or U.S. liquid measure system. This system is a very old English system. It has slowly been replaced by the metric system. A few units of measure in this system are used for medication administration. In the following paragraphs, some basic units for weight and volume in the apothecary system are discussed. Proper notations in the apothecary system are unique. They include common fractions instead of decimals (ss for ½); lowercase Roman numerals instead of Arabic numbers for amounts of 1 to 10, 20, and 30; special symbols for minim and ounce; and units of measure that precede the numeric values.

POINTS TO REMEMBER

The apothecary system of measurement is rarely used in the clinical setting and is one of the oldest of the various measurement systems.

WEIGHT

The basic unit for weight is the **grain**. The abbreviation for grain is gr. **Dram** is also a unit of weight; 1 dr is equal to 60 gr. The dram is usually abbreviated as dr. An **ounce** is larger than a dram; 1 oz is equal to 8 dr. The ounce is usually abbreviated as oz. Also, you should remember that one grain is equivalent to 65 mg.

Example

How many grains are there in 5 dr?

Solution:

Remember that 1 dr is equal to 60 gr, so multiply the 5 dr by 60. Therefore, 300 gr equals 5 dr.

Example

How many fluid ounces are there in 48 fl dr (fluid drams)?

Solution:

You know that 1 fl oz is equal to 8 fl dr. Divide 48 fl dr by 8. The answer is that 48 fl dr equals 6 fl oz.

VOLUME

The basic unit for volume is the **minim**. The abbreviation for minim is a lowercase letter "m." A minim is extremely small, and not able to be accurately measured. It may be considered to be approximately the size of 1 drop. Volume can also be measured by drams and ounces. In summary, the units of the apothecary system are as follows:

Weight:	grain (gr)
Volume:	minim (m)
	dram (dr)
	ounce (oz)

Units of Measure Used for Medications

The quantity of medicine prescribed may also be expressed as four other measurements: international units, units, milliunits, and milliequivalents. Arabic numbers with the appropriate sign are used to indicate an amount. For instance, vitamins and chemicals are measured in international units to establish potency of such items. Likewise, the amount of medication required to produce a standardized desired effect is expressed in units. However, some medications, such as penicillin, heparin, and insulin, are assigned a specific numeral amount in conjunction with the kind of unit to indicate a separate meaning.

INTERNATIONAL UNITS

A **unit** is the amount of medication required to produce a certain effect. The size of a unit varies for each drug. Some medications, such as vitamins, are measured in standardized units called **international units** (IU). These units represent the amount of medication needed to produce a certain effect, but they are standardized by international agreement. As with milliequivalents, you do not need to convert from units to other measures. Medications that are ordered in units will also be labeled in units.

MILLIUNITS

A **milliunit** (mU) represents one thousandth (1/1000) of a unit, thus, 1 unit is equal to 1000 mU. The drug oxytocin (Pitocin®) is measured in milliunits.

MILLIEQUIVALENTS

Some drugs are measured in **milliequivalents** (mEq), which is a unit of measure based on the chemical combining power of a substance. One thousandth (1/1000) of the same amount of a chemical is known as a milliequivalent. The concentrations of serum electrolytes, such as calcium, potassium, sodium, and magnesium, are measured in milliequivalents. Because of the electrical activity of ions, it is impossible to use weight units (e.g., milligrams or grams) to measure quantities of electrolytes. An equivalent (Eq) represents 1000 mEq and is the weight of a substance that combines with or replaces 1 g (atomic weight of hydrogen). Sodium bicarbonate and potassium chloride are examples of drugs that are measured in milliequivalents. You do not need to learn to convert from milliequivalents to another system of measurement.

Example

Heparin 7500 units are ordered, and heparin 10,000 units/mL is the stock drug.

Example

Potassium chloride 10 mEq is ordered, and potassium chloride 20 mEq/15 mL is the stock drug.

Example

Oxytocin (Pitocin) 2 mU (0.002 units) intravenous per minute is ordered, and Pitocin 10 units/mL to be added to a 1000-mL intravenous solution is available.

Note that the international unit, unit, and milliequivalent are measures that require no conversion because the drugs ordered using these units are prepared and given in the same system.

Converting Within and Between Systems

When the pharmacy technician calculates dosages, he or she must often convert between the metric, apothecary, and household systems of measurement. Therefore, the technician will need to know how the measure of a quantity in one system compares to its measure in another system. For example, the relationships between milliliters and liters and between teaspoons and tablespoons were discussed. In pharmacy and medicine, use of the metric system currently predominates over that of the other commonly used systems. Most prescriptions and medication orders are written in the metric system, and labeling on most prefabricated pharmaceutical products has drug strengths and dosages described in metric units, replacing to a great extent the use of other common systems of measurement. Medications are usually ordered in a unit of weight measurement such as grams or grains. Pharmacy technicians must be able to convert and calculate the correct dosage of drugs. The technician can convert between units of measurement within the same system or convert units of measurement from one system to another. He or she must also interpret the order and administer the correct number of tablets, capsules, tablespoons, milligrams, or milliliters.

CONVERSION OF WEIGHTS

Remember that 1000 mg = 1 g and 1000 mcg (micrograms) = 1 mg. To convert grams to milligrams, you should always multiply by 1000 or move the decimal point three places to the right.

Example

$$2\,g = 2000(.)\,mg$$
$$0.2\,g = 200(.)\,mg$$
$$0.02\,g = 020(.)\,mg$$

To convert milligrams to grams, divide by 1000 or move the decimal point three places to the left.

Example

$$250\,mg = 0.250\,g$$
$$50\,mg = 0.050\,g$$
$$5\,mg = 0.005\,g$$

To convert milligrams to micrograms, multiply by 1000 or move the decimal point three places to the right.

Example

$$3\,mg = 3000(.)\,mcg$$
$$0.5\,mg = 500(.)\,mcg$$
$$0.08\,mg = 080(.)\,mcg$$

To convert micrograms to milligrams, divide by 1000 or move the decimal point three places to the left.

Example

$$1500 \text{ mcg} = 1.500 \text{ mg}$$
$$600 \text{ mcg} = 0.600 \text{ mg}$$
$$20 \text{ mcg} = 0.020 \text{ mg}$$

The microgram, milligram, and gram are the most commonly used measurements for medication administration. Tablets and capsules are most often supplied in milligrams. Antibiotics can be provided in grams, milligrams, or units. For small dosages or for very powerful drugs in pediatric and critical care patients, micrograms are used.

CONVERSION OF LIQUIDS

To convert and calculate the correct dosage of liquid medications, remember the units of the metric system for volume.

Example

Convert 0.02 L to mL.

Equivalent: 1 L = 1000 mL.

Conversion factor is 1000.

Multiply by 1000:

$$0.02 \text{ L} = 0.02 \times 1000 = 20 \text{ mL}$$

Or move the decimal point three places to the right:

$$0.02 \text{ L} = 0.020 = 20 \text{ mL}$$

To convert milliliters to liters, one must divide. Remember that the equivalent of 1 L is 1000 mL, and then divide the number of milliliters by 1000.

Example

Convert 3000 mL to L.

Equivalent: 1 L = 1000 mL.

Conversion factor is 1000.

Divide by 1000:

$$3000 \text{ mL} = 3000 \div 1000 = 3 \text{ L}$$

Or move the decimal point three places to the left:

$$3000 \text{ mL} = 3.000 = 3 \text{ L}$$

CONVERSION OF LENGTH

Remember that 2.54 cm = 1 inch, and 25.4 mm = 1 inch. To convert centimeters to inches, or millimeters to inches, see the following examples.

Example

Convert 75.4 cm to inches.

$$\frac{75.4 \text{ cm}}{2.54} = 29.685 \text{ inches}$$

Convert 80 mm to inches.

$$\frac{80 \text{ mm}}{25.4} = 3.150 \text{ inches}$$

CONVERSION OF TEMPERATURES

Temperatures are reported in both the Fahrenheit and Celsius systems. Using the freezing and boiling points of each scale, a conversion formula has been established to calculate equivalent temperatures between them. On the Fahrenheit thermometer, there are 180 degrees between freezing (32°F) and boiling (212°F). On the Celsius thermometer, there are only 100 degrees between freezing (0°C) and boiling (100°C). The ratio equivalent is 180 : 100, which can be reduced to 1.8 : 1.

Therefore, the following formulas are used. To convert Fahrenheit temperatures to Celsius temperatures, the formula is:

$$\frac{°F - 32}{1.8} = °C$$

Example

Convert 97°F to °C.

$$\frac{97°F - 32}{1.8} = \frac{65}{1.8} = 36.1°C$$

To convert Celsius temperatures to Fahrenheit temperatures, the formula is:

$$(1.8 \times °C) + 32 = °F$$

Example

Convert 22°C to °F.

$$(1.8 \times 22°C) + 32 = 39.6 + 32 = 71.6°F$$

CONVERSION OF TIME

Time is measured in two different ways. Throughout the world, except for the United States and some of the English-speaking parts of Canada, the *international clock* is used, which is based on the 24-hour day. It does not use the abbreviations *a.m.* or *p.m.* Instead, each hour and the minutes within a four-digit number identifies it. In the United States and parts of Canada, the 24-hour clock system is referred to as *military time*, since military organizations also utilize it. In the United Kingdom, this system is sometimes referred to as *continental time*. In other places, it is called *railway time*.

The international clock begins at midnight, signified by 00:00, which indicates the hours that have passed in the day, from 0 to 24. Time in the 24-hour format is written as hours:minutes (see Table 8-8). For example, *four twenty a.m.* is expressed as 04:20 in the international clock system, while *four twenty p.m.* is expressed as 16:20. To understand further, once the time reaches noon (12:00), all following hours continue incrementally, with *one p.m.* being 13:00, and so forth.

Table 8-8 24 Hour Clock Chart	
12 Hour Clock (a.m./p.m.)	**24 Hour Clock (HH:MM)**
12:00 a.m. Midnight—start of day	00:00
1:00 a.m.	01:00
2:00 a.m.	02:00
3:00 a.m.	03:00
4:00 a.m.	04:00
5:00 a.m.	05:00
6:00 a.m.	06:00
7:00 a.m.	07:00
8:00 a.m.	08:00
9:00 a.m.	09:00
10:00 a.m.	10:00
11:00 a.m.	11:00
12:00 p.m. Noon	12:00
1:00 p.m.	13:00
2:00 p.m.	14:00
3:00 p.m.	15:00
4:00 p.m.	16:00
5:00 p.m.	17:00
6:00 p.m.	18:00
7:00 p.m.	19:00
8:00 p.m.	20:00
9:00 p.m.	21:00
10:00 p.m.	22:00
11:00 p.m.	23:00
Midnight—end of day	24:00

Summary

Pharmacy technicians are required to have a comprehensive knowledge of the weights and measures used in drug administration. The most commonly used system for measuring medications and solutions is the metric system. Today, pharmacies in the United States use the apothecary system very rarely. The least accurate system of measurement is the household system. When measuring, weight is the most utilized parameter, with milligrams and grams being the most common units of metric weight. For liquids, volume is the most utilized parameter, with the milliliter being the most common unit of metric volume. Volume also includes two additional parameters in dosage calculations: quantity and concentration.

In the Fahrenheit system, freezing is represented by 32 degrees, while boiling is represented by 212 degrees. In the Celsius system, freezing is represented by 0 degrees, while boiling is represented by 100 degrees. In order to convert temperatures between the two systems, conversion formulas are required. Since the ratio equivalent between the two systems is 1.8 to 1, the formulas are as follows. To convert Fahrenheit temperatures to Celsius temperatures, the formula is to subtract 32 from the Fahrenheit temperature, and then divide by 1.8. To convert Celsius temperatures to Fahrenheit temperatures, the formula is to multiply the Celsius temperature by 1.8, and then add 32.

REVIEW QUESTIONS

1. 2 cc is equivalent to _____ L.

2. 760 mcg is equivalent to _____ mg.

3. 4 tbsp are equivalent to _____ tsp.

4. 6 oz are equivalent to _____ tbsp.

5. 0.3 g is equivalent to _____ gr.

6. 4 cups are equivalent to _____ mL.

7. 1 cup is equivalent to _____ tbsp.

8. 2 qt are equivalent to _____ mL.

9. 20 pt are equivalent to _____ fl oz.

10. 26 mcg are equivalent to _____ mg.

11. 0.0546 kg are equivalent to _____ g.

12. An order is presented for 0.15 g of a medication. On hand are 25 mg tablets. The pharmacy technician must dispense _____ tablets to the patient.

13. An order is presented for 10 mg of a medication. On hand are vials containing 20 mg/mL. The pharmacy technician must dispense _____ mL to the patient.

14. An order is presented for 1500 mg of a medication. On hand are 500 mg tablets. The pharmacy technician must dispense _____ tablets to the patient.

15. An order is presented for 75 mg of a medication to be given PO. On hand are 25 mg tablets. The pharmacy technician must dispense _____ tablets to the patient.

16. 63.4°F (Fahrenheit) is equivalent to _____°C (Centigrade).

17. 87.2°F is equivalent to _____°C.

18. 132°F is equivalent to _____°C.

19. 32°F is equivalent to _____°C.

20. 48°F is equivalent to _____°C.

21. 0°C is equivalent to _____°F.

22. 37.4°C is equivalent to _____°F.

23. 100°C is equivalent to _____°F.

24. 32°C is equivalent to _____°F.

25. 55°C is equivalent to _____°F.

26. 1:33 a.m. is equivalent to _____ on the 24-hour clock.

27. Midnight is equivalent to both _____ and _____ on the 24-hour clock.

28. 3:45 p.m. is equivalent to _____ on the 24-hour clock.

29. 7:07 p.m. is equivalent to _____ on the 24-hour clock.

30. 11:11 p.m. is equivalent to _____ on the 24-hour clock.

31. The basic unit of metric weight is the _____

32. The basic unit of metric volume is the _____

33. The basic unit of metric length is the _____

34. Vitamins are examples of substances that are measured in _____ units.

35. The concentrations of serum electrolytes are measured in _____

CRITICAL THINKING

An infant suffering from otitis media is given 5 mL of an antibiotic every 8 hours for 10 days. Her mother is using a household-measuring device to measure the dose of antibiotic.

1. Which household device should the mother use?

2. How much antibiotic should the infant take considering the device that the physician recommends?

WEB LINKS

Convert-me.com: convert-me.com/en

ConvertIt.com: www.convertit.com

OnlineConversion.com: www.onlineconversion.com

Unit Conversion Information: www.convertaz.com

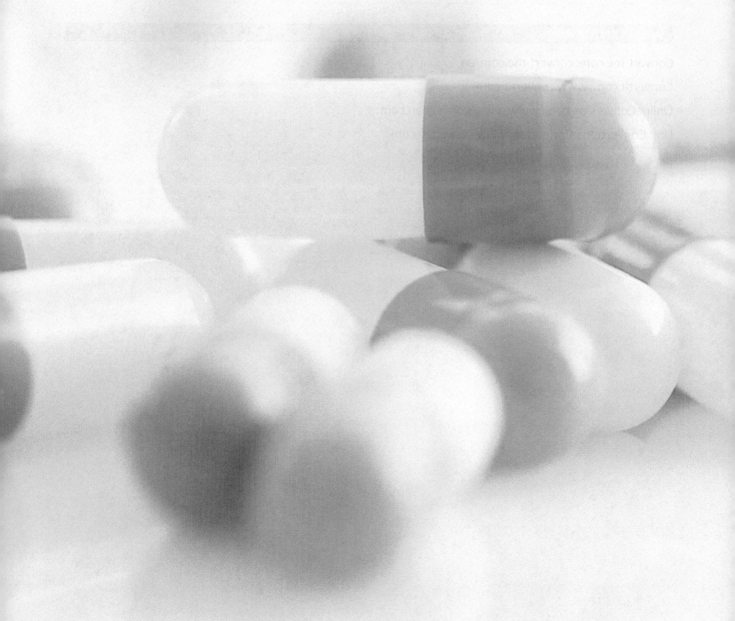

CHAPTER 9

Conversion and Calculations

Pediatric Dosage Calculations
  Clark's Rule
  Young's Rule
  Fried's Rule
  West's Nomogram

OBJECTIVES

Upon completion of this chapter, the reader should be able to:

1. Explain the difference between Arabic numbers and Roman numerals.
2. Change an improper fraction to a mixed fraction.
3. Define ratios, proportions, and percentages.
4. Describe the relationship between decimals and fractions.
5. Define "dimensional analysis."
6. Explain standardized units of drug dosages.
7. State the purpose of using West's nomogram.
8. List the formulas for Clark's Rule, Young's Rule, and Fried's Rule.
9. Explain the formula used to calculate liquid drugs.
10. List the most common types of intravenous solutions.

KEY TERMS

Arabic numbers	drop rate	means	proportion
common fraction	drug label factor	meniscus	ratio
conversion factor	drug order factor	mixed fraction	West's nomogram
decimal	drug order factor	numerator	
decimal fraction	extremes	percent	
denominator	fraction	proper fraction	
	improper fraction		

Overview

The first technical operation that pharmacy technicians must learn is the manipulation of measures of volume, balance, and weights. In this learning process, familiarity with the various systems of weights and measures and their relationships and a mastery of basic mathematics are necessary. The pharmacy technician must learn basic mathematics to be able to calculate the dosage of drugs by weight, measures of volume, and balances. He or she must also be able to convert from one system to another. The technician should also have a working knowledge of fractions, decimals, ratios, and percentages, as well as basic problem-solving skills.

One of the most important functions of pharmacy service is to ensure that patients get the intended drug in the correct amount. The correct dosage of a medication may depend on the patient's age, weight, state of health, or on other drugs the patient may be taking. Often, a pharmacist or technician receives an order for a medication in a dosage that differs from that of the medications in stock. The difference may be in the system of measurement, the strength, or the form of the drug. Formulas and mathematical tables of conversion can be used to calculate the correct dosage of medication to be administered. It is helpful to look at how the correct calculation is arrived at, one step at a time. Learning to correctly calculate drug dosages is an extremely important skill, because it is often the difference between life and death for a patient. Calculating incorrect dosages can lead to undertreatment, resulting in lack of improvement or worsening of the patient's condition. An overdose can cause the patient serious harm.

The ability to calculate drug dosages is a skill that should not be taken lightly. In fact, all health care professionals who deal with the preparation or administration of medications should aim for 100% success in performing this task. To prevent medication errors, the technician should remember the following:

- Right patient
- Right route
- Right drug
- Right technique
- Right dose
- Right documentation
- Right time

The use of calculators is recommended for complex calculations of dosages to ensure accuracy and save time. Basic math skills are needed to use the calculator properly.

Arabic Numbers and Roman Numerals

The system of Roman numerals uses letters to represent number values. Unlike the Arabic system that is commonly used for counting, the Roman system has no symbol for zero. Roman numerals are used less commonly than Arabic numbers in dosage calculation. Still, some physicians and practitioners use this system in prescriptions. The pharmacy technician needs to understand Roman numerals to interpret physicians' orders and drug dosages precisely. In pharmacy settings, the technician usually sees and uses only the Roman numerals that represent the values 1 through 30.

Roman numerals can be written as either uppercase or lowercase letters. In medical usage, "iv," which represents the number 4, is generally written in lowercase to differentiate it from "IV," which is the abbreviation for intravenous.

The building blocks of the Roman system include the letters I, V, X, L, C, D, and M. Only I, V, and X are required to show the values 1 through 30.

Most of the medications administered or ordered should be measured by amounts expressed in **Arabic numbers**. The familiar system of whole numbers (0 through 9), fractions (e.g., ⅕), and decimals (e.g., 0.7) is used widely in the United States and internationally. Table 9-1 shows some examples of Arabic numbers and Roman numerals.

Table 9-1 Examples of Arabic Numbers and Roman Numerals

Arabic Number	Roman Numeral	Arabic Number	Roman Numeral
½	$\overline{SS}$	40	XL
1	I	50	L
2	II	60	LX
3	III	70	LXX
4	IV	80	LXXX
5	V	90	XC
6	VI	100	C
7	VII	500	D
8	VIII	600	DC
9	IX	700	DCC
10	X	800	DCCC
20	XX	900	CM
30	XXX	1000	M

Basic Math Skills

The first technical operation that pharmacy technicians must learn is the manipulation of measures of volume, balance, and weights. In this learning process, familiarity with the various systems of weights and measures and their relationships and a mastery of basic mathematics are necessary. The pharmacy technician must learn basic mathematics to be able to calculate the dosage of drugs by weight, measures of volume, and balances. He or she must also be able to convert from one system to another. To become skilled in math, the pharmacy technician needs extensive practice in solving various types of mathematics problems such as adding, subtracting, multiplying, and dividing whole numbers. The technician should also have a working knowledge of fractions, decimals, ratios, and percentages and basic problem-solving skills. This chapter summarizes these important mathematical operations to support various dosage calculations in the pharmacy.

FRACTIONS

Pharmacy technicians need to understand fractions to be able to interpret and act on practitioners' orders, read prescriptions, and understand patient records and information in the pharmacy literature. Fractions are used in apothecary and household measures for dosage calculations. A **fraction** is an expression of division with a number that is the portion or part of a whole amount. A fraction has two parts (these fractions are known as common fractions). The bottom is referred to as the **denominator**, which represents the whole. It can never equal zero. The **numerator** is the top part of the fraction and represents parts of the whole. See Figure 9-1, which is a diagram representing fractions of a whole. Four parts shaded out of six parts represents:

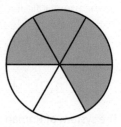

Figure 9-1 Fractions.

$$\frac{\text{Numerator (4 parts)}}{\text{Denominator (6 parts)}} = \frac{4}{6}$$

The fraction ⅔ is read as "two-thirds." It means two parts out of the three parts that make up the whole. The fraction bar also means, "divided by." Thus, ⅔ can be read as "two divided by three" or $2 \div 3$. This definition is important when one changes fractions to decimals.

Classification of Fractions

There are two types of fractions: common fractions and decimal fractions. A **common fraction** usually represents equal parts of a whole. It consists of two numbers and a fraction bar and is shown in the form:

$$\frac{\text{Numerator}}{\text{Denominator}}$$

For example, ¼, ⅖, and ⁹⁄₁₀ are all common fractions. A **decimal fraction** is commonly referred to simply as a decimal (e.g., 0.5). Decimal fractions will be discussed later in the chapter.

There are four types of common fractions: proper, improper, mixed, and complex.

Proper Fractions A **proper fraction** has a numerator that is smaller than the denominator and designates less than one whole unit. Whenever the numerator is less than the denominator, the value of the fraction must be less than 1 (see Figure 9-2).

Example

$$\frac{3}{5} = \frac{\text{Numerator}}{\text{Denominator}} = {} < 1$$

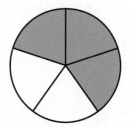

Figure 9-2 Proper fractions.

Other examples of proper fractions are ¾, ⅑, ³²⁄₄₅, and ⁹⁴⁄₁₀₀₀.

POINTS TO REMEMBER

A proper fraction has a numerator that is smaller than the denominator.

Improper Fractions   An **improper fraction** has a numerator that is greater than or equal to the denominator. The value of an improper fraction is greater than or equal to 1 (see Figure 9-3).

Example

$$\frac{6}{4} = > 1$$

More examples of improper fractions are ³⁵⁄₃₀, ²⁸⁄₂₃, and ¹⁵⁵⁄₁₀.

Whenever the numerator and denominator are equal, the value of the improper fraction is always equal to 1 (see Figure 9-4).

Example

$$\frac{6}{6} = 1$$

More examples of improper fractions that equal 1 are ³⁄₃, ¹⁶⁄₁₆, and ⁸⁄₈.

POINTS TO REMEMBER

An improper fraction has a numerator that is equal to or greater than the denominator.

Mixed Fractions   A **mixed fraction** has a whole number and a proper fraction that are combined. The value of the mixed fraction is always greater than 1 (see Figure 9-5).

Example

$$1\frac{3}{5} = 1 + \frac{3}{5} = > 1$$

To convert an improper fraction to a mixed fraction, follow the rule:

1.   Divide the numerator by the denominator. The result will be a whole number plus a remainder.

2.   The remainder is the numerator over the original denominator.

3.   Mix the whole number and the fractional remainder. This mixed fraction equals the original improper fraction.

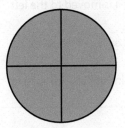 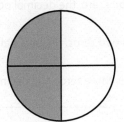

Figure 9-3 Improper fractions.

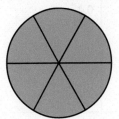

Figure 9-4 When the numerator and denominator are the same, the value of the fraction is equal to 1.

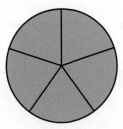 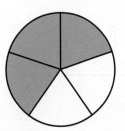

Figure 9-5 Mixed fractions.

Example

Find the mixed fraction for the fraction ¹⁶/₅.

Divide the numerator by the denominator: 16 divided by 5.

The result is 3 ⅕.

To check, convert 3 into ¹⁵/₅. Then add it to ⅕, which leaves the original fraction of ¹⁶/₅.

DECIMALS

Decimal fractions or **decimals** are used with the metric system, which is the system most often used in the calculation of drug dosages. It is very important for the pharmacy technician to be able to manipulate decimals easily and accurately. Each decimal fraction consists of a numerator that is expressed in numerals, a decimal point placed so that it designates the value of the denominator, and the denominator, which is understood to be 10 or some power of 10. In writing a decimal fraction, always place a zero to the left of the decimal point, so that the decimal point can readily be seen. Table 9-2 shows some examples.

For reading and writing decimals, observe Figure 9-6, which shows that all whole numbers are to the left of the decimal point and all fractions are to the right.

Table 9-2 Fractions and Their Related Decimal Fractions

Fraction	Decimal Fraction	Description
⁴/₁₀	0.4	Because 10 has *one* zero, the decimal point of 4 is moved to the left *once*.
¹⁷/₁₀₀	0.17	Because 100 has two zeros, the decimal point of 17 is moved to the left *twice*.
³³⁴/₁₀₀₀	0.334	Because 1000 has three zeros, the decimal point of 334 is moved to the left *three* places.

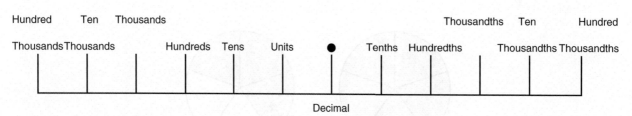

Figure 9-6 Decimal values.

The technician should remember when dealing with decimal fractions (such as 1/10) to always place a zero in front of the decimal, for example, 0.1. This prevents the technician (or anyone else) from mistaking the decimal 1/10 for the whole number 1. It is of vital importance that decimal calculations be double-checked before using them for drug dosages.

MEDICATION ERROR ALERT

The dangers of not carefully checking the existence of a decimal point for an unfamiliar drug are shown in the following example. A dose of 0.30 mg of morphine may be administered for pain. However, if a doctor wrote the order for .30 mg without placing a zero before the decimal point, and the health care worker did not see the decimal point in the .30 mg order or know about the lethal levels of morphine, 30 mg could be administered by error, and the patient would probably die. This situation is potentially disastrous because a 30-mg dose of morphine can kill a healthy person within 5 minutes by slowing breathing to the point that the brain would not receive enough oxygen to live.

POINTS TO REMEMBER

Always write a zero to the left of the decimal point when a decimal has no whole number "part." Using the zero makes the decimal point more noticeable and helps to prevent errors caused by illegible handwriting.

CHANGING COMMON FRACTIONS TO DECIMALS

To obtain a decimal from a common fraction, divide the numerator by the denominator, and place a decimal point in the proper position on the answer line.

Example

$$\frac{3}{5} = 5\overline{)3.0}^{\,0.6}$$

$$\frac{1}{4} = 4\overline{)1.00}^{\,0.25}$$

RATIOS

A **ratio** is a mathematical expression that compares two numbers by division. It is used to indicate the relationship of one part of a quantity to the whole. When written, the two quantities are separated by a colon (:). The use of the colon is a traditional way to write the division sign within a ratio, which is expressed as "3 is to 7."

Example

3/7 may be expressed as a ratio: 3 : 7

Example

1 : 150 may be expressed as a fraction: $\frac{1}{150}$

PROPORTIONS

A **proportion** shows the relationship between two equal ratios. A proportion may be expressed as:

$$4 : 8 :: 1 : 2$$

or

$$4 : 8 = 1 : 2$$

where in the first case (::) is read as "so as." Thus, 4 is to 8 so as 1 is to 2. These ratios are equal because multiplying 1 and 2 by 4 will result in 4 and 8, respectively. In a proportion, the terms have names. The **extremes** are the two outside terms and the **means** are the two inside terms. This relationship is shown in Figure 9-7. In a proportion, the product of the means is equal to the product of the extremes.

To convert a proportion into fractions, use the techniques of cross-multiplying or dividing.

Example

$$1 : 4 :: 3 : 12$$

Convert to fractions: ¼ and ³⁄₁₂.

Cross-multiply first the numerator of the fraction on the left by the denominator of the fraction on the right:

$$1 \times 12$$

and then the denominator of the fraction on the left by the numerator of the fraction on the right:

$$4 \times 3$$

In this formula, the answer is

$$\frac{12}{12}, \text{ which reduces to 1.}$$

It is evident that the term ⁴⁄₂ :: ¹⁶⁄₈ is a proportion because 4 multiplied by 8 is 32 and 2 multiplied by 16 is also 32. Most of the time we know only three terms of a proportion. The term we do not know is the *unknown*, and in this

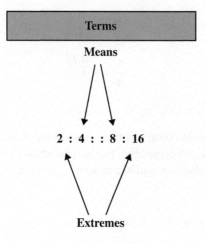

(The *means* are 4 and 8,

while the *extremes* are 2 and 16)

Figure 9-7 Means and extremes.

book, it is labeled *X*. To solve for unknown proportion terms, first multiply the extremes and then multiply the means. Set their products equal. Then, divide both sides of the equation by the number to the left of *X*.

Example

$$2:4 = X:10$$
$$4X = 2 \times 10$$
$$4X = 20$$
$$X = \frac{20}{4} = 5$$

Example

$$\frac{1}{2}:X = 1:8$$
$$1X = \left(8 \times \frac{1}{2} \right)$$
$$1X = 4$$
$$X = \frac{4}{1} = 4$$

PERCENTAGES

The term **percent** and its symbol, %, mean hundredths. A percentage is a fraction whose numerator is expressed and whose denominator is understood to be 100. It may be written in the form of "*x*" with the symbol %, or "*x*%." It can be changed to a decimal by moving the decimal point two places to the left to signify hundredths or to a fraction by expressing the denominator as 100. For example, the ratio of 30 to 100 is 30 percent (30%). This means the same thing as "30 hundredths," or 0.30. Percentages may be expressed as fractions, decimals, or ratios. All of these allow percentages to be expressed as "parts of a whole."

Example

$$7\% \text{ means } \frac{7}{100} \text{ or } 0.07$$

Example

$$\frac{1}{5}\% \text{ means } \frac{1/5}{100} \text{ or } 0.002$$
$$\frac{1}{5} \times \frac{1}{100} = \frac{1}{500} = 0.002$$

When the percentage is unknown, you can use the formula of *X*.

Example

What percent of 10 ounces is 3 ounces? You are looking for a percentage in this case:

$$3 = X \times 10$$
$$3 = 10X \text{ or } 10X = 3$$
$$10X \text{ divided by } 10 = 3 \text{ divided by } 10$$
$$X = \frac{3}{10} \text{ or } X = 30\%$$

Percentages are often used to show strengths of IV solutions, or to indicate medication strengths, such as ointments. For example, a one percent (1%) ointment means one part of 100. A 0.9% solution means 0.9 part (less than one part) of 100.

CHANGING PERCENTAGES TO DECIMALS

To change a percentage to a decimal, move the decimal point two places to the left (to signify hundredths) and add zeros as needed. Another way to do this is to remove the percentage sign and divide by 100.

Example

Convert 35% to a decimal.

Percent   Decimal

$$35\% = 35.\% = .35 = 0.35$$

Example

Convert 115% to a decimal.

$$115\% = 115.\% = 1.15$$

Example

Convert 14 ½% to a decimal.

$$14 \ 1/2 = 14 \ 5/10\% = 14.5\% = 0.145\% = 0.145$$

CHANGING DECIMALS TO PERCENTAGES

To change a decimal to a percentage, move the decimal point two places to the right (to signify hundredths) and add zeros as need. This can also be done by multiplying by 100 and adding the percent sign.

Example

Convert 0.21 to a percentage.

$$0.21 \times 100 = 21\%$$

$$0.21 = 21. = 21\%$$

CHANGING PERCENTAGES TO FRACTIONS

To convert a percentage to a fraction, convert the percentage to a decimal first. Then, convert the decimal to a fraction. Another way to do this is to put the percentage above 100 and reduce.

Example

Change 23% to a fraction.

$$23 \div 100 = 0.23$$

$$\frac{23}{100}$$

Example

Change 0.3% to a fraction.

$$0.3 \div 100 = 0.003$$

$$\frac{3}{1000}$$

CHANGING FRACTIONS TO PERCENTAGES

To change a fraction to a percentage, first convert the fraction to a decimal. Then, convert the decimal to a percentage by multiplying by 100 and adding a percentage sign.

Example

Convert ⅘ to a percentage.

$$\frac{4}{5} = 0.8 = 80\%$$

Example

Convert ⅕ to a percentage.

$$\frac{1}{5} = 0.20 = 20\%$$

Example

Convert ⅗ to a percentage.

$$\frac{3}{5} = 0.60 = 60\%$$

Methods of Calculation

There are four methods for drug dosage calculations: basic formula, ratio and proportion, fractional equation, and dimensional analysis. The ratio and proportion and fractional equation methods are similar. When body weight and body surface area calculations are used, one of the first four methods for calculation is necessary to determine the amount of drug needed from the container. The pharmacist or technician commonly uses these methods when the calculation of drug doses is required.

BASIC FORMULA

The basic formula method is often used to calculate drug dosage. The basic formula that is most commonly used is:

$$\frac{D}{H} \times V = \text{Amount to give}$$

In this equation, *D* stands for desired dose: the drug dose ordered by the prescriber. *H* stands for on-hand dose: the drug dose on the label of the container (ampule, vial, or bottle). *V* stands for vehicle: the form and amount in which the drug is supplied (capsule, tablet, or liquid).

Example

The physician's order is for ampicillin 0.5 g PO tid. The drug available is ampicillin 250 mg capsules.

Both the dosage of the drug ordered and the dosage available are in the metric system; however, the units of measurement are different. They must be converted. To convert grams to milligrams, move the decimal point three spaces to the right (see Chapter 8):

$$0.5 \text{ g} = 0.500 \text{ mg} = 500 \text{ mg}$$

The basic formula is:

$$\frac{D}{H} \times V = \frac{500}{250} = \frac{2}{1} \times 1 \text{ capsule} = 2 \text{ capsules}$$

Example

The physician's order is for Lopressor® 100 mg PO bid. The drug available is Lopressor 50 mg/tablet. No conversion is necessary.

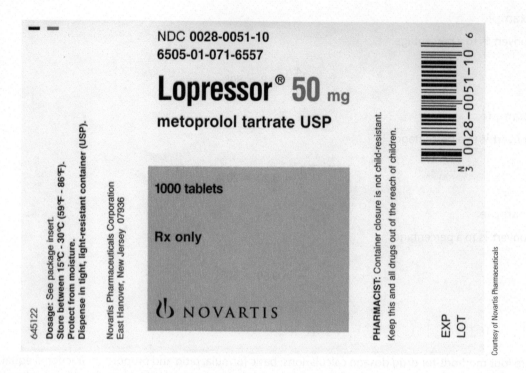

$$\frac{D}{H} \times V = \frac{100}{50} \times 1 \text{ tablet}$$

$$\frac{100}{50} = \frac{2}{1} \times 1 \text{ tablet}$$

$$= 2 \text{ tablets given orally twice daily}$$

Example

You have on hand a dosage strength of 40 mg in 1 mL. A dosage of 30 mg is ordered. How many milliliters are necessary to administer this dosage?

$$\text{Desired dosage } (D) = 30 \text{ mg}$$

$$\text{On hand } (H) = 40 \text{ mg in } (V) \text{ 1 mL}$$

Remember that X must be expressed in the same units of measure as V, which are in milliliters (mL) in this example. Always include the units of measure in the formula:

$$\frac{(D) \text{ 30 mg}}{(H) \text{ 40 mg}} \times (V) \text{ 1 mL} = X \text{ mL}$$

$$\frac{30}{40} \times 1 = X = 0.75 \text{ mL}$$

Therefore, to give a dosage of 30 mg, 0.75 mL must be administered.

Since 30 mg is required, which is a smaller dosage than the strength available of 40 mg in 1 mL, the answer, 0.75 mL, is smaller, and because of this, logical.

Example

A dosage of 0.4 mg is ordered. On hand is 0.35 mg in 1.5 mL. So,

$$D = 0.4 \text{ mg}$$

$$H = 0.35 \text{ mg in } (V) \text{ 1.5 mL}$$

Again, using the conversion formula:

$$\frac{0.4 \text{ mg}}{0.35 \text{ mg}} \times 1.5 \text{ mL} = X \text{ mL}$$

$$\frac{0.4}{0.35} \times 1.5 = X = 1.71 = 1.7 \text{ mL}$$

Therefore, to give 0.4 mg, you must administer 1.7 mL.

Because the dosage of 0.4 mg ordered is larger than the 0.35 mg strength available and the volume containing it must be larger, the answer, 1.7 mL, which is larger, is logical.

Example

The strength available is 1200 mcg per milliliter. A dosage of 800 mcg has been ordered.

$$\frac{800 \text{ mcg}}{1200 \text{ mcg}} \times 1 \text{ mL} = X \text{ mL}$$

$$\frac{800}{1200} \times 1 = X = 0.66 = 0.7 \text{ mL}$$

Therefore, to give a dosage of 800 mcg, you must administer 0.7 mL. The answer must be a smaller quantity than 1 mL, and it is.

RATIO AND PROPORTION

Ratio and proportion is the oldest method used for calculating dosage. It is often referred to as *means multiplied by extremes*. One formula uses ratios based on the dose on hand and the dose desired. The formula is as follows:

$$H : V :: D : X$$

In this formula, H stands for on-hand dose, V stands for vehicle, D stands for desired dose, and X stands for amount to give. H and V are the known quantities. D and X are the desired dose and the unknown amount to give.

V and D are called the means, and H and X are called the extremes. Multiply the means and then the extremes and cross-multiply to solve for X.

Example

Amoxicillin 500 mg PO qid (dose desired) is prescribed by the physician; the dose on hand is 250 mg/5 mL. The formula is as follows:

$$\frac{250 \text{ mg (dose on hand)}}{5 \text{ mL (dose on hand)}} = \frac{500 \text{ mg (dose desired)}}{X \text{ (dose desired)}}$$

Cross-multiply:

$$250X = 5 \times 500$$

$$X = 5 \times \frac{500}{250}$$

$$X = 10 \text{ mL}$$

Example

The ratio formula can be used in calculating dosages. For example, the prescriber orders heparin 10,000 units SC; the dose on hand is 40,000 units/mL.

$$\frac{40,000 \text{ units}}{1 \text{ mL}} = \frac{10,000 \text{ units}}{X}$$

To solve for X, cross-multiply:

$$40,000X = 10,000$$

$$X = \frac{10,000}{40,000}$$

$$X = \frac{1}{4}$$

$$X = 0.25 \text{ mL}$$

Example

A solution strength of 10 mg per milliliter is needed to prepare a dosage of 15 mg. The solution strength available (10 mg/mL) provides the known ratio. The dosage to be given is the incomplete ratio (15 mg). X represents the milliliters that will contain 15 mg. Notice that both numerators are expressed as milligrams while both denominators are expressed as milliliters. The ratios in a proportion must be written using the same sequence of measurement units.

$$\frac{10 \text{ mg}}{1 \text{ mL}} = \frac{15 \text{ mg}}{X \text{ mL}}$$

The first fraction is a complete ratio that expresses the drug strength. The second fraction is an incomplete ratio that expresses the dosage to give. By cross-multiplying, it is easy to see that:

$$10X = 15$$

Therefore, the answer is 1.5 mL. The ordered dosage of 15 mg is contained in 1.5 mL.

It is important to double-check your calculations and to assess whether each answer is logical. In this example, since 1 mL contains 10 mg, you will need a larger volume than 1 mL to obtain 15 mg. The answer, 1.5 mL, is larger, so it is logical. Although this does not verify that the calculation is correct, it indicates that you set up the proportion correctly and cross-multiplied sufficiently.

Example

A dosage of 30 mg has been ordered. The strength available is 35 mg in 2.5 mL.

$$\frac{35 \text{ mg}}{2.5 \text{ mL}} = \frac{30 \text{ mg}}{X \text{ mL}}$$

When you cross-multiply, you find that:

$$35X = 2.5 \times 30$$
$$35X = 75$$

Therefore, $X = 2.14$ mL, which rounds to 2.1 mL.

Because the dosage ordered (30 mg) is smaller than the strength available (35 mg in 2.5 mL), the answer should be smaller than 2.5 mL, and it is. Therefore, it is logical.

Example

The solution strength on hand is 50 mg per milliliter. A dosage of 180 mg is ordered.

$$\frac{50 \text{ mg}}{1 \text{ mL}} = \frac{180 \text{ mg}}{X \text{ mL}}$$

Therefore, $50X = 180$. So, $X = 3.6$ mL.

This answer is logical because 3.6 mL is larger, and the dosage ordered (180 mg) is larger than the solution on hand (50 mg/mL), and must be contained in more than 1 mL.

Example

Shortcuts may be used to simplify the math in these problems. To do this, after cross-multiplying, immediately divide the number in front of X. You can also reduce numbers to their lowest common terms whenever possible. For example, if you have a 200 mg per 1.5 mL solution and need to prepare a dosage of 100 mg:

$$\frac{200 \text{ mg}}{1.5 \text{ mL}} = \frac{100 \text{ mg}}{X \text{ mL}}$$

Cross-multiply and immediately divide by the number in front of X:

$$X = \frac{1.5 \times 100}{200}$$

Reduce the 100 and 200 numbers by 100. Do the final division, and depending on the medication you are using, round to the nearest tenth:

$$X = \frac{1.5 \times 1}{2} = \frac{1.5}{2} = 0.75 \text{ mL}$$

A dosage of 100 mg requires fewer milliliters than the 200 mg per 1.5 mL strength available. Therefore, the smaller answer, 0.75 mL, is logical.

FRACTIONAL EQUATION

The fractional equation method is similar to the ratio and proportion method, except that the calculation is written as a fraction.

$$\frac{H}{V} = \frac{D}{X}$$

H stands for the dosage on hand, V stands for vehicle, D stands for desired dosage, and X stands for the unknown amount to give. Cross-multiply and then solve for X.

Example

The physician's order is for metronidazole (Flagyl®) 1.5 g PO tid × 7 days. The drug available is Flagyl 250 mg per tablet.

Step 1: Convert grams to milligrams:

$$1.5 \text{ g} = 1500 \text{ mg}$$

Step 2:

$$\frac{H}{V} = \frac{D}{X} = \frac{250 \text{ mg}}{1 \text{ tablet}} = \frac{1500}{X}$$

1.5 g of metronidazole = 6 tablets.

Therefore, 6 tablets should be given.

Example

The physician's order is for Motrin® 600 mg PO bid. The drug available is Motrin 300 mg tablets.

Step 1: There is no need to convert.

Step 2:

$$\frac{H}{V} = \frac{D}{X} = \frac{300 \text{ mg}}{1 \text{ tablet}} = \frac{600 \text{ mg}}{X}$$

$$300X = 600$$

$$X = \frac{600}{300} = 2$$

Therefore, 2 tablets should be given.

DIMENSIONAL ANALYSIS

Dimensional analysis is a method that is used for solving complicated pharmaceutical calculations. The dimensional analysis method (the label factor method) is used for calculating dosages with three factors, which include the following:

1. **Drug label factor.** The form of the drug dose (V) with its equivalence in unit (H).

$$\text{Example: 1 tablet} = 250 \text{ mg}$$

2. **Conversion factor.** This can help if the following factor conversions are memorized:

Metric Equivalents	Metric Apothecary Equivalents
1 kg = 1000 g	1 g = 15 gr
1 g = 1000 mg	1000 mg = 15 gr
1 mg = 1000 mcg	1 gr = 60 mg

3. **Drug order factor.** The three factors D, H, and V are set up in an equation that helps to cancel the units, giving the right answer in the right units for delivery.

$$V = V(\text{vehicle}) \times C(H) \times \frac{D \text{ (desired)}}{H \text{ (on hand)}} \times C(D) \times 1$$

(drug label)   (conversion factor)   (drug order)

To set up an equation for dimensional analysis, you must follow these steps:

1. Write the unit of measure being calculated, such as milliliters (mL). This eliminates confusion over which measure is being calculated and determines how the first clinical ratio is entered into the equation.
2. Identify the complete clinical ratio that contains the milliliters, as provided by the dosage strength available. This should be entered as a common fraction.
3. All additional ratios are entered so that each denominator matches with its successive numerator. If the first ratio denominator is milligrams, then the next numerator also must be in milligrams.
4. Cancel the alternate denominator/numerator measurement units (but not their quantities). They must match. If so, all clinical ratios were entered correctly. After cancellation, only the unit of measure being calculated may remain in the equation.
5. Calculate the equation now that all components are in place.

Example

The available drug strength is 500 mg in 2 mL. How many mL are needed to prepare a 300 mg dosage?

$$\text{mL} = \frac{2 \text{ mL}}{500 \text{ mg}}$$

Therefore, based on the desired 300 mg dosage,

$$\text{mL} = \frac{2 \text{ mL}}{500 \text{ mg}} \times \frac{300 \text{ mg}}{1}$$

Therefore, multiplying, 2 mL × 300 mg = 600 mg. This amount, when divided by 500 mg, gives an answer of 1.2 mL, which contains the desired 300 mg of medication. This type of equation works the same way for every calculation, no matter how many ratios are entered. There are no complicated rules to remember.

Example

Because 1 L is equal to 1000 mL, how many fluidounces (fl oz) are in 2.5 L? Approximately 30 mL are in 1 fl oz. Use ratio and proportion as follows:

$$\frac{2.5\ L}{1\ L} = \frac{X\ mL}{1000\ mL}$$

Therefore, X = 2500 mL. So,

$$\frac{1\ fl\ oz}{X\ fl\ oz} = \frac{30\ mL}{2500\ mL}$$

Therefore, X = 83.3 fl oz, which may be rounded to 83 fl oz.

Example

To solve the same equation by dimensional analysis, you would do the following:

$$fl\ oz = \frac{1\ fl\ oz}{30\ mL} \times \frac{1000\ mL}{1\ L} \times 2.5\ L$$

Therefore, the same answer, 83.3 fl oz, can be easily found.

Dimensional analysis allows multiple ratios to be entered into a single equation. It is sometimes easier to do the conversion before the equation is set up. For instance, if a medication is available in milligrams (mg) but is labeled in another unit, such as grams or micrograms, metric conversion must be done.

Example

The IM dosage ordered is 250 mg. The drug available is labeled 1 g per 2 mL. How many mL must you give?

$$mL = \frac{2\ mL}{1\ g}$$

Because the dosage ordered is in milligrams and the drug available is in grams, a conversion ratio is needed: 1 g equals 1000 mg. Therefore, you can change "1 g" to "1000 mg":

$$mL = \frac{2\ mL}{1000\ mg}$$

Next, you must add the dosage ordered into the equation:

$$mL = \frac{2\ mL}{1000\ mg} \times \frac{250\ mg}{1}$$

Then, remove the "milligrams" and carry out the multiplication:

$$mL = \frac{2 \times 250}{1000}$$

This leaves:

$$mL = \frac{500}{1000}$$

The result is ½ mL. Therefore, ½ mL contains the desired dosage of 250 mg.

Example

An intramuscular medication order is for 0.5 mg of medication in solution. The drug label reads "750 mcg in 2 mL." Enter the mL to be calculated followed by an equal sign to the left of the equation. Locate the ratio containing mL, 750 mcg in 2 mL. Enter 2 mL as the numerator to match the mL being calculated. The denominator becomes 750 mcg.

$$mL = \frac{2\ mL}{750\ mcg}$$

Because the medication order was for milligrams, a conversion ratio is needed. Enter the 1000 mcg = 1 mg conversion ratio. The numerator is 1000 mcg, matching the mcg of the previous denominator. The denominator becomes 1 mg.

$$mL = \frac{2\ mL}{750\ mcg} \times \frac{1000\ mcg}{1\ mg}$$

The mg denominator is now matched by the 0.5 mg dosage to be administered, completing the equation.

$$mL = \frac{2\ mL}{750\ mcg} \times \frac{1000\ mcg}{1\ mg} \times \frac{0.5\ mg}{}$$

Cancel the alternate denominator-numerator mcg/mcg and mg/mg units of measure, which checks for the correct ratio entry. Only the mL being calculated should remain. Do the math as follows:

$$mL = \frac{2\ mL}{750} \times \frac{1000}{1} \times \frac{0.5}{} = 1.33$$

To give a dosage of 0.5 mg from the available 2 mL per 750 mcg strength, you must prepare 1.33 mL.

Example

Prepare a 0.5 mg dosage from an available strength of 200 mcg per mL. Enter the mL being calculated to the left of the equation followed by an equal sign. Enter the 1 mL in 200 mcg dosage as the starting ratio, with 1 mL as the numerator to match the mL being calculated; 200 mcg becomes the denominator:

$$mL = \frac{1\ mL}{200\ mcg}$$

An mcg to mcg conversion ratio is needed. Enter 1000 mcg as the numerator to match the mcg in the previous denominator; 1 mg becomes the new denominator.

$$mL = \frac{1\ mL}{200\ mcg} \times \frac{1000\ mcg}{1\ mg}$$

The mg denominator is now matched by the 0.5 mg dosage ordered to complete the equation.

$$mL = \frac{1\ mL}{200\ mcg} \times \frac{1000\ mcg}{1\ mg} \times \frac{0.5\ mg}{}$$

Cancel the alternate mcg/mcg and mg/mg units of measure to double-check for correct ratio entry. Only the milliliter unit being calculated remains in the equation. Do the math.

$$mL = \frac{1\ mL}{200\ mcg} \times \frac{1000\ mcg}{1\ mg} \times \frac{0.5\ mg}{} = 2.5\ mL$$

A 0.5 mg dosage requires a 2.5 mL volume of the 200 mcg per mL strength solution available.

For calculations using dimensional analysis:

- The unit of measure being calculated is written first to the left of the equation.
- The unit of measure is followed by an equal sign.
- All ratios entered must include the quantity and the unit of measure.
- The numerator in the starting ratio must be in the same measurement unit as the unit of measure being calculated.
- The unit of measure in each denominator must be matched in the numerator of each successive ratio entered.
- Incorporating a conversion ratio directly into the dimensional analysis equation can make metric system conversions.
- The unit of measure in each alternate denominator and numerator must cancel. This leaves only the unit of measure being calculated remaining in the equation.
- The numerator of the starting ratio is never cancelled.

Calculation of Oral Medications

Various forms of drugs are commonly administered orally. These include tablets, capsules, powders, and liquids. Oral medications are referred to as "PO" (per os [by mouth]) drugs. They are absorbed by the gastrointestinal tract, mainly from the small intestine.

The advantages of oral drug administration include the facts that the drugs are more convenient to use and cheaper. Disadvantages of oral drug administration are as follows:

- Varied absorption rate
- Irritation of the gastric mucosa
- Retention or inactivation of the drugs in the body (in patients with liver diseases)
- Destruction of drugs by digestive enzymes
- Aspiration of drugs into the lungs
- Discoloration of tooth enamel

MEASURING TABLETS OR CAPSULES

Tablets and capsules are solid medications that are supplied in different strengths or dosages. Their dosages can be expressed in apothecary or metric measures, for example, grains or milligrams.

Conversion Factors

Converting drug measures from one system to another and from one unit to another to determine the dosage to be administered can result in discrepancies, depending on the conversion factor used.

Example

The label for Tylenol® may indicate 325 mg (5 gr). This is based on the equivalent 65 mg = 1 gr. On the other hand, the label for aspirin may indicate 300 mg (5 gr). Here the equivalent 60 mg = 1 gr was used. Both of the equivalents are correct. *Remember that equivalents are not exact.* Use the common equivalents when making conversions, for example, 60 mg = 1 gr.

Rule of 10% Variation

If the precise number of tablets or capsules is determined and administering the amount calculated is unrealistic or impossible, always use the following rule to avoid an error in administration: *No more than 10% variation should exist between the dose ordered and the dose administered.*

Example

One may determine that a patient should receive 0.9 tablet or 0.9 capsule. Administration of such an amount accurately would be impossible. In this case, 1 tablet or 1 capsule could be safely administered.

Administration of Capsules

Capsules are not scored and cannot be divided. They are administered in whole amounts only. Never crush or open a time-released capsule or empty its contents into a liquid or food.

Other Units of Measure

In the calculation of oral doses, measures other than apothecary or metric may be encountered. For example, with electrolytes such as potassium, the number of milliequivalents (mEq) per tablet will be indicated. Another measure that may be seen for oral antibiotics or vitamins is units. For example, the label for vitamin E capsules may indicate 400 units per capsule. Unit and milliequivalent measurements are specific to the drugs for which they are being used. There is no conversion between these and apothecary or metric measures.

MEASURING ORAL LIQUIDS

Liquid medications include elixirs, syrups, tinctures, and suspensions. Certain liquid drugs are irritating to the stomach mucosa and so must be well diluted before administration. An example is potassium chloride (KCl). Tincture medications are always diluted. Any liquid medication that may cause discoloration of the teeth should be diluted and taken through a drinking straw. In general, liquid cough medicines are not diluted. Liquid medications contain a specific amount of drug in a given amount of solution.

When a liquid medication is measured, hold the transparent measuring device at eye level. The liquid curve in the center is called the **meniscus**. All liquid medication is measured at the meniscus level (see Figure 9-8).

For medications in liquid form, calculate the volume of the liquid that contains the ordered dosage of the medication. The label of bottled drugs may indicate the amount of drug per 1 mL or per multiple milliliters of the solution, for example, 20 mg/5 mL, 250 mg/5 mL, or 1.4 g/30 mL. Liquid drugs must be calculated with the formula:

$$\frac{D}{H} \times V = X$$

In this formula, *D* represents the desired dosage or the dosage ordered. *H* represents the dosage you have on hand per a quantity. *V* represents the volume of the drug.

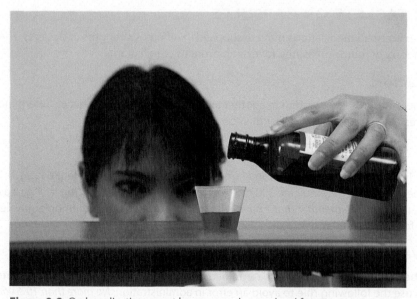

Figure 9-8 Oral medications must be measured at eye level for accuracy.

Example

A prescription is written to give 100 mg of ampicillin with a dosage strength of 125 mg/5 mL. The following formula is used:

$$\frac{D}{H} \times V = \frac{100 \text{ mg}}{125 \text{ mg}} \times 5 \text{ mL} = X$$

$$\frac{4}{5} \times 5 \text{ mL} = \frac{20}{5 \text{ mL}} = 4 \text{ mL}$$

Example

A prescription is written to give 100 mg of ampicillin. The medication is available with a dosage strength of 250 mg/5 mL. The following formula is used:

$$\frac{D}{H} \times V = \frac{100 \text{ mg}}{250 \text{ mg}} \times 5 \text{ mL} = X$$

$$\frac{2}{5} \times 5 \text{ mL} = \frac{10}{5} = 2 \text{ mL}$$

Calculation of Parenteral Medications

Medications administered by injection can be given intradermally (ID, within the skin), subcutaneously (SC, into fatty tissue or under the skin), intramuscularly (IM, into the muscle), and intravenously (IV, into the vein). Injectable drugs are ordered in grams, milligrams, micrograms, grains, or units. The preparations of injectable drugs may be packaged in a solvent (diluent or solution) or in a powdered form. Intramuscular injection is a common method of administering injectable drugs. The volume of solution for an intramuscular injection is 0.5 to 3.0 mL, with the average being 1 to 2 mL. A volume of drug solution greater than 3 mL causes increased muscle tissue displacement and possible tissue damage. Occasionally, 5 mL of certain drugs, such as magnesium sulfate or immunoglobulin (given after exposure to rabies), may be injected in a large muscle, such as the dorsogluteal. Dosages greater than 3 mL are usually divided and given at two different sites. Drug solutions for injection are commercially premixed and stored in vials and ampules for immediate use. At times there may be enough drug solution left in a vial for another dose, and the vial may be saved. The balance of a drug solution in an ampule is always discarded after the ampule has been opened and used. For calculating intramuscular dosage, the following example can be used:

Example

An order is given for gentamicin 60 mg IM. The available dosage strength of gentamicin is 80 mg/2 mL in a vial. The following formula is used:

$$\frac{D}{H} \times V = \frac{60}{80} \times 2 = \frac{120}{80} = 1.5 \text{ mL}$$

or

$$H : V :: D : X$$

$$80 \text{ mg} : 2 :: 60 \text{ mg} : X \text{ mL}$$

$$80X = 120$$

$$X = \frac{120}{80} = 1.5 \text{ mL}$$

Example

The physician's order is for atropine 0.2 mg SC stat. The drug is available at a dosage of 400 mcg/mL (0.4 mg/mL). The following formula is used:

$$\frac{D}{H} \times V = \frac{0.2 \text{ mg}}{0.4 \text{ mg}} \times 1 \text{ mL} = \frac{0.2}{0.4} \times 1 = 0.5 \text{ mL}$$

INJECTABLE MEDICATIONS

Injectable drugs are packaged in ampules or vials (discussed in Chapter 7). The medication is in either liquid or powder form in ampules or vials. Because drugs in solution deteriorate rapidly, they are packaged in dry form and diluent is added before administration. If the medication is in powdered form, mixing directions and dose equivalents such as milligrams per milliliter are usually given; if not, check the drug information insert. After the dry form of the drug is reconstituted with sterile water, bacteriostatic water, or saline, the medication is used immediately or must be refrigerated. Usually, the reconstituted drug in the vial is used within 48 hours to 1 week.

Standardized Units of Drug Dosages

Several drugs that are obtained from animal sources can be standardized in units according to their strengths rather than on weight measures such as milligrams and grams. Some hormones such as insulin are too complex to be completely purified to obtain the exact weight of the drug per unit of volume. Therefore, insulin and many other drugs are measured in units for parenteral administration. The labels of such medications indicate how many units are needed per milliliter.

INSULIN CALCULATIONS

Insulin is ordered and measured in USP units. Most types of insulin are manufactured in concentrations of 100 units/mL. Insulin should be administered with an insulin syringe, which is calibrated to correspond with the U-100 insulin. Insulin bottles and syringes are color-coded. The U-100 insulin bottle and the U-100 syringe are color-coded orange.

Insulin called 70/30 insulin is available for use with U-100 syringes (Figure 9-9). The 70/30 insulin concentration means there is 70% NPH insulin and 30% regular insulin in each unit. Therefore, if the physician orders 10 units of 70/30 insulin, the patient would receive 7 units of NPH insulin (70% or 0.7 × 10 units = 7 units) and 3 units of regular insulin (30% or 0.3 × 10 units = 3 units).

Insulin orders must be written clearly and contain specific information to prevent errors. The order for insulin should include the brand name, supply dosage, number of units to be given, and the route and time or frequency of administration. The two types of insulin used most often are the rapid-acting regular insulin and the intermediate-acting NPH insulin.

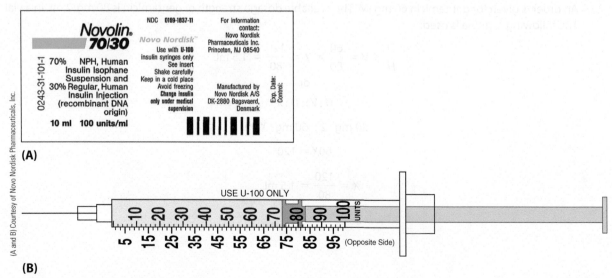

Figure 9-9 Standard dosing of insulin.

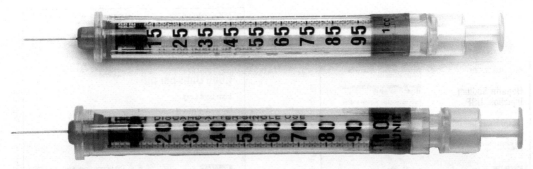

Figure 9-10 Insulin syringe.

Example

An order is given for Humulin R Regular U-100® 14 units SC stat or for Iletin II NPH U-100 24 units SC ½ hour after breakfast.

Insulin is supplied in 10 mL vials labeled with the number of units per milliliter; thus, U-100 insulin means there are 100 units/mL. In the past, insulin was administered in U-40 and U-80 dosage forms. Today, however, the U-100 form has almost totally replaced the weaker strength forms. The smaller volume required per dose decreases local reactions at the injection site, as well as simplifying mathematical calculations. The simplest and most accurate method to measure insulin is within an insulin syringe. The insulin syringe is calibrated in units, and the desired dose may be read directly on the syringe. U-100 insulin should be measured only in a U-100 insulin syringe. It is important to note that for U-100 insulin, 100 units = 1 mL. Two types of insulin syringes are available: Lo-Dose and 1 mL size. Figure 9-10 shows both sides of a standard U-100 syringe. The standard U-100 syringe has a dual scale with even numbers on one side and odd numbers on the other side. Additional types of syringes are discussed in detail in Chapter 7.

If an insulin syringe is not available, a tuberculin syringe may be used, and the unit dosage may be converted to the equivalent number of cubic centimeters, using the proportion method.

Example

Give 40 units of insulin, using U-100 insulin and a tuberculin syringe. The amount administered is calculated as follows:

POINTS TO REMEMBER

The concentration of "U-100" means that 100 units are contained in 1 mL of solution. Likewise, the concentration of "U-500" means that 500 units are contained in 1 mL of solution.

$$\frac{40}{100} \times mL = 0.4\ mL$$

HEPARIN CALCULATIONS

Heparin is a potent anticoagulant derived from animal sources that prevents clot formation and blood coagulation. Heparin dosages are expressed in USP units. The therapeutic range for heparin is determined individually by monitoring the patient's partial thromboplastin time. However, the normal adult heparin dosage is 20,000 to 40,000 units every 24 hours. Heparin can be administered intravenously (IV) or subcutaneously (SC).

When administered intravenously, heparin is ordered in units per hour (units/hr) or milliliters per hour (mL/hr). Usually, heparin is ordered on the basis of units per hour or per day for intravenous administration. Heparin is available in single-dose and multidose vials, as well as in commercially prepared intravenous solutions. Because heparin is available in different strengths, it is important to read labels carefully when it must be administered. Heparin sodium

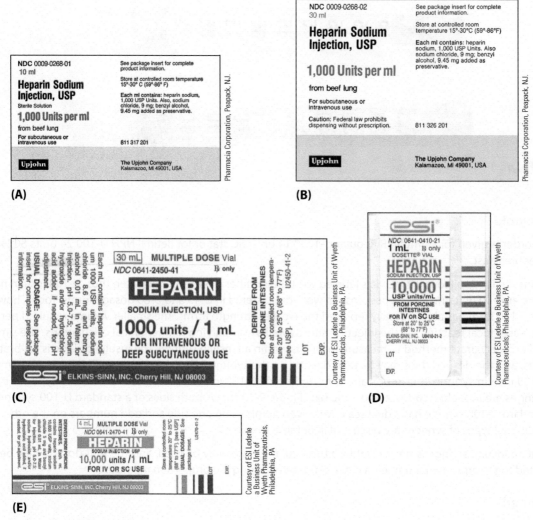

Figure 9-11 Dosage strengths of heparin: (A–C) 1000 units/mL; (D, E) 10,000 units/mL.

for injection is available in several strengths (e.g., 1000, 5000, and 10,000 units/mL). Heparin lock fluid solution (which is used for flushing) is available in 10 units/mL and 100 units/mL. The pharmacy technician must remember that heparin sodium for injection and heparin lock solution are different drugs and can never be used interchangeably. Figure 9-11 shows the various heparin dosage strengths.

Heparin is frequently administered using an electronic infusion device. Patients receiving heparin infusions require continuous monitoring. It may be given intravenously to produce a rapid effect and then given in deep subcutaneous injections in larger and more infrequent doses.

Example

A physician's order is for heparin 7500 units SC. Heparin are available in a dosage of 10,000 units/mL (see Figure 9-11E). The amount administered is calculated as follows:

$$10,000 \text{ units} : 1 \text{ mL} = 7500 \text{ units} : X \text{ mL}$$

$$10,000\, X = 7500$$

$$X = \frac{7500}{10,000}$$

$$X = 0.75 \text{ mL}$$

Example

A physician's order is for D_5W (5% dextrose in water) 1000 mL containing 20,000 units of heparin, which is to be infused at 30 mL/hr. The dose of heparin the patient is to receive per hour is:

$$20,000 \text{ units} : 1000 \text{ mL} = X \text{ unit} : 30 \text{ mL}$$

$$1000\,X = 20,000 \times 30$$

$$\frac{1000\,X}{1000} = \frac{600,000}{1000} = 600 \text{ units/hr}$$

ANTIBIOTIC CALCULATIONS

The dosages of many antibiotics are still standardized in units. These may be prepared for injection in the form of a liquid containing a specified number of units per cubic centimeter (units/cc). Antibiotics are also available in the form of a dry powder in a vial that must first be diluted with water or another diluent. The powder should be diluted so that the desired dose is in 1 or 2 cc (mL) amounts if the dose is to be given intramuscularly. If it is to be given intravenously, a larger amount of diluent may be used.

Example

A vial of powdered penicillin G contains 1,000,000 units. The amount of diluent to be added to obtain a solution containing 100,000 units/mL is:

$$100,000 : 1 \text{ mL} = 1,000,000 : X \text{ mL}$$

$$100,000\,X = 1,000,000 \times 1$$

$$X = \frac{1,000,000}{100,000}$$

$$X = 10 \text{ mL}$$

Example

A physician ordered gentamicin 60 mg IV q8h. In the pharmacy, gentamicin is available 80 mg per 2 mL. The calculation of the amount that should be given intravenously every 8 hours is as follows:

$$\frac{\text{Dosage on hand (80 mg)}}{\text{Amount on hand (2 mL)}} = \frac{\text{Dosage desired (60 mg)}}{\text{Amount desired (}X \text{ mL)}}$$

Cross-multiply to find $80X = 120$:

$$\frac{80X}{80} = \frac{120}{80}$$

$X = 1.5$ mL given intravenously every 8 hours.

Example

A hospital physician ordered clindamycin 0.6 g IV q12h. The hospital pharmacy had clindamycin 300 mg/2 mL on hand. The calculation of the amount that should be given intravenously every 12 hours is as follows:

$$\frac{\text{Dosage on hand (300 mg)}}{\text{Amount on hand (2 mL)}} = \frac{\text{Dosage desired (600 mg)}}{\text{Amount desired (}X \text{ mL)}}$$

Cross-multiply to find $300X = 1200$:

$$\frac{300X}{300} = \frac{1200}{300}$$

$X = 4$ mL given intravenously every 12 hours.

Intravenous Solutions and Calculations

The term *intravenous* literally means "within a vein." Intravenous infusion is the slow introduction of a substance such as a solution, whole blood, plasma, or antibiotics into a vein. Intravenous solutions fall into four functional categories: replacement fluids, maintenance fluids, therapeutic fluids, and agents to keep the vein open. If the patient is dehydrated and unable to eat or drink or if he or she has lost blood, replacement fluids are ordered. Maintenance fluids help patients maintain normal electrolyte and fluid balances. Therapeutic fluids deliver medication to the patient. Some intravenous lines provide access to the vein for emergency situations. Fluids prescribed to keep the vein open include 5% dextrose in water (D_5W). Intravenous fluids and drugs may be administered by two methods: intermittent and continuous infusion. Intermittent infusion, such as intravenous piggyback and intravenous push infusions are used for intravenous administration of drugs and supplemental fluids. Continuous intravenous infusions are used to replace fluid or to help in maintaining fluid levels and electrolyte balance and serve as vehicles for drug administration. Saline or heparin locks are used to maintain venous access without continuous fluid infusion. Thus, the pharmacy technician must learn how to effectively calculate infusion rates and monitor the administration of these agents. Table 9-3 shows common abbreviations for components of intravenous infusions.

Table 9-3 Common Intravenous Component Abbreviations			
Solution Component	**Abbreviation**	**Solution Component**	**Abbreviation**
Dextrose	D	Saline	S
Lactated Ringer's	LR	Ringer's lactate	RL
Normal saline	NS	Water	W

CALCULATION OF INTRAVENOUS HEPARIN FLOW RATE

Units per hour of heparin can be calculated by using the ratio and proportion method. Use the following formula to calculate intravenous heparin flow in milliliters per hour (mL/hr):

$$\frac{D}{H} \times Q = R$$

$$\frac{D \text{ (unit/hr desired)}}{H \text{ (unit available)}} \times Q \text{ (mL available)} = R \text{ (mL/hr)}$$

The ratio of supply dosage is equivalent to ratio of desired dosage rate:

$$\text{unit/mL (supply)} = \frac{\text{unit/hr (desired)}}{X \text{ mL/hr}}$$

This rule also applies to other drugs ordered in mU/hr, mg/hr, mcg/hr, g/hr, or mEq/hr.

Example

An order is given for D_5W 500 mL with heparin 25,000 units IV at 1000 units/hr. What is the flow rate in mL/hr?

$$\frac{D}{H} \times Q = \frac{1000 \text{ units/hr}}{25,000 \text{ units}} \times 500 \text{ mL} = R(\text{mL/hr})$$

The units cancel out to leave mL/hr in the $D/H \times Q = R$ formula.

$$\frac{1000 \text{ units/hr}}{25,000 \text{ units}} \times 500 \text{ mL} = \frac{1}{25} \times 500 \text{ mL} = 20 \text{ mL/hr}$$

Or use the ratio and proportion method to calculate the flow rate that will administer 1000 units/hr in mL/hr:

$$\frac{25,000 \text{ units}}{500 \text{ mL}} = \frac{1000 \text{ units/hr}}{X \text{ mL/hr}}$$

$$25,000X = 500,000$$

$$X = \frac{500,000}{25,000} = 20 \text{ mL/hr}$$

Example

An order is given for D$_5$W 250 mL with heparin 25,000 units IV at 750 units/hr. Calculate the flow rate in mL/hr.

$$\frac{D}{H} \times Q = \frac{750 \text{ units/hr}}{25,000 \text{ units}} \times 250 \text{ mL} = 7.5 \text{ mL/hr}$$

Or use the ratio and proportion method:

$$\frac{25,000 \text{ units}}{250 \text{ mL}} = \frac{750 \text{ units/hr}}{X \text{ mL/hr}}$$

$$25,000X = 187,500$$

$$X = \frac{187,500}{25,000} = 7.5 \text{ mL/hr}$$

INTRAVENOUS SOLUTION CONCENTRATIONS

Solutions may have different concentrations of dextrose (glucose) or 5% dextrose in lactated Ringer's or saline (sodium chloride) solution. For example, 5% dextrose contains 5 g of dextrose per 100 mL. Figures 9-12A and 9-12B show labels for a 5% dextrose solution and a 5% dextrose in lactated Ringer's solution.

Normal saline is 0.9% saline; it contains 900 mg or 0.9 g of sodium chloride per 100 mL (see Figure 9-12C).

EQUIPMENT FOR INTRAVENOUS INFUSION

Equipment used to administer intravenous medications is available in several forms. Administration is either completely manual or electronic.

The primary intravenous line may consist of a bag or bottle of solution and tubing. Bags for intravenous infusion come in different sizes. The solution of fluid to be infused is often 500 or 1000 mL. The tubing, which is the primary line, usually includes a drip chamber, roller clamp, and injection ports (see Figure 9-13). The nurse can regulate the rate manually by either using the roller clamp or placing the tubing in an electronic infusion pump.

The secondary intravenous tubing is used when medications are administered by "piggybacking" into the primary line (see Figure 9-14). This type of tubing generally is shorter and also contains a drip chamber and a roller clamp. The benefit of this technique is that it gives access to the primary intravenous catheter without having to start another line.

To measure the flow rate, the drip chamber must be squeezed until it is half full, making it easier to appropriately count the number of drops falling into the chamber. The roller clamp is used to adjust the speed of the infusion either up or down, as needed. The injection port is available to inject medications into the primary line or to attach a second intravenous line. Two sizes of tubing are available: macrodrop and microdrop. Macrodrop tubing is used for fluids infused at a higher rate, for example, infusions that are set at 80 mL/hr or higher. Microdrop tubing is used for slower infusions for which accuracy of dosage delivery is essential, such as in critical care or pediatric settings.

POINTS TO REMEMBER

In critical care, intravenous medication orders may express an amount of medication to be delivered per minute. You will need to convert this rate into milliliters per hour.

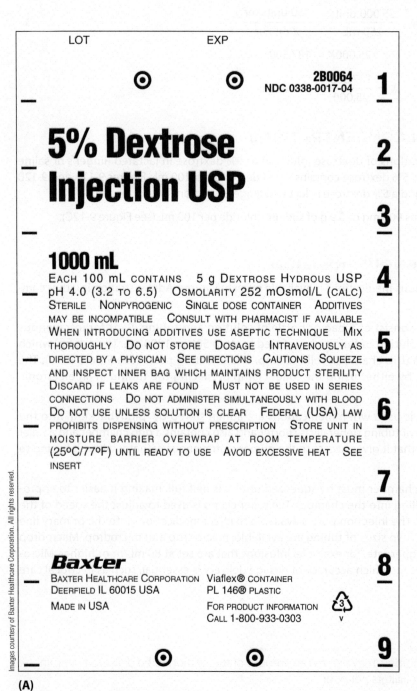

(A)

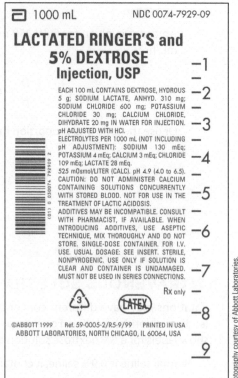

(B)

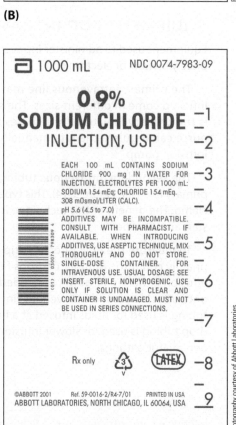

(C)

Figure 9-12 Intravenous solution concentrations: (A) 5% dextrose; (B) 5% dextrose and lactated Ringer's; and (C) 0.9% sodium chloride.

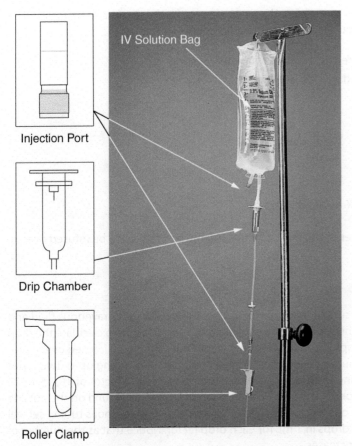

Injection Port

Drip Chamber

Roller Clamp

Figure 9-13 Standard gravity flow intravenous system.

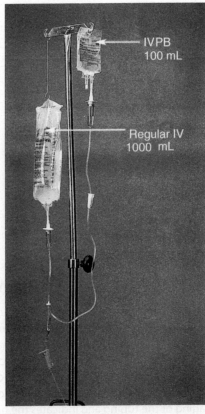

Figure 9-14 Standard intravenous line with piggyback (PB IV).

CALCULATION OF INTRAVENOUS FLOW RATES

A flow rate is the speed at which intravenous fluids are infused into a patient. Allowing the patient to receive a prescribed fluid too fast or too slow can result in adverse reactions. The ability of the pharmacy technician to correctly and efficiently calculate flow rates of intravenous fluids is critical to the well-being of the patient. Flow rates are generally prescribed or written as 125 mL/hr or 500 mL/2 hr, meaning that the fluids should be infused into the patient at a rate of 125 mL over a period of 1 hour or at a rate of 500 mL over a period of 2 hours, respectively. Flow rates can be regulated either by the use of an electronic pump or by manually adjusting the intravenous equipment to achieve the prescribed flow rate. When an electronic pump is used, the flow rate is calculated in milliliters per hour and can be arrived at by using the following formula:

$$\frac{\text{Total amount ordered (mL)}}{\text{Total number of hours (hr)}} = \text{mL/hr}$$

After the flow rate is successfully calculated, the rate is then programmed into an electronic infusion device. For example, Jane Doe is a patient for whom a 500-mL bag of intravenous fluids to be infused over 2 hours has been prescribed. To calculate the flow rate, use the preceding formula:

$$\frac{\text{Total amount ordered (mL)}}{\text{Total number of hours (hr)}} = \frac{500 \text{ mL}}{2 \text{ hr}} = 250 \text{ mL/hr}$$

Therefore, the infusion device is programmed for 250 mL/hr. Another formula is especially helpful when flow rates that have a prescribed infusion time of ½ hour or less are calculated. For example, J. P. Ellen is a patient for whom 500 mg of an intravenous antibiotic in a 100-mL bag of fluid to be infused over 30 minutes has been prescribed. To calculate the flow rate for this patient, use the following formula (remember that 60 minutes = 1 hour):

$$\frac{\text{Total milliliters ordered}}{\text{Total hours ordered}} = \frac{X\ (\text{mL})}{1\ \text{hr}} = \frac{100\ \text{mL}}{30\ \text{min}} = \frac{X\ \text{mL}}{60\ \text{min}}$$

Cross-multiply to get:

$$30X = 6000$$

and dividing both sides by 30 to get:

$$X = 200\ \text{mL/hr}$$

Thus, the electronic infusion pump should be set at 200 mL/hr for the 100-mL bag of fluid to be infused over 30 minutes.

MANUALLY CALCULATING DROP RATES

The pharmacy technician may, depending on the setting, have to calculate a **drop rate** of an intravenous fluid and then manually regulate the equipment to control the speed at which the fluid is being infused. To calculate the drop rate, the technician must determine how many drops (abbreviated as gtt) per minute should be infused over a prescribed time period. The number of drops per minute depends on the type of intravenous tubing used. Two types of tubing are available: standard (or macrodrop) and microdrop. Standard tubing has a drop factor of 10, 15, or 20 gtt/mL, whereas microdrop tubing has a drop factor of 60 gtt/mL. The drop factor is generally found on the outside packaging of the tubing and indicates the number of drops per milliliter that a particular intravenous tubing set will deliver. Figure 9-15 shows the size and number of drops in 1 mL for each drop factor. Notice that as the number of drops per milliliter decreases, the actual drop size increases.

The following formula is used to calculate flow rates in drops per minute:

$$\frac{V\ (\text{total volume to be infused in mL})}{T\ (\text{total time in minutes})} \times C\ (\text{drop factor in gtt/mL}) = R\ (\text{rate of flow in gtt/min})$$

The formula can also be written as:

$$\frac{V}{T} \times C = R$$

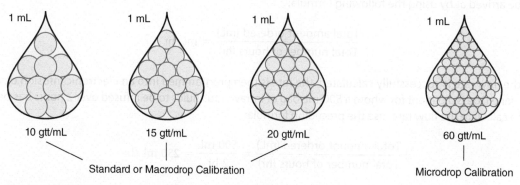

Figure 9-15 Comparison of drop size in macrodrip and microdrip infusions.

Example

John Brown is to receive 200 mL of intravenous fluids over 2 hours. Macrodrop tubing has been selected, which has a drop factor of 20 gtt/mL. The job of the technician is to calculate how many drops per minute are needed so that all 200 mL is infused over 2 hours.

Step 1: Convert 2 hours into minutes (reminder: 1 hour = 60 minutes):

$$2 \times 60 = 120 \text{ min}$$

Step 2: Set up the problem using the formula $V/T \times C = R$

$$\frac{200}{120} \times 20 = 33.3 \text{ gtt/min}$$

Note that the number of drops per minute needs to be rounded to the nearest whole number. In this example, round down to get 33 gtt/min.

Step 3: Set the drop rate by adjusting the roller clamp and counting the amount of drops per minute that fall into the drip chamber.

Example

The order is for 0.9% NS 500 mL with U-200 regular insulin infused at 10 units/hr. The drop factor is 60. Answer the following questions:

Amount of drug/mL: ____

How many mL/hr? ____

How many mL/min? ____

How many gtt/min? ____

1. First, determine the amount of drug in each milliliter. This may be done by using a proportion:

$$\frac{500 \text{ mL NS}}{200 \text{ units insulin}} = \frac{1 \text{ mL NS}}{X \text{ unit insulin}}$$

$$500X = 200$$

$$X = \frac{200}{500}$$

$$X = 0.4$$

$$X = 0.4 \text{ unit insulin/mL}$$

2. Second, determine the flow in mL/hr:

$$\frac{0.4 \text{ unit insulin}}{1 \text{ mL}} = \frac{10 \text{ units insulin}}{X \text{ mL}}$$

$$\frac{0.4}{1} = \frac{10}{X}$$

$$\frac{0.4X}{0.4} = \frac{10}{0.4}$$

$$X = 25$$

$$X = 25 \text{ mL/hr}$$

3. Third, determine the flow in mL/min:

$$\frac{25 \text{ mL}}{60 \text{ min}} = \frac{X}{1 \text{ min}}$$

$$\frac{25}{60} = \frac{X}{1}$$

$$60X = \frac{25}{60}$$

$$X = 0.416$$

$$X = 0.42 \text{ mL/min}$$

4. Finally, determine gtt/min:

$$\frac{60 \text{ gtt}}{1 \text{ mL}} = \frac{X \text{ gtt}}{0.42 \text{ mL}}$$

$$\frac{60}{1} = \frac{X}{0.42}$$

$$X = 25.2$$

$$1 = 25.2 \text{ gtt/min}$$

5. Alternatively, use the following shortcut to determine gtt/min:

$$X \text{ (gtt/min)} = \frac{25 \text{ (volume per hour)}}{60 \text{ (minutes per hour)}} \times \frac{60 \text{ (drop factor)}}{1}$$

$$X = 25/60 \, (60/1)$$

$$X = 25 \text{ gtt/min}$$

   Notice that the answer is slightly different depending on which method is used to solve the problem. Many people may see the ability to adequately calculate and manually adjust drop rates to be outdated because of the improved technology available with electronic infusion pumps, which can be easily programmed. However, the opposite is true. It is important for pharmacy technicians to know the math behind what electronic pumps do because an electronic pump may not be available. In addition, emergency situations require immediate attention, and the ability to correctly determine intravenous infusion drop rates without the aid of an infusion pump is an invaluable skill.

DOSING OF TOTAL PARENTERAL NUTRITION

Total parenteral nutrition (TPN), also called hyperalimentation, is an intravenous infusion that provides a patient with all of his or her daily nutritional requirements in the form of a liquid infusion. TPN is generally prescribed for patients who, because of their disease process or surgical intervention, are unable to eat. It includes fluids such as dextrose, electrolytes, amino acids, trace elements, and vitamins. In some cases, other substances such as fat, insulin, or other drugs can be added to the infusion. The contents of TPN are determined by the patient's individual nutritional requirements. TPN is not infused through a peripheral vein (veins in the hands and arms) but rather through a central vein such as the subclavian vein, superior vena cava, or internal jugular vein.

CONCENTRATION AND DILUTION

Pharmacies often receive prescriptions for liquids or solid medications that are not commercially available in a strength that has been prescribed. The commercial strength is often more than the prescribed strength. Therefore, the pharmacy technician or pharmacist must dilute the commercially available product to one of lower strength. A substance's *concentration* is its strength, which can be expressed as a fraction (such as mg/mL), ratio (such as 1 : 100), or percentage (such as 30% or 60%). The *dilution* of a substance relates directly to its desired concentration. When pharmacy technicians receive an order to prepare a solution of a certain strength and volume, these terms are referred to as its *final strength* (FS) and *final volume* (FV). The process involves choosing a product of an *initial strength* (IS), and then determining the *initial volume* (IV) needed to prepare the compound. If a solid is to be compounded, instead of volume, the terms *final weight* (FW) and *initial weight* (IW) are used. The formula for either type of compounding is as follows:

Initial volume (or weight) × Initial strength = Final volume (or weight) × Final strength

In order to avoid errors, the initial strength must be larger than the final strength. Also, the initial volume (or weight) must be less than the final volume (or weight). The final volume (or weight) minus the initial volume (or weight) equals the amount of *diluent* (*solvent*) that needs to be added. A diluent is an inert substance without a concentration. It is described as having a concentration of 0% and adds volume or mass to a preparation. For solutions, sterile water is commonly used as a diluent. For solids, *petrolatum* is commonly used as a diluent, and it also has a 0% active ingredient. The strengths of preparations are also expressed as percentages, with the volumes using the same units. Most often, volumes are requested in milliliters. Sometimes, the requested volume is in liters or ounces. The most important points that a pharmacy technician must remember, concerning concentration and dilution, are the following:

1. The ratio strengths must be converted to percentage strengths before calculations are made.
2. The initial (stock) strength is always greater than the final strength.
3. The final (desired) weight or volume will be greater than the initial (stock) weight or volume.

ALLIGATION

Alligation is a method, also called *alligation alternate*, that is used to compound solutions and solids when the strength being mixed is different from the strength of the substance or substances in stock. It is the same regardless of whether weight or volume is being dealt with. In the following example, one of the substances is more concentrated than the desired concentration and the other substance is less concentrated than the desired concentration. If the pharmacist receives an order to prepare 5 ounces of a 15% solution using a 30% solution and a 10% solution, how much of each solution should he or she use? Using a table, it is easy to figure out the correct amounts for this mixture:

Highest concentration: 30%		
	Desired concentration (5 ounces of 15%)	
Lowest concentration: 10%		

The next step is to subtract the desired concentration (15%) from the highest concentration (30%) and place the result in the lower right block to show the number of parts needed. Then, subtract the lowest concentration (10%) from the desired concentration (15%) and place the result in the upper right block to show the number of parts needed.

Highest concentration: 30%		5 parts
	Desired concentration (5 ounces of 15%)	
Lowest concentration: 10%		15 parts

Therefore, the total number of parts is: 5 parts + 15 parts, totaling 20 parts.

To determine the final amounts to use, set up a proportion as follows:

$$\text{Highest concentration (30\%)} = \frac{5}{20} \text{ parts} \times 5 \text{ oz}$$

$$= 1.25 \text{ oz of 30\% solution}$$

$$\text{Lowest concentration (10\%)} = \frac{15}{20} \text{ parts} \times 5 \text{ oz}$$

$$= 3.75 \text{ oz of 10\% solution}$$

To verify that the final amounts to use are correct, add the amounts of each concentration to see if they equal the amount to be compounded:

$$1.25 \text{ oz} + 3.75 \text{ oz} = 5 \text{ oz}$$

Pediatric Dosage Calculations

Several rules are used to calculate dosages for infants and children's dosages, including Young's rule, Clark's rule, and Fried's rule. These rules give only approximate dosages; they are not the most accurate methods for determining doses. Even when pediatric drug dosages are calculated on the basis of body surface area, weight, and age of the child, they are based on a proportion of the usual adult dose (approximate).

Because of their age, weight, height, and physical condition, children are more sensitive to medications than are adults. Therefore, children are not able to tolerate adult doses of drugs. Dosage must be measured accurately according to the age and weight of infants and children. When you calculate drug dosages, do not consider a child to be a small adult. The average child does not metabolize drugs the way an adult does. For instance, many organ systems in infants and toddlers are immature. Responses to medications in children are significantly different from those in adults. Several methods are used in calculating dosages for this group of patients. The dosage form per kilogram or pound of body weight is more accurate than dosage calculated by age. The body surface area method is another way to measure the dosage for children. Charts are available to determine the body surface area in square meters, according to height and weight. The amount of medication to be given in 24 hours is calculated and then divided into an equal number of doses. The number of doses is determined by the recommended frequency of administration.

Example

The order is for ampicillin 125 mg PO four times a day for a child weighing 26.44 lb. On hand is ampicillin suspension 125 mg/5 mL. The recommended daily PO dose for a child is 20 to 40 mg/kg/day in divided dosages every 8 hours.

1. Change the child's weight from pounds to kilograms. Remember there are 2.2 lb in each kilogram.

$$\frac{1 \text{ kg}}{2.2 \text{ lb}} = \frac{X \text{ kg}}{26.44 \text{ lb}}$$

$$22.X = 26.44$$

$$X = 12 \text{ kg}$$

$X = 12.01$ kg (which you then round down to 12 kg).

2. Write a proportion(s) using the recommended dosage and the child's weight as your known values to determine the safe recommended dosage or range for this child.

> 20 mg : 1 kg :: X mg : 12 kg
>
> (remember the product of the means equals the product of the extremes)
>
> $X = 240$ mg
>
> 40 mg : 1 kg :: X mg : 12 kg
>
> $X = 480$ mg

The safe recommended range for this child, who weighs 12 kg, is 240 to 480 mg in a 24-hour period.

Many drugs are not advised for administration to children because of their potential for harmful side effects in the growing child or because they have not been sufficiently tested in children to give a recommended dosage range.

CLARK'S RULE

Clark's rule is one of three formulas used to calculate dosages for infants and children. Clark's rule is based on the weight of the child. This system is much more accurate than other pediatric methods, because the size and body weight of children of any age can vary greatly. Clark's rule uses 150 lb (70 kg) as the average adult weight and assumes that the child's dose is proportionately less.

$$\text{Pediatric dose} = \frac{\text{Child's weight in pounds}}{150 \text{ pounds}} \times \text{Adult dose}$$

Example

Find the dose of cortisone for a 30-lb infant (adult dose = 100 mg). The calculation is as follows:

$$\frac{30}{150} \times 100 \text{ mg} = 20 \text{ mg}$$

YOUNG'S RULE

Young's rule is used for children older than 1 year.

$$\text{Pediatric dose} = \frac{\text{Child's age in years}}{\text{Child's age in years} + 12} \times \text{Adult dose}$$

Example

Find the dose of acetaminophen for a 4-year-old child (adult dose = 1000 mg). The calculation is as follows:

$$\frac{4}{4 + 12} \times 1000 \text{ mg} = 250 \text{ mg}$$

Note that Young's rule is not valid after 12 years of age. If the child is small enough to warrant a reduced dose after 12 years of age, the reduction should be calculated on the basis of Clark's rule.

FRIED'S RULE

Fried's rule is a method of estimating the dose of medication for a pediatric patient younger than 24 months.

$$\frac{\text{Age in months}}{150} \times \text{Average adult dose} = \text{Child's dose}$$

Example

Find the dose of phenobarbital for a 15-month-old infant (adult dose = 400 mg). The calculation is as follows:

$$\frac{15}{150} \times 400 \text{ mg} = 40 \text{ mg}$$

Pediatric drug dosages are calculated in three steps. For example, Amoxil® 25 mg/kg/day given every 12 hours is being ordered for a 24-lb baby. The first step in calculating the correct dosage for this baby is to convert pounds to kilograms. The conversion rule is:

$$1 \text{ kg} = 2.2 \text{ lb}$$

$$\frac{1 \text{ kg}}{2.2 \text{ lb}} = \frac{X \text{ kg}}{24 \text{ lb}}$$

Cross-multiply this ratio:

$$2.2X = 24$$

$$X = 10.9 \text{ kg (round up to 11 kg)}$$

The next step is to calculate the drug dosage based on 25 mg/kg of body weight:

$$\frac{25 \text{ mg}}{1 \text{ kg}} = \frac{X \text{ mg}}{11 \text{ kg}}$$

Cross-multiply this ratio:

$$X \text{ mg} = 275$$

$$X = \frac{275 \text{ mg}}{24 \text{ hr}}$$

The third and final step is to calculate how much Amoxil this patient receives per dose. Remember, the patient is to receive a dose once every 12 hours or 2 divided doses in one 24-hour period. The calculation is as follows:

$$\frac{275 \text{ mg}}{2} = 137.5 \text{ mg per dose}$$

Amoxil is available in 250 mg/5 mL dosages so the exact number of milliliters to give the patient per dose needs to be calculated:

$$\frac{250 \text{ mg}}{5 \text{ mL}} = \frac{137.5 \text{ mg}}{X \text{ mL}}$$

Cross-multiply this ratio:

$$250X = 687.5$$

$$X = \frac{687.5}{250}$$

$$X = 2.75 \text{ mL}$$

Therefore, the patient would receive 2.75 mL of Amoxil every 12 hours.

Calculating drug dosages for the pediatric patient is not as time-consuming as it initially appears. After a technician has practiced doing several dosage calculations, he or she will soon become proficient.

WEST'S NOMOGRAM

West's nomogram is a quick reference guide that calculates the body surface area (BSA) of infants and young children based on their height and weight. The nomogram calculates BSA in square meters (m^2). To determine the BSA using West's nomogram, place a dot on the nomogram at the point that corresponds to the patient's height and another dot at the point that corresponds to the patient's weight; then draw a straight line between the two dots. The point where the line crosses the square meter column is the patient's body surface area. Be careful to place the dots correctly, as marking the scales incorrectly will result in calculation of an erroneous BSA. Many physicians use the nomogram as a quick reference in determining body surface area for pediatric doses.

POINTS TO REMEMBER

West's nomogram also displays BSA for children who are of normal height for their weight in the center of the chart. This information is found by using the child's weight in pounds.

BSA is also important for determination of medication doses for burn victims and for patients undergoing open heart surgery, chemotherapy, and radiation therapy. The calculation of the dose to be administered based on BSA and nomogram is as follows:

1. Calculate the patient's BSA.
2. Calculate the desired dose.

$$\text{Dosage ordered} \times \text{BSA} = \text{Desired dose}$$

3. Confirm whether or not the desired dose is safe. If it is unsafe, consult the physician who wrote the order.

4. Calculate the amount to administer, using fractional equation, ratio and proportion, or the formula method. The formula for determining a dose for a child based on the BSA and adult dosage is:

$$\text{Pediatric dose} = \frac{\text{Body surface area (BSA) of child in m}^2}{1.7 \text{ m}^2 \text{ (average adult BSA)}} \times \text{Adult dose}$$

Example

The child's BSA is 0.65 m². The recommended adult dosage is 275 mg. Determine the child's dose.

$$\text{Pediatric dose} = \frac{0.65 \text{ m}^2}{1.7 \text{ m}^2} \times 275 \text{ mg}$$

$$\frac{0.65}{1.7} = 0.38 \times 275 = 105 \text{ mg}$$

$$\text{Pediatric dose} = 105 \text{ mg}$$

Summary

Pharmacy technicians are required to understand basic mathematics in order to be able to calculate drug dosages by weight, volume, and by using balances. They must also be able to convert from one measurement system to another. Correct drug dosage calculations are among the most important factors in the prevention of medication errors. Technicians should have a working knowledge of fractions, decimals, ratios, and percentages, as well as basic problem-solving skills.

The system of Roman numerals uses letters to represent number values and has no letter that represents "zero." In the pharmacy, technicians usually work with Roman numerals between 1 and 50. The building blocks of the Roman system include I, V, X, L, C, D, and M, representing 1, 5, 10, 50, 100, 500, and 1000, respectively. Arabic numbers consist of whole numbers, fractions, and decimals. A fraction is an expression of division with a number that is the portion or part of a whole amount. Decimal fractions, or decimals, are used with the metric system, which is the system most often used in dosage calculation. Each decimal fraction consists of a numerator that is expressed in numerals, a decimal point placed so that it designates the value of the denominator. The denominator is understood to be 10 or some power of 10. In writing a decimal fraction, a zero is placed to the left of the decimal point, so that the decimal point can be readily seen. It is of vital importance that decimal calculations be double-checked before using them for drug dosages.

A ratio compares two numbers by division, with the two numbers separated by a colon, which appears as the symbol ":." A proportion shows the relationship between two equal ratios and is written with a single colon separating each ratio, and a double colon in the middle separating the two ratios from each other (X : Y :: A : B). In a proportion, the two outside terms are called the extremes and the two inside terms are called the means. The term percent, or percentage, means "hundredths" and is expressed using the symbol "%." A percent is a fraction whose numerator is expressed and whose denominator is understood to be 100.

The correct dosage of a medication depends upon the patient's age, weight, state of health, or other drugs that the patient may be taking. Pharmacy technicians among the most important and challenging tasks perform dosage calculations. To prevent medication errors, pharmacy technicians must be skilled in the accurate calculation of dosages. They must follow the seven rights of drug administration. The medication label must be completely read and verified for accuracy three times during the drug dispensing process. There are four methods of drug calculation: the basic formula, ratio and proportion, fractional equation, and dimensional analysis. Calculations of parenteral medications must be precise and accurate because these medications will enter the blood circulation directly. Pediatric dosage calculations differ from adult dosage calculations. There are several methods of calculating pediatric dosages. They include Young's Rule, Clark's Rule, and Fried's Rule, all of which give approximate dosages. The most accurate way of calculating pediatric dosages is by using the child's body surface area (BSA).

REVIEW QUESTIONS

1. The Roman numeral VIII is equivalent to the Arabic number _____.

2. The Roman numeral IX is equivalent to the Arabic number _____.

3. The Roman numeral XII is equivalent to the Arabic number _____.

4. The Roman numeral XIV is equivalent to the Arabic number _____.

5. The Roman numeral XV is equivalent to the Arabic number _____.

6. The Arabic number 19 is equivalent to the Roman numeral _____.

7. The Arabic number 21 is equivalent to the Roman numeral _____.

8. The Arabic number 23 is equivalent to the Roman numeral _____.

9. The Arabic number 25 is equivalent to the Roman numeral _____.

10. The Arabic number 29 is equivalent to the Roman numeral _____.

11. The fraction 1/2 is equivalent to the decimal _____.

12. The fraction 1/6 is equivalent, when rounded to 2 decimal places, to the decimal _____.

13. The fraction 2/15 is equivalent, when rounded to 2 decimal places, to the decimal _____.

14. The fraction 1/158 is equivalent, when rounded to 2 decimal places, to the decimal _____.

15. The fraction 3/200 is equivalent to the decimal _____.

16. The decimal 0.009 is equivalent to the fraction _____.

17. The decimal 0.0033 is equivalent to the fraction _____.

18. The decimal 0.25 is equivalent to the fraction _____.

19. The decimal 0.075 is equivalent to the fraction _____.

20. The decimal 0.84 is equivalent to the fraction _____.

21. The fraction 40/60 is equivalent to the ratio _____.

22. The fraction 6/8 is equivalent to the ratio _____.

23. The fraction 25/200 is equivalent to the ratio _____.

24. The fraction 75/1500 is equivalent to the ratio _____.

25. The fraction 17/170 is equivalent to the ratio _____.

26. 6% is equivalent to the decimal _____.

27. 35% is equivalent to the decimal _____.

28. 0.3% is equivalent to the decimal _____.

29. 0.01% is equivalent to the decimal _____.

30. 0.004% is equivalent to the decimal _____.

31. 1% is equivalent to the ratio _____.

32. 50% is equivalent to the ratio _____.

33. 12.5% is equivalent to the ratio _____.

34. 0.25% is equivalent to the ratio _____.

35. 0.33% is equivalent to the ratio _____.

36. In the proportion 1 : 5 = X : 20, the "X" is equivalent to _____.

37. In the proportion X : 3 = 7 : 21, the "X" is equivalent to _____.

38. In the proportion 1/2 : X = 3 : 12, the "X" is equivalent to _____.

39. In the proportion 1/3 : 2/3 = 1/6 : X, the "X" is equivalent to _____.

40. In the proportion 25 : X = 75 : 1500, the "X" is equivalent to _____.

41. The ordered dosage is 50 mg. The available strength is 60 mg in 1.5 mL. By rounding to the nearest tenth, how many mL, in decimal format, must be supplied? _____

42. The ordered dosage is 300 mcg. The available strength is 0.4 mg per mL. By rounding to the nearest tenth, how many mL, in decimal format, must be supplied? _____

43. The ordered dosage is 0.45 g. The available strength is 300 mg per mL. By rounding to the nearest tenth, how many mL, in decimal format, must be supplied? _____

44. The ordered dosage is 8 mg. The available strength is 5 mg per mL. By rounding to the nearest tenth, how many mL, in decimal format, must be supplied? _____

45. The ordered dosage is 70 mg. The available strength is 250 mg per 5 mL. By rounding to the nearest tenth, how many mL, in decimal format, must be supplied? _____

46. 0.2 g tablets were ordered. The available tablets are 80 mg. By using dimensional analysis, how many tablets must be given? _____

47. A dosage of 85 mg was ordered. The available strength is 0.1 g per 1.5 mL. By using dimensional analysis, and rounding to the nearest tenth, how many mL must be given? _____

48. 0.1 g of an IM medication was ordered. The available strength is 200 mg per mL. By using dimensional analysis, how many mL must be given? _____

49. A dosage of 0.5 mg was ordered. The available strength is 200 mcg per mL. By using dimensional analysis, how many mL must be given? _____

50. A dosage of 0.75 mg was ordered. The available strength is 500 mcg per 1.5 mL. By using dimensional analysis, and rounding to the nearest tenth, how many mL must be given? _____

51. A dosage of 130 mg was ordered. The available strength is 0.1 g per 2 mL. By using dimensional analysis, how many mL must be given? _____

52. A dosage of 1500 mg was ordered. The available strength is 0.5 g per mL. By using dimensional analysis, how many mL must be given? _____

53. 500 mg of an IM medication was ordered. The available strength is 1 g per 3 mL. By using dimensional analysis, how many mL must be given? _____

54. A 0.7 g dosage is ordered. The available strength is 500 mg per 5 mL. By using dimensional analysis, how many mL must be given? _____

55. A 0.75 g dosage is ordered. The available strength is 250 mg per mL. By using dimensional analysis, how many ML must be given? _____

56. Pravachol 20 mg was ordered. The available strength is 10 mg per tablet. How many tablets must be given? _____

57. Quinidine 0.6 g was ordered. The available strength is 200 mg per tablet. How many tablets must be given? _____

58. Prednisone 7.5 mg was ordered. The available strength is 5 mg per scored tablet. How many tablets must be given? _____

59. Aldomet 250 mg was ordered. The available strength is 125 mg per tablet. How many tablets must be given? _____

60. Duricef 0.5 g was ordered. The available strength is 500 mg per tablet. How many tablets must be given? _____

61. Zovirax suspension 400 mg was ordered. The available strength is 200 mg per 5 mL. How many mL must be given? _____

62. Artane elixir 3 mg was ordered. The available strength is 2 mg per 5 mL. How many mL must be given? _____

63. Depakene syrup 125 mg was ordered. The available strength is 250 mg per 5 mL. How many mL must be given? _____

64. Amoxil suspension 100 mg was ordered. The available strength is 125 mg per 5 mL. How many mL must be given? _____

65. Zofran liquid 8 mg was ordered. The available strength is 4 mg per 5 mL. How many mL must be given? _____

66. Demerol 35 mg IM was ordered. The available strength is 50 mg per mL. How many mL must be given? _____

67. Atarax 40 mg IM was ordered. The available strength is 50 mg per mL. How many mL must be given? _____

68. Garamycin 40 mg IM was ordered. The available strength is 80 mg per 2 mL. How many mL must be given? _____

69. Heparin 3500 units SC were ordered. The available strength is 5000 units per mL. How many mL must be given? _____

70. Lasix 60 mg IV was ordered. The available strength is 20 mg per 2 mL. How many mL must be given? _____

CRITICAL THINKING

1. What are the mixed fractions that are equivalent to the improper fractions 24/5, 16/6, and 32/7?

2. The adult dosage of a medication is 250 mg. A child must receive the correct dosage of this medication. His body surface area is 0.65 m^2. Using West's nomogram, what is the correct dose for this child?

3. Using only the most accurate method for pediatric dosage calculations (out of the three rules discussed in this chapter), determine the correct child dose of a medication with an adult dose of 125 mg. The child weighs 65 pounds.

4. Insulin may be administered in U-40, U-80, and U-100 dosage forms. For U-100 insulin, should you use a 1-mL, 5-mL, or 10-mL syringe? Explain why.

5. In case of severe pathologic hypersecretory conditions, a physician may order Zantac® up to 6 g/day. If the patient is to be given 1.5 g/day divided into four doses, what is the amount to administer per dose?

WEB LINKS

AAA Math: www.aaamath.com

A-plus Math: www.aplusmath.com

Math.com: www.math.com

Nursing Math: ncalc.com

DosageHelp.com: www.dosagehelp.com

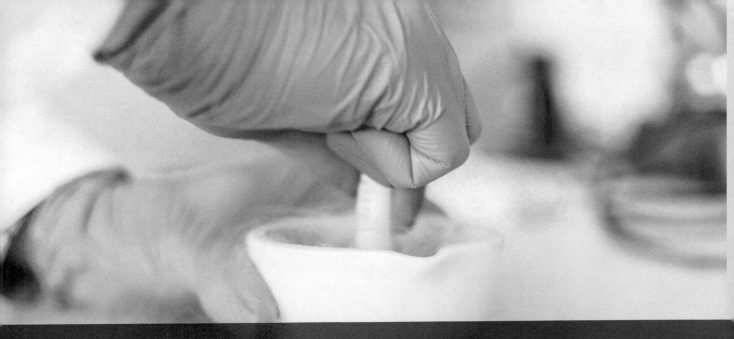

PHARMACY PRACTICE SETTINGS

SECTION II

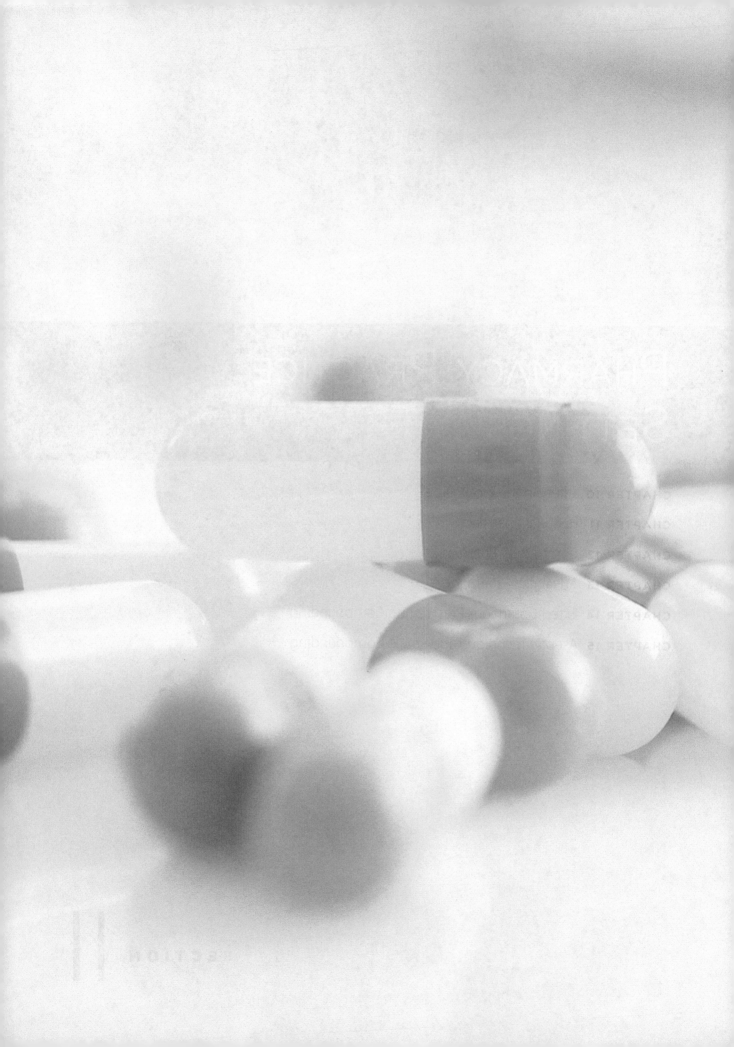

Safety in the Workplace

OBJECTIVES

Upon completion of this chapter, the reader should be able to:

1. Explain the Occupational Safety and Health Administration (OSHA) and its standards.
2. Define ergonomics as related to the workplace.
3. Describe the exposure control plan.
4. Discuss the importance of employee training.
5. Explain safety data sheets (SDS).
6. Describe universal precautions.
7. Explain barrier precautions.
8. Define a hazard communication plan.

9. List four responsibilities of employees for compliance with OSHA regulations.

10. Explain management and disposal of hazardous materials.

KEY TERMS

barrier precautions

biohazard symbol

carcinogenic

caustic

ergonomic

exposure control plan

fire safety and emergency plan

hazard communication plan

safety data sheet (SDS)

teratogenic

universal precautions

Overview

Safety issues are present in any place, and commonsense precautions need to be taken in the workplace, particularly in the pharmacy. The purpose of environmental protection measures is to minimize the risk of occupational injury by isolating or removing any physical or mechanical health hazard in any workplace. In 1970, the federal government passed the Occupational Safety and Health Act, the first national health and safety law, with the goal of ensuring safe and healthful working conditions for all workers in the United States. The act established the Occupational Safety and Health Administration (OSHA) in the Department of Labor. OSHA establishes safety regulations for employers and monitors compliance.

Occupational Safety and Health Administration Standards

OSHA provides for research, information, education, and training in the field of occupational safety and health and authorized enforcement of OSHA standards. OSHA also establishes standards requiring employers to provide their workers with workplaces free from recognized hazards that could cause serious injury or death. In addition, employees must abide by all safety and health standards that apply to their jobs (see Table 10-1).

Table 10-1 Safety Guidelines for the Pharmacy Technician

- Observe warning labels on biohazard containers and equipment.
- Minimize splashing, spraying, and splattering of drops of potentially infectious materials. Splattering of blood onto skin or mucous membranes is a proven mode of transmission of hepatitis B virus.
- Bandage any breaks or lesions on your hands before gloving.
- If exposed body surfaces, such as the eyes, come in contact with body fluids, flush with water, scrub with soap and water, or use both measures as soon as possible.
- Do not recap, bend, or break contaminated needles and other sharps.
- Use hemostats to attach and remove scalpel blades from handles.
- Do not use mouth pipetting or suck blood through tubing.
- Decontaminate contaminated test materials before reprocessing or place in impervious bags and dispose of according to policy.
- Do not keep food and drink in refrigerators, freezers, shelves, or cabinets or on countertops where blood or other potentially hazardous chemical materials could be present.

OSHA regulates all workplace environments by enforcing protocols for the proper removal of hazards and for fire safety and emergency plans. Two specific functions related to the pharmacy, specifically the hospital pharmacy, are protection of employees from exposure to disease and protection from exposure to chemicals. Chemical materials may be flammable, **caustic**, poisonous, **carcinogenic**, or **teratogenic**. Employees can be exposed to these dangers through inhalation, direct absorption through the skin, ingestion, entry through a mucous membrane, or entry through a break in the skin. Information and training on safe work practices must be provided to all workers.

The general health of the employee must be protected, and many standards require plans such as an infection control plan, training of employees, availability of personal protective equipment (PPE), provision of vaccinations such as hepatitis B, and medical intervention after exposure incidents and monitoring of injuries with detailed records. OSHA has the right to inspect private and public work sites to be sure all protocols and guidelines are being followed.

HAZARD COMMUNICATION PLAN

A **hazard communication plan** protects the rights of employees to know what types of hazardous chemicals are present in the workplace and what health risks are associated with those chemicals. All hazardous chemicals must have warning labels as shown in Figure 10-1.

OSHA requires pharmacies to have a **safety data sheet (SDS)** for each hazardous chemical material used. A pharmacy can use sheets provided by the local OSHA area office or by the manufacturer of the hazardous chemical. The pharmacy technician must be familiar with the SDS information and ensure the implementation of proper protective measures for exposure to hazardous materials. Each SDS contains basic information about the specific chemical or product. This includes the trade name, chemical name and synonyms, chemical family, manufacturer's name and address, telephone number for emergencies, hazardous ingredients, physical data, fire and explosion data, and health hazard and protection information (see Figure 10-2).

Containers with chemicals should be tightly sealed and properly labeled. A hazard identification system was developed by the National Fire Protection Association that provides an identification coding method. This consists of four small, colored, diamond-shaped symbols grouped into a larger diamond shape. The top diamond is red and indicates a flammability hazard. The diamond on the left is blue and indicates hazards to health. The bottom diamond is white and provides special hazard information, including radioactivity, special biohazards, and other dangerous situations. Finally, the diamond on the right is yellow and indicates reactivity/stability hazards. The system indicates the severity of the hazard by using numbers from 0 to 4 imprinted in the diamonds, with 4 meaning "extremely hazardous" and 0 meaning "no hazard" (see Figure 10-3).

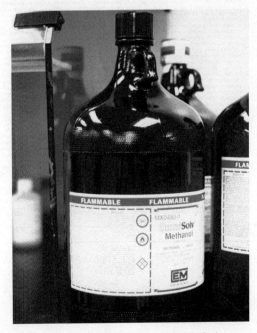

Figure 10-1 Chemicals used in the workplace must be clearly and accurately labeled.

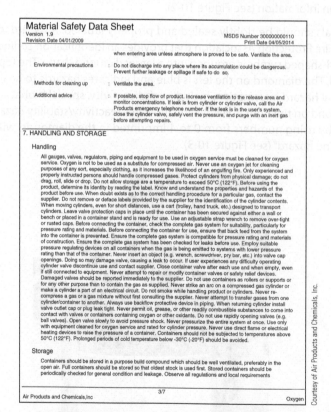

Material Safety Data Sheet
Version 1.9
Revision Date 04/01/2009
MSDS Number 300000000110
Print Date 04/05/2014

1. PRODUCT AND COMPANY IDENTIFICATION

Product name	: Oxygen
Chemical formula	: O2
Synonyms	: Oxygen, Oxygen gas, Gaseous Oxygen, GOX
Product Use Description	: General Industrial
Manufacturer/Importer/Distributor	: Air Products and Chemicals, Inc 7201 Hamilton Blvd. Allentown, PA 18195-1501 GST No. 123600835 RT0001 QST No. 102753981 TQ0001
Telephone	: 1-610-481-4911 Corporate 1-800-345-3148 Chemicals Cust Serv 1-800-752-1597 Gases/Electronics Cust Serv
Emergency telephone number (24h)	: 800-523-9374 USA +1 610 481 7711 International

2. COMPOSITION/INFORMATION ON INGREDIENTS

Components	CAS Number	Concentration (Volume)
Oxygen	7782-44-7	100 %

Concentration is nominal. For the exact product composition, please refer to Air Products technical specifications.

3. HAZARDS IDENTIFICATION

Emergency Overview

High pressure, oxidizing gas.
Vigorously accelerates combustion.
Keep oil, grease, and combustibles away.
May react violently with combustible materials.

Potential Health Effects

Inhalation
: Breathing 75% or more oxygen at atmospheric pressure for more than a few hours may cause nasal stuffiness, cough, sore throat, chest pain and breathing difficulty. Breathing pure oxygen under pressure may cause lung damage and also central nervous system effects.

Air Products and Chemicals,Inc   1/7   Oxygen

Material Safety Data Sheet
Version 1.9
Revision Date 04/01/2009
MSDS Number 300000000110
Print Date 04/05/2014

Eye contact	: No adverse effect.
Skin contact	: No adverse effect.
Ingestion	: Ingestion is not considered a potential route of exposure.

Exposure Guidelines

Primary Routes of Entry	: Inhalation
Target Organs	: None known.

Aggravated Medical Condition

If oxygen is administered to persons with chronic obstructive pulmonary disease, raising the oxygen concentration in the blood depresses their breathing and raises their retained carbon dioxide to a dangerous level.

4. FIRST AID MEASURES

General advice	: Remove victim to uncontaminated area wearing self contained breathing apparatus. Keep victim warm and rested. Call a doctor. Apply artificial respiration if breathing stopped.
Eye contact	: Seek medical advice.
Skin contact	: Seek medical advice.
Ingestion	: Ingestion is not considered a potential route of exposure.
Inhalation	: Consult a physician after significant exposure. Move to fresh air. If breathing has stopped or is labored, give assisted respirations. Supplemental oxygen may be indicated. If the heart has stopped, trained personnel should begin cardiopulmonary resuscitation immediately.

5. FIRE-FIGHTING MEASURES

Suitable extinguishing media	: All known extinguishing media can be used.
Specific hazards	: Most cylinders are designed to vent contents when exposed to elevated temperatures.
Further information	: Some materials that are noncombustible in air will burn in the presence of an oxygen enriched atmosphere (greater than 23.5%). Fire resistant clothing may burn and offer no protection in oxygen rich atmospheres.

6. ACCIDENTAL RELEASE MEASURES

Personal precautions
: Clothing exposed to high concentrations may retain oxygen 30 minutes or longer and become a potential fire hazard. Stay away from ignition sources. Evacuate personnel to safe areas. Wear self-contained breathing apparatus

Air Products and Chemicals,Inc   2/7   Oxygen

Material Safety Data Sheet
Version 1.9
Revision Date 04/01/2009
MSDS Number 300000000110
Print Date 04/05/2014

when entering area unless atmosphere is proved to be safe. Ventilate the area.

Environmental precautions	: Do not discharge into any place where its accumulation could be dangerous. Prevent further leakage or spillage if safe to do so.
Methods for cleaning up	: Ventilate the area.
Additional advice	: If possible, stop flow of product. Increase ventilation to the release area and monitor concentrations. If leak is from cylinder or cylinder valve, call the Air Products emergency telephone number. If the leak is in the user's system, close the cylinder valve, safely vent the pressure, and purge with an inert gas before attempting repairs.

7. HANDLING AND STORAGE

Handling

All gauges, valves, regulators, piping and equipment to be used in oxygen service must be cleaned for oxygen service. Oxygen is not to be used as a substitute for compressed air. Never use an oxygen jet for cleaning purposes of any sort, especially clothing, as it increases the likelihood of an engulfing fire. Only experienced and properly instructed persons should handle compressed gases. Protect cylinders from physical damage; do not drag, roll, slide or drop. Do not allow storage are a temperature to exceed 50°C (122°F). Before using the product, determine its identity by reading the label. Know and understand the properties and hazards of the product before use. When doubt exists as to the correct handling procedure for a particular gas, contact the supplier. Do not remove or deface labels provided by the supplier for the identification of the cylinder contents. When moving cylinders, even for short distances, use a cart (trolley, hand truck, etc.) designed to transport cylinders. Leave valve protection caps in place until the container has been secured against either a wall or bench or placed in a container stand and is ready for use. Use an adjustable strap wrench to remove over-tight or rusted caps. Before connecting the container, check the complete gas system for suitability, particularly for pressure rating and materials. Before connecting the container for use, ensure that back feed from the system into the container is prevented. Ensure the complete gas system is compatible for pressure rating and materials of construction. Ensure the complete gas system has been checked for leaks before use. Employ suitable pressure regulating devices on all containers when the gas is being emitted to systems with lower pressure rating than that of the container. Never insert an object (e.g. wrench, screwdriver, pry bar, etc.) into valve cap openings. Doing so may damage valve, causing a leak to occur. If user experiences any difficulty operating cylinder valve discontinue use and contact supplier. Close container valve after each use and when empty, even if still connected to equipment. Never attempt to repair or modify container valves or safety relief devices. Damaged valves should be reported immediately to the supplier. Do not use containers as rollers or supports or for any other purpose than to contain the gas as supplied. Never strike an arc on a compressed gas cylinder or make a cylinder a part of an electrical circuit. Do not smoke while handling product or cylinders. Never re-compress a gas or a gas mixture from one cylinder/container to another. Always use backflow protective device in piping. When returning cylinder install valve outlet cap or plug leak tight. Never permit oil, grease, or other readily combustible substances to come into contact with valves or containers containing oxygen or other oxidants. Do not use rapidly opening valves (e.g. ball valves). Open valve slowly to avoid pressure shock. Never pressurize the entire system at once. Use only with equipment cleaned for oxygen service and rated for cylinder pressure. Never use direct flame or electrical heating devices to raise the pressure of a container. Containers should not be subjected to temperatures above 50°C (122°F). Prolonged periods of cold temperature below -30°C (-20°F) should be avoided.

Storage

Containers should be stored in a purpose build compound which should be well ventilated, preferably in the open air. Full containers should be stored so that oldest stock is used first. Stored containers should be periodically checked for general condition and leakage. Observe all regulations and local requirements

Air Products and Chemicals,Inc   3/7   Oxygen

Figure 10-2 A safety data sheet must be maintained for each chemical used in a facility. *(Continued)*

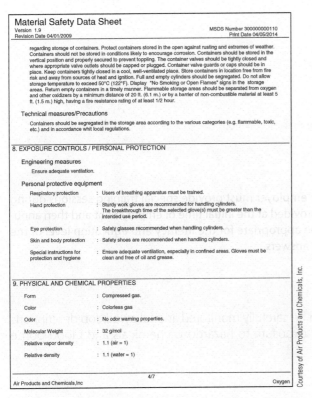

Material Safety Data Sheet

Version 1.9
Revision Date 04/01/2009

MSDS Number 300000000110
Print Date 04/05/2014

regarding storage of containers. Protect containers stored in the open against rusting and extremes of weather. Containers should not be stored in conditions likely to encourage corrosion. Containers should be stored in the vertical position and properly secured to prevent toppling. The container valves should be tightly closed and where appropriate valve outlets should be capped or plugged. Container valve guards or caps should be in place. Keep containers tightly closed in a cool, well-ventilated place. Store containers in location free from fire risk and away from sources of heat and ignition. Full and empty cylinders should be segregated. Do not allow storage temperature to exceed 50°C (122°F). Display "No Smoking or Open Flames" signs in the storage areas. Return empty containers in a timely manner. Flammable storage areas should be separated from oxygen and other oxidizers by a minimum distance of 20 ft. (6.1 m.) or by a barrier of non-combustible material at least 5 ft. (1.5 m.) high, having a fire resistance rating of at least 1/2 hour.

Technical measures/Precautions

Containers should be segregated in the storage area according to the various categories (e.g. flammable, toxic, etc.) and in accordance whit local regulations.

8. EXPOSURE CONTROLS / PERSONAL PROTECTION

Engineering measures

Ensure adequate ventilation.

Personal protective equipment

Respiratory protection	: Users of breathing apparatus must be trained.
Hand protection	: Sturdy work gloves are recommended for handling cylinders. The breakthrough time of the selected glove(s) must be greater than the intended use period.
Eye protection	: Safety glasses recommended when handling cylinders.
Skin and body protection	: Safety shoes are recommended when handling cylinders.
Special instructions for protection and hygiene	: Ensure adequate ventilation, especially in confined areas. Gloves must be clean and free of oil and grease.

9. PHYSICAL AND CHEMICAL PROPERTIES

Form	: Compressed gas.
Color	: Colorless gas
Odor	: No odor warning properties.
Molecular Weight	: 32 g/mol
Relative vapor density	: 1.1 (air = 1)
Relative density	: 1.1 (water = 1)

4/7

Air Products and Chemicals,Inc   Oxygen

Courtesy of Air Products and Chemicals, Inc.

Material Safety Data Sheet

Version 1.9
Revision Date 04/01/2009

MSDS Number 300000000110
Print Date 04/05/2014

Vapor pressure	: Not applicable.
Density	: 0.081 lb/ft3 (0.0013 g/cm3) at 70 °F (21 °C) Note: (as vapor)
Specific Volume	: 12.08 ft3/lb (0.7540 m3/kg) at 70 °F (21 °C)
Boiling point/range	: -297 °F (-183 °C)
Critical temperature	: -180 °F (-118 °C)
Melting point/range	: -362 °F (-219 °C)
Autoignition temperature	: Not applicable.
Water solubility	: 0.039 g/l

10. STABILITY AND REACTIVITY

Stability	: Stable under normal conditions.
Materials to avoid	: Flammable materials. Organic materials. Avoid oil, grease and all other combustible materials.

11. TOXICOLOGICAL INFORMATION

Acute Health Hazard

Ingestion	: No data is available on the product itself.
Inhalation	: No data is available on the product itself.
Skin.	: No data is available on the product itself.

Chronic Health Hazard

Premature infants exposed to high oxygen concentrations may suffer delayed retinal damage that can progress to retinal detachment and blindness. Retinal damage may also occur in adults exposed to 100% oxygen for extended periods (24 to 48 hr). At two or more atmospheres central nervous system (CNS) toxicity occurs. Symptoms include nausea, vomiting, dizziness or vertigo, muscle twitching, vision changes and loss of consciousness and generalized seizures. At three atmospheres, CNS toxicity occurs in less than two hours and at six atmospheres in only a few minutes.

12. ECOLOGICAL INFORMATION

Ecotoxicity effects

Aquatic toxicity	: No data is available on the product itself.
Toxicity to other organisms	: No data available.

5/7

Air Products and Chemicals,Inc   Oxygen

Courtesy of Air Products and Chemicals, Inc.

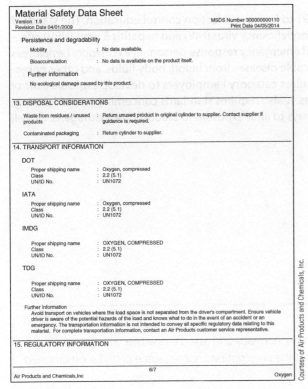

Material Safety Data Sheet

Version 1.9
Revision Date 04/01/2009

MSDS Number 300000000110
Print Date 04/05/2014

Persistence and degradability

Mobility	: No data available.
Bioaccumulation	: No data is available on the product itself.

Further information

No ecological damage caused by this product.

13. DISPOSAL CONSIDERATIONS

Waste from residues / unused products	: Return unused product in original cylinder to supplier. Contact supplier if guidance is required.
Contaminated packaging	: Return cylinder to supplier.

14. TRANSPORT INFORMATION

DOT

Proper shipping name	: Oxygen, compressed
Class	: 2.2 (5.1)
UN/ID No.	: UN1072

IATA

Proper shipping name	: Oxygen, compressed
Class	: 2.2 (5.1)
UN/ID No.	: UN1072

IMDG

Proper shipping name	: OXYGEN, COMPRESSED
Class	: 2.2 (5.1)
UN/ID No.	: UN1072

TDG

Proper shipping name	: OXYGEN, COMPRESSED
Class	: 2.2 (5.1)
UN/ID No.	: UN1072

Further Information

Avoid transport on vehicles where the load space is not separated from the driver's compartment. Ensure vehicle driver is aware of the potential hazards of the load and knows what to do in the event of an accident or an emergency. The transportation information is not intended to convey all specific regulatory data relating to this material. For complete transportation information, contact an Air Products customer service representative.

15. REGULATORY INFORMATION

6/7

Air Products and Chemicals,Inc   Oxygen

Courtesy of Air Products and Chemicals, Inc.

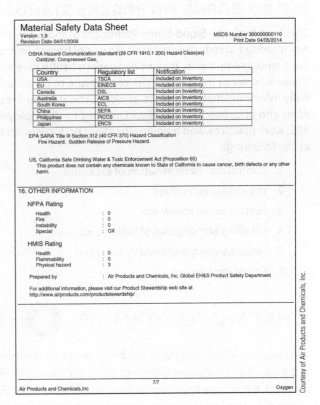

Material Safety Data Sheet

Version 1.9
Revision Date 04/01/2009

MSDS Number 300000000110
Print Date 04/05/2014

OSHA Hazard Communication Standard (29 CFR 1910.1 200) Hazard Class(es)
Oxidizer. Compressed Gas.

Country	Regulatory list	Notification
USA	TSCA	Included on Inventory.
EU	EINECS	Included on Inventory.
Canada	DSL	Included on Inventory.
Australia	AICS	Included on Inventory.
South Korea	ECL	Included on Inventory.
China	SEPA	Included on Inventory.
Philippines	PICCS	Included on Inventory.
Japan	ENCS	Included on Inventory.

EPA SARA Title III Section 312 (40 CFR 370) Hazard Classification
Fire Hazard. Sudden Release of Pressure Hazard.

US. California Safe Drinking Water & Toxic Enforcement Act (Proposition 65)
This product does not contain any chemicals known to State of California to cause cancer, birth defects or any other harm.

16. OTHER INFORMATION

NFPA Rating

Health	: 0
Fire	: 0
Instability	: 0
Special	: OX

HMIS Rating

Health	: 0
Flammability	: 0
Physical hazard	: 3

Prepared by   : Air Products and Chemicals, Inc. Global EH&S Product Safety Department

For additional information, please visit our Product Stewardship web site at
http://www.airproducts.com/productstewardship/

7/7

Air Products and Chemicals,Inc   Oxygen

Courtesy of Air Products and Chemicals, Inc.

Figure 10-2 *(Continued)* A safety data sheet must be maintained for each chemical used in a facility.

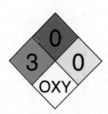

Figure 10-3 The National Fire Protection Association hazard identification symbol.

TRAINING OF EMPLOYEES

Because of the importance of safety in the workplace, the employer must provide special training sessions during working hours at no cost to employees. Training must be provided at the initial time of employment and then annually if there are new procedures. Training material must be appropriate for the literacy and education level of the employee. It must be interactive and permit questions and answers.

POINTS TO REMEMBER

For employee and client safety, safety regulations should be carefully monitored and followed. Job descriptions should identify anything that could potentially cause exposure to hazardous chemicals and blood-borne pathogens.

BLOOD-BORNE PATHOGENS STANDARD

OSHA set forth the Blood-borne Pathogens Standard in 1991 to improve infection control education. The standard was intended to reduce occupational cases of human immunodeficiency virus (HIV) and hepatitis B virus (HBV) infections among employees. It identified various health care and emergency response personnel as *category I employees* (those who are at the greatest risk of exposure to communicable diseases from blood, body fluids, and other potentially infectious materials while at work). The standard requires category I employers to develop *exposure control plans* and offer free hepatitis B vaccinations to all employees. It also requires standards concerning record keeping, PPE, work practices, and training. The standard focuses on ways to limit exposure to blood-borne pathogens, as well as the following:

1. Control and determination of exposure
2. Universal precautions
3. Postexposure follow-up
4. Labeling and disposal of biologic wastes
5. Housekeeping and laundry functions
6. Employee training

WHAT WOULD YOU DO?

A customer who had a cut on his hand came to a community pharmacy and asked a pharmacy technician where the gauze and bandages were kept. While standing in front of the prescription counter, some of his blood dropped onto it. If you were the pharmacy technician, what would you do?

LATEX ALLERGY

Latex, made from Brazilian rubber trees, may cause certain individuals to experience an allergic response to the proteins it contains. Latex gloves are a commonly used product that may transfer the allergen to the susceptible individual. If latex gloves are worn, they should be "low-allergen" and "powder-free." There are three types of allergic reactions to latex:

- Allergic contact dermatitis (the most common reaction)
- Irritant contact dermatitis
- Immediate hypersensitivity (which is a dangerous systemic reaction)

Latex is also present in other products such as blood pressure cuffs, catheters, stethoscopes, wound drains, and more. Approximately 8% to 12% of health care workers are sensitive to latex. Those who are allergic to latex should limit direct contact with other products containing latex and should use "latex-free" or "hypoallergenic" gloves made of either vinyl or nitrile.

FIRE SAFETY AND EMERGENCY PLAN

An OSHA-compliant **fire safety and emergency plan** must include written procedures. Exits must be marked and escape routes published (see Figure 10-4). Fire extinguishers and fire alarm pull boxes must be present, and the employer must provide fire prevention training, conduct fire drills, and test the fire alarm and sprinkler systems.

WHAT WOULD YOU DO?

You are working in the hospital pharmacy when the fire alarm goes off. Along the fire escape route, you see two patients who are trying to leave the building using the elevator. What would you do in this situation?

WORK-RELATED MUSCULOSKELETAL DISORDERS

About one-third of all occupational injuries reported by employers are work-related musculoskeletal disorders. Employers must provide information to their employees about common musculoskeletal disorders and hazards, how to report signs and symptoms of musculoskeletal disorders, the importance of reporting them quickly, and a summary of OSHA requirements and standards.

ERGONOMICS

Ergonomics is the science concerned with designing equipment and environments for human needs. Its goal is to optimize human well-being, comfort, and performance. Ergonomics is also referred to as "human engineering" and "human factors." Good design of chairs and desks, for example, reduces fatigue and discomfort, as well as potential injury. OSHA has its own ergonomics standard that employers should follow when designing work environments for their employees.

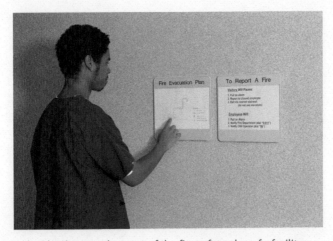

Figure 10-4 Escape routes must be clearly posted as part of the fire safety plan of a facility.

WHAT WOULD YOU DO?

A pharmacy employee lifting a heavy box experienced severe pain in the lumbar area of his back that radiated through his sciatic nerve and left him unable to move. To avoid this type of injury when lifting heavy objects, what would you do?

EXPOSURE CONTROL PLAN

The **exposure control plan** is designed to minimize risk of exposure to infectious material and blood-borne disease. The plan must be written and updated as necessary. OSHA also has regulations for or provides information about hazards associated with radioactive materials (see Figure 10-5).

IMMUNIZATIONS

OSHA regulations require that all health care workers be immunized against hepatitis B, because they are at risk for exposure to blood-borne pathogens. This vaccine must be available free of charge to all who are at risk for occupational exposure to blood-borne pathogens, whether they are full-time or part-time workers, within 10 days of starting employment. Employees may decline the immunization but must sign a declination form that is kept on file as a record of worker refusal. However, the employee may still receive the vaccine at a future date free of charge. For more information about the hepatitis B vaccination, see Chapter 24.

EXPOSURE TO RADIATION

Pharmacy technicians must be very careful to avoid exposure to radiopharmaceutical substances, as used in chemotherapy, which can negatively affect the tissues of the body. Increasing the distance between personnel and radiation sources, decreasing the amount of time personnel are in contact with radiation sources, monitoring radiation exposure with film badges, labeling all potentially radioactive materials, and using appropriate radiation shields can reduce radiation exposure.

MONITORING INJURIES AND RECORD KEEPING

Companies with more than 10 employees must maintain records of all work-related injuries and illnesses. All employees and their representatives have the right to review these records. Minor, work-related injuries must be recorded if they result in a restriction of work or motion, transfer to another job, loss of consciousness, termination of employment, or medical treatment. Employers may keep records on paper or in a computer, utilizing specific record-keeping forms available from OSHA. Record keeping is an important part of an employer's health and safety efforts. Keeping track of work-related injuries can help prevent them in the future. Illness and injury data can be used

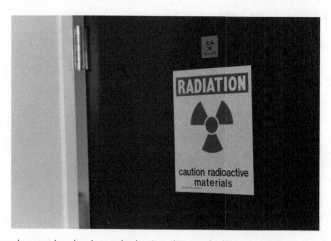

Figure 10-5 Radioactive hazards must be clearly marked using this symbol.

to identify problem areas. Potentially hazardous workplace conditions may be focused on before a serious incident occurs. Company safety and health programs may be administered more effectively when accurate records are kept. Certain establishments are exempt from keeping these types of records, and a list of exempt employers may be found on OSHA's website (www.osha.gov).

Standards and Regulations within the Pharmacy Profession

State boards of pharmacy implement highly specific standards and regulations for the pharmacy profession. Individual facilities may also have certain rules and standards which their employees are expected to uphold. Pharmacy technicians must always follow their employer's policies and procedures for storing, compounding, preparing, and dispensing medications. As a result, they must be familiar with the rules and regulations of their board of pharmacy, as well as those of OSHA.

SAFELY PREPARING MEDICATIONS

Medication errors can be reduced by limiting the amount of medications stored, volumes of medications, and the number of concentrations of each medication. Safely preparing medications is essential in avoiding patient harm. When a pharmacy technician prepares, compounds, or dispenses medications, great care must be taken to avoid contamination with microorganisms that may occur during preparation. Hand hygiene and clean technique are critical. During compounding, injury or harm to the technician or co-workers must be prevented, with employees observing OSHA regulations concerning needle sticks and injury with other sharps. Care should also be taken with medication bags and all other equipment in order to avoid spills, contamination, and transfer of blood-borne pathogens.

SAFE HANDLING OF HAZARDOUS MATERIALS

When cytotoxic or hazardous drugs are prepared and compounded, there is a high potential for skin contact, splashing, and inhalation of toxic elements. The term "cytotoxic" means "toxic to cells" and has been linked to the development of cancer. Therefore, for cytotoxic or hazardous drugs, safe handling during the activities of withdrawal of medications from vials, opening of ampoules, and expelling air from a syringe when measuring medications is essential. In order to minimize exposure, these medications should be prepared within a vertical laminar airflow hood.

Proper protective equipment for these medications includes non-powdered latex or hypoallergenic gloves and a disposable gown with elastic or knit cuffs. In order to reduce internal pressure, vials should be vented prior to use. External surfaces that may have come in contact with a cytotoxic medication should be wiped down with alcohol pads. Ampoules should be snapped open by holding an alcohol pad over the breakage point, offering further protection from injury. Hands should be washed after glove removal and between glove changes.

Proper handling and disposal of cytotoxic and hazardous medications is essential in reducing potential exposures. Disposal guidelines set forth by local, state, and federal agencies must be adhered to. Radiation standards controlled by the state board of pharmacy include limits for radiation doses, levels of radiation in an area, and concentrations of radioactivity in the air and wastewater. Limits also exist for the amount of radioactivity in disposed waste, according to the U.S. Nuclear Regulatory Commission (www.nrc.gov).

In case of contact with cytotoxic medications, the area of contact should be thoroughly washed with soap and water. A scrub brush should not be used because it may compromise the integrity of the skin. Eyes should be immediately flushed with water for at least 15 minutes. Anyone exposed to cytotoxic medications must be taken to the emergency room.

SPILLS AND CLEANUP

Pharmacies have spill cleanup kits in areas where potentially harmful chemicals and substances are used. These kits should be used to clean up most spills. Absorbents and neutralizers in these kits (see Figure 10-6) are designed to clean up acids, alkalis, and other substances. If a biohazard (such as blood) is spilled, bleach is recommended for the cleanup. It will kill any pathogens that may be carried. If an extremely toxic substance is spilled, it is advisable that

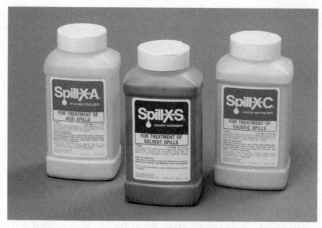

Figure 10-6 Absorbent substances used to clean hazardous chemical spills.

a specially trained hazardous cleanup team be called in. The following steps should be followed when a hazardous material is spilled:

- Put on gloves and PPE.
- Bring appropriate supplies and a hazardous waste container to the area.
- Pick up broken glass with tongs or other equipment—never use your hands.
- Dispose of broken glass in an approved manner.
- Wipe up the spill with appropriate materials from the spill kit, according to the policies and procedures manual.
- Dispose of used cleaning materials in a biohazard container.
- After cleaning the area, disinfect with an approved disinfectant.
- Remove gloves and discard them properly.
- Wash your hands thoroughly.

Universal Precautions

Universal precautions are a set of guidelines for infection control requiring the employer and employee to assume that all human blood and specified human body fluids are infectious for HIV, HBV, and other blood-borne pathogens. Universal precautions should be used if the health care worker is exposed to blood, other body fluids containing visible blood, semen, vaginal secretions, cerebrospinal fluid, pleural fluid, synovial fluid, and any other body fluids. A health care worker should also use universal precautions if exposed to urine, feces, nasal secretions, sputum, breast milk, tears, saliva, and vomitus. In addition, a health care worker should use universal precautions when dealing with broken skin and the mucous membranes inside the mouth, nose, and body cavities.

HAZARDOUS WASTE MANAGEMENT

Hazardous materials include any substance that is not clean, disinfected, or sterilized, or that is corrosive (able to destroy metal), cytotoxic, ignitable (able to create fires), radioactive, reactive (unstable wastes that can cause fumes or explosions), toxic, or caustic (able to burn or otherwise harm people or animals). These materials may be either liquids, gases, sludges, or solids. The EPA categorizes hazardous wastes into three groups:

- F-list: nonspecific source wastes
- K-list: source-specific wastes
- P-list or U-list: discarded commercial chemicals

Safe handling of hazardous materials is essential at all times. Proper protective equipment should be worn to minimize potential contact with hazardous materials. Proper hazardous waste management includes regulations that concern the following:

- Air emissions
- Closure of containers
- Monitoring of ground water
- Proper cleanup
- Restrictions on land disposal
- Strict permitting procedures

DISPOSAL OF HAZARDOUS WASTE

Any materials that have come into contact with blood or body fluids are treated as hazardous waste. Various containers are used to collect hazardous material. Waste containers are labeled with the **biohazard symbol** to ensure that all employees are aware of the contents (see Figure 10-7). Plastic bags are used for gloves, paper towels, dressings, and other soft material; rigid containers are used for sharps such as needles, glass slides, scalpel blades, or disposable syringes (see Figure 10-8). Most facilities contract with a company that specializes in removal and disposal of hazardous waste. Cleaning staff should be instructed not to empty hazardous waste containers. When health care workers change hazardous waste bags, they must wear gloves, masks, and protective eyewear; close the bags securely; and put the bag inside a second hazardous waste bag (double bag) if there is any chance of leakage.

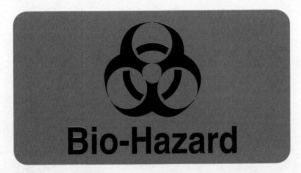

Figure 10-7 Biohazard symbols alert the pharmacy technician to hazardous materials.

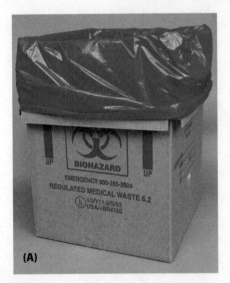
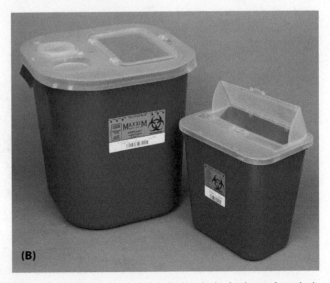

Figure 10-8 (A). Hazardous materials must only be disposed of in the containers properly labeled with the biohazard symbol. (B). Any sharp items must be disposed of in a hard plastic "sharps" container.

USE OF PERSONAL PROTECTIVE EQUIPMENT

A health care worker must use appropriate PPE, such as gloves, gowns, masks, and surgical gowns with cuffs, hair covers, shoe covers, and possibly face shields or goggles, to protect himself or herself from exposure to pathogens (disease-causing microorganisms). These items serve as **barrier precautions**. This equipment is used to place a barrier between the employee and blood or bodily fluids along with other methods of compliance to prevent exposure that can contaminate skin, mucous membranes, or nonintact skin. Gloves must be worn when there is a possibility of hand contact with blood or bodily fluids, mucous membranes, or nonintact skin. Masks, face shields, and goggles must be used if there is a risk of splashing or splattering of blood or bodily fluids. Gowns, laboratory coats, or scrubs must be worn to protect against exposure and must be left at the work site in an area set aside for their storage. Eyewash stations are required in each facility by law for emergencies. If an employee is exposed to chemicals or body fluids at work, he or she must be able to flush out the eyes at the eyewash station and flush mucous membranes with water as soon as possible after contact of the eyes with blood or chemical substances (see Figure 10-9). Proper PPE

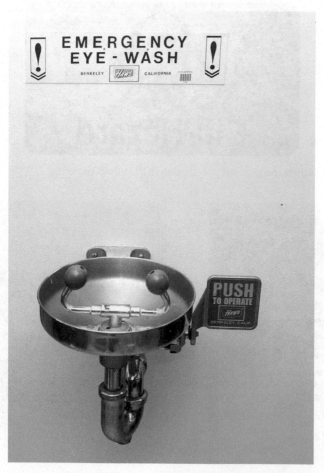

Figure 10-9 Eyewash stations must be available for emergency decontamination if a worker is exposed to chemicals or blood substances.

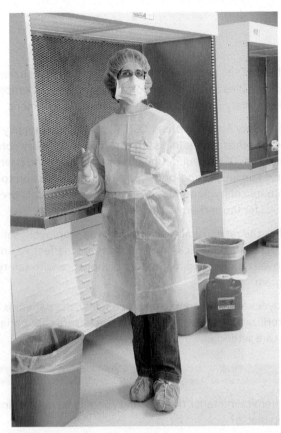

Figure 10-10 Proper personal protective equipment must be worn at all times. This photo shows a pharmacy technician who is ready for sterile compounding.

for compounding sterile medications is required by USP Chapter <797>. Technicians must comply with the proper use of PPE while compounding to prevent microbial contamination of sterile products due to human exposure. Figure 10-10 shows a pharmacy technician who is ready for sterile compounding.

Employee Responsibilities

Although OSHA does not cite employees for violations of their responsibilities, each employee shall comply with all occupational safety and health standards and all rules, regulations, and orders issued under the act that are applicable. Employee responsibilities and rights in a state that has its own occupational safety and health programs are generally the same as those for workers in states using federal OSHA regulations. An employee should do the following:

- Read the OSHA poster at the job site.

- Comply with all applicable OSHA standards.

- Follow all employer safety and health rules and regulations, and wear or use prescribed protective equipment while working.

- Report hazardous conditions to the supervisor.

- Report any job-related injury or illness to the employer and seek treatment promptly.

- Cooperate with the OSHA compliance officer conducting an inspection if he or she inquires about safety and health conditions in the workplace.

- Exercise rights under the act in a responsible manner.

Summary

Workplace safety is a responsibility of the employer and the employee. It is a shared responsibility that protects the employer from noncompliance penalties and, more importantly, protects the employee's health. Patient health and safety are also protected by sound safety practices in the health care environment.

The Occupational Health and Safety Administration (OSHA) is the federal agency that is responsible for workplace safety rules and the enforcement of those rules. In health care, OSHA's primary concern is protection of employees from biological and chemical hazards. OSHA requires health care employers to have a written exposure control plan that outlines protective measures against blood-borne pathogen transmission to employees. OSHA also requires employers to have a written chemical hygiene plan that outlines chemicals present in the workplace and safe handling and disposal procedures for those chemicals.

The health care employee has the responsibility to abide by the employer's safety policies and procedures. The best-written exposure control plans and chemical hygiene plans are ineffective unless employees understand and follow the written plans. Employee training and mandatory compliance with safety procedures are essential for an effective workplace safety program.

When employers and employees are attuned to workplace safety, the patient is also protected. Closely followed procedures for disinfection, sterilization, and aseptic technique ensure that patients are not exposed to harmful biological agents in the health care setting.

REVIEW QUESTIONS

1. For each hazardous chemical material, the pharmacy should be able to find a safety data sheet (SDS) from which of the following places?

   A. Office depot
   B. Post office
   C. Manufacturer
   D. Government authority

2. Universal precautions should be followed if the pharmacy technician is exposed to which of the following?

   A. Radioactive substances
   B. Chemical materials
   C. Dangerous gases
   D. Human body fluids

3. The Occupational and Safety and Health Act established the:

   A. Department of Labor.
   B. OSHA.
   C. DHHS.
   D. HIPAA.

4. Employers must provide safety training to employees:

   A. upon hiring them.
   B. upon firing them.
   C. if they are expectant mothers.
   D. at least once a month.

5. Exits must be marked and escape routes published on a(n):

   A. exposure control plan.
   B. hazard communication plan.
   C. fire safety and emergency plan.
   D. OSHA poster.

6. OSHA requires that employers with more than 10 employees:

    A. maintain vacation records.
    B. must record injuries that happen to their employees at home.
    C. keep records only if they feel it necessary.
    D. maintain records of all work-related injuries and illnesses.

7. Universal precautions are a set of guidelines for infection control requiring the employer and employee to assume that all human blood and specified human body fluids are:

    A. radioactive.
    B. infectious for HIV, hepatitis B, and other blood-borne pathogens.
    C. viral.
    D. disease-causing.

8. Any materials that have come into contact with blood or body fluids are treated as:

    A. sterile.
    B. aseptic.
    C. hazardous waste.
    D. disposable.

9. Hazardous waste should be disposed of by:

    A. certified pharmacy technicians only.
    B. licensed pharmacists only.
    C. only a licensed hazardous waste disposal company.
    D. none of the above.

10. Splattering of blood onto skin or mucous membranes is a proven mode of transmission of:

    A. hepatitis B virus.
    B. hepatitis A virus.
    C. influenza.
    D. tuberculosis.

11. Which of the following should be done if you have a known sensitivity to latex gloves?

    A. Do not wear gloves at all.
    B. Put powder in the gloves.
    C. Wrap gauze on your hands and then put on the gloves.
    D. Ask for non-latex gloves.

12. OSHA is part of which of the following departments?

    A. Department of Law
    B. Department of Safety
    C. Department of Labor
    D. Department of Human Rights

13. "Carcinogenic" is defined as able to:

    A. destroy metal.
    B. cause burns.
    C. cause fires.
    D. cause cancer.

14. Which of the following refers to the designing of equipment to maximize productivity by lessening the discomfort and fatigue of employees?

    A. Universal precautions
    B. Barrier precautions
    C. Ergonomics
    D. Exposure control

15. What is the minimum amount of time that a pharmacy technician should allow for the rinsing of the eyes after contact with a potentially hazardous substance?

    A. 5 minutes

    B. 10 minutes

    C. 15 minutes

    D. 20 minutes

CRITICAL THINKING

A pharmacy technician was sent to a hospital for his externship. The pharmacist at the hospital pharmacy asked him to review the policies and procedures manual concerning OSHA standards to familiarize himself with them.

1. Describe the importance of safety precautions in the pharmacy setting. How do these needs differ in the hospital and retail pharmacy?

2. What vaccinations must a pharmacy technician maintain to protect himself or herself while on the job? Are there pros and cons to these vaccines? Would you choose to obtain the vaccines or opt not to get the vaccine? Why or why not?

WEB LINKS

Allergy Home: www.allergyhome.org

American Red Cross: www.redcross.org

Centers for Disease Control and Prevention: www.cdc.gov

Ergonomics.org: ergonomics.org

Immunization Action Coalition: www.immunize.org

National Fire Safety Protection Association: www.nfpa.org

Occupational Health & Safety Administration: www.osha.gov

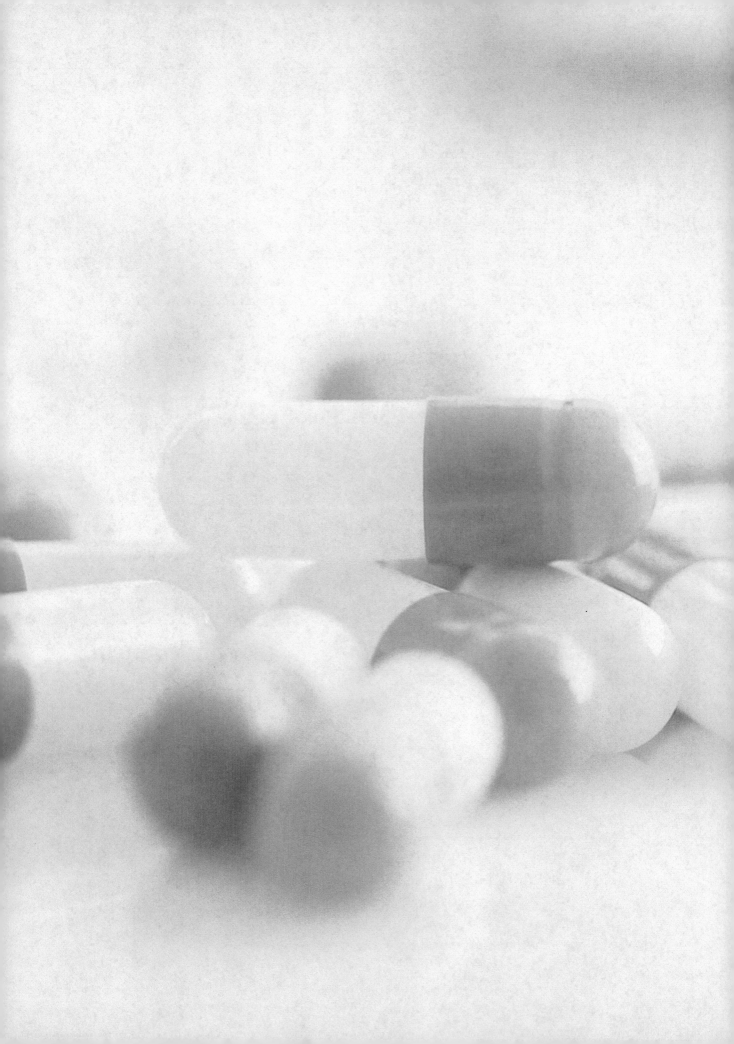

Hospital Pharmacy

OUTLINE

Maintaining Privacy
Auditing and Reporting of Medication Processes
Communication Skills
Working Safely and Cooperatively
Regulatory Agencies That Oversee Hospital Pharmacy
Future of Hospital Pharmacy

OBJECTIVES

Upon completion of this chapter, the reader should be able to:

1. Describe various services of the hospital pharmacy.
2. Explain medication orders.
3. Define the terms "floor stock" and "point-of-entry system."
4. Explain the advantages of computerized physician order entry (CPOE) systems.
5. Describe the patient prescription system.
6. Explain the unit-dose drug distribution system and its advantages.
7. Describe the use of unit-dose liquids.
8. Explain the entering of medication orders into the hospital information system.
9. List the duties of pharmacy technicians in the hospital pharmacy.
10. Describe the information included in a hospital patient record.

KEY TERMS

ASAP medication order	**demand/stat medication order**	**The Joint Commission**	**standing order**
automation		**medication order**	**State Board of Pharmacy (BOP)**
Centers for Medicare & Medicaid Services (CMS)	**emergency medication order**	**patient prescription system**	
		PRN (as needed) medication order	**sterile product**
computerized physician order entry system (CPOE)	**floor stock system**		**unit-dose drug distribution system**
	group purchasing	**scheduled intravenous (IV)/ total parenteral nutrition (TPN) solution order**	
controlled substance medication order	**hospital pharmacy**		
Department of Public Health (DPH)	**investigational medication order**	**scheduled medication order**	

Overview

In the hospital setting, the practice of pharmacy combines support, product, clinical, and educational services to provide all-encompassing medical care. Dispensing processes have become much more sophisticated than in the past in response to the need to handle a variety of different types of medication orders. The unit-dose system of drug distribution has become the preeminent method used by hospital pharmacies, reducing errors, cost, unused medication, and drug inventories. Hospital pharmacies control the cost of their inventories either by purchasing directly from pharmaceutical manufacturers or by using **group purchasing**, which involves many hospitals negotiating volume purchases together. The advent of pharmacy automation has increased the volume of medication transactions while maintaining accuracy. Robots are being used for many of the dispensing activities formerly done only by pharmacists or pharmacy technicians (see Figure 11-1). Many of the duties once exclusively performed by pharmacists, including compounding medication and inspecting the drug stocks of the nursing units, can now be performed by the pharmacy technician. With increased numbers of older adults requiring care, and an ever-increasing number of new medications being introduced to treat complex conditions, the future of the hospital pharmacy looks very bright.

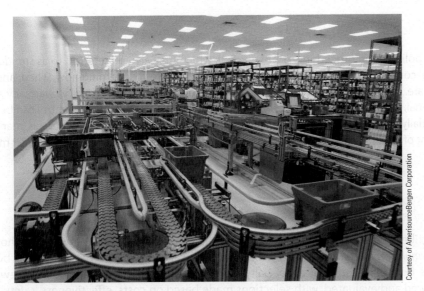

Courtesy of AmerisourceBergen Corporation

Figure 11-1 Automated dispensing unit.

What Is Hospital Pharmacy?

In the simplest terms **hospital pharmacy**, in today's practice setting, can be defined as the provision of pharmaceutical services within an institutional or hospital setting. The practice of pharmacy within an institution comprises several types of services:

- Support services—ordering and properly storing medications and maintaining an inventory of pharmaceuticals and associated medical supplies, billing for services, and installing and maintaining computer systems

- Product services—dispensing, preparing, and processing medication orders for inpatients and maintaining required patient records and drug control records

- Clinical services—managing the formulary system, evaluating drug use, and reviewing drug orders for appropriateness

- Educational services—providing education about medications to pharmacy staff, other health care professionals, the public, and patients and their caregivers

Hospital pharmacy practice now encompasses all aspects of drug therapy through the total continuum of medical care.

MEDICATION ERROR ALERT

According to the United States Library of Medicine and National Institutes of Health, studies have shown that an average of 3.6% of medication doses filled by hospital pharmacy technicians contain errors. However, of these errors, only 79% were detected during routine verification, meaning that 0.75% of incorrect doses filled left the hospital pharmacy to be administered to patients.

POINTS TO REMEMBER

The principal organization associated with accreditation of hospitals is The Joint Commission. The Joint Commission standards address services provided in organized health care settings.

Policies and Procedures

Every pharmacy has a policies and procedures (P&P) manual, which may also be referred to as *standard operating procedures*. The manual contains the facility's polices, rules, and procedures concerning how, when, and why things are done the way they are. This forms the *protocol* of the facility, and the rules apply to every pharmacy employee. By following the P&P manual, patients are kept safe, and both quality assurance and quality control can be maintained. The manual describes daily work routines, responsibilities, benefits, emergency situation protocols, mandatory training, and a large amount of vital information. The pharmacy technician must be familiar with the P&P manual for his or her hospital.

Hospital Protocol

The term *protocol* describes hospital guidelines. This includes the *formulary medications*, which are those approved for use, and the *non-formulary medications*, which are not approved. Each formulary is developed by a board of pharmacists and physicians, from different medical specialty areas, who do not work for the hospital. New and current medications are reviewed and evaluated, with selections made based on costs, effectiveness, safety, and patient demographics. When recommended criteria are not met, the medication is considered non-formulary and will not be included in the approved formulary list.

There is constant updating and enforcement of hospital protocol. Regularly, potential changes in protocol are discussed by the Pharmacy and Therapeutics Committee, made up of pharmacists, physicians, nurses, other health care professionals, and administrators. The committee chooses the best medications at the best costs. A *drug education coordinator* is a pharmacist who educates health care providers about protocol changes related to drug coverage. He or she assists the hospital pharmacy in implementing these changes. Sometimes, the drug education coordinator role is simply part of the duties of staff pharmacists or pharmacy managers.

Medication Orders

The practice of hospital pharmacy begins with the **medication order** generated by the physician. In the hospital pharmacy, the medication order is the equivalent to the prescription in the retail pharmacy. All medications, including prescription and over-the-counter (OTC), ordered in a hospital require a medication order. The medication fulfillment process begins in the pharmacy department when a copy of the original medication order is received in the department. The original physician's order can be a carbon copy or an electronically scanned copy.

The medication order must contain the following information (see Figure 11-2):

- Patient's name, height, weight, date of birth, medical record number, medical condition, and known allergies
- Drug and dosage schedule
- Instructions for preparing the drugs
- The exact dosage form of the drug
- The dosage strength
- Directions for use
- Route of administration

POINTS TO REMEMBER

A medication order is one part of a patient's chart. The other parts include the patient's diagnosis, imaging orders, laboratory orders, dietary requirements, and prescribed physical therapies. Pharmacy technicians should be familiar with patient charts to understand the medication order for each patient.

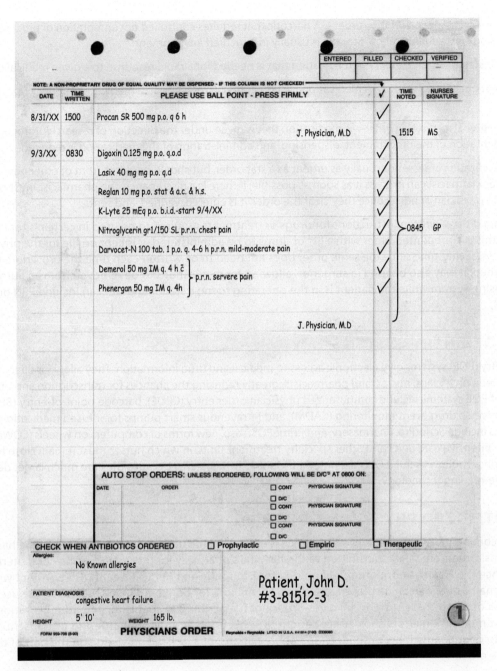

Figure 11-2 Sample physician's order.

Pharmacy technicians must be able to distinguish between various types of orders that are written on the medication order because there may be many orders on this document that do not pertain to the pharmacy. Medication orders may be stat orders, ASAP orders, or standing orders. Diet, laboratory, radiology, and physical activity orders are a few examples of non-medication orders. A variety of types of medication orders may also be encountered. The types of orders are the following:

- **Scheduled medication order**—A medication that is given on a continuous schedule according to the medication order.

- **Scheduled intravenous (IV)/total parenteral nutrition (TPN) solution order**—A medication that is given by the injectable route and must be prepared in a controlled environment.

- **PRN (as needed) medication order**—A medication that may be given in response to a given parameter or condition defined in the medication order. If the defined situation does not occur, the medication is not given.

- **Controlled substance medication order**—A narcotic that requires controlled documentation of procurement, dispensing, and administration. Storage is usually in a secured environment.

- **Demand/stat medication order**—A medication that is needed for a rapid response to a given medical condition.

- **Emergency medication order**—A medication that is needed in response to a medical emergency (e.g., cardiac arrest).

- **Investigational medication order**—A medication that is given under the direction of research protocols. Strict documentation of the procurement, dispensing, and administration of the medication is required.

- **ASAP medication order**—not usually as urgent as a stat order, but should be put in front of other new orders so that the pharmacist can process it as soon as possible; if there is a discrepancy, the pharmacist must contact the patient's physician or nurse; once they clear the order, it is entered, verified, and sent.

- **Standing order**—written instructions for drugs or treatments required to be used in certain situations; often, this is a preprinted order with a list of drugs to be administered; it is kept on file for the physician to access, saving time since the same order does not need to be written each time the procedure is performed; it may also be used in surgeries, allowing for medications to be removed from an automated dispensing system while the patient is in the operating room; a standing order can include PRN orders (see earlier).

POINT-OF-ENTRY SYSTEMS

Point-of-entry (POE) systems give electronic access to medical and drug information. They allow for direct communication between physicians, nurses, and pharmacists, greatly reducing the chances for transcription and other errors. Examples of POE systems include computerized physician order entry (CPOE), barcode point-of-entry (BPOE), computerized adverse drug event monitoring (CADM), and intravenous smart pumps for infused medications. Popular POE systems include ScriptPro, Pharmaserv, and PrimePOS. Also, new forms of computers on wheels (COWs) are used primarily in intensive care units and other specialty treatment units, in which nurses must remain close to patients for monitoring. Though useful, COWs are not as efficient as POE systems because they are much larger devices and lack barcode-reading technology.

COMPUTERIZED PHYSICIAN ORDER ENTRY

CPOE is becoming more popular in hospitals since it eliminates the need to read and interpret the handwriting of physicians. Orders are safely transmitted to the hospital's pharmacy for processing, using computerized entry of data. Since the Health Information Technology for Economic and Clinical Health (HITECH) Act was passed in 2009, penalties have been instituted, of up to $1.5 million, for noncompliance regarding the use of CPOE. The process of using these systems involves ordering, transcribing, dispensing, and administration. Studies of inpatient medication errors showed that about 90% occurred at either the ordering or transcribing stage, often due to poor handwriting, misunderstood abbreviations, or a lack of knowledge on the part of the person creating the order.

Medication errors are greatly reduced by use of these systems, which can check a patient's new medications against those already being administered, for contraindications or interactions. The computer alerts the user about possible problems between medications, and the order is not allowed to continue until the problem is handled appropriately. Using patient diagnoses and parameters, CPOE systems check for correct dosage selection. Providers enter laboratory results, medications, dietary needs, and special notes. All patient information is accessible immediately. Medication orders are directly transmitted to the pharmacy, meaning that no orders are lost. Also, the CPOE system allows codes to be created if the product does not have a code from the manufacturer. This system is usually paired with some type of clinical decision support system (CDSS), which helps prevent errors during the ordering and dispensing stages and also improves safety of orders. Most CDSS systems suggest default values for medication doses, routes of administration, and dosage frequency. They check for drug allergies, drug–drug interactions, and even drug–laboratory problems, such as warning against the use of a nephrotoxic medication for a patient who has elevated creatinine. They prevent against excessive doses, failing to order a medication that is needed as prophylaxis for a condition, and against overuse of radiologic studies and other procedures.

BARCODE POINT-OF-ENTRY

BPOE systems allow nurses and other service providers to be electronically connected to the hospital pharmacy. Medication dosages are checked for accuracy right at the patient's bedside. There is a barcode on every unit-dose medication. The barcode is scanned using a handheld device. The information is linked to the pharmacy and the electronic medication administration record (E-MAR). As the dose is verified, the nurse is alerted to special warnings or notes. Any problems between a current medication order and the scanner will detect a medication sent from the pharmacy, with an alert given to the nurse. This includes a medication order that has been recently discontinued, so that the nurse cannot administer a dose that is no longer supposed to be given, according to the physician. The nurse must verify each order prior to medication administration. If there is a discrepancy, the nurse can communicate with the pharmacy for clarification. This *real-time*, constant communication increases the quality of patient care. BPOE systems are designed to ensure medication administration that is safe, correct, timely, effective, and thoroughly documented.

In the E-MAR, there is complete documentation of vital signs and other chart notes, which are directly entered onto the E-MAR from the patient's bedside. Information may include blood pressure, levels of pain, respiration rate, and many other parameters. Verifying dosages at the bedside helps ensure the *five rights of medication safety*: the *right person*, the *right dose*, the *right time*, the *right medication*, and the *right route*. Time needed for charting is reduced, less paperwork is generated, and more time can be spent between the nurse and patient. Examples of E-MAR systems include ChartMeds, HCS-eMAR, and CareSuite.

COMPUTERIZED MONITORING FOR ADVERSE DRUG REACTIONS

Computerized monitoring for adverse drug reaction is a system allowing for detection and monitoring of adverse drug events. These CADM systems have been used by pharmacies for many years, but today they have become integrated into CPOE and electronic health record (EHR) systems. Difficulties in integration of these systems include the need to barcode each and every medication for identification and ensuring that computerized information correctly shows how each dosage form is to be administered. There must be accurate training of pharmacists, physicians, and nurses to become used to these systems, and continued analysis is required for accuracy and interactions between other systems in use. It is important that the chosen CADM system is not too complicated to use. Today, more hospitals are using CADM systems because of improved simplicity and accuracy. Examples include DoseEdge, Omnicell, and Grifols-IV, which are designed for pharmacy technicians to prepare intravenous medications with scans and barcoding of each ingredient prior to the final product being compounded. This allows the supervising pharmacist to accurately assess whether the final product contains the exact amounts of required medications.

Medication Dispensing Systems

The role of the pharmacist has changed from being a product dispenser to having expanding responsibility for the entire medication process. Medication dispensing systems have changed to support this increasing responsibility. In the past, medications were stored in the pharmacy in bulk quantities. The medications were then dispensed in bulk quantities and multidose containers to "mini" pharmacies located on the patient care units. Nurses prepared doses for administration to patients. This system has evolved into sophisticated unit-dose and automated dispensing processes to allow pharmacists and their support personnel to concentrate on the final preparation of the medications for administration to the patient and the monitoring of the proper use of medications.

THE FLOOR STOCK SYSTEM

In the **floor stock system**, the role of the pharmacy in the medication process is product related, only. Drugs are purchased in bulk and multidose dosage forms. The drugs are issued to patient care units using a bulk drug order form and are stored in medication rooms. Once placed in the medication room, drugs for administration to patients are prepared by a nurse. A medication could be used for more than one patient. In this system, the nurse is responsible for most of the steps in the medication process.

The disadvantages of this system are the following:

- Potential for medication errors
- Potential for drug diversion and misappropriation, resulting in economic loss

- Increased inventory needs
- Inadequate space for medication storage on the patient care unit

PATIENT PRESCRIPTION SYSTEM

In an attempt to improve on the floor stock system, the **patient prescription system** was developed. In this system, the nurse orders medications on a specific patient form. The information is transcribed by the nurse from the medication order prepared by the physician to this medication order form. The pharmacy then dispenses a three-day supply of medication. The nurse still prepares the medications for administration to the patient. The pharmacy still has little patient information and cannot properly monitor medication utilization. The system is an improvement over the floor stock system but is an inefficient method of drug distribution.

UNIT-DOSE MEDICATIONS

In response to the increasing availability of new and more complex medications, pharmacists are expected to play an expanded role in the medication process. The distribution system that evolved as a result is the **unit-dose drug distribution system**. It is considered to be the safest, most efficient, most effective medication system for distributing medications. The features of the unit-dose system are the following:

- A copy of the original physician's order is received by the pharmacy and is used as the dispensing document.
- Medications, including liquid and injectable medications, are prepared by the pharmacy technician or pharmacist in ready-to-use forms and are dispensed per individual patient.
- Individual doses of medications are labeled (see Figure 11-3).
- The pharmacy receives more patient information, including drug allergies, weight, and, usually, a medication history.
- No more than a 24-hour supply of medication is dispensed.

The advantages of using the unit-dose drug distribution system are the following:

- Reduction in medication errors
- Improved medication control
- Decreased overall cost of medication distribution
- More precise medication billing
- Reduction in medication credits (medications returned unused)
- Reduced drug inventories

MEDICATION ERROR ALERT

Medication errors in hospitals that adversely affect patient care can be reduced through the following steps: increased staffing of clinical pharmacists, drug therapy monitoring that is pharmacist supervised, drug information services provided by pharmacists, adverse drug reaction management that is pharmacist assisted, drug histories of patients taken during admission by pharmacists, and drug counseling by pharmacists at the time of hospital discharge.

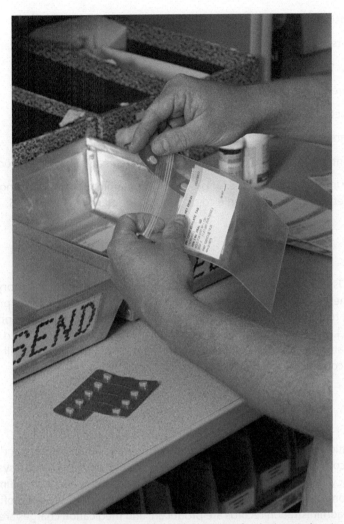

Figure 11-3 The pharmacy technician prepares a single dose of medication for the hospital patient in the unit-dose system.

UNIT-DOSE LIQUIDS

Because of improved standards designed to reduce medication errors (see Chapter 18), The Joint Commission now requires hospitals to make all medications specific to each dose for each patient. Therefore, every liquid dose is required to be prepared in a unit-dose package, and labeled, prior to being sent to the patient's room. There may be a separate room in the hospital, in which the preparation of all oral liquid medications is performed, often using oral syringes in the process. Some pharmacies make their own unit-dose cups from a bulk stock, with the pharmacy technician following specific repackaging guidelines. Prior to today's standards, bulk liquid items were sent to the patient's floor of the hospital in a bulk container, which would remain there until it was empty. These reduced the need to place several unit-dose cups into a small cassette drawer but meant that errors were more likely to occur.

Sterile Products

The term **sterile product** is usually associated with drugs that are administered by injection or are intended for oph-thalmic use. A sterile product contains no living microorganisms. When a product of this nature that is not available commercially is required, the responsibility for preparing the medication resides in the pharmacy department. The pharmacy department will do the following:

- Ensure that the person preparing these products is properly and carefully trained in the use of aseptic technique.

- Prepare the product in an environment (clean room and laminar flow hood) that will prevent contamination.

- Prepare the product using aseptic technique to prevent contamination.
- Ensure that all contents of the preparation are chemically, physically, and therapeutically compatible.
- Ensure that the product is stable over the time it is to be used.
- Ensure that the prepared product is stored under proper conditions.
- Ensure that the product is labeled properly.
- Keep records of preparation.
- Use proper quality control processes to ensure that a proper preparation has been produced.

Hand washing is a very important procedure for preventing contamination. In preparing sterile products, the primary concern must be safety and accuracy. Sterile compounding is detailed in Chapter 15.

Inventory Control

The director of pharmacy is responsible for maintaining an adequate medication inventory and establishing specifications for the procurement of all drugs, chemicals, and biologic agents related to the practice of pharmacy. This duty is usually delegated to a pharmacy buyer or pharmacy technician. Customers of pharmacy services expect drugs to be available quickly and cheaply, to be of high quality, and to have been stored properly. In the hospital pharmacy, the pharmacy and therapeutics committee determines which medications will be purchased and maintained in stock. Inventory control is discussed in detail in Chapter 17.

Automation

Automation is the automatic control or operation of equipment, processes, or systems, and it often involves robotic machinery controlled by computers. The advent of automation (pharmacy information systems) has improved the efficiencies of the pharmacy. Automation provides the ability to rapidly process large volumes of medication orders accurately and quickly. From the automated processing of medication orders, patient profiles are generated; medication labels, fill lists, and administration records are produced; and medication charges are processed. Some disadvantages of the increased involvement of the pharmacy in the medication process are the need for massive amounts of information and the need to process many transactions quickly. No matter how efficient automation may be, however, it always requires someone to supervise because it is not a perfect system (see Figure 11-4).

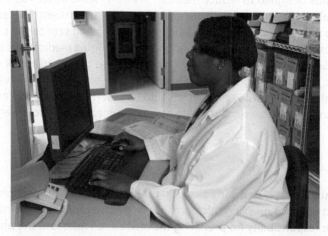

Figure 11-4 Pharmacy information systems within the hospital allow processing of massive amounts of information, resulting in quicker and more efficient service.

Clinical screening can occur to check for drug interactions, drug allergies, and dosage ranges. Reports can also be generated to produce data to monitor appropriate drug utilization. Utilization and usage data from the pharmacy information system can be used to order and maintain a medication inventory. One of the problems identified with this process is the medication order. It is a document handwritten by the physician, nurse practitioner, or physician's assistant that is prone to error because the handwriting may be illegible. Currently, in many facilities, the physician rather than the pharmacy staff is responsible for entering medication orders into the hospital information system. This type of system is generically called a **computerized physician order entry system (CPOE)**.

POINTS TO REMEMBER

Automation has the ability to simplify narcotic drug inventory and tracking records.

Many unit-dose systems use the 24-hour medication cart exchange process. These carts contain a 24-hour supply of medication for each patient on a patient care unit. The carts are usually filled by a pharmacy technician and checked by a pharmacist. A robotic device interfaced with the pharmacy information system will fill each patient medication tray in the cart. This robotic device is also capable of returning credited medication to proper stock locations. Automation is also used to create point-of-service storage cabinets that are interfaced with the pharmacy information system. Use of these cabinets eliminates the medication cart-filling process. An example of this type of automation is the automated dispensing cabinet. Many fear that the use of automation will decrease the need for pharmacy personnel. However, these devices require human intervention for appropriate use. The pharmacy technician of the future will be controlling these machines and providing proper maintenance, repair, and quality assurance processes. If mechanical failure occurs, manual backup processes must be in place, and human intervention will be needed to repair failed mechanical systems. Human intervention can never be replaced.

WHAT WOULD YOU DO?

A hospital physician quickly wrote a medication order for a cardiac medication, stat. Because of poor handwriting, the hospital pharmacy technician entered the wrong amount into the hospital pharmacy computer system. Fortunately, a dosage-checking component of the software alerted the pharmacy technician that the dosage was extremely high. If you were this pharmacy technician, what would you do?

The Responsibilities of Pharmacists in Hospitals

Hospital pharmacists have two major areas of responsibilities—dispensing and general responsibilities. A pharmacist's dispensing responsibilities include checking for accuracy of dispensed medications, medication control, ensuring proper compounding techniques, reviewing medication orders, supervising medication administration, and monitoring medication use. General responsibilities include documentation, training, education, establishment of policies and procedures, and evaluations of medical use.

MEDICATION ERROR ALERT

Hospital medication errors often occur because of miscommunication between a pharmacist and a physician or a nurse. When a pharmacist determines there is a risk to a patient if a certain prescription is filled, it is his or her job to consult with the physician. Often, a patient has more than one physician to treat multiple coexisting health conditions. In such cases, the pharmacist may be the only individual who knows all the medications the patient is being given.

The Roles and Duties of Pharmacy Technicians in Hospitals

The increasing complexity of health care in the modern hospital is creating ever-greater demands for the hospital pharmacy to broaden its scope of services. New health care legislation and rapid changes in health care technology are imposing new demands on hospital pharmacies, which result in a need for increased manpower. The scope of pharmaceutical services being provided in most hospitals is limited largely by personnel shortages. The time of the hospital pharmacist can be freed to a great extent by delegation of routine tasks to the pharmacy technician, under the supervision of the pharmacist. Supportive hospital pharmacy personnel are used in most hospitals today. Therefore, it is essential to understand the roles and duties of the technician in the hospital setting, as summarized in the following list:

- Following policies and procedures
- Maintaining medication records
- Maintaining competence
- Preparing unit doses
- Compounding medications
- Packaging
- Preparing all parenteral IV mixtures, including large-volume drips and parenteral nutrition
- Preparing and delivering prescriptions to nursing homes, hospice, and rehabilitation facilities
- Transporting medications throughout the hospital; including filling medication drawers in pharmacy carts
- Performing nursing floor inspection and pharmacy supply inspections
- Preparing cytotoxic agents and other medications accompanying these agents as part of chemotherapy
- Gathering controlled substance inventory sheets; filling and delivering controlled substances to the nursing floor, after review by the pharmacist
- Filling prescription orders as patients are discharged from hospitalization
- Filling all requisitions sent to the pharmacy
- Filling unit-dosing bulk medications
- Inputting computer data and answering phone calls
- Transcribing and retrieving medication orders
- Using automated medication dispensing systems
- Ensuring billing accuracy; handling invoices
- Inspecting nursing unit drug stocks to monitor medication control, security, and controlled substance accountability
- Stocking and ordering pharmacy inventory
- Controlling narcotic inventory and auditing narcotics when required
- Inventory maintenance including ordering specialty items, handling returns and recalled items
- Medication reconciliation for completeness and correctness, including for interactions, duplications
- Preparing labels
- Maintaining privacy
- Auditing and reporting of medication processes
- Communication skills

- Helping to train new technicians and pharmacist interns
- Working safely and cooperatively
- Participating in hospital committees relevant to work responsibilities, as required

FOLLOWING POLICIES AND PROCEDURES

Pharmacy technicians must follow the policies and procedures of the hospital in which they work. Policy and procedures manuals focus on general responsibilities, technical responsibilities, documentation, and reporting duties of pharmacy technicians and other pharmacy personnel. It is essential for pharmacy technicians to understand and follow these standards because they are accountable for all outcomes, including those that result from the failure to follow procedures.

MAINTAINING MEDICATION RECORDS

An important part of the job of the pharmacy technician is to accurately maintain the patient records on the pharmacy information system. Records should include the patient's weight, height, diagnosis, treatment, therapy, diet plans, blood and laboratory test results, and the name of the primary physician. Maintaining up-to-date records allows the pharmacist to provide better care and counseling of the patient.

MAINTAINING COMPETENCE

Pharmacy technicians must improve their skills and knowledge because the practice of pharmacy is growing and evolving more quickly than ever. To keep up with changing demands, it is essential to attend continuing education lectures, courses, and seminars. In fact, pharmacy technician recertification requires 20 continuing education credits (with one hour being focused on pharmacy law) every two years.

PREPARING UNIT DOSES

The pharmacy technician is responsible for preparing the unit doses for individual patients each day. The technician will prepare each day's doses of medication for all patients and place them in a unit-dose cart to be delivered to the patient care areas of the hospital. The pharmacist must check the cart before delivery to the patient care floors.

COMPOUNDING MEDICATIONS

In some circumstances, a drug may need to be created from a prepared recipe or formula (see Figure 11-5). If a written procedure exists for preparation of a drug, then the pharmacy technician can prepare it. This process is called compounding. To create a compound drug, the technician must be able to clearly understand the formula and be able to adjust it to increase or decrease amounts as necessary. A sound understanding of mathematical principles is required. Extemporaneous prescription compounding is discussed in detail in Chapter 14.

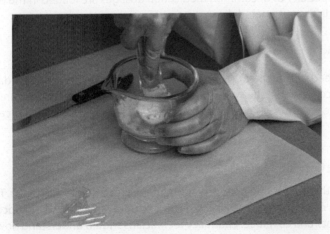

Figure 11-5 To compound a drug, the pharmacy technician must be able to accurately follow written procedures and formulas.

PACKAGING

Many drugs have to be placed in proper containers to remain active and potent. The pharmacy technician must be aware of these characteristics of drugs to properly choose the appropriate containers for dispensing and storing them. Packaging can also refer to packaging medications as unit doses.

PREPARING ALL PARENTERAL IV MIXTURES, INCLUDING LARGE-VOLUME DRIPS AND PARENTERAL NUTRITION

Pharmacy technicians prepare all types of parenteral intravenous mixtures. These include large-volume drips and parenteral nutrition. The pharmacy technician and the pharmacist who work in the IV room must update all changes in IV medication information. They must have specialized training and wear appropriate garb and equipment. Preoperative (preop) medications are usually ordered early in the morning, while postoperative (postop) medications are usually ordered later in the morning. Usually, the same pharmacy technician will prepare all IV medications.

Contamination of various types of admixtures by microorganisms may harm, permanently damage, or even cause the death of patients. As a result, pharmacy technicians must always utilize aseptic technique when preparing these products. Aseptic technique and admixtures are discussed in detail in Chapter 15.

PREPARING AND DELIVERING PRESCRIPTIONS TO NURSING HOMES, HOSPICE, AND REHABILITATION FACILITIES

Some hospitals are affiliated with facilities outside of the hospital itself, such as nursing homes and rehabilitation centers. The pharmacy technician is responsible for preparing the medications these facilities need, and for delivering them to the facilities in a timely manner.

TRANSPORTING MEDICATIONS THROUGHOUT THE HOSPITAL, INCLUDING FILLING MEDICATION DRAWERS IN PHARMACY CARTS

Pharmacy technicians often transport medications of all types throughout the hospital. Their duties also include filling medication drawers in pharmacy carts. Patient cassette drawers must be regularly loaded with the correct medications. Medications needed for the next day are loaded into the patient cassette drawer. Each morning, the pharmacy technician reads the daily medication record that is printed and fills the necessary medications into medication cassettes. Normally, routine medications are placed into these drawers in front, with the as-needed (prn) doses put in the back, separated by a divider. Patient cassette drawers are held in large pushcarts so that they can be delivered to various hospital floors every day. All medications are delivered to patient floors using two carts, which are rotated daily. All previous medications are emptied from the drawer before the next 24-hour supply is loaded into it. This helps reduce the likelihood of errors. Many hospitals use patient cassette drawers along with an automated dispensing system. Specialty or uncommon medication dosages are loaded in the cassettes, while commonly used medications are stock in the automated dispensing systems.

INPUTTING COMPUTER DATA

Data entry is an important part of the pharmacy technician's job. Accurate entry of new data into the computer system and maintenance of records within the system are important. The pharmacy then can be run efficiently because patient records are accurate, inventory is maintained at appropriate levels, and billing can be done in an accurate and timely manner.

ENSURING BILLING ACCURACY

During the billing process, there are many potential areas where inaccuracies can occur. This is due to the involved process of insurance claims, coding, and related forms. Failure to understand how this process works will cause errors in payments, reimbursements, and coverage. Pharmacy technicians should understand how Medicare, Medicaid, and other common insurance providers are correctly billed for the coverage of their patients. Accurate billing procedures must always be followed, and pharmacy technicians often handle invoices. Therefore, they must be trained in the procedures that affect what is included on each invoice and understand how to process the paperwork. See Chapter 16 for detailed information on health insurance billing.

INSPECTING NURSING UNIT DRUG STOCKS

Nursing unit drug stocks must be maintained by the pharmacy. The technician is responsible for inspection of unit drug stocks for proper storage conditions, appropriate inventory, and replacement of expired or damaged stock. The Drug Enforcement Administration (DEA) monitors the use of scheduled drugs and those who prescribe them. Proper security measures are vital because of the increase in crimes involving controlled substances and prescription medications. Medication controls should be in place so that any misappropriation of these substances can be discovered and dealt with as quickly as possible. This task is one of the most important responsibilities of pharmacy technicians and pharmacy personnel in general, because their ability to practice may be threatened by inefficient medication control policies. According to the DEA, a hospital that keeps large quantities of controlled substances on hand may need a safe or locked cabinet, similar to the requirements for a drug distributor. Factors that are evaluated in relation to controlled substances include the number of people, whether employees, customers, or patients, who have access to the controlled substances, along with the location of the hospital, in a high crime or low crime area. There must be an effective alarm system in place, a predetermined quantity of controlled substances that can be kept in the hospital, and consideration of any prior theft or diversion of these substances.

INVENTORY MAINTENANCE, INCLUDING ORDERING SPECIALTY ITEMS

Ordering and maintenance of stock levels is often the responsibility of the pharmacy technician. The technician must ensure that stock levels are appropriate to allow the pharmacy to operate efficiently without having to borrow stock or order stock at higher prices. When a stock is delivered, it must be checked and verified against the order. Receipt of the order must be clearly marked on the invoice. All orders must be appropriately stored within the pharmacy (see Figure 11-6). Any damaged goods or expired drugs must be returned or properly disposed of.

During inventory control processes and maintenance, the pharmacy computer system should prompt the pharmacy staff when it is time to reorder specific medications and supplies. Pharmacy technicians must follow their organization's policies and procedures for reordering. They must know when to notify the pharmacist or pharmacy supervisor that specific drugs need to be reordered that technicians are not allowed (by law) to order themselves. The same is true for specialty items that are needed, such as medical equipment and other supplies.

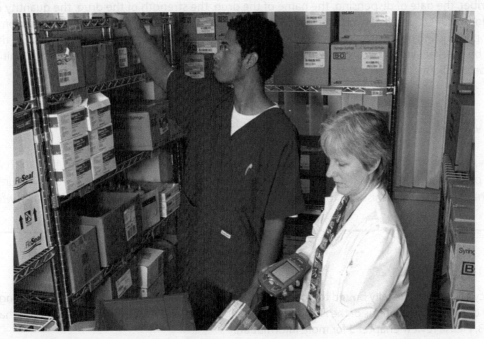

Figure 11-6 Proper maintenance of inventory levels is necessary to allow the pharmacy to run efficiently.

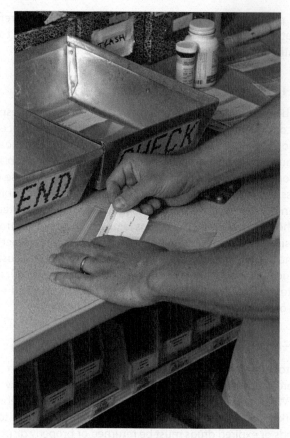

Figure 11-7 Each filled medication order must be appropriately labeled.

PREPARING LABELS

Each filled medication order must be appropriately labeled (see Figure 11-7). The label should contain the name of the patient the drug is prescribed for, the patient's medical record number, the patient's room number, the name of the prescriber, the date of dispensing, the name of the drug, the strength of the drug, the quantity of the drug dispensed, dosage directions, and expiration date. The label should also contain the initials of the person dispensing the drug. Proper labeling on medications is critically important. A great deal of care should be taken in this task. The label should be checked and rechecked against the medication order. All labels must be checked and initialed by the pharmacist before the medication leaves the pharmacy.

WHAT WOULD YOU DO?

You are a hospital pharmacy technician and receive a medication order for a patient in Room 436, which you know is a single-patient room. However, the medication order says it is for the patient in bed "B." To make sure that the medication order will be administered to the correct patient, in the correct room, in the correct bed, what would you do?

MAINTAINING PRIVACY

The pharmacy technician is legally bound to uphold the privacy of all patients. Standards for maintaining a patient's privacy were detailed in regulations of the Health Insurance Portability and Accountability Act (HIPAA) that went into effect in 2003. Please review Chapter 3 for more information.

AUDITING AND REPORTING OF MEDICATION PROCESSES

Pharmacy technicians must keep complete records of orders, reorders, and dispensations of all drugs (with scheduled drugs being most important) in their hospital pharmacy. For scheduled drugs, federal law requires records be kept on file for two years, and many state laws may require them to be kept for up to five years. Medication records may be audited by different federal and state agencies, as well as insurance companies.

COMMUNICATION SKILLS

Communication skills are very important in the field of pharmacy. The pharmacy technician will need to accurately communicate with patients as well as other health care workers. Communication skills are discussed in detail in Chapter 4.

WORKING SAFELY AND COOPERATIVELY

For the health and safety of pharmacy personnel, a safe working environment must be maintained. Work areas should be clean, and accidental exposures to harmful substances should be avoided. Emergency and exposure treatment plans should be in place. The pharmacy technician should be aware of and quickly be able to respond to any unsafe condition. Workplace safety is discussed in more detail in Chapter 10.

REGULATORY AGENCIES THAT OVERSEE HOSPITAL PHARMACY

The agencies that oversee all aspects of hospital operations, including the pharmacy department, are as follows:

- **The Joint Commission:** This organization surveys and accredits health care services. All health care organizations must undergo this accreditation process every three years. The Joint Commission identifies specific guidelines for every department within the hospital.

- **State Board of Pharmacy (BOP):** This agency licenses pharmacists and pharmacy technicians. Currently, only 20 states require that pharmacy technicians be certified and registered with the BOP. Over 40 states require registration or licensing and many require certification if the pharmacist/pharmacy technician ratio is greater than a set number. Each state BOP governs everything involved in pharmacy practice within that state's boundaries. Aside from the 50 states, there are also boards of pharmacy in the District of Columbia and U.S. territories such as Guam, Puerto Rico, and the Virgin Islands.

- **Centers for Medicare & Medicaid Services (CMS):** The CMS inspects and approves hospitals that provide care for Medicaid patients. Approval by this organization is required to receive reimbursement for any patients covered by Medicaid and Medicare.

- **Department of Public Health (DPH):** This organization oversees hospitals, including the pharmacy department. Hospitals undergo inspections by the DPH to assure compliance with laws concerning hospital practice.

WHAT WOULD YOU DO?

The Joint Commission has arrived at your hospital for an unannounced survey. You are aware that several expired medications were missing from the return paperwork over the last few months and believe they were diverted for illegal use by someone on the hospital staff with access to the pharmacy. When you previously alerted a supervisor about this, you were told not to worry about it and that it would be taken care of. A representative from The Joint Commission questions you, as well as other staff members, about the hospital pharmacy's operations and includes questions about drug diversion. If you were this pharmacy technician, what would you do?

Future of Hospital Pharmacy

With the aging of the population and the increasing number of medications being produced by research, an increasing need for pharmacy services in all settings will be seen. Trends for the future include the following:

- Continuing expansion of the responsibilities of pharmacy technicians to allow pharmacists to concentrate on direct patient care activities.

- An increasing need for education of both pharmacists and pharmacy technicians.

- An increasing need for pharmacists and pharmacy technicians to obtain the skills necessary to work directly with patients.

- An increasing multiprofessional approach to providing patient care, thus requiring better communication skills.

- Increasing use of automation to perform routine tasks and to handle the massive amounts of information and documentation that must occur as a result of providing patient care. Automation will also be used to make patient information available in the multiple settings in which patient care will be delivered.

The future of pharmacy is bright for those who choose pharmacy as a profession. It is the responsibility of those in the field now to prepare for the requirements of the future directions of pharmacy.

Summary

Pharmacy practice in the institutional setting includes support, product, clinical, and educational services. Automated machines may do medication dispensing, and technical personnel such as pharmacy technicians must finalize the preparation of the medications. Today, hospital pharmacy routinely uses computerized systems to ensure better patient care, with the goal of eliminating medication errors. Systems that are used include point-of-entry, computerized physician order entry, barcode point-of-entry, and computerized monitoring for adverse drug reactions. The Joint Commission now requires all hospitals to make all medications specific to each dose, for each patient, including unit-dose liquid medications. The term *sterile product* is usually associated with drugs that are administered by injection. The pharmacy director is responsible for maintaining an adequate medication inventory. This duty is usually delegated to a pharmacy buyer or pharmacy technician.

REVIEW QUESTIONS

1. Which of the following statements is critically important about medication orders?

   A. The pharmacy technician must initial them.
   B. They must be properly labeled.
   C. The technician's hands must be washed before dispensing.
   D. The order must contain the patient's medical record number.

2. The disadvantages of the floor stock system include all of the following, *except*:

   A. the potential for drug diversion and misappropriation resulting in economic loss.
   B. decreased inventory needs.
   C. inadequate space for medication storage on the patient care unit.
   D. the potential for medication errors.

3. Which of the following are not point-of-entry order systems?

   A. Computers-on-wheels
   B. Computerized physician order entry
   C. Barcode POE
   D. Computerized adverse drug event monitoring

4. Which of the following types of computerized systems in the hospital is able to detect levels of pain, blood pressure, and can verify dosages?

    A. CPOE
    B. COW
    C. E-MAR
    D. CADM

5. The patient prescription system is designed to supply medication for how many days?

    A. One day
    B. Two days
    C. Three days
    D. Seven days

6. Which of the following is a disadvantage of the unit-dose drug distribution system?

    A. Decreased costs of medications
    B. It dispenses only a 24-hour supply of medication
    C. More precise medication billing
    D. Reduced drug inventory

7. Preparing unit-dose medications is a responsibility of the:

    A. pharmacy technician or pharmacist.
    B. nurse or pharmacy director.
    C. medical assistant or nurse.
    D. pharmacy manager.

8. The unit dose is considered to have all of the following characteristics, *except:*

    A. it is safest.
    B. it is the most efficient.
    C. it is designed to be administered over one month.
    D. it is the most effective.

9. Creating a medication from a formula is called:

    A. compounding a medication.
    B. administering a medication.
    C. a responsibility of all pharmacy services.
    D. inventory maintenance.

10. Which of the following equipment is often used to prepare a unit-dose liquid?

    A. Pipette
    B. Graduate
    C. Oral syringe
    D. Beaker

11. Which of the following, in many facilities, are currently responsible for entering medication orders into the hospital information system?

    A. Physicians
    B. Nurses
    C. Pharmacy technicians
    D. Pharmacy managers

12. Which of the following is not a role of the hospital pharmacy technician?

    A. Gathering controlled substance inventory sheets
    B. Delivering controlled substances to the nursing floor
    C. Preparing parenteral IVs
    D. Advising a nurse when to inject a parenteral IV

13. Which of the following is not included in a patient's hospital record?

- **A.** Weight and height
- **B.** Patient's level of education
- **C.** Diet plan and blood test results
- **D.** Name of the primary physician

14. In the hospital, how long must scheduled drugs records be kept on file?

- **A.** One year
- **B.** Two years
- **C.** Three years
- **D.** Five years

15. How often must a hospital undergo the accreditation process by The Joint Commission?

- **A.** Every year
- **B.** Every two years
- **C.** Every three years
- **D.** Every five years

CRITICAL THINKING

A pharmacy technician began an inventory of the pharmacy. Using bar coding, each item was able to be quickly recorded into the computer system.

1. Why is inventory control so vital in the hospital pharmacy?

2. In today's pharmacy, how do pharmacy technicians know when to order items?

WEB LINKS

Look up the website of your state's board of pharmacy. Become acquainted with various policies and procedures of the state in which you practice.

Centers for Medicare and Medicaid Services: www.cms.gov

The Joint Commission: www.jointcommission.org

National Association of Boards of Pharmacy: nabp.pharmacy

U.S. Department of Health & Human Services: www.hhs.gov

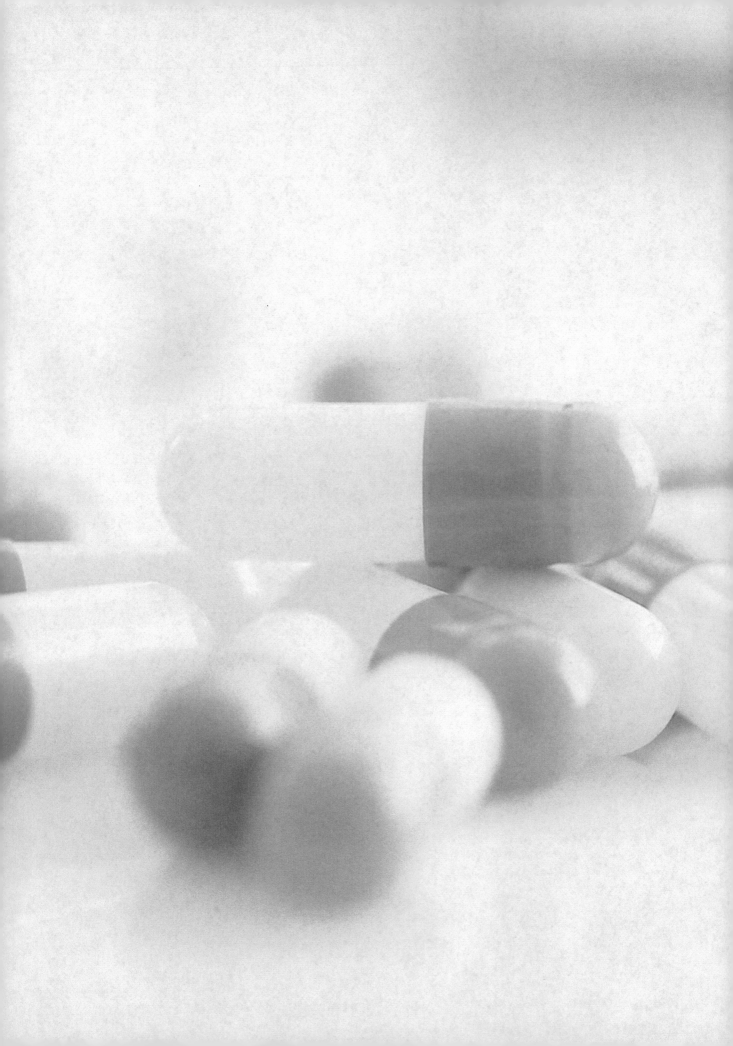

Community Pharmacy

OUTLINE

OBJECTIVES

Upon completion of this chapter, the reader should be able to:

1. Explain the important functions of the community pharmacy.
2. Discuss the various roles and responsibilities of pharmacy technicians in community pharmacies.
3. Explain the importance of understanding *behind-the-counter* (BTC) *medications*.
4. Identify the advantages of e-prescribing.
5. Identify how completed prescriptions are stored and organized prior to being picked up by patients.
6. Discuss how schedule II medications should be secured in the community pharmacy.
7. List the most important character traits of a good pharmacy technician.
8. Describe the role of the pharmacy technician regarding immunizations in the community pharmacy.
9. Differentiate between durable and nondurable supplies and equipment.
10. Explain *strip packaging*, as used when a community pharmacy supplies medications for long-term care services.

KEY TERMS

behind-the-counter (BTC) medications	community pharmacy	e-prescribing	professionalism
chain pharmacy	drive-through	franchise pharmacy	short dating

Overview

According to the National Council for Prescription Drug Programs, there are more than 67,000 community pharmacies across the United States. They are the primary providers of pharmaceuticals and pharmaceutical care services to patients. Community pharmacies are found in a variety of locations such as shopping centers, grocery stores, department stores, and medical office buildings. They are classified into two main categories: independent pharmacies and chain pharmacies. Independent pharmacies are owned by local individuals. Chain pharmacies such as Walgreens and CVS are usually regionally or nationally based. Giant regional or national mass merchandisers such as Walmart or Target also have pharmacies inside most of their stores. Pharmacists in the community pharmacy provide several important functions:

- They provide distribution of prescribed drug products.
- They are caretakers of the nation's drug supply.
- They compound prescriptions to meet the specific needs of individual patients.
- They educate the public to maximize the intended benefits of drug therapy while minimizing unintended side effects and adverse reactions.

Recent studies indicate that pharmacy technicians of today are involved in more areas of pharmacy practice than ever before. In addition to assisting with outpatient prescription dispensing, many community pharmacy technicians participate in purchasing, inventory control, billing, and repackaging products. Today, community pharmacies in the United States regularly use computers and online claims processing. Many also use automated dispensing systems to count doses, fill medication containers, and print patient information and labels.

POINTS TO REMEMBER

More than 7 billion prescriptions are dispensed each year in the United States, including all types of pharmacy settings.

Community Pharmacy

The term **community pharmacy** is also referred to as *retail pharmacy* or *ambulatory care pharmacy*. Many independent pharmacies offer compounding services, the sale or rental of durable medical equipment, and immunizations. A **franchise pharmacy** is one in which an individual or group purchases the name, branding, and use of an identified *franchisor*, such as Medicine Shoppe or Health Mart. A **chain pharmacy** is a group of pharmacies owned by a corporation, with shared branding and centralized management. They usually have standardized business practices, with a headquarters overseen by a board of directors. Walgreens and CVS are the two largest chain pharmacies in the United States. According to the statistical analysis company called Statista, there were 4.13 billion prescriptions filled in the United States in 2017. Of these, about 75% were filled by chain pharmacies.

In the community pharmacy, the pharmacy technician assists the pharmacist, prepares prescription medications, gives customer support, and performs many administration tasks. They receive most prescription requests, input prescriptions into the pharmacy computer system, count the correct amount of doses required, label prescription bottles, update patient files, prepare insurance claims, answer phones, stock shelves, and "check out" customers on cash registers. The pharmacy technician must be appropriately trained, with a large range of knowledge applicable to the community pharmacy.

The Role of the Pharmacy Technician

In the community pharmacy, the primary role of the pharmacy technician is to assist the pharmacist. This is similar to pharmacy technician roles in hospitals or any other types of pharmacy settings. The most common duties of the community pharmacy technician include customer service, taking information from customers or health professionals concerning prescriptions to be filled, checking prescriptions to make sure they are complete in regard to the information they contain, answering phones, and obtaining refill information from patients. The pharmacy technician performs a large variety of general, administrative, and technical duties. One of the most important tasks of a pharmacy technician is to know when to refer a patient directly to the pharmacist, such as when the patient requires counseling about a medication.

The pharmacy technician regularly inputs data into the pharmacy computer system. He or she may add prescribers, new patients, drugs, or insurance plans to the database. Every day, there are usual updates to patient profiles and prescriber information. New prescriptions must be entered and processed for prior drug approvals. Refill authorizations must be obtained, and prescriptions must be refilled, filed, reversed, and with the pharmacist's assistance, transferred. Various types of productivity reports must be run. Regarding the compounding of prescriptions, pharmacy technicians perform calculations prior to actual compounding, weight or measure medications, and clean equipment after compounding. Daily duties include package and labeling of prescriptions, including counting prescribed quantities and selecting appropriate containers. Technicians apply prescription and auxiliary labeling to containers in an area where customers cannot view any information contained on the labels. They print literature that accompanies each prescription, which will also be given to the patient, and return medications to appropriate areas of shelving. Technicians often have to apply pricing to medications. They organize inventory and alert pharmacists when there are shortages of medications and supplies.

The pharmacy technician is also responsible for reordering medications and supplies, checking ordered medications against their packing slips, placing medications where they belong on the correct shelves, and check the pharmacy stock for medications that may have **short dating**. Technicians accept payments, process insurance claims, alert the pharmacist to customer questions and other needs, perform basic housekeeping duties in the pharmacy, and generally anything else that the pharmacist asks them to assist in doing.

MEDICATION ERROR ALERT

Nearly 250,000 senior citizens are hospitalized every year because of reactions between prescription and OTC medications. Another related danger is that many OTC products contain ingredients such as acetaminophen that may also be present in the prescription medications a patient is taking, leading to a potential overdose.

Prescription Processing

In the community pharmacy, as well as other types of pharmacies, most medications are either *prescription* (*legend*) *drugs* or *over-the-counter* (OTC) *drugs*. However, in the community pharmacy, because of the Combat Methamphetamine Epidemic Act of 2005, there is a new subclassification of OTC drugs called **behind-the-counter** (BTC) **medications**. These are OTC drugs that contain *ephedrine*, which is one of the ingredients used to make *methamphetamine*, a schedule I controlled substance. People wanting to purchase products containing ephedrine must do so at the pharmacy counter, supervised by the pharmacist. The purchaser must provide proper identification and be at least 16 years of age. Each individual may purchase up to 3.6 g of products with ephedrine, such as *pseudoephedrine*, per day. They can purchase no more than 9 g in a 30-day period.

When a physician writes a prescription for a patient, the prescription is often taken directly by the patient to a community pharmacy. The physician can also choose to have someone at his or her practice call a prescription into a pharmacy for a specific patient. When this occurs, the pharmacist at the pharmacy must create a written form of the received telephone order. The physician can also fax a patient's prescription to the pharmacy. Some states allow patients to fax their own prescriptions to the pharmacy, but they must then provide the pharmacy with the original prescription before they can receive the medication.

Prescriptions today are regularly sent electronically to pharmacies via computer technology, or **e-prescribing**. This is electronic transfer of prescription data directly from a prescriber's computer system to a pharmacy's computer system and does not use e-mail or fax machines. Electronic prescribing may involve new prescriptions, changed prescriptions, requests for refills, fill status notifications, cancellation of a prescription, and medication history of the patient. Many individual practitioners, hospitals, clinics, provider associations, software manufacturers, pharmacies, trade associations, professional associations, ancillary services, laboratories, state or federal governments, terminology and code set organizations, standards development organizations, health plans, payers, and processors are involved. The advantages of e-prescribing include the following:

- Prescribers can receive prompts on their computer screens about drug-specific dosing information.
- Refills are expedited quickly.
- Data can be exchanged between physicians, pharmacists, and patients.
- The patient's medical file can be linked to his or her prescription file easily.
- The prescriber can be notified if the drug is covered by the patient's insurance plan as soon as the order is generated, instead of when it reaches the pharmacy.
- Illegible handwriting errors are eliminated or greatly reduced.

Disadvantages of e-prescribing include a longer time needed to process prescriptions, software incompatibilities, and the fact that smaller chain pharmacies may experience increased costs implementing e-prescribing. Detailed information about prescriptions and processing can be found in Chapter 6.

Organization of the Retail Pharmacy

Most retail pharmacies have a consistent layout and floor plan. Specific areas are designated for a particular task to be performed. There are also areas for interaction between the patient and the pharmacist or pharmacy technician. All areas of the pharmacy are designed to achieve a particular goal in providing services.

PRESCRIPTION COUNTER AND CONSULTING AREA

Almost all community pharmacies have similar floor plans and are generally organized into two areas: the front area and the prescription processing area. OTC drugs, cosmetics, and other merchandise items are located in the front area. Only authorized individuals are able to enter the prescription processing areas. The prescription counter is an area that a pharmacist or a technician can use to prepare prescriptions. The consultation area is strictly for the pharmacist's use to counsel patients privately. The technician must always remember that he or she is not legally permitted to counsel patients about medications. This is the role and responsibility of the pharmacist.

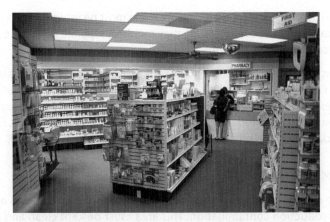

Figure 12-1 The front area of the retail pharmacy.

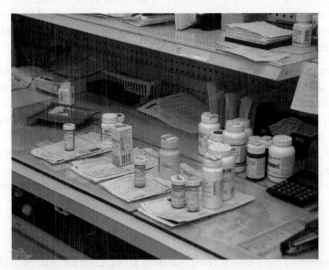

Figure 12-2 The dispensing area of the retail pharmacy.

By state regulations, a description of the space and equipment is required. Figures 12-1 and 12-2 show the front and prescription dispensing areas of community pharmacies.

TRANSACTION WINDOWS

Customers drop off prescriptions, new hard copy or refill, or verbally ask for a refill at the transaction window. The technician should obtain all personal information that is required for a hard copy prescription. This information must be entered into the computer before starting the order. When the information for the prescription has been entered, the order is filled. The community pharmacy is different from the hospital pharmacy. Technicians in the community pharmacy interact with patients as customers. Therefore, customer service is one of the most important aspects in the community pharmacy, and technicians must have strong interpersonal skills. Customers can also pick up their prescription in this area.

PHARMACY STOCK AREA

In a community pharmacy, many different dosage forms are stocked, usually arranged alphabetically. Sometimes, medications are arranged alphabetically by brand name or generic name. Many pharmacies have certain areas for oral dosage forms, oral liquids, reconstituted liquids such as antibiotics, inhalation products, oral contraceptives, ophthalmic products, otic products, topical agents, vaginal and rectal products, and products requiring refrigeration. Some community pharmacies have special areas for the most commonly dispensed medications in the pharmacy, which sell and are restocked quickly. For refrigerated drugs, there must be refrigerators with monitoring thermometers. When controlled substances must be refrigerated, they require a separate refrigerator. Nothing must be kept in medication refrigerators except actual medications.

The community pharmacy staff must continually check for expired medications. This is often stated in the pharmacy's *Standard Operating Procedure* (SOP) manual. If a medication is found to be expired, it must be removed from the shelf and placed in a designated area where expired and recalled medications are kept. The medication cannot be dispensed or sold and must be separated from all other pharmacy stock medications. Expired and recalled medications are kept in this special area of the pharmacy until they can be properly discarded.

NONSTERILE COMPOUNDING AREA

The pharmacy's nonsterile compounding area should be separated from other areas of work to reduce distractions and possibilities of production contamination. This area must be kept clean and uncluttered, with proper ventilation and temperature control. All equipment and supplies needed for nonsterile compounding must be easily accessible. All equipment is regularly checked for cleanliness prior to use; the equipment is then washed immediately after use to prevent cross-contamination between ingredients and the final compounded product. Isopropyl alcohol (70%) is usually used to clean the compounding area, and a log should be kept that shows when the equipment was cleaned.

All state boards of pharmacy require community pharmacies to have sinks with hot and cold running water and proper drainage. Sponges, various brushes, and other needed cleaning products, as well as disposable paper towels, must be kept next to the sink. Trash container must be kept away from compounding areas. All trash must be disposed of properly and safely, especially personal protective equipment (PPE) and hazardous wastes. Equipment used for nonsterile compounding includes balances, containers (such as beakers, graduated cylinders and other graduates), brushes, evaporating dishes, funnels, metric weights, weighing papers or boats, mortar and pestles, pipettes, stirring rods, spatulas, spray bottles, and sharps containers. All pharmacy technicians should be experienced with the *United States Pharmacopeia* Chapter <795> (USP <795>), and with the equipment and techniques used for nonsterile compounding.

STERILE COMPOUNDING AREA

Some community pharmacies also have sterile compounding areas, used for intravenous medications, and sometimes, for the administration of vaccines. The sterile compounding area must comply with *United States Pharmacopeia* Chapter <797> (USP <797>), which has specific guidelines for the maintenance of sterility in compounding and the addressing of medication errors. The American Society of Health-System Pharmacists (ASHP) and National Coordinating Committee on Large Volume Parenterals (NCCLVP) have also released guidelines on the conditions and practices required for *compounded sterile preparations* (CSPs). Their goals are to prevent harm or death because of cross-contamination of components used in sterile compounding.

STORAGE

When prescriptions are completed and customers do not pick them up right away, they should be placed in a specific area or on shelves. For storage, prescriptions should be alphabetized by the name of the patient (see Figure 12-3). Most community pharmacies utilize patient bins in a secured area outside the prescription department, which are not accessible to patients. Access is restricted only to those individuals allowed to work with prescriptions by the pharmacist. The patient bins are usually in alphabetical order as well as the actual prescriptions themselves. It is of utmost importance to place each prescription in the correct bin matching the last name of the patient. Each state regulates whether pharmacy technicians can provide a patient with his or her medication if the pharmacist is not present.

COMPUTER SYSTEMS

The use of computers is now standard in pharmacy practice because of the expanded informational needs of the pharmacist. Another factor is the increased amount of paperwork required in practice. Computer systems are essential for promoting efficiency, offering technological advantages and expansive databases that provide needed support. Most chain pharmacies are linked together by dedicated telephone lines or satellites, thus facilitating the sharing of information between pharmacies.

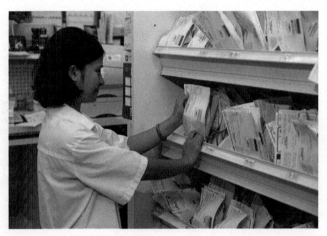

Figure 12-3 Prescription storage area.

There are three areas in the pharmacy in which computerized systems can be used:

- Prescription dispensing and associated record maintenance
- Clinical support and accounting
- Business management

Many insurance and prescription plans now require online verification and authorization before the dispensing of any medication. Pharmacists and pharmacy technicians can now use the Internet to obtain and download information about disease states and drug therapy for their patients.

POINTS TO REMEMBER

If a pharmacy technician receives a new prescription from a prescriber by telephone, he or she must consult with the supervising pharmacist.

CUSTOMER PICKUP (DRIVE-THROUGH)

Today, the majority of community pharmacies have **drive-through** windows that allow customers or patients to drop-off prescriptions or purchase their medications (see Figure 12-4). Pharmacy technicians need to make sure that the correct person is receiving his or her order and not another person's order. The technician must ask if the patient has any questions about the prescription for the pharmacist. The pharmacist should be available for consultation.

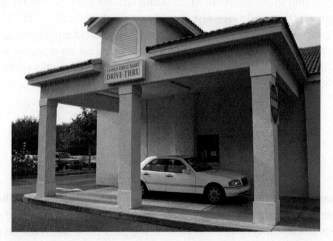

Figure 12-4 Drive-through window.

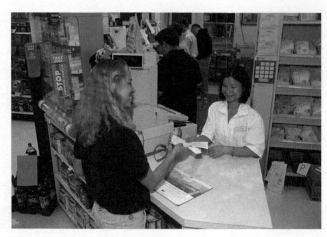

Figure 12-5 Pharmacy technicians must also be able to operate the cash register to take customers' payments.

CASH REGISTER

The technician may ring up prescriptions and other items such as OTC products into the cash register and accept payment for their purchase. Cash register machines are connected into the pharmacy's computer and can provide prices automatically by using bar code scanners. The pharmacy technician must handle payments properly (see Figure 12-5). For cash payments, he or she must count the payment in the presence of the customer, confirming the amount verbally.

CONTROLLED SUBSTANCE PRESCRIPTIONS

A prescription for a controlled substance (Schedules II through V) must be handled carefully. The lower the number of the drug schedule, the higher the potential for abuse of the drug. The most dangerous scheduled drugs are called controlled substances, and they are kept in a locked storage cabinet under the pharmacist's supervision. Locks may have numerical combinations or keys, and today there are *biometrically protected locks* that use the fingerprints of authorized pharmacy staff members in order to gain access. The pharmacy technician must take direction from the pharmacist about which controlled substances he or she may handle in preparation of distribution to customers. All controlled substances require prescriptions, and repeated checking of the products, labeling, packaging, and the customer who receives them must be performed for error-free handling.

PURCHASING AND INVENTORY CONTROL

The pharmacy technician often orders products for use or sale. He or she may work alone with a purchasing agent or deal directly with pharmaceutical or medical supply companies on matters such as price. The technician must complete a purchase order that includes the product name and amount. The order is then transmitted directly to manufacturers. Although selection of drugs must always remain the responsibility of the pharmacist, a pharmacy technician may prepare purchase orders. When pharmaceutical products are received, the technician must carefully check the product against the purchase order. Damaged products must be reported without delay and returned to the manufacturer. The pharmacy technician must check all products for expiration dates. The term *inventory* refers to all drugs available for sale. Inventory is discussed further in Chapter 17.

The Professional Characteristics of Pharmacy Technicians

The pharmacy technician must maintain a professional manner in all aspects of the job. A professional is held accountable for his or her actions while on the job, must maintain an ethical standard of behavior, must clearly and concisely communicate with customers and other health care providers, and must be able to work as a team member and in a fast-paced environment.

ACCOUNTABILITY

Pharmacy technicians must understand the boundaries of what they can and cannot do legally. They must be accountable for their performances and also their mistakes. An error, even a small one, can have disastrous consequences for a patient, a customer, or the pharmacy itself. The pharmacy technician must develop work habits to ensure accuracy and expect to be held responsible for what he or she does on the job. The technician must always double-check everything to avoid mistakes.

ETHICAL STANDARDS AND PROFESSIONAL BEHAVIOR

Ethics is the study of moral values or principles, and a professional is an individual qualified to perform the activities of a specific occupation. **Professionalism** goes beyond the knowledge, skills, and abilities required to perform those activities. The pharmacy technician, as a professional, represents the profession of pharmacy. He or she must always be courteous and listen with focus. The technician must respect the privacy of patients and keep all information confidential. The most important character traits of a good pharmacy technician are honesty, organization, reliability, and dependability. The pharmacist must be able to count on the technician to maintain confidentiality and privacy of patients and behave ethically, even when not under direct supervision, because of the higher level of trust needed to provide excellent patient care. The Health Insurance Portability and Accountability Act (HIPAA) privacy rule became effective on April 14, 2001, and all health care facilities were required to become compliant by April 14, 2003. This rule sets national standards for the protection of health information of patients. To become compliant, the covered entities must implement standards to protect individually identifiable health information and guard against the misuse of that information. HIPAA was drafted to help ensure the confidentiality of medical records, which was discussed in Chapter 3. The privacy rule does not replace federal, state, or other laws that grant individuals even greater privacy protection. Therefore, pharmacy technicians must always keep in mind that they must maintain confidentiality and privacy of patients.

COMMUNICATION SKILLS

One of the fundamental skills that the pharmacy technician must acquire to function successfully in the pharmacy is effective verbal communication. Verbal communication is either oral (spoken) or written. Written communication has traditionally been thought of as being more formal than oral conversation. Today, however, with the increasing use of e-mail, written communication is often as informal as oral communication.

Nonverbal communication is generally easy to understand, if one pays attention to the other party. Facial expression, eye contact, and body position are all methods of communicating without using words. Listening to the words and the tone of voice is important. The pharmacy technician must always use a nonjudgmental expression and tone of voice. Communication skills are covered in more depth in Chapter 4.

INTERACTING WITH THE PHARMACIST

Communication between pharmacy technicians and pharmacist must be clear and brief. Proper terminology should be used, and the pharmacy technician must carefully listen to the pharmacist. The pharmacist should check that the technician understood what was being communicated, and the technician should ask for clarification if he or she is unsure of anything. Feedback is essential to ensure good communication. The pharmacist should also listen carefully to how the technician responds about the information being communicated.

TEAMWORK

A pharmacy technician needs to be genuinely interested in helping people and be warm and caring. He or she should be able to put the needs of others first. An effective health care team working together does not just happen. To be effective, team members work together to provide appropriate care for each patient. Each member of the team must be committed to problem solving, focusing on the patient, and communicating. A team approach to patient care ensures comprehensive service without expensive duplication of effort. Teamwork is also necessary for the smooth operation of the entire pharmacy. Technicians work closely with others to perform their duties.

INTERACTING WITH THE PATIENT

Pharmacy communication may be delayed because of challenges created by unique patient obstacles. There are a large variety of barriers to good communication. When a pharmacy technician senses that a patient has a certain problem, he or she should consider the perception being made of the patient. If the patient is elderly, having memory problems, visually impaired, or hearing impaired, these obstacles can be barriers to proper communication. The pharmacy technician, along with the pharmacist, must never make any assumptions about the patient, because these are also barriers to good communication.

ELDERLY PATIENTS

Today, elderly patients are a larger part of the population because of medical advances and better lifestyles. However, they regularly experience more chronic conditions than younger people and usually require a larger regimen of medications. Communication skills are often poorer with advanced age. Information processing may be slower, and it may be difficult to communicate or understand information that is occurring too quickly, or in distracting environments. Elderly persons may have problems with attention, recall, and short-term memory processing. They may also have different perceptions and expectations than younger individuals. Physical changes linked to aging may impair communication skills. It is often necessary to explain how to take medications or how to store medications when talking with elderly patients.

Hearing loss is a common problem, and it varies from individual to individual. Such individuals may need to read the lips of someone speaking to them, use facial expressions for better communication, and use certain gestures. Therefore, when speaking with hearing-impaired individuals, it is important to stand 3 to 6 feet away and avoid speaking directly into the patient's ear, since this may distort the sounds of speech. Instead of repeating a sentence that was not understood, break it down into shorter, simpler phrases. Some people have speech impairments that harm communication. These people may need to use notes or sign language to communicate. Therefore, it is good to keep a pad of paper nearby for anyone who needs to communicate by writing. Some individuals may have problems understanding speech, but they may not have any hearing impairment. This *aphasia* can involve difficulty with certain names or words or in putting words into the correct order. Since they may be able to hear normally, speaking loudly is not helpful. Because of this specific communication barrier, it is best to speak with the patient's caregiver in order to give proper information to the patient.

PATIENTS WITH MENTAL DISORDERS

According to National Institute of Mental Health, nearly one in five adults in the United States lives with a mental illness. As of 2016, this totaled 44.7 million people. It may be difficult or uncomfortable trying to communicate with a patient with a mental disorder. The patient may not want to communicate with a pharmacy staff member. This may be due to a reluctance in wanting to interact with others or due to poor self-esteem. Others simply do not trust health care providers of any type. Another factor is when a pharmacy technician or pharmacist does not know what the patient's physician has actually told the patient about his or her condition. Therefore, for patients with mental disorders, it is best to use open-ended questions and attempt to treat them the same as any other patient, showing dignity and respect. As much as possible, it is good to offer support if the patient responds positively to this; ask if there is anything he or she has questions or worries about, show compassion, and be very professional in how you listen as well as speak.

PATIENTS WITH HEALTH LITERACY ISSUES

The term *health literacy* is defined as the ability to read, understand, and act upon health care information. Many minorities and immigrants may have literacy problems, including Hispanics, African Americans, Asians, and the elderly of all ethnic groups. Poor health literacy results in much higher health care costs, increased problems with care that is received, worsened outcomes, inability to act upon available modes of care, inability to understand terminology used in paperwork that accompanies prescriptions, more hospitalizations, and an inability to take medications correctly. Often, patients with health literacy issues are uncomfortable, failing to inform their pharmacist or pharmacy technician about their situation. If this occurs, the pharmacy staff cannot correctly assess if the patient is understanding the information being provided. Therefore, the USP has created *pictographs*, which are illustrations used to demonstrate common medication instructions and precautions. They include how to take a medication by mouth, how to store it in a refrigerator, when to take it (such as at bedtime), avoiding taking a medication with milk or other dairy products, how to place drops into an ear, when to avoid drinking alcohol in relation to a medication, and how to use an inhaler properly.

IMMUNIZATIONS

Immunizations are often provided by community pharmacies, including those for influenza, hepatitis A and B, pneumococcal infection, herpes zoster, and varicella. In most states, only pharmacists are allowed to administer immunizations, not pharmacy technicians or other staff members. However, pharmacy technicians are allowed to draw the correct amount of vaccine into a syringe for the pharmacist to use. Pharmacy technicians assist with immunization programs by providing billing, documentation, reporting of adverse events, and in fostering good communication between staff and patients. Pharmacy technicians also participate in training and certification for cardiopulmonary resuscitation.

DURABLE AND NONDURABLE SUPPLIES AND EQUIPMENT

Patients often need to purchase certain supplies and equipment to use at home for continuing self-care following hospitalization. Many community pharmacies supply these products, which are called *durable and nondurable supplies and equipment*. Durable equipment is reusable and used for the treatment of illnesses or injuries. It includes wheelchairs and hospital beds. Nondurable products must be discarded after use. They include diabetic or ostomy supplies and compression stockings. The reasons that community pharmacies often supply these products include the fact that there are more elderly patients than ever before, with many patients preferring to be in their homes for recovery, and because at-home recovery is less expensive than hospitalization or other institutional settings. These products help patients remain independent because of evolving technologies. Managed care advocates for the discharge of patients for recovery at home.

Community pharmacies may also supply canes, crutches, and walkers for their patients. Additional supplies and equipment include bedpans, first aid supplies, various medical instruments, nutrition therapies, braces, incontinence products, oxygen tanks, prescription respiratory drugs administered by in-home visiting nurses, prosthetic devices, and products for decubitus ulcers and wound care. Pharmacy technicians should be trained in the use of these products in order to provide the best possible care.

LONG-TERM CARE SERVICES

Community pharmacies may work with long-term care facilities to provide medications for residents. These facilities include correctional facilities, assisted living facilities, subacute care facilities, and board-and-care homes. Pharmacy technicians may assist in these services. For long-term care, medication packaging is different. It utilizes blister cards or strip packaging. This makes it easier to dispense and when orders are changed. Long-term care facilities utilize 30-day cards that have individual medication pockets. Therefore, each dose can be separated and administered individually. Unopened blisters or pockets can be returned for order changes when necessary. Also, each patient receives the contents of a blister or pocket, ensuring that the correct dose was obtained. This is better than counting doses from standard bulk medication containers. Some community pharmacies have a special area focusing only on packaging for contracted long-term care facilities.

Strip packaging refers to a method of packaging performed by a machine or robot. Canisters are kept stocked by pharmacy technicians, who operate the tray for specific medications. Each *pouch* contains a medication that is to be administered at a specific time of the day: breakfast, lunch, or dinner. The pouch lists medications that are contained, and are perforated, but are in a roll form. The roll is placed into a box, and the patient tears the pouch off when it is time to take that medication during the day. The packages are delivered to the patient once per month. In one pouch, there can be several different medications together, which are supposed to be taken at the same time.

In long-term care, the pharmacy technician is involved in many activities that are similar to those in the community pharmacy. These include billing for all types of medications and nondrug products. They enter computer data for all types of orders, maintain the drug library, and maintain patient profiles and drug information requests, along with delivery records and repackaging equipment. Pharmacy technicians order, receive, and stock medications and supplies. They package and label prescriptions and perform general housekeeping activities. Additionally, they process returned medications so that they can be reused, provide required paperwork to long-term care facilities, repackage and label medications, and transport medications to the facilities. There will be additional employment opportunities for pharmacy technicians in community pharmacies, including long-term care areas, because of the increasing elderly population.

DISEASE PREVENTION

Many community pharmacies offer disease prevention and wellness programs. These often focus on heart conditions, diabetes, and other illnesses. Pharmacy technicians, for example, can assist patients in choosing transdermal patches, other drug forms, meters to measure blood glucose, test strips, lancets, and other related products. Pharmacy technicians may be needed to assist with choices of OTC medications, vitamins, and herbal supplements. They must understand which of these can interact with other medications that each patient may be taking. Maintaining an electronic record of all of these substances is crucial to creating a complete patient medication profile.

ABILITY TO HANDLE A BUSY WORK ENVIRONMENT AND STRESS

A pharmacy technician's ability to learn new ideas, modify his or her thinking, adapt to new situations, and handle stress in the pharmacy is an increasingly important skill in today's evolving and complex health care delivery system. Most difficult problems can be solved after an individual steps back and looks at the situation from the other person's point of view. Team members should try to see obstacles and then work together to move past the problem. A team member in the pharmacy should expect to work in a high-stress environment. The pharmacy technician must handle any workload and other specific situations in a professional manner.

MEDICATION ERROR ALERT

Information that is not kept up to date in the patient profile can lead to medication errors. These can occur during prescribing, dispensing, or administration of medications. One in four prescribing errors is directly associated with inadequate patient information. Without an up-to-date patient profile, indicating all current health conditions, patients can be given medications that may be contraindicated.

Summary

A community pharmacy is also known as a retail or ambulatory care pharmacy. Primary duties of pharmacy technicians in these settings are to assist the pharmacist in providing customer service, handling prescriptions in all forms, answering phones, updating computer information, and keeping the pharmacy properly stocked with supplies. Some community pharmacies offer nonsterile and/or sterile compounding services. Community pharmacy organization includes separate areas for storage of controlled substances and for the pharmacist to counsel patients. Community pharmacy technicians must be of good moral character and always display high ethics and professionalism. Their communication skills must be excellent with all individuals, including the pharmacist, other staff members, health care professionals, and customers of all ages and conditions.

REVIEW QUESTIONS

1. The Medicine Shoppe is classified as which type of pharmacy?

    A. Chain
    B. Franchise
    C. Hospital
    D. Ambulatory

2. The pharmacy technician may do which of the following?

    A. Count or pour medications
    B. Empty returned medications into stock containers
    C. Take prescriptions over the phone
    D. Counsel a patient

3. Which of the following OTC drugs is classified as "behind-the-counter"?

    A. Ibuprofen
    B. St. John's wort
    C. Acetaminophen
    D. Ephedrine

4. Which of the following is a disadvantage of e-prescribing compared to traditional prescribing?

    A. Refills are expedited quickly.
    B. It eliminates handwriting errors.
    C. It may be more expensive for smaller pharmacy chains to implement.
    D. Prescribers can find drug dosage information.

5. Which of the following is not a daily duty of the community pharmacy technician?

    A. Counting prescribed quantities
    B. Packaging prescriptions
    C. Labeling prescriptions
    D. Cooperating with board of pharmacy inspections

6. Which of the following scheduled drugs must be stored in a locked safe?

    A. Schedule IV
    B. Schedule III
    C. Schedule II
    D. Schedule V

7. Which of the following USP chapters is used for nonsterile compounding?

    A. USP <794>
    B. USP <795>
    C. USP <797>
    D. USP <800>

8. Which of the following is a nondurable supply or equipment?

    A. Hospital bed
    B. Compression stocking
    C. Wheelchair
    D. Cane

9. How often should pharmacy technicians deliver medication packages to long-term care centers?

    A. Every day
    B. Every week
    C. Every two weeks
    D. Every month

10. Products that are damaged at the time they arrive at the pharmacy must be:

    A. destroyed immediately.
    B. reported without delay and returned to the manufacturer.
    C. repackaged after removing the damaged portion.
    D. tested to see if they are still able to be sold.

11. What do most community pharmacies use to temporarily store completed prescriptions before patients pick them up?

    A. Locked cabinets
    B. Prescription receptacles
    C. Alphabetized bins
    D. Computerized safes

12. All of the following are important character traits of a good pharmacy technician, *except*:

    A. reliability.
    B. honesty.
    C. judging patients.
    D. accountability.

13. Which of the following cannot be performed by a pharmacy technician regarding immunizations?

    A. Drawing the correct amount of vaccine into a syringe
    B. Administering subcutaneous vaccinations
    C. Providing billing and documentation of immunizations
    D. Reporting adverse events concerning immunizations

14. For how many days is strip packaging, or blister cards, used for long-term care pharmacy services?

    A. 3 days
    B. 7 days
    C. 15 days
    D. 30 days

15. Which of the following is not a duty of a community pharmacy technician?

    A. Ordering medications
    B. Stocking pharmacy shelves
    C. Making decisions during drug utilization evaluation
    D. Compounding nonsterile products

CRITICAL THINKING

Cheyene has finished her externship and has been hired to work in a retail pharmacy. Prior to starting work, she reads the policies and procedures manual of the pharmacy to become more familiar with her job's duties and responsibilities.

1. Why are privacy and confidentiality so important in the field of health care and pharmacy?

2. Describe the characteristics that a pharmacy technician should possess. Why are these important?

WEB LINKS

Community Pharmacy Foundation: communitypharmacyfoundation.org

Community Pharmacy Online: communitypharmacy.org

National Community Pharmacists Association: www.ncpanet.org

PharmCatalyst: www.pharmcatalyst.com

Virtual Library Pharmacy: www.pharmacy.org

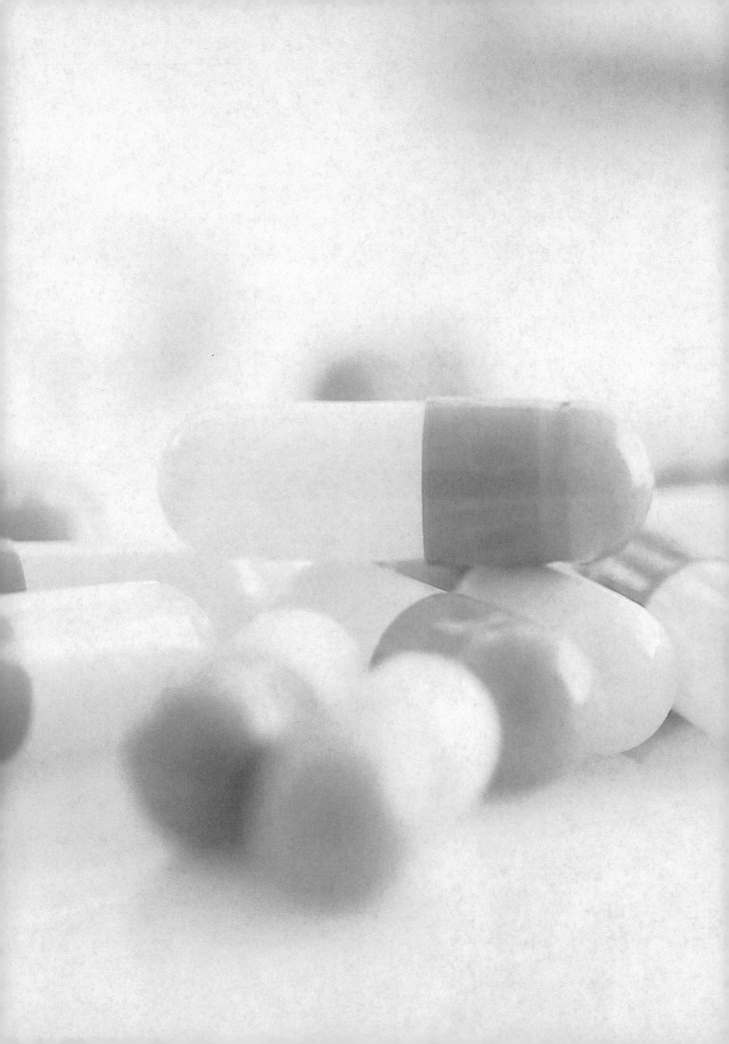

CHAPTER 13

Advanced Pharmacy

OUTLINE

Long-Term Care Pharmacy Services
   Drug Distribution Systems
Home Health Care Pharmacy
Home Infusion Pharmacy
Hospice Pharmacy
Ambulatory Care Pharmacy
Mail-Order Pharmacy
Central Fill Pharmacy
Internet Pharmacy
Nuclear Pharmacy
   Equipment and Supplies
   Guidelines for Practice of Nuclear Pharmacy

OBJECTIVES

Upon completion of this chapter, the reader should be able to:

1. Define long-term care.
2. Explain long-term care pharmacy organization.
3. Describe home health care and the responsibility of the pharmacy.
4. Identify common types of medication packaging used in home health care and long-term care facilities.
5. Explain total parenteral nutrition (TPN).
6. Describe hospice and ambulatory care.
7. Explain the differences between home health care and hospice.
8. Name the advantages of mail-order pharmacy.
9. Explain the importance of health and safety in nuclear pharmacy.
10. Describe the roles of the pharmacy technician in home infusion pharmacy.

KEY TERMS

automated dispensing system	drug distribution system	Internet pharmacy	mail-order pharmacy
blended-dose system	home health care pharmacy	long-term care	modified unit-dose system
central fill pharmacy	hospice	long-term care pharmacy organization	modular cassette

multiple medication package	**parenteral nutrition**	**reagent kit**	**starter kit**
	radiopharmaceutical	**specialty mail-order pharmacy**	**unit-dose system**
nuclear pharmacy			

Overview

Today the role of the pharmacist is expanding. The rapid development of new drugs and drug delivery systems, changes in the health care delivery system, an increase in the acuity of illness of institutionalized patients, and increased emphasis on patient outcomes and quality of health care have contributed to the evolution of pharmacy practice. The primary goal is to reduce health care costs and increase the overall quality of life for the patient. Pharmacy technicians must be trained, skilled, and knowledgeable in these areas, because many of the drug preparation and distribution tasks formerly performed by pharmacists have been delegated to pharmacy technicians working under the direct supervision of a pharmacist. Trained pharmacy technicians have an opportunity to work in various care delivery areas, including inpatient care, home care, ambulatory care, mail-order pharmacy, and more advanced areas such as nuclear medicine and chemotherapy.

Long-Term Care Pharmacy Services

Long-term care is defined as a range of health and health-related support services, and it has become an important component in the total health care system. There are now more long-term facility beds than acute care beds. Future emphasis on this sector will result in increased numbers of facilities and beds designated for long-term care, whereas those designated for acute care will be reduced. With advances in medical sciences and technologies, people are living longer. Prolongation of life expectancy has created a new set of problems for the health care system. At the same time, there has been a rapid rise in the number of people with chronic disease conditions and associated social and emotional problems that require a different management approach. The recipients may be people of any age, such as children with congenital anomalies, young adults experiencing lengthy recovery periods from trauma, or frail elderly adults with chronic diseases and multifaceted changes associated with aging (e.g., mental or physical impairment). The goal of long-term care is to enable a person to maintain the maximal possible level of functional independence. The same forces affecting acute care also have had an impact on the growth of long-term care.

The numbers and size of long-term care facilities have increased. Various types of long-term care facilities exist, with nursing homes, including skilled-nursing facilities and intermediate-care facilities being among the most common. Increasing numbers of alternative-care sites are also available, such as those that offer board and nursing care. Many patients in these facilities are treated with long-term and multiple drug therapy. Because of this, it is vital to maintain a *medication administration record* (MAR) for each patient. Today, these are usually in electronic form and are known as an *eMAR*. An MAR or eMAR is a report that serves as a legal record of medications administered to a patient at any type of facility. It is part of the patient's permanent record on his or her medical chart. The health care professional treating the patient signs off on the record at the time when a drug or device is administered. Commonly, these records are referred to as *drug charts*.

Increasing numbers of patients being admitted to long-term care facilities require high-technology pharmacy services. Because of limited resources, most long-term care facilities contract out dispensing and clinical pharmacy services, meaning that they pay another company to take care of most patient medications. The licensed professional pharmacy or practice that provides medications and clinical services to long-term care facilities and their residents is called a **long-term care pharmacy organization**. A pharmacist or pharmacy technician does not have to present physically at the facility during all hours; however, pharmacy services must be made available 24 hours a day.

Pharmacists perform two types of functions for long-term care facilities: distributive and consultant. The distributive pharmacist is responsible for ensuring that patients receive the correct medicines that were ordered. This job is mainly done outside the long-term care facility. The impact and savings of the use of consultant pharmacist services in long-term care have been documented. The role of the pharmacist has been shown to decrease overall medication costs, adverse drug reactions and interactions, medication errors, the length of hospitalization, and mortality rates of long-term care patients. The consultant pharmacist in long-term care is, in many ways, like a hospital pharmacy director, because he or she must supervise all aspects of the comprehensive pharmaceutical services delivered to patients. The consultant pharmacist interacts with doctors, nurses, and other health professionals. The consultant pharmacist is responsible for several different nursing homes or other facilities and may only visit each at certain weekly or monthly intervals. Standards, such as the Omnibus Budget Reconciliation Act of 1990 (OBRA '90), and various national health care reform initiatives require the pharmacist to assume greater responsibility and participation in long-term care facility. In addition to maintaining a safe drug distribution and control system, pharmacists are asked to apply this knowledge by reviewing drug regimens, providing cost containment, participating in patient care and related committees, and developing pharmacy policies and procedures.

MEDICATION ERROR ALERT

In many long-term care facilities, nurses are responsible for at least 25 residents at a given time. The chances for medication errors are significant but advances in automation, computer records, and the use of bar codes to track all medications help to prevent them from occurring. Electronic medical records have "checks and balances" built in to maintain extremely accurate control of where medications are being dispensed, and to whom.

DRUG DISTRIBUTION SYSTEMS

In the long-term care pharmacy, a **drug distribution system** is the container or other type of packaging that holds a drug while it is transferred from a pharmacy to a patient. These containers are required to meet light and moisture resistance standards by the United States Pharmacopeia and the National Formulary (USP–NF) and are designed to help reduce medication errors. Pharmacy technicians should be familiar with the various types of drug distributions used in the long-term care pharmacy setting.

Unit-Dose System

The **unit-dose system** was originally created for use in hospitals and other acute health care settings (see Chapter 11). The unit-dose system provides medications in their final "unit-of-use" form that is safe for use in a long-term care facility. In the unit-dose system, a single-unit package of a medication is dispensed just before it is needed by a patient. The medication is contained in a small packet with a thermal paper/foil laminate side and a transparent or slightly colored side (in the case of medications that are sensitive to light). The paper/foil laminate side features medication information printed upon it that describes the contained medication (see Figure 13-1). Unit doses are packaged by automated machinery designed specifically for this purpose. These machines drop the medication into an

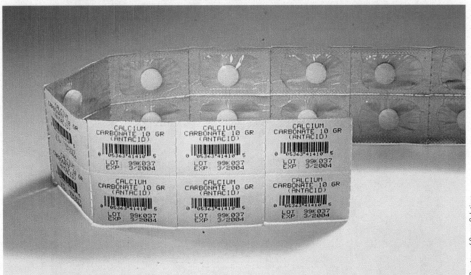

Figure 13-1 Individual unit-dose packages.

open package, seal the package, and print the medication information onto the package. The pharmacy technician may place packaged medications in drawers in a medication cart by patient and then deliver the cart to the patient care floor. It is important to understand that only medications used on a regular basis are made into unit doses. For medication orders or unusual dosage strengths that are not common, pharmacy technicians must prepare individual dosages as they are needed for the patient.

Modified Unit-Dose System

The **modified unit-dose system** features unit doses that are "blister" packaged on a multiple-dose card instead of being packaged individually. A single medication dose is contained in each blister on cards that can hold between 30 and 90 blisters. These cards are also known as *blister cards, punch cards*, or *bingo cards* (see Figure 13-2). The steps used to fill and seal the multiple-dose cards are similar to those used for single-unit packaging. After the medication is dropped in each blister, it is sealed with a thermal paper/foil laminate, upon which the medication information is printed. The blister portion may be transparent, amber-colored, or made of light-resistant plastic. The blisters may be sealed either by heat-sealing or cold-sealing methods.

Blended Unit-Dose System

A **blended-dose system** combines non–unit-dose drug distribution systems with a "unit-of-use" medication packaging system. Of the two types of blended unit-dose systems available, the **multiple medication package** (also known as an *adherence package* or a *pouch package*) contains all medications that are to be administered to a single patient at a specific time during a given day (Figure 13-3). Each of the patient's scheduled drug administrations is placed in a package on a "strip" of these packages, with the time for administration of each package printed on one side. Automated strip packaging machines are used to create these medication strips.

A **modular cassette** offers the combined advantages of both blister-packaged and unit-dose medications along with hospital-type drawer or cassette exchange systems. These cassettes contain either one-week or two-week medication strips that also contain reserve doses in a narrow plastic slide-tray design. These systems are often used in long-term care settings to decrease the chance of medication errors, minimize waste, and simplify record keeping.

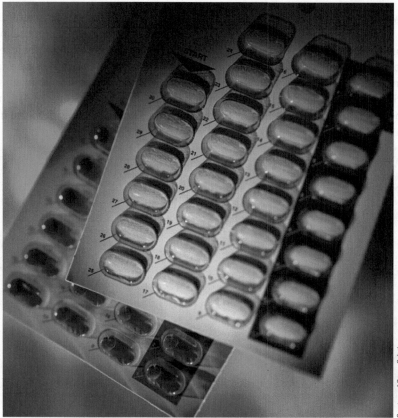

Courtesy of Capsa Solutions

Figure 13-2 Punch cards.

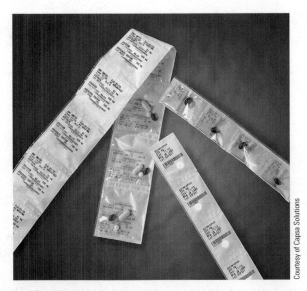

Courtesy of Capsa Solutions

Figure 13-3 Multiple medication package.

Automated Dispensing System

An **automated dispensing system** features a dispensing cabinet that stores and dispenses medications somewhere outside of the long-term care pharmacy. This cabinet is linked to the pharmacy's computer, and it releases medications upon individual pharmacist's approval. Nurses can gain access to medications within by using fingerprint scans or passwords. It is a process that reduces medication errors and automates billing, reordering, and record keeping; however, these systems are expensive, require significant amounts of space, and have been prone to computer connectivity problems. Automated dispensing systems are most often used in larger long-term care facilities.

WHAT WOULD YOU DO?

You discover that a nurse has obtained a controlled substance by falsifying an automated dispensing record as well as a medication administration record. What would you do?

Home Health Care Pharmacy

Home health care pharmacy is one of the fastest growing segments of the health care market. Today, most serious medical conditions and problems are treated outside the hospital setting, often at home. Home health care is an important part of the continuum of care. The growth of this system is related to several factors, including the increase in the number of elderly adults, patient preference, lower costs, improvements in technology, focus on managed care, and physician acceptance. The services rendered are performed under the supervision of individuals licensed to provide such services or care in accordance with the laws of the state in which the care is given. A state-licensed administrator assumes responsibility for facility operations, including the quality of health care rendered to patients. Nursing procedures require the professional skills of a registered nurse or a licensed practical nurse. These skills include administering medication, giving injections, placing catheters, and performing other procedures ordered by the physician. Posthospital care after strokes, heart disease, or orthopedic procedures is available.

Several types of home health care services may be available. These include the following:

- Pharmaceutical services
- Nursing services
- Personal care services
- Rehabilitation services
- Home medical supply services

Table 13-1 Sources of Payment for Home Care

Payment Source	Percent
Medicare	39.0
Medicaid	27.2
Private insurance	12.0
Out-of-pocket	20.5
Other and unknown	1.3
Total	100.0

The use of home care is a viable alternative that is safe and cost effective. It is also mutually satisfying to the patient and caregiver. The major sources of payment for home health care services are Medicare and Medicaid (see Table 13-1).

Many home health care products and services are provided by pharmacies. These services include provision of durable medical supplies, orthopedic supplies, oxygen therapy, wound care, artificial limbs, medical devices, prescription medications, and infusion therapy (intravenous [IV] and nutritional therapy). For patients with multiple conditions that require monitoring of treatment beyond high-technology therapy, the home care providers and the patient's regular physician will continue to be involved. The technician can assist the pharmacist in these services. The most common high-technology therapies include the following:

- IV antibiotic therapy
- Chemotherapy
- Pain medication
- Total parenteral nutrition
- Enteral nutrition
- Renal dialysis
- Respiratory and ventilation therapy

High-technology home care requires close collaboration of the physician, the pharmacist, the registered nurse, and, depending on the type of therapy, the medical supply company.

MEDICATION ERROR ALERT

Unfortunately, studies have shown that as many as one-third of home health care patients have received incorrect dosages of medications or have been given inappropriate medications for their conditions. With better patient and caregiver education, medication errors can be dramatically reduced for these patients and better treatment outcomes can be achieved.

Home Infusion Pharmacy

Home infusion pharmacy is a unique practice for pharmacists and pharmacy technicians. In this type of practice, infusion therapies are prepared and dispensed to patients in the home. In the acute care and home IV therapy environment, substantial pharmacy effort is devoted to the preparation of sterile products for IV and other parenteral administration (see Figure 13-4). Home infusion pharmacy service includes preparation of IV solutions, other injectable drugs, and enteral nutrition therapy. This type of service involves the safe compounding of an IV solution and its delivery to the patient. Equipment and supplies needed to infuse the solution are also provided. Home infusion pharmacies may be used in different areas, such as community pharmacies, long-term care pharmacies, and hospital pharmacies.

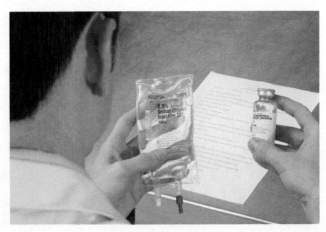

Figure 13-4 Home infusion therapy is one of many expanding areas of pharmacy practice in which the pharmacy technician can work.

Several types of infusion therapies are prescribed for home infusion, depending on the conditions of patients. These therapies include antibiotic therapy, pain management therapy, hydration therapy, total parenteral nutrition therapy, and cytotoxic cancer chemotherapy agents. Drugs added to IV solutions can be degraded by the diluting solution and by the effects of light, heat, and the storage environment. Drugs mixed in an IV solution also can interact with each other, leading to decreased effectiveness or to toxicity. The IV admixture itself may be contaminated through manipulation, leading to bacterial growth and transmission of bacteria to the patient. Some new biotechnology-derived drugs have very short periods of stability and may require special techniques for dilution and dispersion. Accuracy of preparation supports delivery of the labeled amount and ensures consistency from dose to dose and from patient to patient. In the past, IV solutions were prepared by nurses on the patient care units, but this practice is no longer recommended.

POINTS TO REMEMBER

Home infusion pharmacy is a sterile compounding practice that is similar (but not identical) to a hospital pharmacy practice.

Among the various types of equipment used in home infusion pharmacy are automated compounding and dispensing devices, horizontal and vertical laminar flow hoods, a refrigerator with a locked compartment for storage of drugs, computer hardware, and printers. Supplies used in home infusion pharmacy include syringes, needles, dispensing pins, IV solution containers, filters, transfer sets, IV tubing, alcohol preparation pads, gloves, masks, gowns, beard and shoe covers, and others.

One of the main duties of the pharmacy technician in home infusion pharmacy is the processing of equipment and supply orders. The pharmacy technician must be familiar with vascular access and vascular access devices, infusion devices, and other IV delivery systems. The pharmacy technician performs the compounding of sterile products and handling of home infusion equipment and supplies (see Figure 13-5).

He or she must have knowledge and skills specific to home infusion therapies and nutritional products, sterile compounding, aseptic technique, pharmaceutical calculations, and computer use, and an understanding of the laws and regulations pertaining to home infusion pharmacy. The pharmacy technician may be responsible for compounding, managing equipment and supplies, and monitoring computer functions in home infusion pharmacy. Pharmacy technicians also must be familiar with nutrition therapy. Two types of nutritional therapy are provided by home infusion pharmacy: parenteral and enteral.

In **parenteral nutrition** therapy, nutrients are delivered directly into the bloodstream. Total parenteral nutrition (TPN) consists of amino acid (protein), dextrose (carbohydrate), fats, electrolytes, vitamins, trace elements, and medication (e.g., insulin and heparin) (see Figure 13-6). Parenteral and TPN formulas both provide necessary nutrients. While parenteral nutrition is often used as a supplemental therapy, the goal of TPN is to provide compete replacement for patients who cannot take nutrition by any other route. TPN formulations are highly complex, and proper

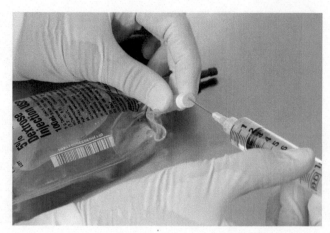

Figure 13-5 Preparation of intravenous medications within a sterile environment is one of the primary responsibilities of the pharmacy technician working in home infusion pharmacy.

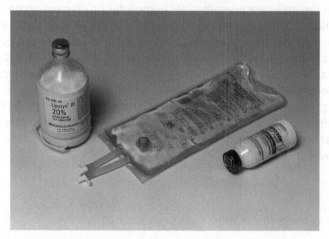

Figure 13-6 Total parenteral nutrition (TPN) consists of amino acid (protein), dextrose (carbohydrate), fats, electrolytes, vitamins, trace elements, and medication (e.g., insulin and heparin).

mixing is important. A safe and effective order of mixing ingredients should be followed. TPN formulations for home infusion are usually prepared several days before they are administered.

In enteral nutrition therapy, foods and nutrients are delivered into the gastrointestinal tract through a tube. This process is called tube feeding and is the most common home infusion nutritional therapy. Enteral nutrition can be used to supplement oral or parenteral nutrition, or it can be used to meet the patient's entire nutritional needs. Patients with swallowing problems resulting from conditions such as stroke, dementia, trauma, cancer, or acquired immunodeficiency syndrome (AIDS) are candidates for home enteral nutrition. Feeding tubes placed into the stomach through the nose are used for short-term therapy of up to three to four weeks.

Feeding tubes placed into the stomach or small intestine through the skin are used for long-term enteral therapy. Various enteral feeding routes are shown in Figure 13-7.

POINTS TO REMEMBER

There are many activities that a pharmacy technician may perform in the home infusion pharmacy, including compounding, computer data entry, and working with equipment and supplies.

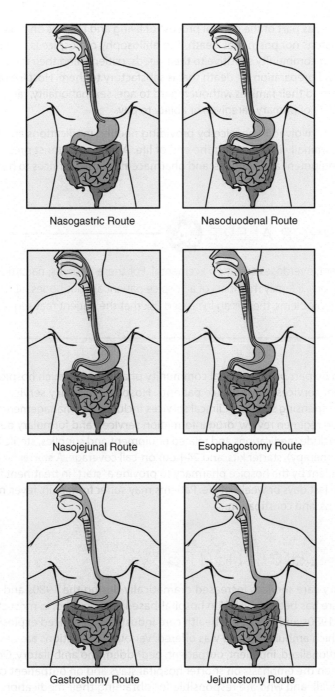

Nasogastric Route

Nasoduodenal Route

Nasojejunal Route

Esophagostomy Route

Gastrostomy Route

Jejunostomy Route

Figure 13-7 Enteral feeding routes.

Hospice Pharmacy

Hospice is an organized program of services to meet the medical, physical, emotional, spiritual, and social needs of a patient who is terminally ill, in both the hospital and home setting. Hospice care focuses on the patient's comfort rather than on a cure for the disease. Hospice care allows the patient to live the remainder of his or her life as free from pain and other symptoms as possible. Hospice serves all types and ages of patients. Hospice services are provided in various settings. The preferred setting is in the patient's home. An inpatient hospice facility may provide a safe and comfortable alternative. Funding for hospice programs comes from Medicare, Medicaid, and private insurance. For a patient to be eligible for hospice care under Medicare, a physician must certify that death is expected within six months. The average length of stay in hospice is 51 days. Hospices are licensed by the state department of health.

Hospice care recognizes dying as part of the normal process of living and focuses on maintaining the quality of life; it affirms life and neither hastens nor postpones death. The philosophy of hospice is that through appropriate care and the promotion of a caring community sensitive to their needs, patients and their families may be free to attain a degree of mental and spiritual preparation for death that is satisfactory to them. Hospice offers palliative care to terminally ill people and support to their families without regard to age, sex, nationality, race, creed, sexual orientation, disability, diagnosis, availability of primary caregiver, or ability to pay.

Pharmacists have become involved in hospice by providing needed medications and pharmaceutical care services to patients who are terminally ill or nearing the end of life. A pharmacy must prepare and dispense medications, medication-related equipment and supplies, and pharmaceutical care services to hospice patients at home or in an inpatient facility.

MEDICATION ERROR ALERT

In the hospice environment, overdoses are often accidental. For these patients, narcotics are examples of commonly prescribed medications. If family members of a hospice patient are not honest about the patient's previous history of substance abuse problems, there is an increased risk that the patient may request increased dosages of narcotics.

A hospice pharmacy can be part of a traditional community pharmacy, in which hospice is a part of its business, or it can be a pharmacy that services only hospice patients. Hospice pharmacy services can be divided into two areas: clinical services and dispensing services. Clinical services include pain management, symptom management, medication monitoring, drug regimen review, drug information services, and formulary development and management. Dispensing services include medications and related equipment and supplies, sterile IV infusion compounding (pain, hydration, and chemotherapy), starter kits, and 24-hour on-call coverage. A **starter kit** is a group of medications that is given to a hospice patient by the hospice pharmacy to provide a "start" in treatment for most urgent problems that can develop during the last days or weeks of life. Patients may suffer from pain, fever, nausea, vomiting, anxiety, agitation, increased secretions, and constipation.

Ambulatory Care Pharmacy

The provision of ambulatory care services increased dramatically during the 1980s and mid to late 1990s. Traditionally, most outpatient care has been provided in hospital-based facilities and, in most cases, on the campuses of such hospitals. During the 1980s and 1990s, the health care industry experienced explosive growth in the type of ownership of facilities in which ambulatory care was offered. Various designations are used to categorize patients: institutionalized, noninstitutionalized, inpatient, outpatient, bedridden, and ambulatory. One of the most significant trends in health care has been the emphasis on shorter hospital stays and on outpatient care. Ambulatory patients are those who are able to walk and who are responsible for obtaining their medication, storing it, and taking it. Ambulatory care has become the standard for health care delivery. The term *ambulatory care* includes a range of services such as outpatient pharmacies, emergency departments, primary care clinics, specialty clinics, ambulatory care centers, and family practice groups. At present, ambulatory care services provide radiation therapy, dialysis centers, diagnostic imaging, mobile imaging, rehabilitation, free-standing ambulatory surgery, urgent care, wound care, sleep study laboratories, infusion therapy, chemotherapy, ambulatory clinical pharmacy, and endoscopy centers.

The increase in ambulatory care services has greatly expanded the opportunities for ambulatory care pharmacy practitioners. Clinical pharmacists practice in various clinic settings; their involvement in these settings improves drug therapy documentation and patient adherence, decreases duplicate prescriptions, and reduces the risk of overdosage. The pharmacy clinic provides refills to drop-in patients. Patients are referred by physicians to clinical pharmacists, who provide physical assessment, order laboratory tests, alter dosages, and change medications. One of the most successful types of pharmacist-managed ambulatory care clinics is the anticoagulation clinic. The advantages of including clinical pharmacists in the chronic management of patients with preexisting conditions (e.g., hypertension, diabetes, and allergies) who are receiving anticoagulation therapy should be obvious. One of the most important features of ambulatory care practice is the involvement of the clinical pharmacist in drug therapy decisions. This requires that the pharmacist be available and accessible when the patient is being seen. It is clear that successful ambulatory care pharmacy services must be comprehensive and continual. Clinical pharmacy services must be provided 80% to 90% of the time.

WHAT WOULD YOU DO?

Your pharmacy provides medications for ambulatory care patients, and you are aware of the medications listed as "high alert." These include carbamazepine, warfarin, and methotrexate. You are given a prescription to fill for methotrexate, and you notice that the patient is not being treated for cancer, but for rheumatoid arthritis, and the dosage seems excessive. Based on methotrexate's high-alert status when not used as an oncology medication, what would you do?

Mail-Order Pharmacy

Mail-order pharmacy is defined as a pharmacy that dispenses maintenance medications to patients through mail delivery. It is one of the fastest growing areas in pharmacy practice. It is offered by most health plans today as an option to the traditional retail pharmacy for obtaining prescriptions. Medications are sent to patients through mail or delivery services, and many mail-order pharmacies offer online ordering through the Internet (see "Internet Pharmacy" later in the chapter). Mail-order pharmacy is a unique setting for pharmacists and pharmacy technicians. Staff members consist of licensed pharmacists, registered nurses, and technicians. Pharmacy technicians in these pharmacies perform almost all the dispensing functions involved with filling prescriptions. They are responsible for more data entry and production tasks than in a traditional retail pharmacy.

POINTS TO REMEMBER

The advantages of mail-order pharmacy include cost savings, patient convenience, and privacy.

Mail-order pharmacies provide services to all 50 states. They operate at a high volume, which results in discounts and is more economical for patients. Mail-order pharmacies can serve more patients, particularly those who have chronic illnesses such as diabetes, high blood pressure, depression, heart disease, asthma, arthritis, or gastrointestinal disorders. The need for medication can be predicted, and the supply can be easily maintained by mail delivery. Medication that is required regularly for the treatment of a chronic condition is called a maintenance medication. In most cases, mail-order pharmacies contract with health insurers and fill prescriptions at discounted rates for members of those plans. Both the Food and Drug Administration (FDA) and the National Association of Boards of Pharmacy (NABP) estimate that there are more than 200 combination mail-order/online pharmacies located within the United States.

POINTS TO REMEMBER

Disadvantages of mail-order pharmacy include medication waste, lack of personal contact, increases in medication errors, and time delays.

A traditional mail-order pharmacy usually fills prescriptions requiring maintenance medications. The patient pays a copayment, with the prescriptions usually covered by a single payer. A **specialty mail-order pharmacy** handles many different types of prescriptions, including those for patients with chronic diseases such as cancer, diabetes, multiple sclerosis, hepatitis, infertility, or rheumatoid arthritis. Commonly, these "specialty" medications are packaged for injection and are not easily found in the average retail community pharmacy. These prescriptions are often covered by several different payers, including Medicaid, Medicare, and private insurers. Specialty mail-order pharmacies have more complicated billing, pricing, processing, and reporting activities than traditional mail-order pharmacies.

Central Fill Pharmacy

A **central fill pharmacy** is usually located near individual pharmacies in a specific area and provides services to varying numbers of these individual pharmacies. For example, retail chain pharmacies often use central fill pharmacies to provide prescriptions to many different retail pharmacy locations. These pharmacies mostly handle refills of prescriptions, utilizing automation due to the large volume of prescriptions filled. Central fill pharmacies may deliver filled prescriptions to the individual pharmacies they serve or to patients' homes. Other activities handled by a central fill pharmacy include resolving problems with insurance claims, performing drug use reviews, and interfacing with physicians. Central fill pharmacies reduce costs, provide patients with more options concerning their prescriptions, and allow local pharmacists at individual pharmacies to have more time for patient counseling.

Internet Pharmacy

An **Internet pharmacy** utilizes commercial websites to allow patients to order prescription and over-the-counter medications, as well as supplements over the Internet. They bill each patient's insurance and charge the patient a copay amount via their credit card. Delivery costs are usually reduced in order to be competitive with traditional retail pharmacies, and overnight delivery is available. Internet pharmacies usually provide e-mail and toll-free phone numbers so that patients can communicate directly with them. These pharmacies usually provide comprehensive websites and links to other online sites that offer complete, detailed information about the medications they offer. Legitimate Internet pharmacies operate with extremely rigid safeguards to ensure that their customers receive the best quality pharmacy care and counseling. However, there are many illegitimate Internet pharmacy websites, frequently operating outside of the United States, that have been charged with selling unsafe medications and dispensing medications to customers who have not provided a proper prescription. The government regularly seeks out these operations for prosecution. Overall, Internet pharmacy is expected to play a growing role in the future of pharmacy.

WHAT WOULD YOU DO?

You are working for an Internet pharmacy and find that other pharmacy technicians who fill orders are routinely giving out advice to patients, through e-mails and online "chat" services, in place of actual pharmacists handling all patient counseling. These activities are actually encouraged by the owners of the business, because customers don't know whom they are interacting with, and the company employs only a few pharmacists. What would you do?

Nuclear Pharmacy

Nuclear pharmacy is a branch of pharmacy that deals with the provisions of services related to **radiopharmaceuticals**. A radiopharmaceutical is a radioactive drug that is used in the diagnosis and treatment of disease. A radiopharmaceutical consists of both a drug component and a radioactive component. The drug component is responsible for localization in specific organs or tissues. The radioactive component contains radioactive elements. The three types of radiation that can be released by a radionuclide are alpha, beta, and gamma. Gamma radiation is the most penetrating type of radiation. It differs from alpha and beta radiation, because it is electromagnetic, whereas they are particulate. Gamma radiation differs from x-rays, ultraviolet rays, and visible light only in wavelength (or frequency).

Nuclear medicine uses very small quantities of radionuclides for the diagnosis and treatment of disease. Radiopharmaceuticals are used as tracers for assessing the structure, function, secretion, excretion, and volume of a particular organ or tissue. They are also used to analyze biological specimens; to treat specific diseases such as hyperthyroidism, thyroid cancer, and polycythemia vera; and to alleviate bone pain. Most radiopharmaceuticals are prepared as sterile, pyrogen-free intravenous solutions or suspensions to be administered directly to the patient. An important component of nuclear medicine is imaging, which involves administering radiopharmaceuticals to a patient orally, intravenously, or by inhalation to localize a specific organ or system and its structure and function. Nuclear pharmacy is a sterile compounding practice. The most commonly used radionuclides are iodine and technetium compounds. Technetium-99m (^{99m}Tc) is used in about 80% of radioactive drugs. Most technetium compounds are used for diagnosis. Manufacturers develop compounds that can be labeled with ^{99m}Tc, which are used for imaging various organ systems or tissues. These compounds are often available in a form that is known as a **reagent kit**. Reagent kits are vials containing the particular compounds, usually in freeze-dried form. The kit is a multidose vial that contains the compound (ligand) as it is labeled.

Iodine-131 (^{131}I) is used for treatment of hyperthyroidism or, more recently, for ovarian and prostate cancer. There are numerous other radionuclides used in medicine. These include xenon (a gas used to image the lungs), thallium, gallium, cobalt, chromium, indium, and strontium. A radiopharmaceutical used more recently for treatment is strontium-89 (^{89}Sr) as strontium chloride. This radionuclide emits beta radiation. ^{89}Sr, an analog of calcium, localizes in areas of metastatic disease of bone and reduces pain through the effect of the beta radiation at the tumor site. Unlike the use of ^{131}I to destroy thyroid cancer, this agent is not used to cure cancer, but rather as a palliative agent to provide relief from pain.

Some radiopharmaceuticals are prepared in their final form at the manufacturing site, whereas others are compounded in a nuclear pharmacy or nuclear medicine department. There are several levels of sophistication to the compounding of these agents, ranging from simple addition of radioactive pertechnetate to the reagent kit vial to radiolabeling of autologous blood cells, custom radiolabeling of peptides and antibodies, and rapid hot laboratory chemical compounding of short-lived positron-emitting radiopharmaceuticals. Because the radionuclides commonly used in radiopharmaceuticals have short half-lives, most radiopharmaceuticals must be prepared on the day of use. Nuclear pharmacy involves the procuring, storage, compounding, dispensing, and provision of information about radiopharmaceuticals and is one possible area of specialization for both pharmacists and pharmacy technicians (see Figure 13-8). To practice nuclear pharmacy, pharmacists must have specialized training in several areas, such as nuclear physics, radiation detection instrumentation, radiochemistry, and radiation protection.

POINTS TO REMEMBER

Pharmacy technicians are commonly sent for radiopharmaceutical training by the nuclear pharmacy that employs them. Experience with sterile IV compounding is generally required for this type of position.

Experience in a practice site is essential as well. The level of knowledge and experience necessary, as well as services provided, vary with the practice site. Most nuclear pharmacists practice in a centralized commercial nuclear pharmacy. Most practitioners in this setting have a professional degree, whereas nuclear pharmacists in an institutional site commonly have received an advanced degree (MS). The basic functions are similar; however, the pharmacist in the larger hospital may be more involved with clinical service, investigational products, and teaching. The pharmacist in a centralized nuclear pharmacy inherently spends considerable time preparing and dispensing radiopharmaceuticals, because one pharmacy generally services 10 to 15 hospitals and clinics.

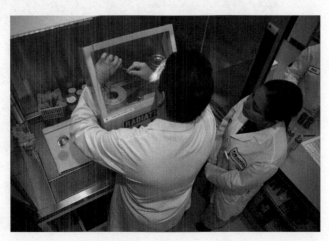

Figure 13-8 Nuclear pharmacy is another area of specialization in which pharmacy technicians may choose to work.

EQUIPMENT AND SUPPLIES

Though many pieces of equipment and other supplies in the nuclear pharmacy are the same as those used in other types of pharmacy, these pharmacies also have very specialized equipment designed for the radioactive materials they deal with on a regular basis. Specialized nuclear pharmacy equipment includes the following:

- Autoclaves—for sterilization
- Centrifuges—used to spin whole blood samples for separation of elements or for combining with a radionuclide
- Dose calibrators—used to measure radioactivity of radionuclides (see Figure 13-9)
- Dosimeters—used to measure radiation exposure to individuals
- Fume hoods—laminar airflow hoods adapted to vent air outward in order to release radiation rather than recycle it back into the hoods (see Figure 13-10)
- Geiger counters—used to measure low-level radiation in an area
- Glove boxes—laminar airflow hoods designed so that a worker's hands may be inserted through special gloves allowing access into them
- Heating devices—dry heat ovens, incubators, and hot water baths
- Refrigerators and freezers—lead-lined units designed for radioactive compounds
- Respirators—used to prevent the inhalation of radioactive substances
- Shields—lead barrier shields used to protect workers from radioactivity
- Showers—used to remove radioactive substances from workers
- Sinks—deep stainless steel sinks used to prevent splashing of radioactive compounds onto workers
- Storage boxes—lead-lined boxes for storage and decay of radioactive materials
- Testing equipment—instruments such as chromatographs, microscopes, and pH meters used for quality control procedures

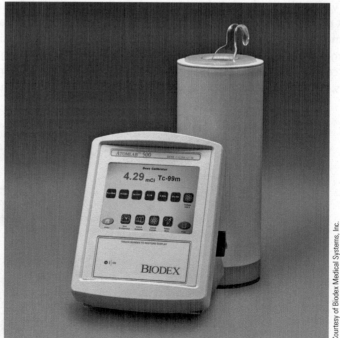

Courtesy of Biodex Medical Systems, Inc.

Figure 13-9 Dose calibrator.

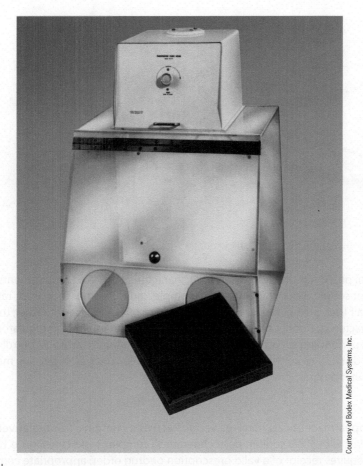

Courtesy of Bodex Medical Systems, Inc.

Figure 13-10 Fume hood.

Specialized nuclear pharmacy supplies include lead-lined aprons and gloves, leaded protective eyewear, leaded syringe and vial shields (see Figures 13-11A and 13-11B), long tweezers or tongs, ammonia, cushioning materials, specialized labels and shipping containers, and vehicles used to deliver products.

GUIDELINES FOR PRACTICE OF NUCLEAR PHARMACY

The practice of nuclear pharmacy is a specialized field of pharmacy that requires specific guidelines and regulations. The nine general areas involved in nuclear pharmacy practice are the following:

1. Procurement
2. Compounding
3. Quality assurance
4. Dispensing
5. Distribution
6. Health and safety
7. Provision of information and consultation
8. Monitoring patient outcome
9. Regulations

Procurement

Procurement of radiopharmaceuticals and other drugs, supplies, and materials necessary for nuclear pharmacy practice involves determining product specifications, initiating purchase orders, receiving shipments, maintaining inventory, and storing materials under proper conditions. Although these tasks appear similar to those involved in

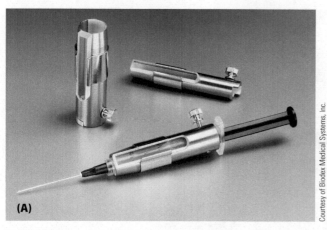

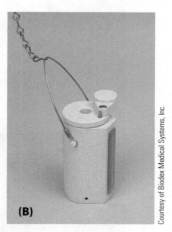

Figure 13-11 Leaded shields include (A) syringe shields, and (B) vial shield.

community and hospital pharmacy practice, the special characteristics of and requirements associated with radio-pharmaceuticals present some unique demands. For example, radiopharmaceuticals or radioactive components, because of their short half-lives, are not available through conventional wholesalers; rather, they typically are ordered directly from the manufacturers. Receipt of radioactive materials involves following regulatory procedures for opening packages, including performing surveys for radioactive contamination. Inventory control of radioactive materials is complicated by their distinctive, continuous radioactive decay. Fortunately, repetitive manual calculations have been replaced by computer programs developed for this purpose.

Compounding

Compounding of radiopharmaceuticals involves various activities ranging from relatively simple tasks such as reconstituting reagent kits with ^{99m}Tc sodium pertechnetate to complex tasks (see Figure 13-12). Compounding of radiopharmaceuticals requires receipt of a valid prescription or drug order; appropriate components, supplies, and equipment; a suitable environment, especially for sterile dosage forms; appropriate record keeping; and verification of the compounding procedure, storage conditions, and expiration.

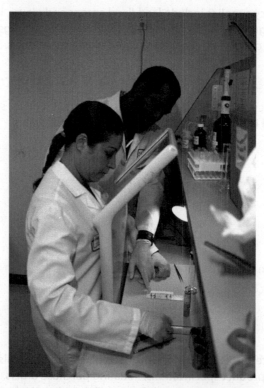

Figure 13-12 One of the primary duties within nuclear pharmacy is that of compounding radiopharmaceuticals.

Quality Assurance

Quality assurance of radiopharmaceuticals involves performing the appropriate chemical, physical, and biological tests on radiopharmaceuticals to ensure the suitability of the products for use in humans.

Dispensing

Dispensing radiopharmaceuticals occurs upon the receipt of a valid prescription or drug order. In contrast to traditional pharmacy practice, radiopharmaceuticals are rarely dispensed directly to patients; rather, they are dispensed to hospitals or clinics for administration to patients by trained health professionals. Radiopharmaceuticals generally are dispensed in unit doses ready for administration to the patient. In addition to radiopharmaceuticals, certain other drugs, such as those used in pharmacological intervention studies, often are dispensed by nuclear pharmacists.

Distribution

Distribution of radiopharmaceuticals within an institution is subject to institutional policies and procedures, generally involving lead-lined boxes or other shielded containers labeled with identifying information (see Figure 13-13).

Distribution of radiopharmaceuticals from a centralized nuclear pharmacy to other institutions is subject to local, state, and federal regulations, including those promulgated by state boards of pharmacy, the U.S. Department of Transportation, and the U.S. Nuclear Regulatory Commission (NRC). These requirements generally relate to packaging, labeling, shipping papers, other record keeping, and personnel training.

Health and Safety

Health and safety are crucial elements of nuclear pharmacy practice. Radiation safety standards, including limits for radiation doses, levels of radiation in an area, concentrations of radioactivity in air and waste water, waste disposal,

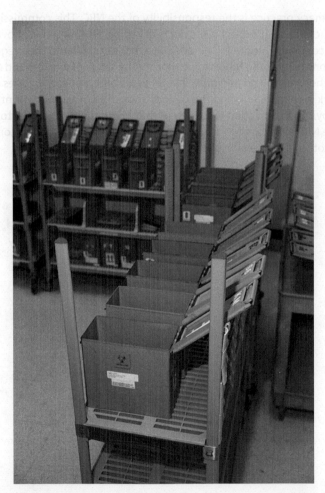

Figure 13-13 Special precautions must be taken in the handling, care, storage, and distribution of radioactive materials.

and precautionary procedures, have been established and are enforced by the NRC. Although radiation protection may be the most visible and most regulated, other aspects of health and safety are also important. Hazardous chemicals, such as chromatography solvents, must be stored, handled, and disposed of using proper techniques, personal protective devices, containers, and environment. Biological specimens, such as blood samples obtained for preparation of labeled red and white blood cells, must be handled as potentially infectious, using standard precautions. Last, physical exertion, such as lifting heavy lead shields, must be done with appropriate care.

Provision of Information and Consultation

Provision of information and consultation is a highly important function of nuclear pharmacists. Using both oral and written communication skills, nuclear pharmacists convey their expert knowledge to physicians, technologists, pharmacy technicians, patients, and others. The nuclear pharmacist should provide appropriate types of information, including the biological effects of radiation, radiation physics and radiation protection, radiopharmaceutical chemistry, radiopharmaceutical compounding, and quality assurance.

Monitoring Patient Outcome

Monitoring patient outcome is an important component in pharmaceutical care. A nuclear pharmacist can assist in ensuring that patients are referred to appropriate nuclear medicine procedures. Evaluating the safety and efficacy of radiopharmaceutical and ancillary medications is important, as is ensuring that patients receive proper preparation before receiving radiopharmaceuticals. A nuclear pharmacist must be sure that clinical problems associated with the use of the radiopharmaceuticals are prevented or recognized, investigated, and rectified. He or she must be administering therapeutic or diagnostic radiopharmaceuticals and ancillary medications and performing nuclear medicine procedures.

Regulations

Regulation of nuclear pharmacy practice is the responsibility of the NRC. This commission issues licenses and has regulatory authority for functions relating to by-products of radioactive materials; however, individual states are responsible for regulating accelerator-produced materials in a manner similar to their regulation of x-ray–producing machines. The primary responsibility of the NRC is to provide for the safety of workers and the general public exposed to radiation and to protect their health and minimize danger to life and property. Badges must be worn by all health care professionals who work with radiation, and the badges should be monitored monthly (see Figure 13-14). The responsibility of the employing organization is to ensure that no worker is exposed to higher levels of radiation than those approved by the NRC, maintain a radiation safety committee, monitor and control patient exposure, and provide lead shielding to protect all vulnerable body parts.

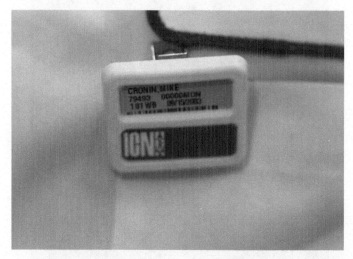

Figure 13-14 Staff within the nuclear pharmacy must wear devices to monitor the amount of radiation they are exposed to while on the job.

Summary

Because of advances in medical science and technology, people are living longer, resulting in a greater need for long-term care than ever before. Long-term pharmacy organizations have been created to provide medications and clinical services to the increasing numbers of long-term care facilities. In addition, home health care services have expanded to include pharmaceutical, nursing, personal care, rehabilitation, and home medical supply services. High-technology home care includes administration of IV antibiotics, chemotherapy, pain medications, TPN, and enteral nutrition; renal dialysis; respiratory and ventilation therapy; and even hospice services for the terminally ill. Clinical pharmacists are routinely involved in drug therapy decisions for ambulatory care practices. Mail-order pharmacies, which dispense medications through mail delivery, have become one of the fastest growing areas in pharmacy. One possible area of specialization is nuclear pharmacy, which involves the procuring, storage, compounding, dispensing, and provision of information about radiopharmaceuticals. With so much growth in advanced pharmacy, it is essential that pharmacy technicians be trained in all areas that reflect the growing needs of the public.

REVIEW QUESTIONS

1. NRC is the abbreviation for:

   A. Nuclear Regulatory Commission.
   B. Nuclear Registry Center.
   C. nuclear remission cancer.
   D. nuclear register consulting.

2. The major services provided in nursing homes include:

   A. assuring the patient's comfort rather than caring for their disease.
   B. satisfying Medicare requirements for palliative care to the terminally ill.
   C. meeting the physical, emotional, and spiritual needs of a patient.
   D. nursing care.

3. Compounding of radiopharmaceuticals requires:

   A. payment in advance.
   B. a patient's insurance card.
   C. receipt of a valid prescription.
   D. technicians who are nationally certified.

4. One of the fastest growing areas in pharmacy is:

   A. health care administration.
   B. mail-order.
   C. traditional.
   D. None of the above.

5. A container that is required to meet light and moisture resistance standards by the USP–NF in the long-term care pharmacy is called a(n):

   A. individual unit-dose package.
   B. modified unit-dose system.
   C. unit-dose system.
   D. drug distribution system.

6. Home infusion pharmacy includes:

   A. radiography.
   B. enteral nutrition therapy.
   C. physical therapy.
   D. hydrotherapy.

7. At present, ambulatory care services provide:

    A. surgery.
    B. sleep study laboratory.
    C. pharmacy.
    D. All of the above.

8. Which of the following patients are often the candidates for home enteral nutrition therapy?

    A. Those who have diabetes
    B. Those who are in shock
    C. Those who have cancer
    D. Those who have bone fractures

9. Which of the following is the most penetrating type of radiation?

    A. Beta
    B. Gamma
    C. Alpha
    D. X-ray

10. An "adherence package" or a "pouch package" is also known as a:

    A. multiple medication package.
    B. single medication package.
    C. modular cassette.
    D. unit-dose system.

11. Modular cassettes are often used in long-term care settings for all of the following, *except*:

    A. to simplify record keeping.
    B. to minimize waste.
    C. to decrease chances of medication errors.
    D. to decrease the workload of the pharmacist.

12. Which of the following activities is not allowed to be performed by pharmacy technicians in home care settings?

    A. Working with chemotherapeutics
    B. Working with pain medications
    C. Working with IV antibiotics
    D. Consulting patients

13. The main duties of the pharmacy technician in home infusion pharmacy include:

    A. performing the compounding of sterile products.
    B. handling home infusion equipment and supplies.
    C. processing equipment and supply orders.
    D. All of the above.

14. Total parenteral nutrition (TPN) formulations for home infusion are usually prepared how long before they are administered?

    A. Less than 1 hour
    B. Several hours
    C. Several days
    D. Several years

15. Which of the following is one of the fastest growing parts of the health care market?

    A. Home nuclear pharmacy
    B. Home health care services
    C. Home mental care services
    D. All of the above

CRITICAL THINKING

Greg has been working for six months in a pharmacy that compounds chemotherapeutics. He has been trained and certified for this specialized work.

1. Research the educational requirements and duties for a pharmacy technician working in this type of pharmacy.

2. Compare mail-order pharmacy with long-term care pharmacy.

WEB LINKS

Advanced Pharmacy Technician Roles: www.ashp.org/pharmacy-technician/about-pharmacy-technicians/advanced-pharmacy-technician-roles

American Pharmacists Association: www.pharmacist.com

American Society of Health-System Pharmacists: www.ashp.org

Hospice Foundation of America: hospicefoundation.org

National Association of Boards of Pharmacy: nabp.pharmacy

CHAPTER 14

Extemporaneous Prescription Compounding

OUTLINE

OBJECTIVES

Upon completion of this chapter, the reader should be able to:

1. Explain the use of a Class-A prescription balance and a counter balance.
2. Describe extemporaneous compounding.
3. Describe the difference between a solution, a suspension, an elixir, and an emulsion.
4. Identify how capsule sizes are classified.
5. Define a "Class-A prescription balance."
6. Name the most common and important equipment for extemporaneous compounding.
7. Discuss which liquid ingredients are used to mix with powders in the compounding of tablets.
8. Identify methods in which graduates are correctly used for compounding.
9. Describe the indications of spatulas and pipettes in compounding.
10. Explain the terms *levigate* and *meniscus*.

KEY TERMS

Class-A prescription
balance

compounding slab

conical graduates

counter balance

cylindrical graduates

electronic balance

extemporaneous
compounding

geometric dilution

levigate

master formula sheet

mortar

pestle

pipette

solvent

tablet triturates

tare

triturate

Overview

Compounding has always been a basic part of pharmacy practice. The equipment or techniques, drugs, and dosage forms used are the variables. Manufacturing is the mass production of compounded prescription products for resale to pharmacies and is regulated by the Food and Drug Administration (FDA). Good manufacturing practices are the standards of practice used in the pharmaceutical industry and are regulated by the FDA. Extemporaneous compounding addresses the needs of patients who require pharmaceutical products that are not available through mass production manufacturing.

Community pharmacists must comply with state board of pharmacy regulations and guidelines to ensure a quality product, which includes using proper materials, weighing equipment, documented technique, and dispensing and storage instructions. The liability of compounding is no greater than the risk of filling a prescription for a manufactured product, because the pharmacist must ensure that the correct drug, dose, and directions are provided. A **master formula sheet** is used for extemporaneous compounding (see Figure 14-1). It lists all of the ingredients needed for a specific formulation, listing amounts of ingredients, manufacturers of each ingredient, lot numbers, the actual compounding procedure, and expiration dates. The individual performing the compounding must initial the master formula sheet to confirm his or her actions during the process.

Extemporaneous Compounding

Extemporaneous compounding is the preparation, mixing, assembling, packaging, and labeling of a drug product based on a prescription order from a licensed practitioner for the individual patient. The pharmacist is responsible for preparing a quality pharmaceutical product, providing proper instructions about its storage, and advising the patient of any adverse effects. Compounding may have different meanings for different pharmacists, including the following:

- The preparation of oral liquids, topical preparations, and suppositories
- The conversion of one dose or dosage form into another
- The preparation of select dosage forms from bulk chemicals
- The preparation of intravenous admixtures, parenteral nutrition solutions, and pediatric dosage forms from adult dosage forms
- The preparation of radioactive isotopes
- The preparation of cassettes, syringes, and other devices with drugs for administration in the home setting

Extemporaneous compounding can be done in a dedicated facility that focuses on these types of activities, or other pharmacy settings when these activities are required. The reasons for extemporaneous compounding today include the following:

- Unavailable dosages, routes, and strengths of commercial products
- Dilution of adult doses to pediatric or geriatric strengths
- Converting solid dosage forms to suspensions or solutions
- Combining topical products for dermatological use that are not already available
- Inactive ingredients in commercial drug products that can cause allergic reactions

MASTER FORMULA SHEET – NON-STERILE MANUFACTURING

PRODUCT: **HYDROCHLOROTHIAZIDE** 5 mg/mL AND **SPIRONOLACTONE** 5 mg/mL SUSPENSION

Date Prepared: ____________________ **FINAL PRODUCT CHECKED BY:** ____________________

EXPIRY DATE: ____________________

INGREDIENT	MANUFACTURER	LOT #	MAN. EXPIRY DATE	FORMULA QUANTITY	QUANTITY USED	MFG BY	CHK BY
Hydrochlorothiazide 25 mg Spironolactone 25 mg tablet				20			
Ora-Blend®	Paddock			qs to 100 ML			

EQUIPMENT

- Mortar and pestle
- Graduated Cylinder

MANUFACTURING DIRECTIONS

1. Crush tablets to make a fine powder in a mortar.
2. Levigate powder with a small amount of the vehicle to make a fine paste.
3. Continue to add vehicle until product liquid enough to transfer to a graduated cylinder.
4. Rinse mortar several times with vehicle and add to product in graduated cylinder.
5. QS to final volume with vehicle.
6. Dispense in amber plastic bottles. May be refrigerated or stored at room temperature.

FINAL APPEARANCE

Opaque white suspension

SAMPLE LABEL

HYDROCHLOROTHIZIADE 5 mg/mL
and SPIRONOLACTONE 5 mg/mL Suspension
Shake well. Refrigerate. Take with Food.
Date Prepared: Date Expired:

STABILITY

60 days in fridge or at room temperature.

REFERENCE(S)

- Nahata MC, Hipple TF, Pediatric Drug Formulations, 4th ed. 2000, pp 115
- Allen LV, Erickson MA. AJHP 1996, 53: 2304-9

MASTER Sheet Revision Dates: ____________________ ***Final Approval By:***

The non-sterile manufacturing formulas are provided for informational purposes for qualified health care professionals. The hospital will not assume responsibility for the continued currency of the information, any errors or ommissions, and/or any consequences arising from the use of the information outside of CHEO.

Figure 14-1 Master formula sheet.

Regulations concerning compounding pharmacies were heightened in 2013 with the passage of the Drug Quality and Security Act (see Chapter 3). It reclassified compounding pharmacies as "outsourcing facilities" and required them to comply with *current good manufacturing practices*, to be inspected by the FDA according to a risk-based schedule, to report adverse events, and to provide the FDA with certain information about compounded products. However, the majority of extemporaneous compounding activities are regulated by each state's board of pharmacy.

MEDICATION ERROR ALERT

Like other areas of pharmacy, extemporaneous compounding can be vulnerable to medication errors. A pharmacist who was refilling a compounded suspension of *primidone*, an anticonvulsant, decided to improve the formulation by using bulk powder instead of primidone tablets. Mistakenly, he or she used stock *baclofen* bulk powder, and the young child who received the newly compounded suspension had to be taken to the emergency department, but fortunately the child survived.

EQUIPMENT

The correct equipment is important when compounding. Therefore, pharmacy technicians should be familiar with those pieces of equipment that are necessary for compounding drugs. Many state boards of pharmacy have a required minimum list of equipment for compounding prescriptions. These pieces of equipment vary according to the amount of material needed and the type of compounded prescription. There are several conventional pieces of equipment and instruments that a pharmacist or pharmacy technician may use for the operation of compounding. These include balances, forceps, spatulas, compounding slabs, mortars and pestles, graduates, and pipettes.

Class A Prescription Balances

Each pharmacy is required to have a **Class-A prescription balance** or an **electronic balance** (see Figure 14-2), or both. Class A balances have a sensitivity requirement of 6 mg. An electronic balance is an instrument used to electronically weigh small amounts of drugs; the measurement is indicated on a digital screen.

Counter Balances

A **counter balance** is capable of weighing larger quantities, up to about 5 kg. It is a double-pan balance. A counter balance is not indicated for prescription compounding. It is used for measuring bulk products.

Weights

Good-quality weights are essential, and they should be stored appropriately. Weights made from corrosion-resistant metals, such as brass, are preferred (see Figure 14-3). Metric weights are positioned in the front row and apothecary weights are in the back row. When transferring weights, you should always be careful not to drop them, and you should always use forceps (see Figure 14-4). Handling of the weights with bare hands may cause a buildup of oils on the weights that will alter their accuracy.

Spatulas

Spatulas are available in stainless steel, plastic, or hard rubber (see Figure 14-5). Spatulas are used to transfer solid ingredients, such as ointments and creams, to weighing pans. Spatulas are also used to mix compounds on an ointment slab. They must be clean and have indented edges.

Compounding Slabs

The **compounding slab** is a plate made of ground glass with a hard, flat, and nonabsorbent surface for mixing compounds (see Figure 14-6). Compounding slabs are also called ointment slabs.

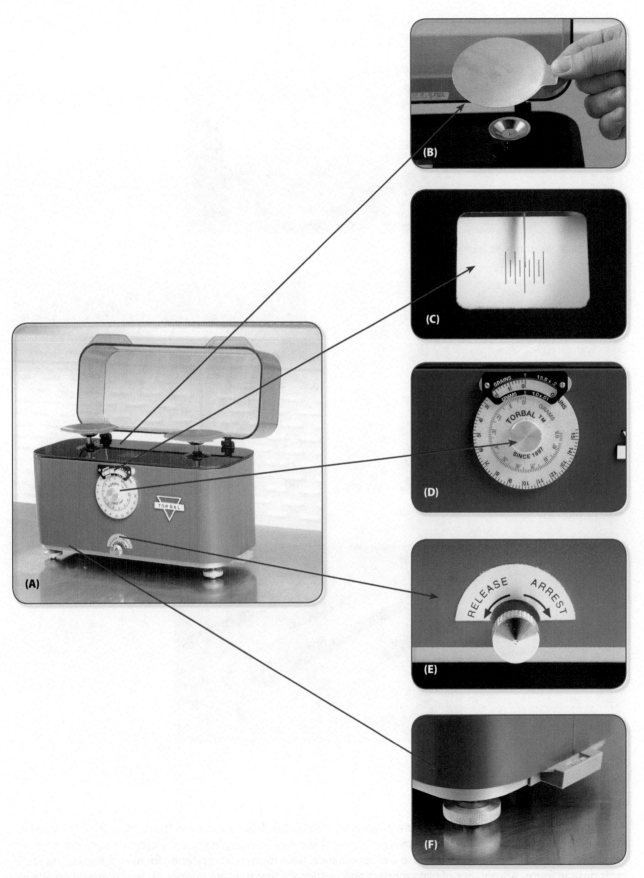

Figure 14-2 (A) Class-A prescription balance. (B) Weighing pans. (C) Index plate. (D) Graduate dial. (E) Locking or arrest mechanism. (F) Leveling feet.

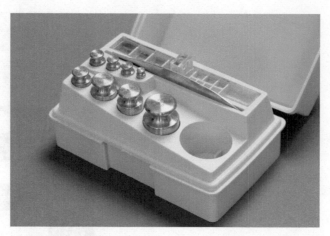

Figure 14-3 Weights used in pharmacy practice.

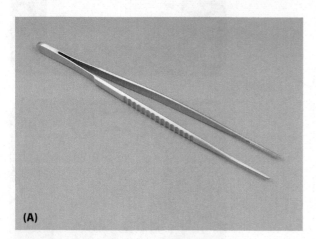

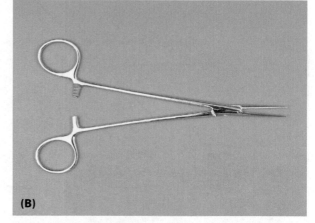

Figure 14-4 Forceps: (A) Tissue. (B) Hemostatic.

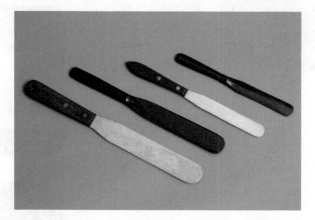

Figure 14-5 Spatulas.

Mortars and Pestles

A **mortar** is a cup-shaped vessel in which materials are ground or crushed by a **pestle** in the preparation of drugs. Mortars and pestles are available in three types: glass (see Figure 14-7A), Wedgwood, and porcelain (see Figure 14-7B), which is quite similar to Wedgwood in use and appearance. Glass mortars are preferred for mixing liquids and semi-soft dosage forms. Advantages of glass mortars and pestles are that they are nonporous and nonstaining. Wedgwood and porcelain mortars and pestles are coarser and best used when triturating crystals, granules, and powders. They will produce a finer trituration.

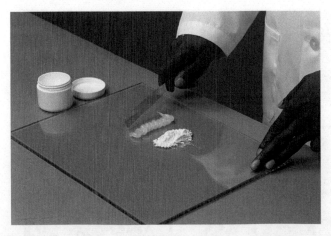

Figure 14-6 Compounding slab.

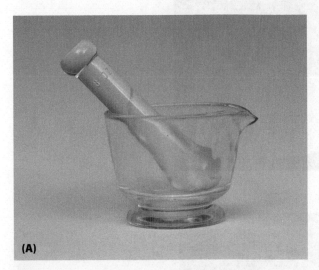

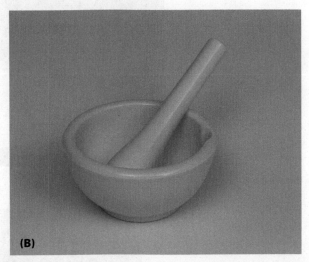

Figure 14-7 (A) Glass mortar and pestle. (B) Porcelain mortar and pestle.

Electronic Mortars and Pestles

Electronic mortars and pestles (EMPs) have the ability to produce quality ointments, creams, and oral liquids. They use a spinning blade and moving arm to mix products, which can be weighted, mixed, and dispensed all in the same jar (see Figure 14-8). Electronic mortars and pestles are easily cleaned with alcohol or detergents but should be maintained by an authorized service company.

Heat Guns

Heat guns are commonly used to shrink bands onto vials. They resemble hair dryers (see Figure 14-9) and are used in a similar way, by turning the end of the heat gun that emits heat slightly in order to thoroughly apply heat to the vial's shrink band. They may also be used for drying tablets during compounding.

Hot Plates

Hot plates are used for quick heating of substances, and they resemble weight scales. They have flat ceramic or aluminum surfaces and front panels with controls (see Figure 14-10). Some hot plates offer automated stirring technology. They vary in design, either intended for low-heat or high-heat use. A common use for hot plates is in melting cocoa butter or other substances used as bases in compounding ointments or suppositories.

Heat Sealers

Heat sealers are commonly used to seal packages without damaging the chemicals, drugs, or other substances that these packages contain. Various types of heat sealers exist, which may offer controls that affect temperature, sealing pressure, processing time, and automatic sample loading.

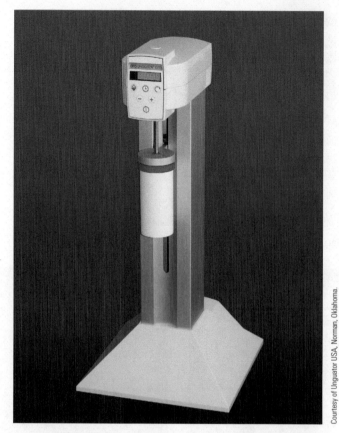

Courtesy of Unguator USA, Norman, Oklahoma.

Figure 14-8 Electronic mortar and pestle.

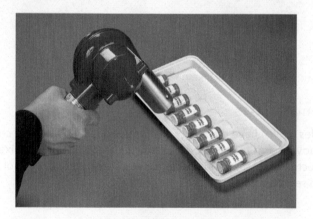

Figure 14-9 Heat gun.

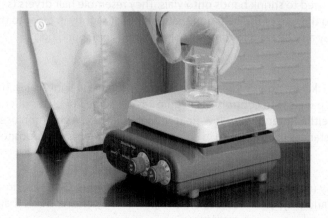

Figure 14-10 Hot plate.

Tongs

Laboratory tons include crucible tons with or without ridges, beaker tongs, flask tongs, and test tube holders (Figure 14-11). They are used for the sterile grasping and maneuvering of a variety of different types of laboratory equipment. Tongs can be easily cleaned with alcohol or detergents, and may be autoclaved.

Crimpers

Crimpers resemble pliers (see Figure 14-12A) and may be designed for manual use or for use with robotic machinery. Crimpers are common pieces of equipment found in pharmacies that handle extemporaneous compounding. Crimpers are commonly used to seal vials and other containers (see Figure 14-12B). Also, some crimpers are designed to be able to be used as decappers (see the following section).

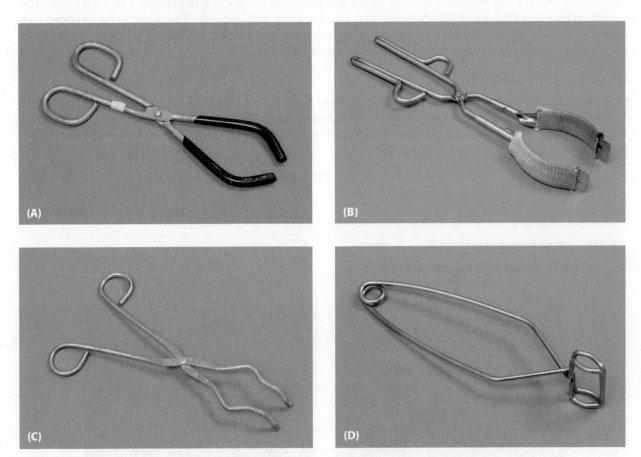

Figure 14-11 Laboratory tongs. (A and B) Beaker tongs. (C) Crucible tongs. (D) Test tube holder.

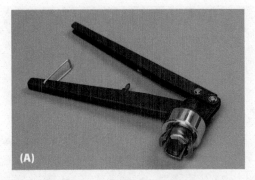
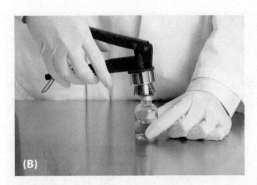

Figure 14-12 (A) Crimper. (B) Can also be used as a decapper.

Decappers

Decappers are also known as "decrimpers." They are used to remove seals placed onto vials and other containers. They may also be used manually or with robotic machinery.

Tablet Molds

Tablet molds are commonly made of metal, with various sizes of plate cavities (ranging between 60 and 100 mg). They are used by pressing a prepared, moistened powder mixture into the tablet cavities (see Figure 14-13A). After the cavities are filled (see Figure 14-13B), pressure is applied, forcing the formed tablets out of the cavities so that they can dry.

Suppository Molds

Suppository molds come in various types of aluminum, plastic, or rubber, and range from 1 to 2.5 g in size. The aluminum type (see Figure 14-14A) is held together with screws or nuts and bolts. The plastic or rubber types (see Figure 14-14B) are commonly used if the suppositories need to be refrigerated, and they allow the suppositories to be easily pushed out of each cavity once they have become firm.

Ultrasonic Cleaners

Ultrasonic cleaners are also known as *ultrasonic baths* and can clean metal and plastic equipment (Figure 14-15). They effectively remove blood, proteins, contaminants, grease, waxes, and oils. They work by moving sound waves through a heated solution to create *cavitation*, which is the rapid swelling and collapsing of microscopic bubbles. Advantages of ultrasonic cleaners are as follows:

- Faster, safer, and more thorough than other clearing methods
- Powerful enough to remove heavy oils
- Consistent enough to manage difficult lab cleanups
- Safe enough for delicate electronic components
- Designed to be functional, reliable, and easy to use

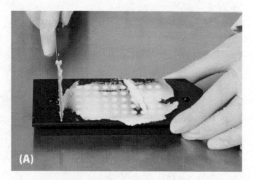
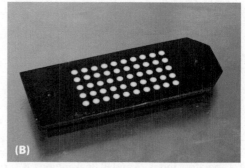

Figure 14-13 Tablet mold: (A) Pressing in mixture. (B) Applying pressure to force out tablets.

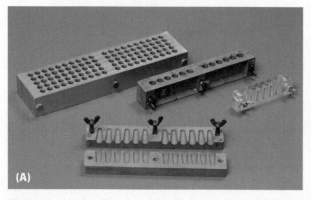
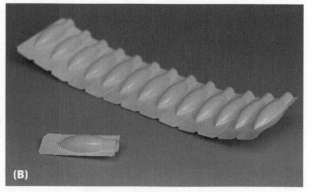

Figure 14-14 Suppository mold: (A) Aluminum type. (B) Plastic type.

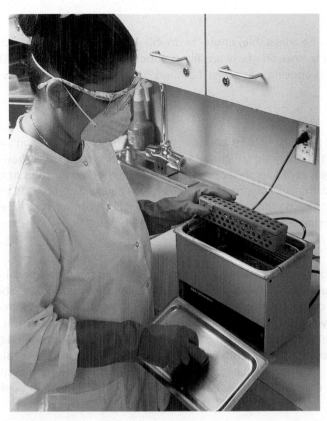

Figure 14-15 Ultrasonic cleaning unit.

Ultrasonic cleaners may be easily cleaned with alcohol or detergents, but they should be maintained by an authorized service company.

Pipettes and Pipette Fillers

A **pipette** can be used for measurement of volumes of liquids less than 1.5 mL, and offer extreme accuracy. This device is a long, thin, calibrated, hollow tube that is made of glass. There are two types of pipettes: auto-pipettes and mouth pipettes (not often used). They are durable and easy to clean. A *pipette filler* is a bulb that draws a solution into the pipette. Pipette fillers are commonly made of rubber with stainless steel valves. They do away with the hazardous practice of pipetting by mouth, which is never recommended. Pipette fillers are very simple to use and offer the advantage of fitting with all sizes of pipettes, making them a must for every laboratory. Pipettes and pipette fillers are usually cleaned with deionized water, detergents, or isopropyl alcohol. Pipettes and pipetting aids are shown in Figure 14-16.

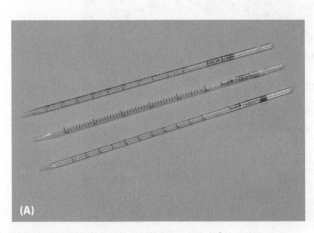
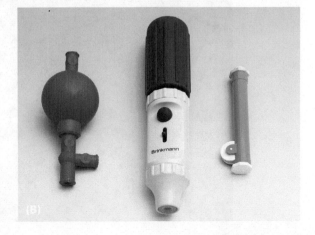

Figure 14-16 (A) Pipettes. (B) Pipetting aids.

Spray Bottles

Laboratory spray bottles may be adjustable, single- or double-headed, and virtually unbreakable. They are commonly used in the laboratory to rinse off glassware, filters, tubes, and other equipment. They can vary the flows of solutions they contain, even producing a fine mist if desired. Spray bottles may be easily rinsed and cleaned with detergents.

Stirring Rods

Stirring rods may be made of glass, as well as rubber, polypropylene, or bendable Teflon®, and are used to stir a variety of solutions or mixtures in the laboratory (Figure 14-17). Glass stirring rods usually have polished, rounded ends, and they may have rubber sleeves fit over their tips. They should be checked for chips or cracks prior to use and be discarded if they are visibly damaged. Polypropylene stirring rods have a flattened end that may also be used as a scoop or small spatula. Teflon stirring rods are flexible yet unbreakable, containing a wire insert that bends to any shape. Stirring rods are easily cleaned by isopropyl alcohol or detergents.

Graduates

Standard equipment used to measure liquids consists of conical graduates, cylindrical graduates, pipettes, and syringes. **Conical graduates** have wide tops and wide bases and taper from the top to the bottom (see Figure 14-18). They are easier to clean than cylindrical graduates. **Cylindrical graduates** are designed with a narrow diameter that is the same from top to base. Cylindrical graduates are more accurate than conical graduates (see Figure 14-19). These types of graduates are generally calibrated in metric units (cubic centimeters), and conical graduates are mostly calibrated in both metric and apothecary units. Both types of graduates are used in different sizes, ranging from 5 mL to more than 1000 mL (1 L). The smallest graduate available should always be used to measure a particular volume of liquid. Measuring of volumes that are less than 20% of the capacity of the graduate should be avoided, because the accuracy is unacceptable.

Beakers

Beakers are usually cylindrical containers with flat bottoms that are used to hold liquids. They commonly range in size from 25 to 600 mL and may be made of glass, plastic, or other materials specifically designed for laboratory use. They differ from flasks in that their sides are straight rather than sloped. Beakers are designed for mixing and melting substances (see Figure 14-20).

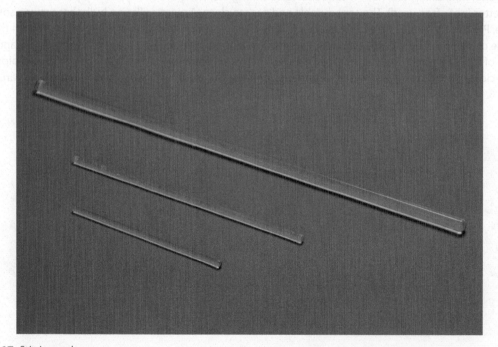

Figure 14-17 Stirring rods.

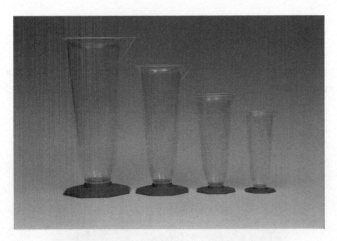

Figure 14-18 Conical graduates.

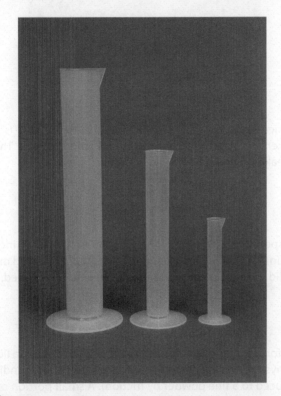

Figure 14-19 Cylindrical graduates.

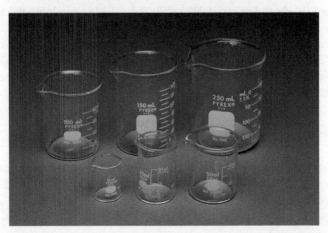

Figure 14-20 Beakers.

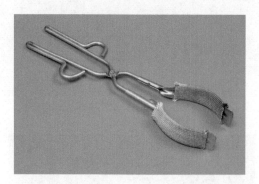

Figure 14-21 Beaker tongs.

Beaker Tongs

Beaker tongs resemble ordinary ice tongs, but may have either two or three "jaws" (see Figure 14-21). They are used in the laboratory for lifting beakers onto and off of hot plates and other surfaces. These tongs are usually made of stainless steel and can handle beakers ranging from 50 to 2000 mL in size.

Compounding of Liquid Drugs

Liquid dosage forms include suspensions, solutions, elixirs, and emulsions. Active ingredients are dissolved in a liquid vehicle known as a **solvent**. Liquids are the most common form of compounded medications. Liquid volumes are much easier to measure than solid volumes because they do not have to be weighed. The following sections discuss liquid dosage forms in detail.

SUSPENSIONS

A suspension is a liquid dosage form that contains solid drug particles floating in a liquid medium. Suspensions are easy to compound; however, physical stability of the final product after compounding is problematic. The insoluble powders are **triturated** (reduced to a fine powder by friction). A small portion of liquid is used to **levigate** the powder (grind into a smooth surface with moisture), and the powders are triturated until a smooth paste is formed. The levigating agent is added slowly and mixed deliberately. The vehicle containing the suspending agent is added in divided portions. A high-speed mixer greatly increases the dispersion, and the final mixture is transferred to a "light-resistant" bottle for dispensing to the patient. All suspensions should be dispensed with an auxiliary label reading "Shake well before use." Suspensions are not filtered. The water-soluble ingredients, including flavoring agents, are mixed in the vehicle before mixing with the insoluble ingredients. The steps performed to compound a suspension are illustrated in Figures 14-22 through 14-28.

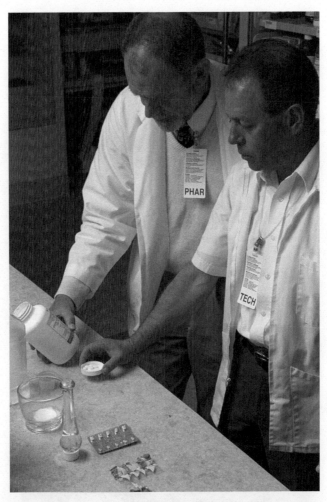

Figure 14-22 The technician and pharmacist are checking the dosage of tablets for compounding.

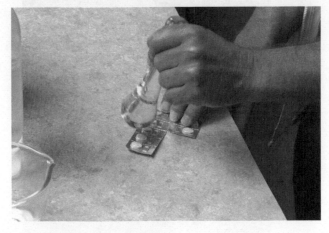

Figure 14-23 The technician is grinding the tablets into a powder.

SOLUTIONS

A solution is similar to a suspension but does not require shaking before use. Common types of solutions include sterile parenteral and ophthalmic solutions. Nonsterile types include oral, topical, and otic solutions. When compounding solutions, the solubility characteristics of each active ingredient must be known so that they can be dissolved in the most soluble solvents. The compounding of solutions should not be rushed so that the proper mixing

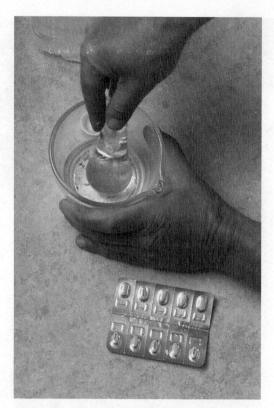

Figure 14-24 The technician is further grinding the powdered tablets.

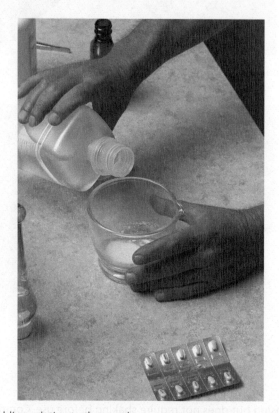

Figure 14-25 The technician is adding solution to the powder.

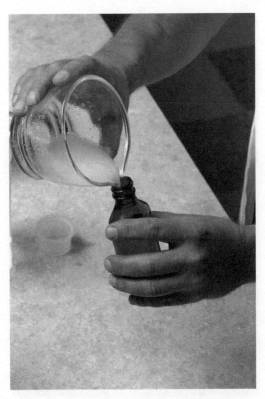

Figure 14-26 The compounded suspension is being poured into the patient's bottle.

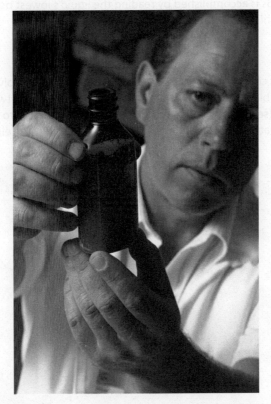

Figure 14-27 The technician is verifying the amount of the solution at eye level.

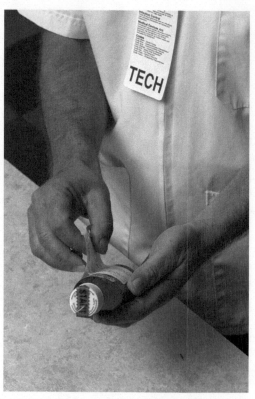

Figure 14-28 The technician is labeling the bottle.

can occur. Measuring of solutions is accomplished by reading the liquid's lowest point or center, the edges appear slightly higher than its center—this is known as the meniscus (see Figure 14-29).

ELIXIRS

Elixirs are sweetened liquids that contain alcohol and water. They are made by dissolving alcohol-soluble ingredients in ethanol, dissolving water-soluble ingredients in water, and then combining the two solvents by adding the water solvent into the alcohol solvent (see Figures 14-30 through 14-32). It is important to keep the alcohol concentration as strong as possible; thus, the water solvent is added into the alcohol solvent. The elixir should be stirred constantly.

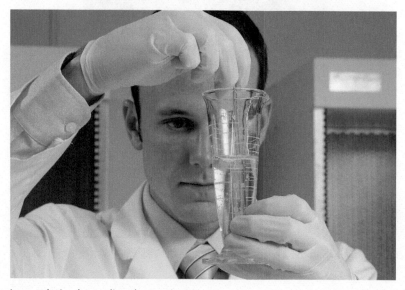

Figure 14-29 Measuring a solution by reading the meniscus.

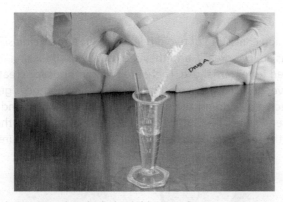

Figure 14-30 Compounding a solution: Dissolve alcohol-soluble ingredients.

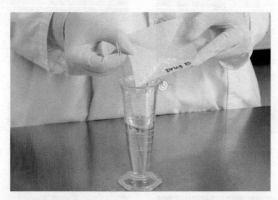

Figure 14-31 Dissolve water-soluble ingredients.

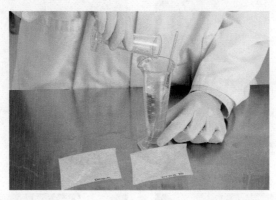

Figure 14-32 Add the two and triturate.

WHAT WOULD YOU DO?

Your hospital pharmacy sometimes compounds medications extemporaneously when required but has strict rules that this type of compounding is only done during daytime shifts when there are plenty of people working who can double-check accuracies. Another reason for daytime compounding is to avoid fatigue during these procedures if compounding is requested after workers have been on duty for a full shift. As you are getting ready to leave work one day, you see a pharmacist getting ready to compound a medication. You know the pharmacist has worked the same amount of hours as you did, and there is no rush for the medication. What would you do?

EMULSIONS

An emulsion is a type of suspension consisting of two different liquids and an *emulsifier*—an agent that holds them together. Oil-in-water emulsions are nongreasy, and they are usually used for oral use. Water-in-oil emulsions are greasy, and they are usually used for external use. There are two methods for creating emulsions: the "dry gum" (Continental) method and the "wet gum" (English) method. The dry gum method is generally preferred and involves mixing gum acacia into the selected oil, adding all the desired amount of water, and triturating until the color and sound of the mixture change (see Figures 14-33 through 14-38). The wet gum method involves mixing water into gum acacia, and then adding in the selected oil plus additional ingredients (see Figures 14-39 through 14-44).

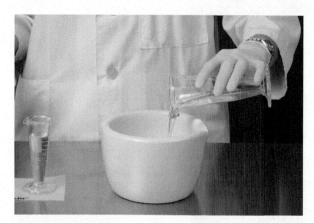

Figure 14-33 Compounding an emulsion—dry gum method: Place oil into the mortar.

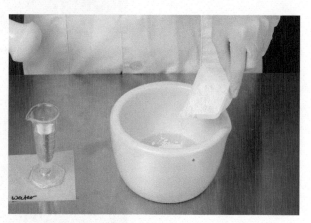

Figure 14-34 Place gum into mortar.

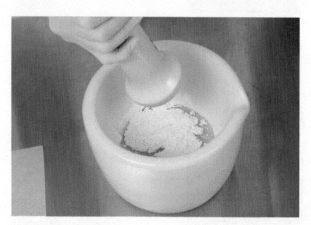

Figure 14-35 Triturate.

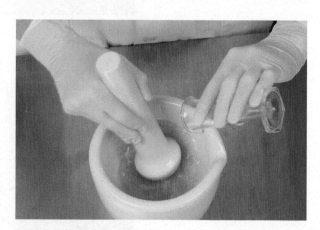

Figure 14-36 Add water.

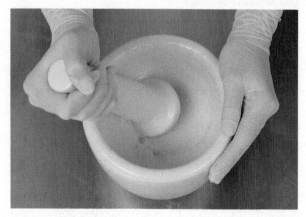

Figure 14-37 Triturate.

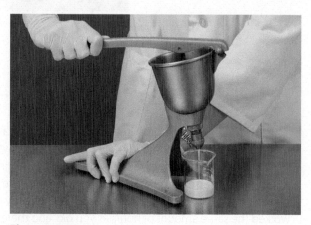

Figure 14-38 Homogenize.

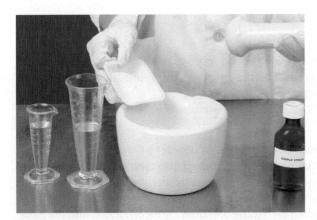

Figure 14-39 Compounding an emulsion—wet gum method: Place gum into mortar.

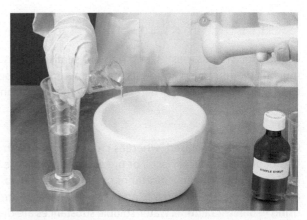

Figure 14-40 Add water and triturate.

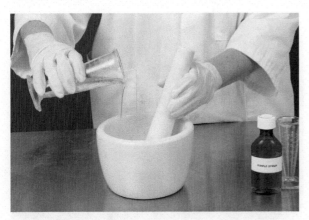

Figure 14-41 Add oil and triturate.

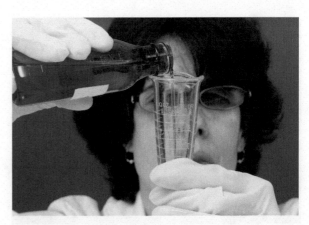

Figure 14-42 Measure syrup and active ingredient.

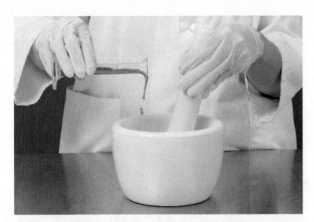

Figure 14-43 Add other ingredients.

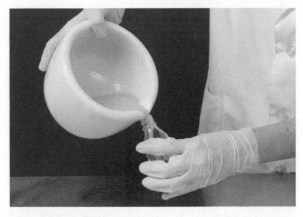

Figure 14-44 Place in appropriate container.

Compounding of Semisolid Drugs

Ointments, creams, pastes, and gels are semisolid dosage forms intended for topical application to the skin or mucous membranes. Ointments are characterized as being oily. Creams are generally oil-in-water or water-in-oil emulsions, and pastes are characterized by their high content of solids.

OINTMENTS

Ointments are oil-based, whereas creams are water-based. Drugs that are in powder or crystal forms, such as hydrocortisone, salicylic acid, or precipitated sulfur, are often ordered to be mixed into ointment or cream bases. Mixing can be done in a mortar or on an ointment slab. Liquids are incorporated by gradually adding them to an absorption-type base and mixing. Insoluble powders are reduced to a fine powder and then are added to the base, using **geometric dilution**. Water-soluble substances are dissolved with water and then are incorporated into the base. The final product should be smooth and free of any abrasive particles. The steps followed to compound an ointment are shown in Figures 14-45 through 14-50.

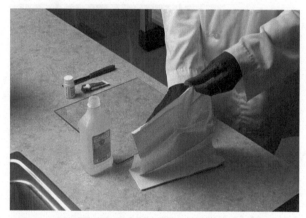

Figure 14-45 The technician is cleaning the glass slab for compounding an ointment.

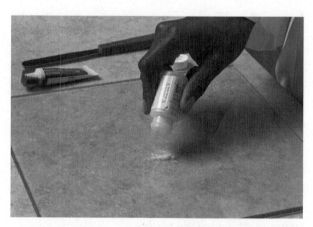

Figure 14-46 The technician is pouring the desired amount of powder to compound into ointment.

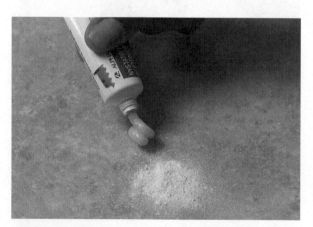

Figure 14-47 The technician is adding a partial amount of the cream needed to make the ointment.

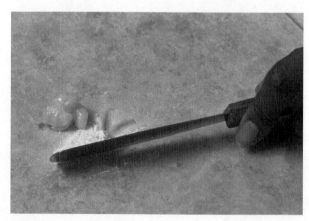

Figure 14-48 The technician is mixing the powder into the cream.

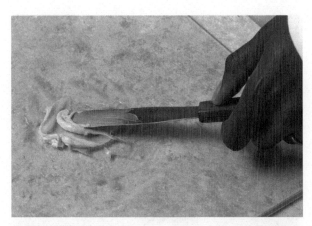

Figure 14-49 The technician is blending the powder and cream.

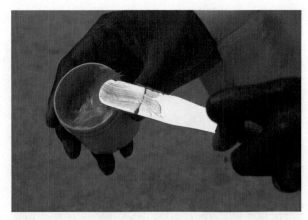

Figure 14-50 The technician is putting the blended ointment into the patient's ointment container.

CREAMS

Creams are usually used topically, and they are combinations of oil with water. Creams are thicker than lotions and may or may not contain a medication. They may be dispensed from either a jar or a tube. Creams are compounded in the same manner as ointments.

PASTES

Pastes are intended for external use (except for toothpaste), and may or may not contain a medication. They do not melt or soften at body temperature. Though similar to ointments, creams, and gels, they contain a higher amount of solids. Pastes are compounded in the same way as ointments.

GELS

Gels consist of suspensions made up of either small inorganic particles or large organic molecules interpenetrated by a liquid. These dosage forms are generally applied externally. They may act solely on the surface of the skin to produce a local effect (e.g., an antifungal agent), or they can release a medication that penetrates into the skin (e.g., cortisol cream). These semisolid dosage forms also may release medication for systemic absorption through the skin (e.g., nitroglycerin).

Compounding Suppositories

Suppositories are solid bodies of various weights, sizes, and shapes. They are adapted for introduction into the rectal, vaginal, or urethral orifices of the human body. Suppositories are used to deliver drugs for local or systemic effects. There are three common suppository bases:

- Cocoa butter (theobroma oil), which melts at body temperature. It is a fat-soluble mixture of triglycerides that is most often used for rectal suppositories.

- Polyethylene glycol (Carbowax) derivatives are water-soluble bases suitable for vaginal and rectal suppositories.

- Glycerinated gelatin is a water-miscible base often used in vaginal and rectal suppositories.

The first step in preparing suppositories is to choose a proper mold. Remember that suppository molds can be made of rubber, plastic, brass, stainless steel, or other suitable material. If appropriate, a "Refrigerate" label should appear on the container. Regardless of the base or medication used in the formulation, the patient should be instructed to store the suppositories in a cool, dry place. Steps for compounding suppositories are highlighted in Figures 14-51 through 14-56.

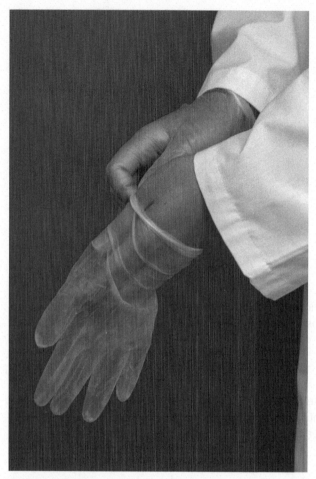

Figure 14-51 The technician is putting on gloves for the procedure of compounding suppositories.

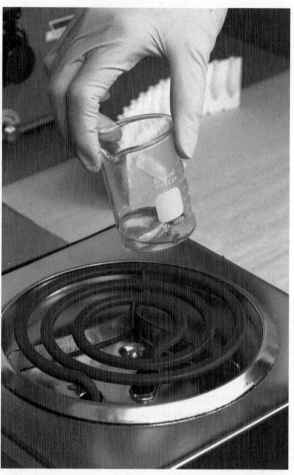

Figure 14-53 The technician is melting the base material that will be combined with the powder.

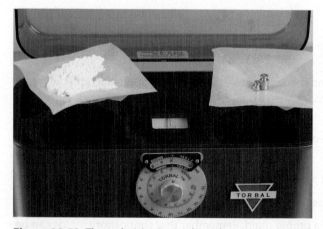

Figure 14-52 The technician is weighing the powder that will be compounded into suppositories.

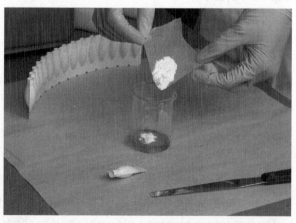

Figure 14-54 The technician is adding the powder to the melted base material.

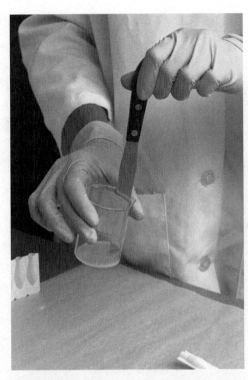

Figure 14-55 The technician is mixing the two ingredients together.

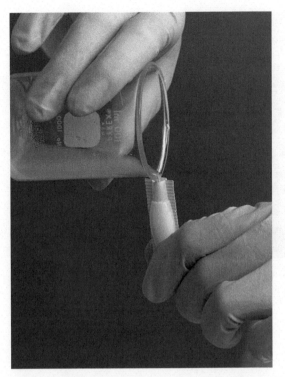

Figure 14-56 The technician is pouring the mixture into the suppository mold.

Compounding of Solid Drugs

Solid drugs include capsules, tablets, and powders. They are generally made using compression or trituration. Diluents used in compounding these types of drugs include various sugars and moistening agents.

CAPSULES

Capsules are solid forms in which the drug is enclosed within either a hard or soft soluble container or a shell. The shells are usually made from a suitable gelatin. Hard gelatin capsules may be manually filled for extemporaneous compounding. Capsule sizes for oral administration in humans range from number 5, which is the smallest, to number 000, the largest. Number 0 is usually the largest oral size suitable for patients. Figure 14-57 shows various capsule sizes and indicates the amount of milligrams they hold.

For preparation of hard and soft capsules, the correct size must be determined by trying different sizes, weighing, and choosing the appropriate size. Before capsules are filled with the medication, the body and cap of the capsule are separated. Filling is accomplished by using the "punch" method. The powder formulation is compressed with a spatula on a pill tile. The empty capsule body is repeatedly pressed into the powder until full. The capsule is then weighed to ensure an accurate dose. An empty **tare** capsule (the weight of an empty capsule used to compare to the full capsule) of the same size is placed on the pan containing the weights. The capsules are wiped clean of any powder or oil and dispensed in a suitable prescription container. Figures 14-58 through 14-66 illustrate the steps involved in compounding a capsule.

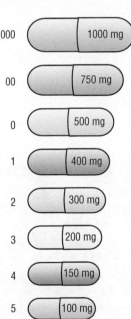

Figure 14-57 Capsule sizes.

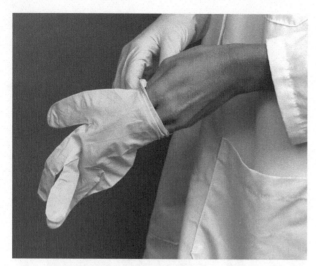

Figure 14-58 The technician is putting on gloves for the capsule compounding procedure.

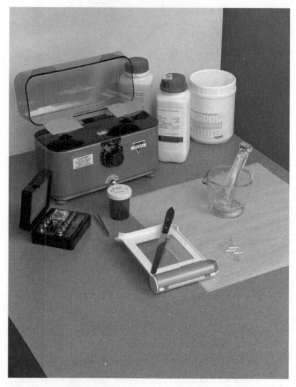

Figure 14-59 The technician has prepared all the materials needed to compound capsules.

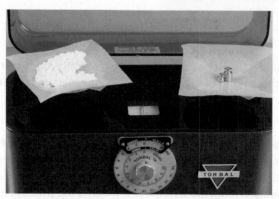

Figure 14-60 The material for the capsules is being weighed.

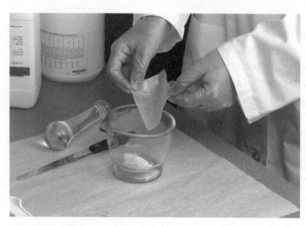

Figure 14-61 The technician is putting the weighed material into a mortar for grinding.

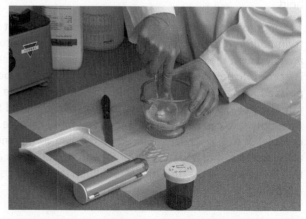

Figure 14-62 The technician is grinding the material into a fine powder inside the mortar with the pestle.

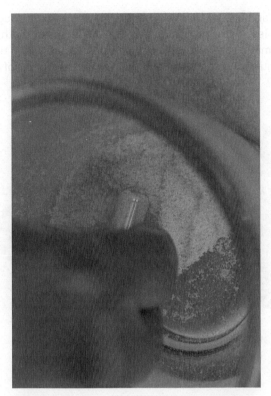

Figure 14-63 The technician is "punching" the powdered mixture into the empty capsule shell.

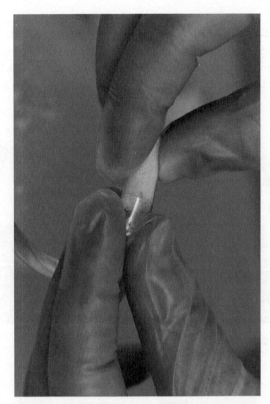

Figure 14-64 The technician is putting the two capsule halves together.

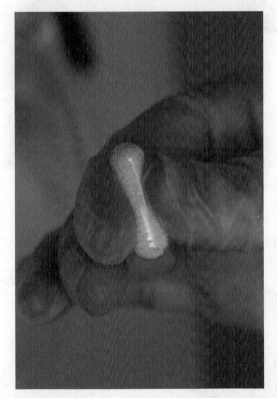

Figure 14-65 The technician is checking to see that the capsule is full of powdered mixture.

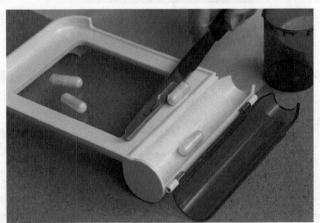

Figure 14-66 The technician is counting the compounded capsules for dispensing.

For a large number of capsules, capsule-filling machines can be used to save time (see Figures 14-67 through 14-72). They allow preparation of larger quantities of capsules, distributing powdered medications and other ingredients uniformly into empty capsules. They are not automatic and still require the compounder to weigh the finished capsules to check for accuracy within 10%. Weights must be recorded on a formula worksheet for proof of accuracy.

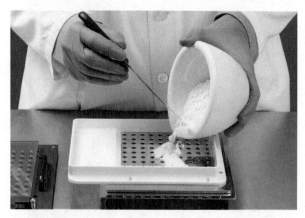

Figure 14-67 Compounding capsules using a capsule-filling machine: Add active ingredients.

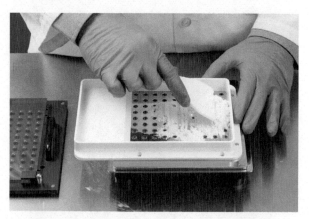

Figure 14-68 Use a spatula or tool to fill capsules.

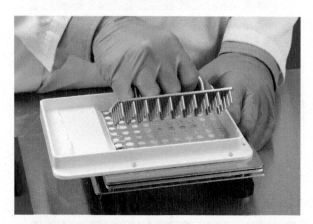

Figure 14-69 Align top of machine with capsule slots.

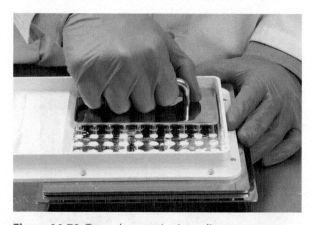

Figure 14-70 Tamp down active ingredients.

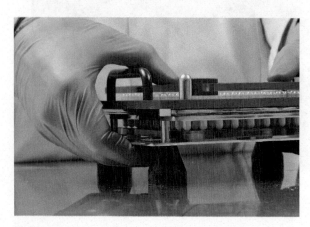

Figure 14-71 Squeeze top and bottom of machine together.

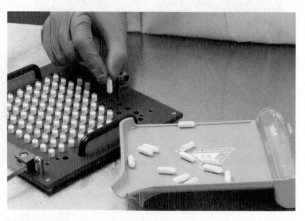

Figure 14-72 Remove completed capsules and ensure they are locked.

TABLETS

Tablet triturates are solid and small and are usually cylindrically molded or compressed tablets. Tablets are made of powders created by moistening the powder mixture with alcohol and water. They are used for compounding potent drugs in small doses. Tablet triturates are made in special molds consisting of a pegboard and a corresponding perforated plate. In addition to the mold, a diluent, usually a mixture of lactose, sucrose, and a moistening agent, is used. Moistening agents are usually a mixture of ethyl alcohol and water. The diluent is triturated with the active ingredients, and then a paste is made by using the alcohol and water mixture. This paste is spread into the mold, and the tablets are punched out and remain on the pegs until dry.

POWDERS

Powdered dosage forms are used when drug stability or solubility is a concern. These dosage forms may also be used when the powders are too bulky to make into capsules and when the patient has difficulty swallowing a capsule. Powdered dosage forms may be unpleasant-tasting medications. Blending of powders may be accomplished by using trituration in a mortar, stirring with a spatula, and sifting (see Figures 14-73 through 14-77). Geometric dilution should be used if needed. When heavy powders are mixed with lighter powders, the heavier powder should be placed on top and then blended (combined into one substance). When two or more powders are mixed, each powder should be pulverized (reduced in particle size by crushing or grinding) separately to about the same particle size before they are blended together.

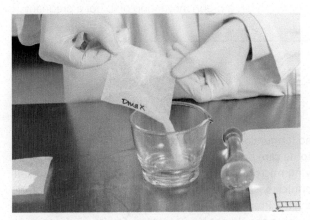

Figure 14-73 Compounding powders: Place drug in mortar.

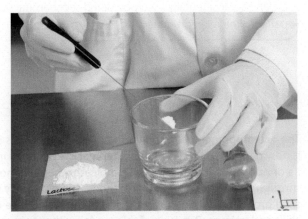

Figure 14-74 Place an equal amount of powder in mortar with drug.

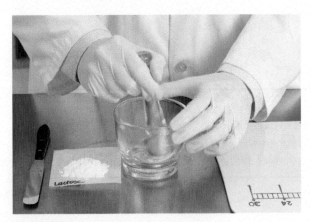

Figure 14-75 Triturate.

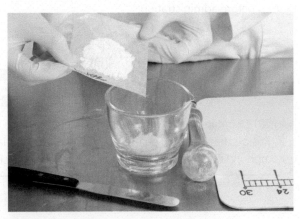

Figure 14-76 Combine powders in mortar by doubling each time.

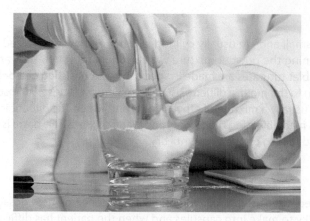

Figure 14-77 Triturate.

WHAT WOULD YOU DO?

Use of powdered medications when mixing extemporaneous compounds is common. However, not paying strict attention to the powdered agent to be used can have dangerous results. If you discovered that a pharmacy technician had accidentally used powdered secobarbital sodium, which has a pregnancy rating of "D," for a pregnant patient, what would you do?

Compounding Parenteral Products

The extemporaneous compounding of sterile products is no longer confined only to the hospital environment. It is now performed by community pharmacists engaged in home care practice. There are two types of product: sterile or nonsterile. The term "sterile" indicates there are no living microorganisms present. Sterility can be achieved through heat, gas, or filtration methods. The pharmacy technician is an integral part of the production of parenteral products, both in hospitals and in the home care industry. Preparation of sterile products requires special skills and training. Provision of this service without proper training should not be attempted. Sterile products must be prepared in a clean room, using aseptic technique (discussed in **Chapter 15**). Dry powders of parenteral drugs for reconstitution are used for drug products that are unstable as solutions. It is important to know the correct diluents that can be used to yield a solution. Drug solutions for parenteral administration may also be further diluted before administration.

MEDICATION ERROR ALERT

In 2012, contaminated epidural steroid injections were linked to more than 700 illnesses, including a fungal meningitis outbreak, and 60 deaths. The failure of individuals to adhere to regulations concerning extemporaneous compounding of parenteral products has led to increased scrutiny of this type of compounding in recent years.

Summary

Extemporaneous compounding provides pharmacists with a unique opportunity to practice their time-honored profession. This service is expected to become an even more important part of pharmacy practice in the future, including community, hospital, nursing home, home health care, and specialty practices. The pharmacy technician must be trained and skilled to compound medication under the supervision of the pharmacist. Procedures vary for preparation of different extemporaneous compounds, such as powders, capsules, solutions, suspensions, suppositories, ointments, and creams. The extemporaneous compounding of sterile products is no longer confined only to the hospital environment. It is now performed by community pharmacists engaged in home care practice. Quality control and proper documentation of all products are essential. Preparation of sterile products requires special skills and training. A clean room and the use of aseptic technique are very important to minimize contamination.

REVIEW QUESTIONS

1. When measuring the amount of liquid in a graduate, at what level of the meniscus do you read?

   A. Bottom
   B. Front
   C. Back
   D. Top

2. A liquid dosage form in which active ingredients are dissolved in a liquid vehicle is known as a:

   A. solute.
   B. solution.
   C. suspension.
   D. precipitate.

3. Which of the following equipment can be used for weighing large quantities?

   A. Counter balance
   B. Class A prescription balance
   C. Slab
   D. Graduate

4. Avoid measurement of volumes that are less than 20% of the capacity of the graduate, because:

   A. contamination is more likely.
   B. this percentage is not sufficient for measurement.
   C. the type of graduate may be incorrect.
   D. accuracy is unacceptable.

5. A semisolid, external dosage form with an oily base is called:

   A. a suppository.
   B. a cream.
   C. a lotion.
   D. an ointment.

6. Capsule sizes for oral administration in humans range from number 0 to 5. Which of the following capsule sizes is the smallest?

   A. 000
   B. 00
   C. 0
   D. 5

7. The powders in tablets are moistened by mixing with:

    A.   water.
    B.   water and alcohol.
    C.   oil.
    D.   water, oil, and alcohol.

8. Spatulas are used to:

    A.   measure bulk products.
    B.   transfer solid ingredients for weighing.
    C.   grind materials in the preparation of drugs.
    D.   measure volumes of liquid.

9. A pipette is used for volumes less than:

    A.   15 mL.
    B.   10 mL.
    C.   5 mL.
    D.   1.5 mL.

10. The preparation of a drug product for an individual patient, based on a prescription order from a licensed practitioner, defines:

    A.   trituration.
    B.   conversion.
    C.   extemporaneous compounding.
    D.   bulk materials.

11. A piece of equipment that consists of a two-pan balance used for weighing small amounts of drugs is a:

    A.   Class-A prescription balance.
    B.   counter balance.
    C.   weight.
    D.   mortar and pestle.

12. The preferred type of mortar for mixing liquids and semisoft dosage forms is:

    A.   porcelain.
    B.   glass.
    C.   aluminum.
    D.   Wedgwood.

13. When compounding liquid drugs, active ingredients are dissolved in a liquid vehicle known as a:

    A.   solution.
    B.   suspension.
    C.   solvent.
    D.   medium.

14. Heat guns are often used to:

    A.   heat a substance.
    B.   shrink a seal on a vial.
    C.   melt a waxy substance.
    D.   sterilize equipment.

15. The term used to indicate that there are no living microorganisms present is:

    A.   extemporaneous.
    B.   nonsterile.
    C.   clean.
    D.   sterile.

CRITICAL THINKING

A pharmacy technician was asked to compound 20 capsules for a prescription. The prescription required a combination of three substances.

1. Explain why it is important to follow the order precisely when compounding medications.

2. What are the dangers of carelessness in compounding?

WEB LINKS

Carie Boyd's Prescription Shop: www.carieboyd.com/stevens

Fallon Wellness Pharmacy: www.fallonpharmacy.com/

International Academy of Compounding Pharmacists: www.iacprx.org/default.aspx

Lorraine's Pharmacy: lorrainespharmacy.com

University Compounding Pharmacy: www.ucprx.com

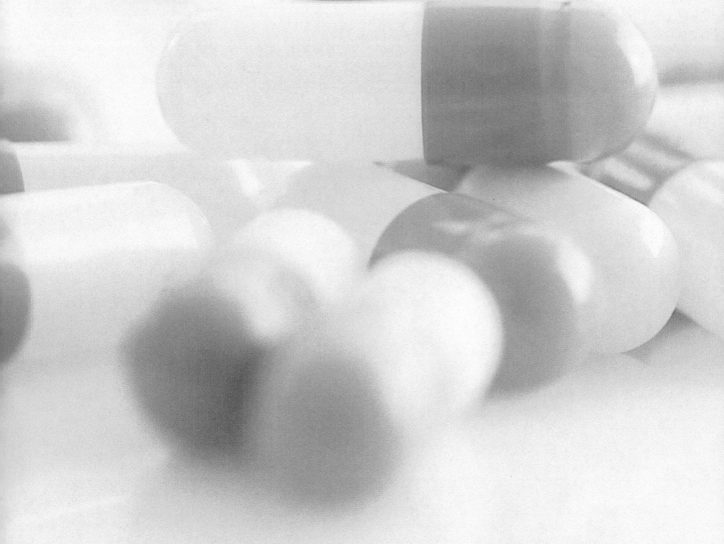

Aseptic Technique and Sterile Compounding

OBJECTIVES

Upon completion of this chapter, the reader should be able to:

1. List six categories of injections.
2. Define *sanitizing* and *disinfection*.
3. Explain the uses of laminar airflow hoods.
4. Explain the control methods used for the compounding of parenteral products.
5. Describe TPN products.
6. Explain an intravenous piggyback.
7. Discuss the preparation of large-volume parenteral (LVP) preparations.

8. Define the term *intravenous admixture*.

9. Explain the use of refrigeration for high-risk compounding products.

10. Explain the indications of sterile irrigations.

KEY TERMS

aseptic technique	conjunctiva	medical asepsis	sanitization
beyond-use date	dry heat sterilization	piggyback	surgical asepsis
chemical sterilization	laminar airflow hood		

Overview

When preparing sterile products, it is important to remember certain facts concerning microorganisms. Contamination must be expected when pharmacy technicians prepare materials for sterilization. Most raw materials will rarely be sterile, and improper storage of these materials may increase microbial content. Since raw materials are not usually handled in a sterile (or protected) environment, the manufacturing area's air, surfaces, water, and other environmental factors should be expected to contribute to contamination of prepared products.

Parenteral products are injected directly into body tissue through the skin and veins. Therefore, parenteral products must be produced in a sterile environment to reduce the risk of infection that administration of these products may impose. Sterile preparations must be kept pure and free from biological, chemical, and physical contaminants. The pharmaceutical industry strives to maintain good manufacturing practices of parenteral dosage forms as a result. Likewise, pharmacists and technicians must practice good aseptic technique when working with these products.

Parenteral Preparations

Parenteral preparations are given when a medication is rendered inactive in the gastrointestinal (GI) tract or when a patient is unable to take medication by mouth (due to vomiting or unconsciousness). Fluids, electrolytes, and nutrients are often administered parenterally. Irrigations used in surgery and ophthalmics are also examples of parenteral preparations.

Parenteral products must have the following unique qualities:

- They must be sterile.

- They must be free from contamination by endotoxins.

- They must be free from visible particles, which includes reconstituted sterile powders.

- They should be isotonic; the correct level of isotonicity depends on the route of administration.

- They must be chemically, physically, and microbiologically stable.

- They must be compatible with intravenous (IV) delivery systems, diluents, and other drug products to be coadministered.

For administration, injections may be classified in the following six categories:

- Solutions ready for injection

- Dry and soluble products ready for combination with a solvent just prior to use

- Suspensions ready for injection

- Dry, insoluble products ready for combination with a vehicle just prior to use

- Emulsions

- Liquid concentrates ready to be diluted prior to administration

Formulation modifications, or different routes of injection, can be used to slow a drug's onset, and thus prolong its action. Parenteral products are commonly administered by intravenous "push" (a one-time, rapid injection), by continuous infusion, or using an intravenous "piggyback" (IVPB). Parenteral administration more readily controls the therapeutic response of a drug because intestinal absorption is bypassed. Disadvantages of parenteral administration, however, include the following:

- Asepsis required at administration
- Risk of tissue toxicity from local irritation
- Pain
- Difficulty in correcting errors

Pharmacy technicians must follow the policies and procedures of the pharmacy concerning sterile compounding. The goal is to handle and prepare parenteral preparations in a manner that is as free from biological, chemical, and physical contaminants as possible. This requires proper aseptic technique because parenteral preparations are often unstable and highly potent—their characteristics must be preserved without contaminating them.

POINTS TO REMEMBER

Important properties of parenteral preparations that must be considered include compatibility, osmolality (concentration of particles or substances), osmolarity (concentration of diffused, active particles), pH, stability, and tonicity (the tone or tension of a substance).

Types of Asepsis and Ways to Achieve It

The most effective way to eliminate transmission of disease from one host to another is through asepsis, which means "being completely sterile (free from microorganisms)." There are two types of asepsis: medical asepsis and surgical asepsis.

MEDICAL ASEPSIS

Medical asepsis is the removal of pathogens to reduce transfer of microorganisms by cleaning any body part or surface that has been exposed to them. Medical asepsis benefits both the patient and the health care worker by preventing exposure to pathogens from other patients, from each other, or from other staff. Medical asepsis is also called *clean technique*.

Hand Hygiene

The single most important means of preventing the spread of infection is frequent and effective hand hygiene by all health care workers. Hands must be washed, using the correct technique. An extended scrub is not needed each time hands are washed, but the first scrub of the day should be extensive, lasting 2 to 4 minutes, unless the hands are excessively contaminated. A good antimicrobial soap with chlorhexidine, such as Hibiclens®, which has antiseptic residual action that will last several hours, should be used. Even with this technique, the hands are still not sterile, because skin cannot be sterilized. Normal flora (nonpathogens) remain, but most pathogens have been removed. Proper hand washing depends on two factors: running water and friction. The water should be warm, because water that is too cold or too hot will cause the skin to become chapped. Friction involves the firm rubbing of all surfaces of the hands and wrists. Figures 15-1A through 15-1H shows the steps of hand washing that a technician should use.

WHAT WOULD YOU DO?

You observe the pharmacist insufficiently washing his hands in between sterile compounding procedures. He is talking with another pharmacist and is distracted while washing his hands. You are aware that poor hand hygiene is linked to inadequate aseptic technique. What would you do?

Cleaning and Sanitizing

Equipment and instruments need to be cleaned promptly and carefully after every use to remove visible residue before proceeding with the steps of disinfection or sterilization. Microorganisms may hide under residue and survive the disinfection or sterilization process if residue is not removed. **Sanitization** is the cleansing process that decreases the number of microorganisms to a safe level as dictated in public health guidelines. This cleansing process removes debris such as blood and other body fluids from instruments or equipment. Blood and debris must be removed so that when instruments are later disinfected or sterilized, chemicals (disinfection) or steam, heat, or gases (sterilization) can penetrate to all surfaces of the instruments. Items that cannot be cleaned at once are usually rinsed with cold water and placed in a soaking solution to prevent anyone from touching them and to prevent the residue from hardening. When instruments are sanitized, the soaking solution is drained off, and each instrument is rinsed in cold, running water. The sharp instruments should be separated from the others because other metal instruments may damage the cutting edges, and the sharp instruments may damage the other instruments or injure someone. All the sharp instruments are cleaned at one time, to avoid the dangers of injury. Instruments are rinsed in hot water. The items should be hand-dried with a towel to prevent spotting. The use of *disposable* instruments when working with human blood or giving injections minimizes the need for sanitization, disinfection, and sterilization.

POINTS TO REMEMBER

Sanitization is a very important step, and it cannot be overlooked or done carelessly. All instruments and items must be sanitized after each use.

Disinfection

Disinfection is the ability to kill microorganisms on the surface of various items (see Figure 15-2). Disinfection can be accomplished by use of a chemical disinfectant or by boiling. Boiling is used for items that enter body cavities such as the mouth or anus, which are not sterile. Disinfection is also used for items that are sensitive to heat such as glass thermometers or rubber materials. Large equipment and counter surfaces that cannot fit into an autoclave for sterilization should be disinfected by use of chemical disinfectants. Boiling kills many microorganisms but does not kill bacterial spores. Directions for proper use are provided on labels of disinfectant solutions, including the proper length of time to soak items. Many pharmacies use commercial solutions or prepare solutions containing household bleach. A 1:10 solution of household bleach (1 part bleach to 10 parts water) provides disinfection. Small spills of blood or body fluids on counter surfaces can be cleaned with bleach solution and paper towels (see Figure 15-3).

SURGICAL ASEPSIS

Surgical asepsis is the destruction of all microorganisms, pathogenic, and nonpathogenic, on an object or instrument. Therefore, all equipment used are sterile. The goal of surgical asepsis is to prevent any microorganisms from entering the patient's body through an open wound, especially during surgery. It is used when sterility of supplies and the immediate environment is required. Any item that will come into contact with the sterile field (the area in which the sterile procedure will be performed or where sterile supplies will be maintained during the procedure) must be sterilized using physical or chemical agents. Once the surfaces are sterilized, every precaution must be taken to prevent contamination of the sterile areas from a nonsterile surface or from airborne contamination.

Living tissue surfaces such as skin cannot be sterilized but can be rendered as free of pathogens as possible with the use of a sterile covering. One example is the use of surgical hand washing technique before sterile gloves are applied. Another example is the use of a **laminar airflow hood** in the pharmacy whenever a sterile working environment is needed; this is discussed later in the chapter. Surgical asepsis requires sterile hand washing (surgical scrub), sterile gloves, special handling procedures, and sterilization of materials. Most dangerous microorganisms are destroyed at a temperature of 50 to 60°C (122 to 140°F).

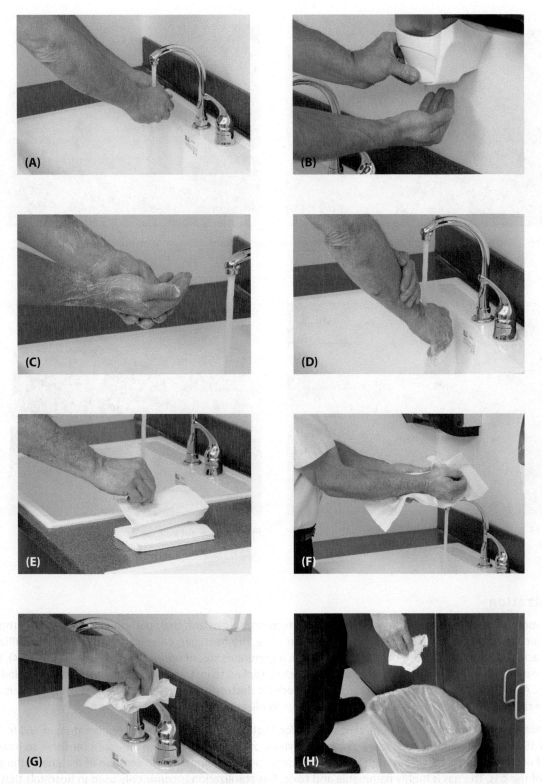

Figure 15-1 Hand washing: (A) thoroughly wet hands in a flowing stream of water; (B) apply soap; (C) work soap into a lather; (D) rinse in flow of water letting water run down arms and fingertips; (E and F) pat dry with clean paper towels; (G) turn off the running water using the paper towel, don't touch clean hands to faucets; (H) dispose of paper towel in trash.

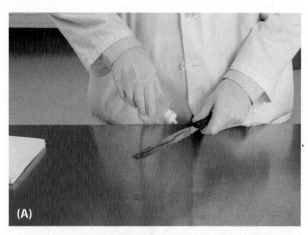

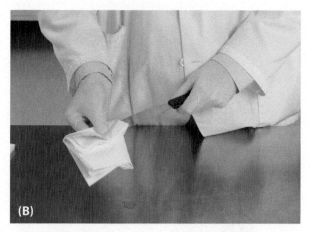

Figure 15-2 Proper technique for disinfection: (A) use back-and-forth motion to cleanse instruments and surfaces; (B) immediately rinse and dry.

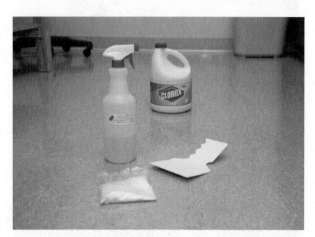

Figure 15-3 Blood and spills can be cleaned with a bleach solution.

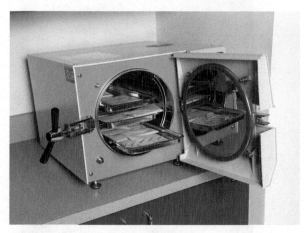

Figure 15-4 An autoclave.

Sterilization

Sterilization is the process of killing or destroying all microorganisms and their pathogenic products. Methods of sterilization include the application of steam under pressure, dry heat, gas, chemicals, and radiation. Sterilization can be achieved through the use of an autoclave, which generates steam under pressure (see Figure 15-4). When moist heat of 132°C (270°F) under pressure of 30 pounds is applied to instruments, all organisms will be killed in 20 minutes. Autoclaving is one of the most effective methods for destroying all types of microorganisms. The autoclave must be cleaned after each load. Indicator strips used for sterilization are shown in Figure 15-5.

Dry heat sterilization is another method of sterilization that uses heated dry air at a temperature of 160 to 180°C (320 to 356°F) for 90 minutes to 3 hours. The gas ethylene oxide is used for items that are sensitive to heat; this method of sterilization is called gas sterilization. It requires special equipment and aeration of materials after application of the gas. The gas is highly flammable and toxic. Gas sterilization is commonly used in hospitals that have room-sized gas sterilization chambers. Many prepackaged products for intravenous infusion and bandages are sterilized using this method. **Chemical sterilization** is used for instruments, and chemicals can be applied topically to the body for disinfection. Iodine, household bleach, Mercurochrome®, and alcohol are examples of disinfectants that can be used in this manner.

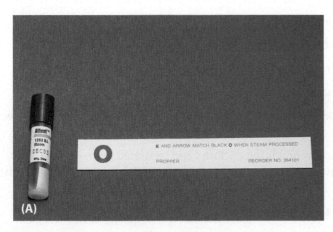
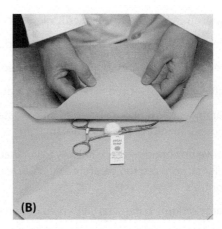

Figure 15-5 Indicator strips used for sterilization.

Equipment and Supplies

Parenteral products must be prepared so that contamination is avoided. The following equipment is used in sterile compounding:

- Administration sets—disposable tubing that connects intravenous (IV) administration sets to injection sites (see Figure 15-6)

- Ambulatory pumps—small pumps worn by patients

- Ampule breakers—used to break necks of ampules

- Ampules—long glass containers with breakable necks (see Figure 15-7)

- Catheters—inserted into veins for direct vascular system access

- Clamps—adjust flow rates of solutions

- Drip chambers—hollow areas where IV solutions drip without allowing air bubbles to enter IV tubing (see Figure 15-8)

- Filters—used to remove particulates and microorganisms from solutions

- Filtered needles—used to prevent glass from ampule breakage from entering final solution withdrawn from the ampule (see Figure 15-9)

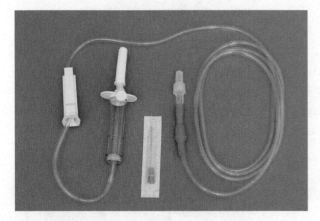

Figure 15-6 IV administration set.

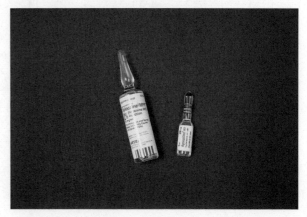

Figure 15-7 Ampules.

- Filter straws—used to pull medication out of ampules

- Flexible bags—plastic containers that hold 50 to 3000 mL of solution

- Heparin locks—short tubing filled with heparin, attached to a needle or catheter; they prevent clotting

- Infusion pumps—used to regulate medication flow into patients (see Figure 15-10)

- Laminar airflow hoods—used to prepare sterile compounds by circulating air through HEPA filters to remove more than 99% of possible contaminants

- Glove box hoods—used similarly to laminar airflow hoods but enclosed and separated from workers; they offer customized temperature and particle control, static safety, humidification or dehumidification, and other controls

- Large-volume parenteral (LVP) preparations—those greater than 100 mL

- Male/female adapters—used to mix two substances by attaching to syringes

- Minibags—containing between 50 and 100 mL of solution

- Needles—used to inject substances; consist of a hub and a shaft, they attach to syringes

- Piggybacks—a small volume of solution added to a LVP preparation

- Sharps container—a rigid plastic container used for sharps such as needles, glass slides, scalpel blades, or disposable syringes

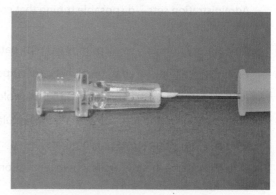

Figure 15-9 Filtered needle.

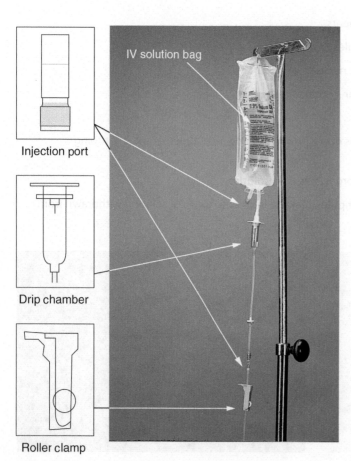

Figure 15-8 Drip chamber on IV administration set.

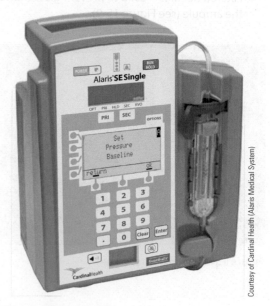

Figure 15-10 Infusion pump.

Courtesy of Cardinal Health (Alaris Medical System)

- Small-volume parenteral preparations—those that are smaller than or equal to 100 mL (see Figure 15-11)

- Spikes—rigid pieces of plastic that insert into IV bags

- Syringes—the most common syringe sizes used in pharmacy for sterile compounding include 1, 3, 6, 12, 20, 35, and 60 mL

- Syringe caps—used to prevent contamination of syringes when they are moved between locations

- Tubing—used to conduct solutions between a container and a patient

- Vials—containers with rubber stoppers that contain medications (see Figure 15-12)

The following supplies are used in sterile compounding:

- ¼ NS—0.225% sodium chloride

- $D_5\frac{1}{2}NS$—5% dextrose and 0.45% sodium chloride (for injection, United States Pharmacopeia [USP])

- 70% isopropyl alcohol—for cleaning surfaces

- Alcohol pads—for cleaning ports, stoppers, skin surfaces, and so on

- $D_{10}W$—10% dextrose in water

- D_5NS—5% dextrose in normal saline with 0.9% sodium chloride (for injection, USP)

- D_5W—5% dextrose in water

- LR—lactated Ringer's solution with 5% dextrose (for injection, USP)

- NS—normal saline solution with 0.9% sodium chloride (for injection, USP)

- SW—sterile water for injection (SWFI)

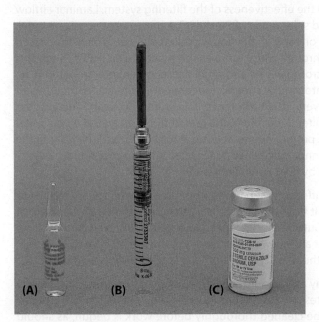
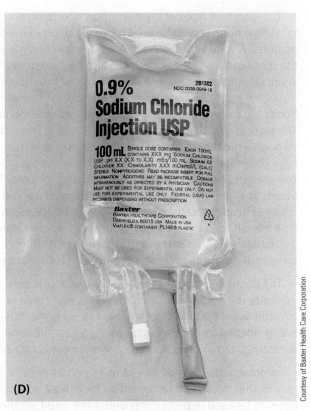

Figure 15-11 Small-volume parenteral products: (A) ampule; (B) prefilled syringe; (C) vial; and (D) piggyback minibag.

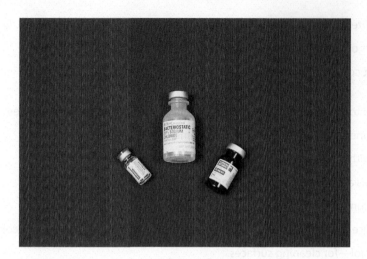

Figure 15-12 Vials.

Laminar Airflow Hoods

A laminar airflow hood is a piece of equipment designed for the handling of materials whenever a sterile working environment is required (see Figure 15-13). This device uses a system of circulating filtered air in parallel flow planes. Because room air may be highly contaminated, the system reduces the risk of bacterial contamination or exposure to chemical pollutants in surgical theaters, hospital pharmacies, laboratories, and food preparation areas. Sneezing, for example, produces up to 200,000 aerosol droplets, which can attach to dust particles and stay in the air for weeks! Laminar airflow hoods are very effective for providing a clean area, if they are operating properly.

There are two types of laminar airflow hoods: vertical and horizontal (see Figures 15-14A and 15-14B). A horizontal airflow hood should be used for preparation of numerous types of parenteral medications and sterile product mixtures. A vertical airflow hood is used for all chemotherapeutic agents, because of the direction of the airflow and the specifications of the hood. It can also be used to mix nonchemotherapeutic agents. However, chemotherapeutic agents should not be mixed in a horizontal airflow hood. The horizontal hoods used in hospital pharmacies must be inspected each year by an authorized inspector to ensure the effectiveness of the filtering system. Laminar airflow hoods basically have a box-like structure, with the top and sides made of Plexiglas®, a transparent acrylic material. The work area is bathed by positive pressure (horizontal or vertical) flowing air called *laminar*, which has passed through a prefilter that removes lint and dust and then through a high-efficiency particulate air (HEPA) filter. This filter, the most important part of the system, removes microorganisms and small particles of matter from room air, compressing and redistributing the now ultra-clean air into airflow streams that are parallel to each other. The air moves at a rate of 90 to 120 linear feet per minute, with very little turbulence, at a uniform velocity. This process removes nearly all of the bacteria from the air. The HEPA filter is located at the rear of the work area in a horizontal flow hood (top in a vertical flow hood), with a removable, perforated metal diffuser further toward the front in the horizontal hood (top in the vertical hood). HEPA filters cannot be cleaned or recycled and must be replaced every three to five years on average. The work area is illuminated by fluorescent lights.

The controlled area should be a limited-access area sufficiently separated from other pharmacy operations to minimize the potential for contamination that could result from the unnecessary flow of materials and personnel into and out of the area. The controlled air is a buffer from outside air that is needed because strong air currents from briefly opened doors, personnel walking past the laminar airflow workbench, or the air stream from the heating, ventilating, and air conditioning system can easily exceed the velocity of air from the laminar airflow workbench.

Laminar airflow hoods should be left on 24 hours a day and require regular maintenance. If turned off for any reason, the unit should be turned on for at least 30 minutes and then thoroughly cleaned before reusing. Also, all items to be used in procedures under the hood should be cleaned thoroughly before work is begun, as should the operator's hands and arms. Excess dust must be avoided at all costs. The operator should remove any jewelry from the hands and wrists. Technicians should use gowns with knit cuffs and rubber gloves while working inside

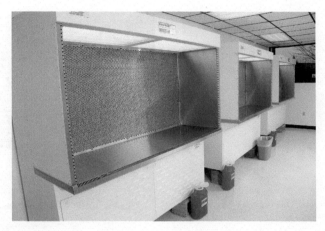

Figure 15-13 Laminar airflow hood.

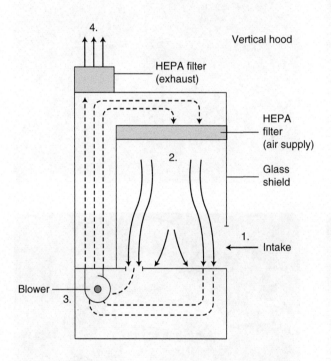

1. Room air enters the laminar airflow. This makes up about 30% of the air in the hood.

2. HEPA-filtered air enters and makes up 70% of the air in the hood.

3. Air from the work area is drawn down into the base and pulled back through the unit.

4. Air is exhausted after being filtered through carbon or HEPA filters.

(A)

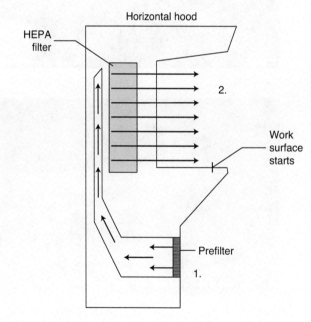

1. Room air enters, is filtered and drawn up to the top of the hood, where it is filtered through a HEPA filter.

2. Filtered air is directed out over the work surface.

(B)

Figure 15-14 (A) Vertical laminar airflow hood. (B) Horizontal laminar airflow hood.

laminar airflow hoods. The steps required to correctly put on a gown are shown in Figure 15-15. Face masks are recommended because most personnel talk or may cough or sneeze (see Figure 15-16). Personnel who have sensitivity to latex should use powder-free, low-latex protein gloves, or, if the allergy is severe, latex-free (synthetic) gloves are recommended. This minimizes the shedding of skin flora into the work area. Conventional laboratory coats are

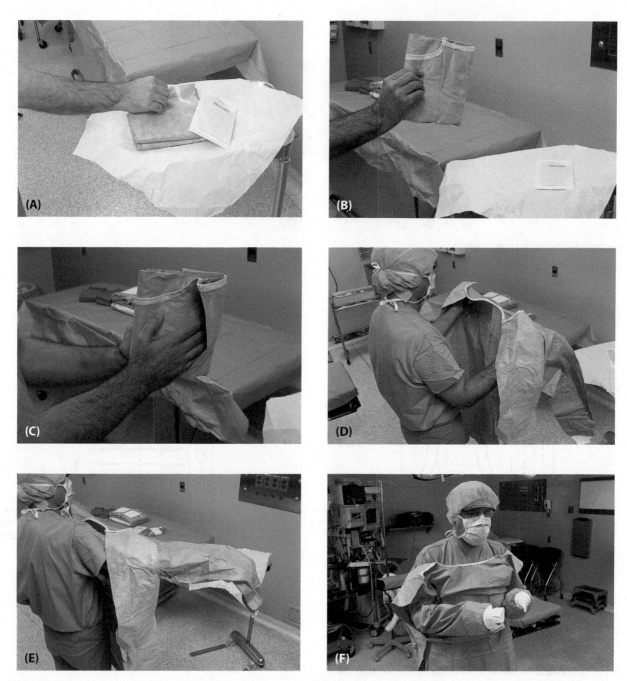

Figure 15-15 Donning a gown: (A) pick gown up by center without touching sterile packaging; (B) lift gown away from packaging and keep from touching any other items; (C) allow gown to unfold; (D) position gown so that you are able to slide your arms into it; (E) slide arms into gown without putting hands through cuffs; and (F) allow assistant to secure gown in back.

not sufficient, because their open cuffs allow entrapment of contaminated air between the technician's wrist and forearms and inside the sleeves.

It is important for operators to keep their hands within the cleaned area of the hood as much as possible and not touch hair, face, or clothing. Only materials essential for preparing the sterile product should be placed in the laminar airflow workbench or barrier isolator (see Figure 15-17).

The surface of ampules, vials, and container closures (e.g., vial stoppers) should be disinfected by swabbing or spraying with alcohol before placement in the workbench. All aseptic procedures should be performed at least 6 inches inside the front edge of the laminar airflow workbench, in a clear path of unidirectional airflow between the HEPA filter and work materials (e.g., needles or closures). The operator should avoid spraying or squirting solutions

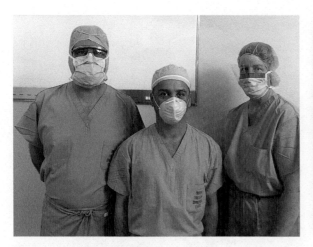

Figure 15-16 Face masks.

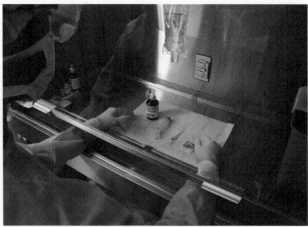

Figure 15-17 All materials used in the laminar airflow hood must be placed within the workbench clean area.

onto the HEPA filter, always aiming away from the filter when opening ampules or adjusting syringes. In a horizontal hood, items should be placed away from the sides and HEPA filter, and nothing should touch the filter. Large objects should never be placed near the back of the hood, because they will contaminate everything downstream from them and disrupt the flow pattern of air.

Work areas should be cleaned after each use. Before and after a series of intravenous admixtures are prepared (the preparation of sterile products) or anytime something is spilled, the work surface of the laminar airflow hood should be thoroughly cleaned with 70% isopropyl alcohol. A long side-to-side motion should be used, starting at the ceiling of the hood. If it is a vertical flow hood, the cover over and around the filter should be cleaned at this time. The next step is to clean the back of the hood if it is a horizontal airflow hood. It is important to never touch the actual HEPA filter itself. Next, sides should be cleaned, working from the back of the hood to the front. Finally, the bottom of the hood should be cleaned, working from the back to the front (see Figure 15-18A to 15-18G).

POINTS TO REMEMBER

When cleaning a laminar airflow hood, you must use a new piece of gauze (or lint-free cloth) wetted with 70% isopropyl alcohol for each separate surface of the hood—never use the same piece for multiple surfaces.

If the sides of the laminar airflow hood are acrylic plastic, they should also be cleaned periodically with solutions that can be used on them and by following the directions closely. Disinfectants should be alternated periodically to prevent development of resistant microorganisms. The HEPA filter should be serviced and certified every six months. Active work surfaces in the controlled area (e.g., carts, compounding devices, and counter surfaces) should be disinfected. Refrigerators, freezers, shelves, and other areas where pharmacy-prepared sterile products are stored should be kept clean. The floors of the controlled area should be nonporous and washable to enable regular disinfection.

Aseptic technique (preparing and handling sterile products in a manner that prevents microbial contamination) must be strictly applied when preparing parenteral products. The work area must be tightly controlled to assure cleanliness in order to prevent contamination from any source. Clean areas may be easily provided by the use of laminar airflow hoods, used in conjunction with proper aseptic technique. As previously described, laminar airflow hoods filter air through HEPA filters that flow through the hood in straight and parallel lines; 99.97% of all particles larger than 0.3 μm in size, and therefore all microbial contaminants and particulate matter, are removed by HEPA filters. Laminar airflow moves fast enough to keep the work area from becoming contaminated, in either a horizontal or a vertical direction.

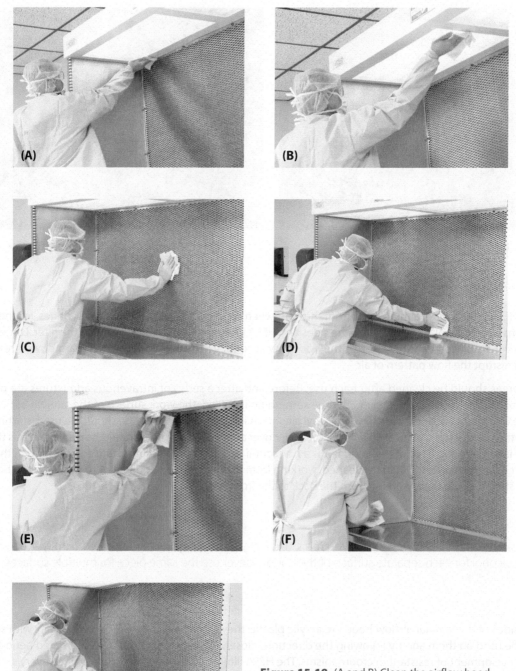

Figure 15-18 (A and B) Clean the airflow hood with long strokes from left to right; (C and D) working down from the top clean the back of the airflow hood; (E and F) then clean each side of the airflow hood; and (G) last, clean the countertop of the airflow hood.

Glove Box Hoods

Also known as *glove boxes*, these hoods separate workers from the areas in which they are performing various procedures. Glove box hoods can be configured or customized for temperature and particle control, static safety, humidification, dehumidification, and other important operating conditions. There are two general forms: *isolation glove box hoods* and *containment glove box hoods*. Isolation glove box hoods allow for controlled environments, protecting

Table 15-1 Compounded Medications—Storage and Stability

Risk Level	Room Temperature (68 to 77°F) (20 to 25°C)	Refrigerator (36 to 46°F) (2 to 8°C)	Freezer (13 to 14°F) (5 to 10°C)
High	24 hours	3 days	45 days
Medium	30 hours	9 days	45 days
Low	48 hours	14 days	45 days
Lowest	12 hours or less	12 hours or less	Not applicable

contamination-sensitive materials from ambient conditions. Containment glove box hoods allow for safe processing environments, protecting operators from biohazards inside their chambers. Glove box hoods resemble laminar airflow hoods in their construction, but the work areas are entirely contained and feature a glass barrier through which the worker can visualize the work area. There are holes lined with rubberized materials in the shapes of gloves into which workers insert the hands to manipulate materials.

Storage and Stability

There is an increased risk for bacterial growth the longer a compounded IV is exposed to room temperature. Also, to ensure constant temperatures, refrigerators must be monitored at least once per day. Table 15-1 summarizes guidelines for temperature ranges and the expiration dates of compounded medications, based on risk levels. The limits shown are for aseptically prepared products that have not passed a sterility test. These limits are not applicable to batches that have been tested. There may be longer expiration dates for products tested for sterility. Storage requirements include training of the patient and his or her caretaker about the proper use and storage of compounded products. All adverse events must be monitored and reported using the proper channels, consistently, and with thorough documentation.

Compounding of a Parenteral Product

Parenteral products must be prepared with strict controls to avoid contamination (see Figure 15-19). Parenteral products can be contaminated by contact with health care personnel, supply air, particle infiltration, and contaminants on equipment. Giving a patient a contaminated product can cause serious adverse effects, including death. After compounding a parenteral product, it should be visually inspected for correct labeling and any hazing, cloudiness, or particulates in the solution (see Figure 15-20).

Parenteral medications account for more than 40% of all medications administered in institutional practice. The following factors control the choice of a parenteral product's formulation and dosage form:

- Route of administration—Intravenous, subcutaneous, intradermal, intramuscular, intra-articular, and intrathecal; the type of dosage form will determine the route of administration, and the route of administration will place requirements on the formulation.

- Pharmacokinetics—Rates of absorption for any routes of administration besides intravenous or intra-arterial, rates of distribution, rates of metabolism, and rates of excretion will have an effect on the selected route of administration and type of formulation.

- Solubility—Solubility dictates the concentration of a drug in its dosage form; if the drug is insufficiently soluble in water at the required dosage, the formulation must contain a co-solvent or a solute that increases and maintains the drug in the solution.

- Stability—Stability is sometimes affected by drug concentration; if the drug has significant degradation problems in solution, then a freeze-dried or other sterile solid dosage form must be developed.

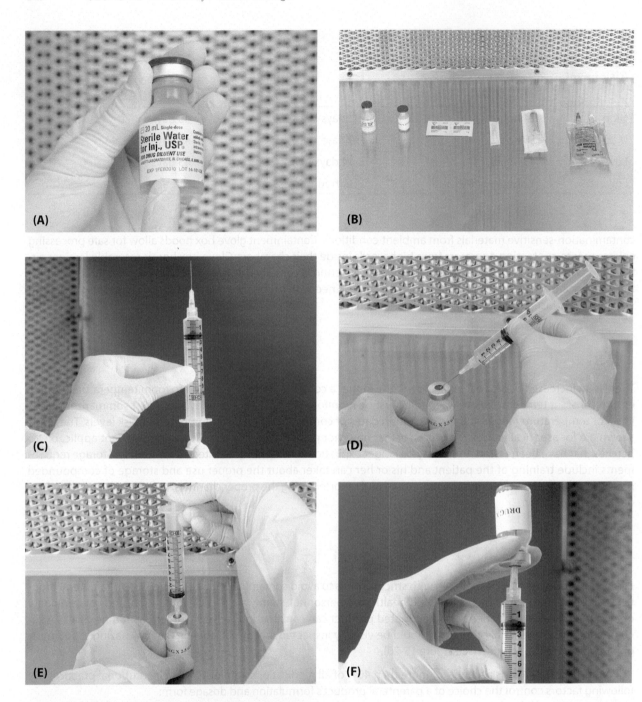

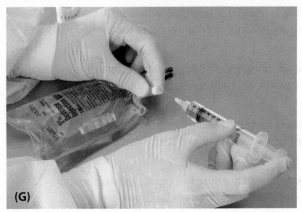

Figure 15-19 Compounding a parenteral product: (A) check the expiration dates on all products to be combined; (B) position the supplies in the laminar airflow hood; (C) draw air into the syringe; (D) insert the syringe at a 45-degree angle; (E) move the syringe to a 90-degree angle; (F) invert the vial and fill syringe with medication; and (G) instill medication into the final container.

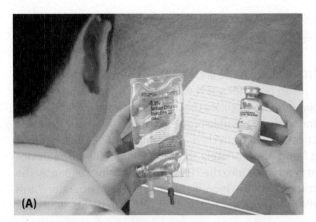
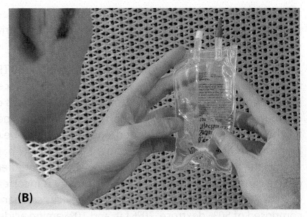

(A)   **(B)**

Figure 15-20 Visual inspection of a parenteral product: (A) read the label and verify that it is the correct medication and (B) turn the container upside down and look for hazing, cloudiness, and particulates in the solution.

- Compatibility—A drug must be compatible with potential formulation additives; this requires preformulation screening studies to ensure that additives will not cause additional problems with the preparation.

- Packaging—The desired type of packaging is often based on marketing preferences and competition; formulation scientists should know the intended type of packaging early in the developmental process so that the correct formulation may be accomplished.

POINTS TO REMEMBER

The pharmacy technician involved in sterile compounding works under the direct supervision of the pharmacist.

Compounding of a TPN Product

Total parenteral nutrition (TPN) provides lipids, proteins, electrolytes, sugars, salts, vitamins, and essential elements designed to meet the entire nutritional needs of the patient. It is indicated for patients with severe GI distress, those with poor nutrient absorption, and those who cannot eat. This system of nutrition may be used for patients who have acquired immunodeficiency syndrome (AIDS), cancer, Crohn's disease, severe diarrhea, hyperemesis gravidarum, or surgical removal of the intestines. Premature neonates and comatose patients may also receive TPN. This method of nutrition is infused directly into a vein, usually over a 10- to 12-hour period. Careful compounding procedures must be followed when working with TPN solutions. Levels of added ingredients must be carefully balanced to ensure that no harm will come to the patient. After the pharmacist or pharmacy technician has made the pertinent mixture calculations, they must be double-checked by a pharmacist. TPN solutions are compounded in laminar airflow hoods or in biological safety cabinets. The base solution is composed of dextrose, amino acids, SWFI, and sometimes lipids. Additives that are mixed into the base solution may include electrolytes, minerals, vitamins, and other prescribed substances. TPN solutions may be compounded either by hand or by using automated mixing devices.

When choosing a bag to contain the TPN solution, the bag that is the closest size in which the entire finished mixed solution will fit should be chosen. The base components must be mixed in the following order to ensure proper formulation: dextrose, amino acids, lipids, and SWFI. The additives are then injected separately into the TPN bag after the pharmacist performs a final check as to their accuracy. The bag should be gently mixed in between the addition of each additive. Lipids should always be added last, because they can mask particulates or precipitation in the final solution. After all additives have been injected, gently rotate or shake the bag to blend all the ingredients evenly.

A standard TPN solution is as follows: 42.5 g of amino acid and 250 g of dextrose (500 mL of an 8.5% amino acid solution and 500 mL of 50% dextrose) per liter. This formula provides 1000 calories per liter, with a non-protein-calorie–to–nitrogen ratio of 150:1. To prevent essential fatty acid deficiency, IV lipids are usually provided separately twice per week. Before administering the TPN solution, verify with the facility's procedures whether any inline filters should be used.

Automated filling devices may be used to compound TPN solutions. These are linked to computers to help control accuracy. When a pharmacist or pharmacy technician receives an order for a TPN solution, the information from the prescription is entered into the automated filling device's computer to calculate the amounts of each ingredient. The computer has automatic warning software to alert the operator of any possible problems. Labels are then generated for the solution to be compounded, and these should be checked and rechecked. The compounding device should be programmed for the correct patient and the TPN bag hung appropriately so that it can be filled. The device weighs the filled bag to ascertain accuracy. Each ingredient is pumped into the TPN bag in a specific sequence. The device can detect whether the specific gravity is incorrect for any of the ingredients and alert the operator if this occurs. Newer types of automated filling devices can handle more complex mixtures of TPN ingredients, which are composed of 50% dextrose, 20% fat, and 10% amino acids.

POINTS TO REMEMBER

It is wise to have a different pharmacist double-check TPN calculations prior to compounding these solutions.

WHAT WOULD YOU DO?

Contaminated TPN bags have resulted in an outbreak of *Serratia marcescens* bacteremia, resulting in many patient deaths. You witness the compounding of a TPN solution, and believe that the compounding technician accidentally switched dextrose for sterile water—a commonly occurring mistake. What would you do?

Preparing an Intravenous Piggyback

Intravenous **piggybacks** (IVPBs) may be prepared in several ways based on the type of equipment used. In the traditional method, a vial of medication is added to an IV medication by removing the contents of the vial using a syringe and injecting it into the IV bag of medication. Before any medication is added to an IVPB, its expiration date must be checked. The steps required to remove a medication from a vial prior to adding to an IVPB are shown in Figure 15-21.

Many antibiotics are prepared as IVPBs. Other types of piggybacks, called Add-a-Vial and Add-Vantage systems, are not activated and are mixed immediately before administration. These systems include a powdered vial of antibiotic connected to a small-volume parenteral preparation and are labeled "Activate when you want to administer"—therefore, they do not require refrigeration before being activated. However, once activated, if they are not used immediately, they should be refrigerated with a label stating "Do not freeze." This technique usually allows for longer expiration dates than in the traditional method.

Large-Volume Parenteral Preparations

LVP preparations are able to deliver large quantities of electrolytes, TPN solutions, chemotherapy, and other fluids. Popular LVPs include 0.9% sodium chloride, 5% dextrose in water (D_5W), and 5% dextrose and lactated Ringer's (D_5LR) (Figure 15-22). Magnesium, lidocaine, aminophylline, nitroglycerin, dopamine, and potassium are other ingredients that may be present in premixed solutions. In the pharmacy, it is important that the pharmacist ensure the stability, compatibility, and safety of the mixture. The pharmacist should verify *high doses of drugs or electrolytes* with the physician who orders an LVP to be compounded.

Types of water that are commonly used when compounding LVPs include the following:

- Bacteriostatic water for injection USP—sterile, with antimicrobial agents
- Sterile water for injection USP—sterile but has no antimicrobial agents

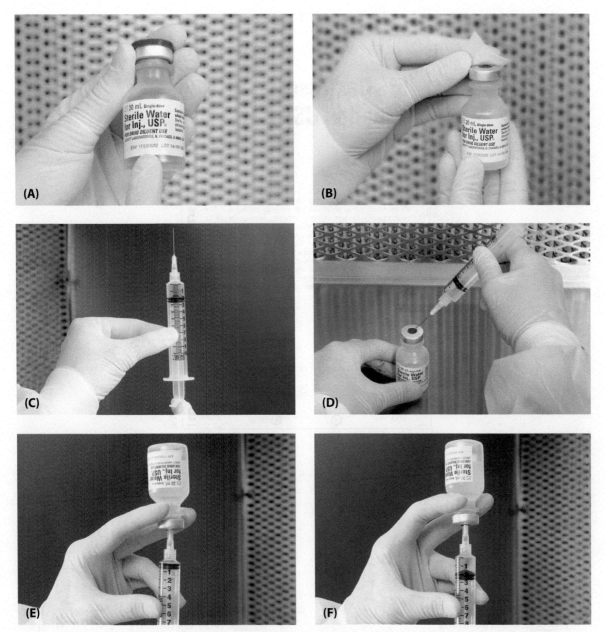

Figure 15-21 Removing medication from a vial: (A) check the expiration date; (B) swab the top of the vial with alcohol; (C) draw air into the syringe; (D) insert the syringe into the vial; (E) inject air into the vial; and (F) withdraw fluid from the vial.

POINTS TO REMEMBER

There are other types of water that have a variety of medical uses; however, they should not be used for sterile compounding. These types include purified water USP, water for injection USP, and sterile water for irrigation USP.

MEDICATION ERROR ALERT

The need for complete sterility when compounding many types of medications cannot be stressed enough. In 1990, four patients died of a bacterial infection from a nonsterile cardioplegia solution compounded in a Nebraska hospital.

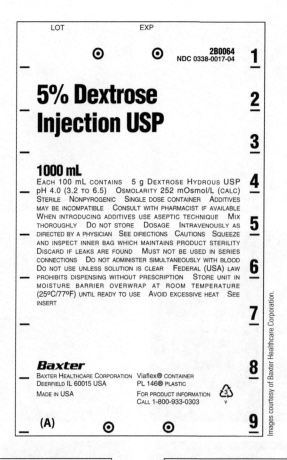

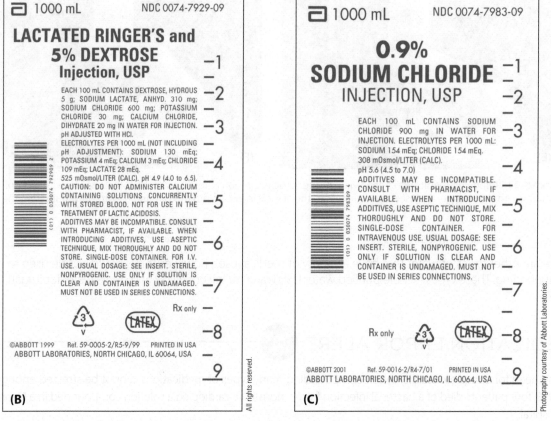

Figure 15-22 (A) 5% Dextrose. (B) 5% Dextrose and lactated Ringer's. (C) 0.9% Sodium chloride.

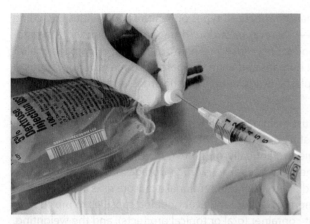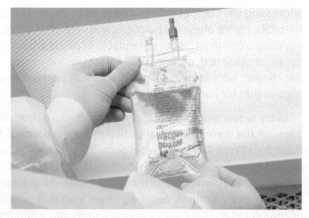

Figure 15-23 Preparing an IV admixture: (A) insert the syringe into the port on the IV bag and (B) check the medication in the bag.

Preparation of Intravenous Admixtures

Intravenous admixtures consist of several sterile products added into an IV fluid for administration (see Figure 15-23). They must be mixed using aseptic technique. This may be accomplished by mixing them inside of a laminar airflow hood. Each sterile product should be added into the IV fluid with a fresh disposable syringe.

POINTS TO REMEMBER

It is possible for certain antibiotics to be frozen after being mixed in an IV bag, thawed, and then used within 24 hours. These antibiotics include penicillin G potassium, cefazolin sodium, and nafcillin. However, this practice is not commonly performed today.

United States Pharmacopeia (USP) Chapter <797>

Chapter <797> of the *United States Pharmacopeia* has set the standards for compounding, preparing, and labeling of sterile drug preparations. It has provisions that are required and enforced by the FDA and the state boards of pharmacy. Some of these standards that relate to sterile compounding include beyond-use dating and the maintenance of quality sterile drug preparations once they leave the pharmacy.

A **beyond-use date** is calculated from the time that a sterile drug product is compounded until it is administered to a patient. There are three risk levels for contamination of sterile products under the USP:

Risk	Time at Room Temp	Refrigerate for
High	24 hours	3 days
Medium	30 hours	7 days
Low	48 hours	14 days

All risk levels can be frozen for up to 45 days. Compounded sterile products should not be shaken, exposed to excessive light, or exposed to excessive heat. Patients and caregivers should be trained about the proper storage of sterile drug products if they need to keep them for use at home.

United States Pharmacopeia (USP) Chapter <800>

Chapter <800> of the USP is a new, general chapter that was created to identify requirements for the receipt, storage, mixing, preparing, compounding, dispensing, and administration of *hazardous drugs*. It was designed to protect the patient, health care personnel, and the environment. Before USP <800>, there was no existing USP chapter addressing the compounding of hazardous drugs. This chapter affects all types of health care facilities, including hospitals, clinics, physician practices, and veterinary offices—wherever hazardous drugs are compounded. A hazardous drug is one that has the potential to impair human reproduction, cause fetal harm, cause cancer, damage or alter genes, or cause toxicity, even at low doses, in the organs of humans and animals. There are three groups of drugs in this chapter, with some overlap. They include non-antineoplastic drugs, antineoplastic drugs, and drugs with reproductive risks for humans.

Every organization that compounds hazardous drugs must maintain a complete list of them, which must include items on the current National Institute for Occupational Safety and Health (NIOSH) *List of Antineoplastic and Other Hazardous Drugs in Healthcare Settings*. The list must be reviewed annually, or more frequently, when new agents or dosage forms become available. Each facility must record the type of hazardous drugs, dosage form, risk of exposure, packaging, and manipulation for all hazardous drugs it handles. Areas of unintentional exposure risks include receiving or unpacking orders, counting doses from bulk containers, crushing tablets or opening capsules to mix in food or compound an oral liquid, pouring liquids into a different container (oral or topical products), and the weighting, mixing, diluting, or reconstitution of hazardous drugs. Additional risk areas include expelling air from syringes containing a hazardous drug, expelling a hazardous drug from a syringe, touching work surfaces that have hazardous drug residues present, and inhalation aerosolized hazardous drugs (such as by a patient or visitor sharing a room with another patient). Additionally, risks include handling body fluids with hazardous drugs as well as contaminated clothing, linens, and other materials, and maintaining equipment and devices.

Personal protective equipment (PPE) such as gloves, gowns, hair covers, face covers, beard covers, and shoe covers is required for handling damaged or broken containers, all types of compounding, routine cleanup, and collection and disposal of wastes and spills. Also, eye, face, and respiratory protection is required for receiving damaged or broken contains, and for the collection and disposal of wastes and spills. Staff training must be imparted to ensure competency and responsibility when personnel handle hazardous drugs. Upon receiving these drugs, there must be a visual inspection with a plan for follow-up action if damage is suspected to the packaging and/or external shipping containers. If safety strategies do not support shared storage, hazardous drugs must be stored separately in a room with negative or neutral pressure, with at least 12 air changes per hour (ACPH). There must be a written hazard communication program that describes how hazardous drugs are identified, defining the process of supplying safety data sheets for each hazardous drug available in the workplace. To promote safety, there must be administrative, environmental, and engineering controls in three specific categories: primary, secondary, and supplementary. For all compounding, there must be externally vented rooms with restricted access, which utilize minimum negative pressures.

Noninjectable Products

There are certain noninjectable products that must be sterile for use. These include irrigations and ophthalmic products.

OPHTHALMICS

Ophthalmics are sterile preparations intended for direct administration into the **conjunctiva** of the eye. Ophthalmic drops contain filtered elements that are safe to use. Ophthalmics are compounded in laminar airflow hoods in aseptic conditions, and then autoclaved for sterilization. They are then cultured to ensure that they contain no contaminants. The process for compounding ophthalmics properly takes from one to two weeks.

MEDICATION ERROR ALERT

Sterile compounding is of great importance with ophthalmics. Patients have lost their vision after becoming infected by *Pseudomonas aeruginosa* found in indomethacin eye drops compounded in a community pharmacy, even though commercial nonsteroidal drops were available at the time.

IRRIGATIONS

The most common sterile irrigations include gentamicin irrigation solution and surgical antibiotic solution (SAS). These agents, which include sterile water or saline, are used during surgery to irrigate open surgical sites. While not truly aseptic in nature, they must be compounded in a sterile environment using sterile IV bottles or bags. The labels of these types of irrigations state that they are to be used *for irrigation only*, and they are never to be used intravenously.

MEDICATION ERROR ALERT

Even prefilled containers of saline are liable to become contaminated. In California, 11 children became septic, with 10 of them testing positive for **Enterobacter cloacae** bloodstream infections, associated with contaminated prefilled saline syringes.

Compounding Records

Compounding records are also known as "mixing reports" and may be computerized or paper records (see Figure 15-24). They are used to document the activities undertaken during the compounding process and should be stored along with patient charts. A compounding record includes expiration dates of the substances used, lot numbers, stability information about the final mixture, and specific compounding instructions for the mixture.

WHAT WOULD YOU DO?

You notice that several of your pharmacy's compounding records of last week did not include expiration dates of substances used. Concerned that the compounding pharmacist did not check these dates, you ask him to verify that all of the substances he had used were not expired. He says he cannot remember because he had compounded so many different medications that week. Concerned that someone will receive expired ingredients in their medications, what would you do?

Policies and Procedures for Sterile Product Preparation

Health care personnel should read their facility's policies and procedures, and verify by signature that they have done so, prior to any sterile compounding procedures. The following topics should be covered by the policies and procedures manual concerning sterile product preparation:

- Job description—education level; certification; registration; experience; lifting various weights; pushing carts; handling rapid, repetitive, and accurate manipulations; work shifts; environment; garb; compounding pharmaceutical products that are free of contaminants

- Job orientation—roles of employees; garb; facilities; equipment; area-specific techniques; reference materials

- Training and education—aseptic technique; quality control; properties of drugs; good manufacturing practices; equipment operation; product handling

- Competency evaluation—observation and testing methods; intervals between evaluations; aseptic technique; new equipment; written math tests

MIXING REPORT

Stability:	Patient Name:
Reference: *Handbook of Inj. Drugs*	Origin Rx Number:
Other:	
Calculations:	Place copy of Rx label here:
Checked By	

Refill Date	Ingredients (one per line)	Volume used	Units used	Prepared date–time	MFG lot no.	Exp. date	Prep. by:

Figure 15-24 Compounding report.

- Acquisition—ingredient selection; bulk substance dating procedures; repackaging guidelines; ingredient testing; purchasing equipment, containers, and closures
- Storage—monitoring of temperatures, light, ventilation, and humidity; stock rotation and inspection; locations of quarantined products

- Handling—proper removal of outer packaging; handling pouched supplies; decontaminating ampules and vials; disposal of used items, hazardous wastes, and sharps; inspection of sterile ingredients and containers; handling expired drugs and supplies; handling product recalls

- Facilities—cleaning procedures; traffic control; safety

- Equipment—location; use; cleaning; allowable cart usage areas; laminar airflow hoods; traffic

- Personal conduct and garb—eating; drinking; smoking; makeup and jewelry; hand washing and drying; infectious conditions; garb policies and procedures

- Other important areas include product integrity, aseptic technique, work sheets, batch preparation records, sterilization methods, environmental monitoring, process validation, expiration dating, labeling, end-product valuation, quality of compounded products, patient monitoring, housekeeping, quality assurance, and documentation records

Summary

Noninjectable products include irrigations (used for open surgical sites) and ophthalmics (intended for direct administration into the conjunctiva of the eye). Parenteral products include intravenous (IV) products (either small-volume or large-volume parenteral preparations) and total parenteral nutrition (TPN). Small-volume parenteral preparations consist of secondary or "piggyback" IVs, which are added to large-volume parenteral (LVP) preparations (also known as primary IVs). A parenteral product may be chosen based on its route of administration, pharmacokinetics, solubility, stability, compatibility, and packaging. TPN is designed to meet the entire nutritional needs of a patient who cannot eat, cannot absorb nutrients properly, or has severe gastrointestinal (GI) distress. Parenteral products are commonly administered by IV push, infusion, or an intravenous piggyback (IVPB).

Parenteral products must be prepared using strict control measures to avoid contamination, commonly in laminar airflow hoods. Standards for the correct procedures of compounding, preparing, and labeling of sterile drug preparations are set forth in the *United States Pharmacopeia* (USP) Chapter <797>. This includes beyond-use dates, which are calculated from the time a sterile drug product is compounded until it is administered to a patient. USP Chapter <800> concerns the handling and usage of hazardous drugs.

REVIEW QUESTIONS

1. The most important characteristic of an injectable solution is:

   A. viscosity.
   B. dispensability.
   C. sterility.
   D. color.

2. Which of the following are most commonly used for the compounding of IV antibiotics?

   A. Intravenous piggybacks
   B. Large-volume bags
   C. Irrigations
   D. Syringes

3. Which of the following is/are the base solution(s) for compounding TPN?

   A. Sterile water
   B. Amino acid
   C. Dextrose
   D. All of the above

4. According to the USP, high-risk compounding products can be kept in a refrigerator for:

   A. 6 hours.
   B. 24 hours.
   C. 48 hours.
   D. 72 hours.

5. Which of the following base components must be mixed last into a TPN bag?

   A. Dextrose
   B. Lipids
   C. Sterile water
   D. Amino acids

6. LVP preparations can deliver large quantities of all of the following, *except*:

   A. chemotherapy.
   B. antibiotics.
   C. electrolytes.
   D. TPN solutions.

7. Ophthalmics are compounded in laminar airflow hoods for which of the following purposes?

   A. Sterilization
   B. Destruction of spores
   C. Aseptic conditions
   D. Nonsterile products

8. Sterile irrigations are used for:

   A. intravenous injections.
   B. rehydration.
   C. surgical sites.
   D. cleaning nasal cavities.

9. Medications given by the parenteral route may be administered using which of the following?

   A. Rapid direct injection
   B. Continuous infusion
   C. Intermittent infusion
   D. All of the above

10. Parenteral products must be prepared with strict controls to avoid:

    A. expiration.
    B. contamination.
    C. lysation.
    D. None of the above.

11. The laminar airflow hood should be cleaned with:

    A. 95% ethyl alcohol.
    B. 95% isopropyl alcohol.
    C. 70% isopropyl alcohol.
    D. 70% methyl alcohol.

12. A pharmacy technician is compounding a prescription that the order indicates should be composed of 50% dextrose, 20% fat, and 10% amino acids in 1000 mL of normal saline. What type of compounding is being done in this example?

    A. Total peripheral nutrition
    B. Total parenteral nutrition
    C. Peripheral parenteral nutrition
    D. Partial parenteral nutrition

13. HEPA filters must be certified every:

    A. three months.
    B. six months.
    C. nine months.
    D. year.

14. Small spills of blood or body fluids on counter surfaces can be cleaned with:

    A. 70% wood alcohol.
    B. 95% isopropyl alcohol.
    C. 95% household bleach.
    D. 1:10 solution of household bleach.

15. Many IV admixtures (antibiotics), after activation, are commonly stored in:

    A. shelves at room temperature.
    B. refrigerators.
    C. freezers.
    D. microwaves.

CRITICAL THINKING

A pharmacy technician was sent to do an externship in a hospital pharmacy. He or she was anxious to observe sterile compounding procedures.

1. Explain vertical laminar airflow hoods and when they should be used.

2. Describe the basics of USP Chapter <797>.

WEB LINKS

American Society of Health-System Pharmacists: www.ashp.org

B&B Pharmacy & Health Care Center: bbpharmacy.com

Laminar Airflow Hoods: www.nuaire.com

SCA Pharmaceuticals: scapharma.com

United States Pharmacopeial Convention: www.usp.org

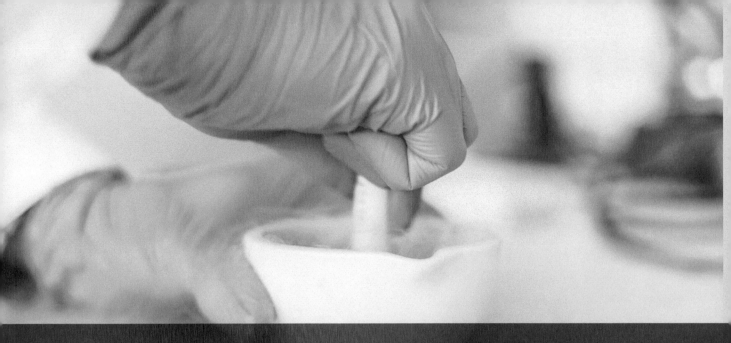

ADMINISTRATIVE SKILLS

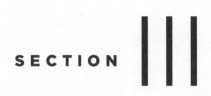

SECTION III

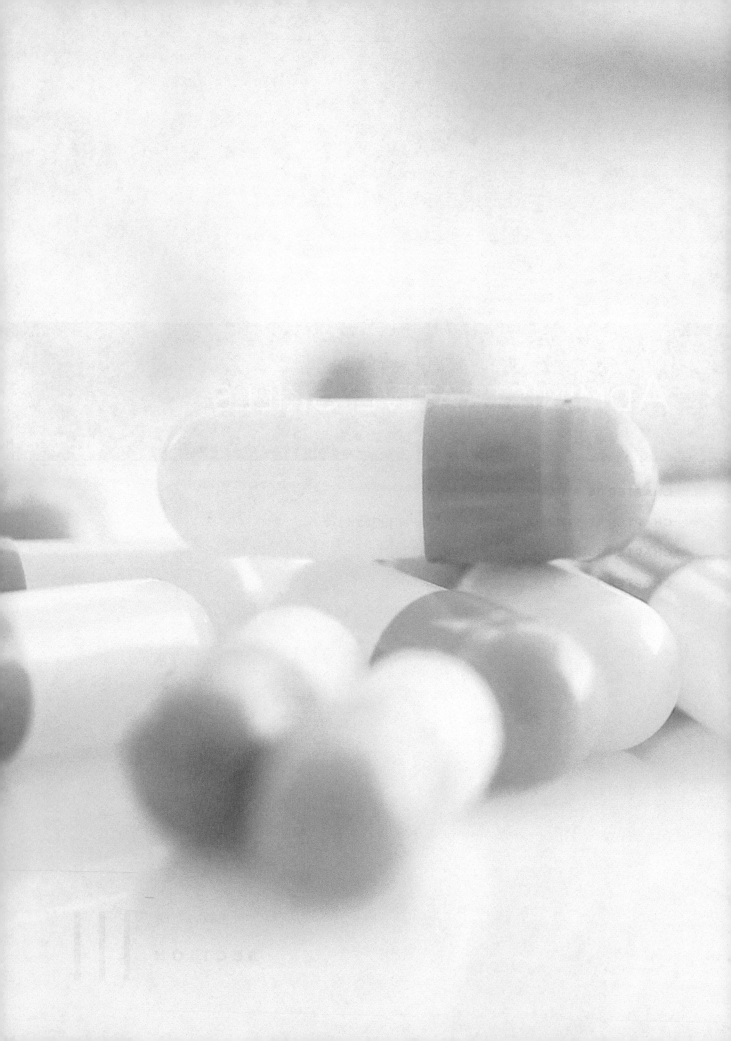

CHAPTER 16

Insurance and Billing

OUTLINE

Group Plan

Prepaid Health Plan

Individual Contract

Types of Health Insurance
- *Private Health Insurance*
- *Managed Care Programs*
- *Government Plans*

Insurance Policy

Patient Profiles

Prior Authorization

Claims Processing
- *Billing Secondary Payers*
- *Problems with Claims*
- *Claim Rejection*

Special Billing
- *Immunizations*
- *Durable Medical Supplies*
- *Clinic and Inpatient Billing*
- *Medication Therapy Management*
- *Healthcare Common Procedure Coding System*

Payments
- *Claim Adjudication*
- *Monitoring Claim Status*

Third-Party Audits
- *Dispensed Quantity Exceeds Authorized Quantity*
- *Higher Than Expected Usage*
- *Inconsistent Days Supply*
- *Wrong Package Size*
- *Inappropriate Dispense-as-Written Code*
- *Missing or Incomplete Original Prescription*

Role of the Insurance Billing Pharmacy Technician

OBJECTIVES

Upon completion of this chapter, the reader should be able to:

1. Explain the terms *deductible, premium,* and *copay.*

2. Define group plans and prepaid health plans.

3. Explain and list various types of private health insurance.

4. Discuss government insurance plans.

5. Explain eligibility criteria for Medicare.

6. Discuss Medicaid benefits.

7. Describe the process of adjudication regarding coverage.

8. Identify the information required by various types of insurance claims.

9. Differentiate between ICD-10, NDC, and HCPCS codes.

10. Describe the various types of coverage rejections and their causes.

KEY TERMS

audits	deductible	Medicare Advantage plan	refill too soon
beneficiary	dependents	overpayment	subscriber
CHAMPVA	desk audits	patient identification number	third-party payer
coinsurance	eligibility		time limit
contract	field audits	plan limitations exceeded	TRICARE
coordination of benefits	health insurance	policy limitation	waiting period
copayment	Medicaid	preauthorization	
days supply exceeded	Medicare	premium	

Overview

Health care costs are continually increasing. According to the Centers for Disease Control and Prevention (CDC), health expenditures in the United States, in 2016, totaled $3.3 trillion. In the year 2000, this total was much lower, at $1.37 trillion. By the year 2025, total expenditures are expected to reach $5.6 trillion. Prescription costs are also increasing. In 2000, they totaled $121 billion, but in 2016, they were over $457 billion. As a result of these increases, citizens are looking for help in paying for health care and prescriptions. Pharmacy technicians and other staff members must understand how to correctly bill prescription insurance, ensuring payments for the pharmacy, protection against audits, and for the correct copay amounts for patients.

Group Plan

Any insurance plan by which a group of employees is insured under a single policy issued to their employer, with individual certificates given to all insured individuals or their families, is classified as a group plan or policy. A group policy usually provides better benefits and offers lower premiums than individual plans.

Prepaid Health Plan

In a prepaid health plan, a policyholder or an enrolled group of policyholders (subscribers) pay a yearly fee or fixed periodic payments. Providers of services are paid by capitation, which is a system of payments used by managed care plans in which physicians and hospitals are paid a fixed, per capita amount for each patient who registers for a specific period of time, regardless of the type and number of services provided.

Individual Contract

An insurance plan issued to an individual (the **beneficiary**) and his or her **dependents** is considered an individual **contract**. While the insured individual is usually the beneficiary, he or she may select other individuals to also be beneficiaries. This kind of policy includes a higher **premium** and the benefits are fewer. This type of insurance may also be called *personal insurance*.

Types of Health Insurance

Many forms of **health insurance** coverage are available in the United States. The majority of patients, approximately 84%, have coverage from some type of insurance policy or other third-party payer. A **third-party payer** is an individual or corporation that makes a payment on an obligation or debt but is not a party to the contract that created the obligation or debt. To understand third-party payers better, let us first discuss first- and second-party payers. The first party is the person designated in the contract to receive a contracted service, whereas the second party is the person or organization providing the service. There are three major third-party payers: third-party full-payment groups (private insurance companies), third-party contractual payment groups (Blue Cross®, Medicare, and Medicaid), and the cash payment group. Health insurance may include private insurance, government plans, managed care contracts, and worker's compensation—all referred to as third-party payers.

Pharmacy technicians must understand the different types of insurance coverage, obtain required information from insurance cards, determine if each patient has prescription coverage, which entity should be billed, and how to correctly transmit claims. Commonly used types of insurance plans and cards include CHAMPVA cards, drug discount cards, Medicaid cards, Medicare or Medicare Advantage cards, medical insurance ID cards, Medigap cards, pharmacy benefits cards (which have the Rx symbol and the word YES printed on them), prescription coupon cards from drug manufacturers (provided to patients as incentives to try medications or to help patients in certain income groups), TRICARE cards, and workers' compensation, which requires no card to be presented.

The majority of health insurance companies contract with pharmacy benefit managers (PBM) to handle claims for prescriptions. These individuals contract with pharmacy providers, process claims from pharmacies, provide payments to pharmacies for the submitted claims, administer and recommend member copays, formularies, and restrictions or limitations on prescription coverage (on behalf of insurance plans), manage clinical pharmacy programs, and negotiate rebate contracts with pharmaceutical manufacturers.

PRIVATE HEALTH INSURANCE

Numerous private insurance companies across the United States offer health insurance to individuals and groups. Health insurance is the coverage of policyholders by insurance carriers or government programs. Third-party health insurance plans are often provided by employers as employment benefits but can also be purchased by individuals when they lack other types of insurance coverage. In the United States, the five largest health insurance companies are WellPoint, CIGNA, Aetna, Humana, and United Healthcare. They all offer many different types of prescription coverage. Pharmacy claims are unique compared to medical claims. Some information contained in prescription medication claims, such as the patient's name, date of birth, address, and certain demographic information, are identical to information found in medical claims. However, pharmacy claims also require other information, including name of product written and dispensed, National Drug Code (NDC), quantity dispensed, usage instructions, and day's supply.

Blue Cross®–Blue Shield® Association

The Blue Cross®–Blue Shield® Association (BCBS) is a nationwide federation of local insurance organizations that offer health care services to subscribers, requiring them to pay a fee in advance of services. BCBS is a private insurer and not a government-run entity. Under a prepaid health coverage plan, the carrier will pay for specified medical expenses if premiums are paid in advance. Previously, the Blue Cross® part of BCBS covered hospital services, outpatient and home care services, and other institutional care and the Blue Shield® plan covered medical services, dental services, vision, and other outpatient benefits. Now, however, both offer full health care coverage for their subscribers. In most states, they have become a single corporation, although in some they remain separate. Various plans are offered through BCBS, including individual, family, group, preventative care, and managed care plans. Some local BCBS organizations help the government administer Medicare, Medicaid, and TRICARE programs. There are 36 local BCBS plans in the United States, each with its own claim form. Plans make direct payments to member health care providers, but payments may be made to the **subscriber** (patient) if the provider is a nonmember. Many small groups and individuals who may not be able to get coverage elsewhere can join a BCBS plan. Some plans offer coverage regardless of medical condition during special periods of time. Plans must get permission from the state to raise their rates. Pharmacies submit claims to BCBS electronically, and usually it is the pharmacist who must do this. Up to six receipts per patient may be submitted on one claim form. BCBS claim forms must include the pharmacy's contract number, group number, contract/service code, enrollee/subscriber's name, complete health care provider information, complete patient information, additional insurer information, date of service, prescription number, quantity, number of days the medication should last, dispensing indicator, NDC number, explanatory information, and signatures of the person receiving the prescription as well as the pharmacist. BCBS claim forms will be returned if information is missing or incorrect. A response or payment from BCBS may take up to 45 days, and BCBS requires that pharmacies wait to submit any follow-up to a claim form until this period has expired.

Health Maintenance Organizations

Health maintenance organizations (HMOs) were the first type of managed care organizations developed to control the expenditure of health care dollars and to manage patient care. The HMO contracts with employers to provide health service for their employees. The member of an HMO selects a primary care physician (PCP) from the medical group. The HMO is responsible for all but limited administrative needs of a PCP, including processing of capitation and fee-for-service checks. The HMO remains a challenging and exciting setting for developing the optimum contribution of drug services to good medical care.

Kaiser Foundation Health Plan

The Kaiser Foundation Health Plan is a type of prepaid group practice HMO. The Kaiser Foundation was a pioneer of the nonprofit prepaid group practice, beginning in California in 1933. The plan owns its own medical facilities and directly employs physicians and other providers.

Workers' Compensation

All state legislatures have passed workers' compensation laws to protect wage earners against the loss of wages and the cost of medical care resulting from occupational accidents or disease. Compensation benefits include medical care benefits, weekly income replacement benefits for temporary disability, permanent disability settlements, and survivor benefits, when applicable. The providers of service, such as doctors, hospitals, therapists, or pharmacies, accept the workers' compensation payment as payment in full and do not bill the patient. Time limitations are set forth for the prompt reporting of workers' compensation cases. The employee is obligated to promptly notify the employer; the employer, in turn, must notify the insurance company and must refer the employee to a source of medical care. Individuals entitled to workers' compensation insurance are private business employees, state employees, and federal employees such as postal workers, coal miners, and maritime workers. Workers' compensation insurance coverage provides benefits to employees and their dependents if employees suffer work-related injuries, illnesses, or death. When a claim is made, a workers' compensation claim form is completed and sent to the insurance carrier or to the state fund for reimbursement. The injured worker receives no bills and pays no **deductible** or **coinsurance**; 100% of medical expenses related specifically to that injury are covered.

MANAGED CARE PROGRAMS

During the past six decades, there have been many reforms of the health care system. Medical practices have made transitions from rural to urban, from generalist to specialist, from solo to group practice, and from fee-for-service to capitated reimbursement. The expansion of health care plans to encompass a number of different types of delivery systems that try to manage the cost of health care resulted in managed care. Managed care organizations manage, negotiate, and contract for health care with the goal of keeping costs down. Managed care organizations sign up health care providers who agree to charge a fixed fee for services. These fixed fees are set by the managed care organization or by the governmental agency responsible for managed care.

Independent Practice Association

An independent practice association (IPA) is a closed-panel HMO. Instead of maintaining its own staff and clinic buildings, the IPA contracts with independently practicing physicians. The IPA may pay each doctor a set amount per patient in advance (capitation), or the fees charged for services to group members may be billed directly to the IPA rather than to the patient. Fees for services to nonmember patients are handled the same as any other fee for service. The physician may be contracted with several IPAs.

Preferred Provider Organization

In a preferred provider organization (PPO), a type of managed care plan, enrollees receive the highest level of benefits when they obtain services from a physician, hospital, or other health provider designated by their program as a preferred provider. Enrollees receive reduced benefits when they obtain care from a provider who is not designated as a preferred provider by their program. PPO patients may see specialists without **preauthorization** (prior authorization) from their PCPs. HMOs offering point-of-service options are more like PPOs. Prescriptions that must be preauthorized include those for nonpreferred drugs, specific preferred drugs, drugs for which the prescribed quantity exceeds the quantity limit, drugs within a therapeutic class not included in the preferred drug list (PDL), and multisource brand name drugs with A-rated generic equivalents available for substitution. The classes of drugs for which many insurance plans require preauthorization vary greatly. Some examples include antihyperglycemic agents, growth hormones, antirheumatic agents, and certain drugs used for specific conditions. These include drugs that treat benign prostatic hypertrophy, erectile dysfunction, hepatitis C (interferon A), irritable bowel syndrome, multiple sclerosis, narcolepsy, pulmonary arterial hypertension, certain types of cancer, and antirejection drugs for transplant patients.

GOVERNMENT PLANS

Government plans sponsor insurance coverage for eligible individuals. The federal government provides coverage under Medicare, Medicaid, TRICARE or CHAMPUS, and CHAMPVA.

Medicare

Medicare is the largest single medical benefits program in the United States. Medicare is a federal program authorized by Congress and administered by the Centers for Medicare & Medicaid Services (CMS). It became a law in 1965 as Title 18 of the Social Security Act. Medicare is a nationwide program that offers the same benefits in all 50 states. It provides health insurance to citizens aged 65 and older and to younger patients who are blind or widowed or who are disabled because of serious long-term illnesses such as kidney failure. There are four distinct parts (A, B, C, and D) to the Medicare program.

Medicare Part A

Medicare Part A covers hospital, nursing facility, home health, hospice, and inpatient care. Those who are eligible for Social Security benefits are automatically enrolled in Medicare Part A, including the aged, disabled, and blind.

Medicare Part A provides the following benefits to applicants:

- A patient bed in a hospital (up to 90 hospital days per benefit period)
- A patient bed in a nursing facility (up to 100 extended-care days per benefit period)
- Home health care services
- Care in a psychiatric hospital (up to 190 days in a person's lifetime)
- Hospice care to a terminally ill patient diagnosed as having six months or less to live

Medicare Part B

Medicare Part B covers outpatient health care services, services by physicians, durable medical equipment, and other services and supplies. Medicare Part B also covers certain prescription medications, nebulizer solutions, antirejection medications, some vaccines, and oral anticancer drugs. It also covers oral antiemetic drugs, immunosuppressants, and end-stage renal disease-related medication. Additionally, it covers diabetic testing strips, control solutions, lancets, and blood glucose monitor batteries. Under Medicare Part B, claims are submitted by using the CMS 1500 form, which must be completely correct or it will be rejected. Medicare Part B coverage is optional.

Medicare Part B provides Supplementary Medical Insurance (SMI) benefits for aged and disabled patients. It is paid for equally by the insured and the federal government. Monthly automatic premium deductions are taken out of monthly Social Security checks, railroad retirement checks, or civil service checks. Some patients pay the premium directly to the Social Security Administration. Patients (in certain states) who are eligible for Medicare Part B and Medicaid may have their monthly Medicare Part B premiums paid for by Medicaid.

Everyone eligible for Medicare Part A can choose to enroll in Part B by paying monthly premiums. Deductibles must be met in Parts A and B before payment benefits begin. Medicare pays only a portion of a patient's hospitalization expenses. Some federal employees and former federal employees who are not eligible for Social Security benefits and Medicare Part A may still enroll in Part B. Many Medicare enrollees also carry private supplemental insurance that pays the deductible and the 20% coinsurance.

Medicare Part C

Medicare Part C is known as the **Medicare Advantage plan**, which was created to offer a number of health care options in addition to those available under Medicare Part A and Part B. This plan receives a fixed amount of money from Medicare to spend on their Medicare members. Some varieties of this plan may require members to pay a premium similar to the Medicare Part B premium. If the patient chooses coverage under Part C, he or she will not need coverage under Part A and Part B. Part C plans can include Part D coverage, which are referred to as MA-PD plans, but not all Part C plans include this coverage. Patients eligible for both Medicare and Medicaid, often referred to as *Dual Eligibles*, receive their prescription benefits through a Medicare Part D plan. Premiums, deductibles, and copays are usually lower for dual eligible patients than for people who are only covered by Medicare. Plans available under this program may include the following:

- Health maintenance organization (HMO)
- Point-of-service (POS) plan
- Private fee-for-service (PFFS)
- Provider-sponsored organization (PSO)
- Religious fraternal benefit society (RFBS)
- Medicare medical savings account (MSA) (pilot program)

If a patient has both Medicare and Medicaid, charges must be filed with Medicare first, and Medicaid is the secondary payer.

Medicare Part D

Medicare Part D is offered to all Medicare recipients to cover the costs of their medications. This plan was designed to give patients greater access to required drugs so that they can obtain medications in a retail setting. In order to be eligible for Part D, you must first join a plan run by an insurance company or another private company approved by Medicare. Medicare Part D requires a separate enrollment by the members, in addition to his or her Part A and Part B coverage. Plans vary in cost and the actual drugs that are covered. Monthly premiums usually apply. When you first become eligible for Medicare, you may choose to join or not join into Part D—but if you later change your mind, you may have to pay a penalty in order to join. Individuals with limited finances may qualify for additional financial assistance in paying for their Part D coverage. Medicare Part D, like many outpatient drug plans, uses the "cost plus fee" technique. Under Medicare, a drug's cost is combined with a dispensing fee of approximately $4.50 to determine the final price of the drug product.

Medicaid

In 1965, Congress passed Title 19 of the Social Security Act, setting up a combined federal-state medical insurance program to provide medical care for persons with income below the national poverty level. **Medicaid** is a health benefits program designed for low-income people (those receiving welfare payments or other forms of public assistance) and at-risk populations such as the blind, the disabled, and the members of families with dependent children deprived of the support of at least one parent and financially eligible on the basis of income and resources. Each state decides what services are covered and what the reimbursement will be for each service. Two types of **copayment** requirements may apply to the Medicaid patient. Federal money is given to each state, with the states being responsible for paying providers. Approximately 20% of Americans had coverage through Medicaid in 2015. Some states require a small fixed copayment paid to the provider at the time of service (e.g., $1.00 or $2.00). This policy was instituted to help pay some of the administrative costs of physicians participating in the Medicaid program. Certain groups of patients may be exempt from this copayment requirement (e.g., persons younger than 18 years or women receiving prenatal care). To determine whether a Medicaid patient is required to make a copayment, a pharmacy technician should use the pharmacy computer system that is linked with Medicaid. Copayment information is listed for each state on the linked Medicaid website.

Another requirement is the share of cost copayment. Some Medicaid recipients must meet this copayment requirement monthly before Medicaid benefits can be claimed. The amount may change from month to month, so the copayment should be verified each time it is collected. Fee-for-Service Medicaid coverage involves the states directly reimbursing providers for every provided service. In many locations of the country, this is being replaced by Managed Medicaid, in which the state contracts with health insurance providers, or managed care organizations (MCOs), to provide needed services to beneficiaries. Usually, each state pays the MCO a per-member, per-month rate. The MCO determines rates paid to providers, copays and coinsurance charged to members, formularies, and various covered services.

TRICARE

TRICARE is a comprehensive health benefits program offering three types of plans for dependents of men and women in the uniformed services (military). Under the basic TRICARE program, individuals have the following three options:

- TRICARE Standard: fee-for-service (cost-sharing plan)
- TRICARE Extra: preferred provider organization plan
- TRICARE Prime: health maintenance organization plan with a point-of-service option

TRICARE is a new program that replaced CHAMPUS (Civilian Health and Medical Program of the Uniformed Services). CHAMPUS was a health care benefit for families of uniformed personnel and retirees from the uniformed services (the Army, Navy, Air Force, Marines, Coast Guard, Public Health Service, and National Oceanic and Atmospheric Administration). TRICARE runs a military pharmacy as well as a mail-order pharmacy. The TRICARE mail-order pharmacy can fill limited types of prescriptions for military personnel while they are stationed overseas. TRICARE requires that prescriptions be filled with generic products if they are available.

CHAMPVA

CHAMPVA (Civilian Health and Medical Program of the Veterans Administration) was created in 1973. CHAMPVA covers the expenses of the families of veterans with total, permanent, service-connected disabilities. It also covers the expenses of surviving spouses and dependent children of veterans who died in the line of duty. **Eligibility** is determined and identification cards are issued by the nearest Veterans Affairs medical center. The insured persons are then free to choose their own private physicians. Benefits and cost-sharing features are the same as those for TRICARE beneficiaries who are military retirees, dependents of military retirees, or dependents of deceased members of the military.

Insurance Policy

An insurance policy is a legally enforceable agreement. It is also called an insurance contract, regardless of whether the contract is a group, individual, or prepaid contract. There is no standard health insurance contract; however, state laws regulate the way policies are written and the minimum requirements of coverage. A policy might also include dependents of the insured, which means the spouse and children of the insured. However, under some contracts, parents and other family members may be covered as dependents. The policy becomes effective only after the company offers the policy and the person accepts it and pays the initial premium. Some insurance policies have an exclusion (**policy limitation**), or exclusions, for certain types of coverage. Some types of exclusions include acquired immunodeficiency syndrome (AIDS), attempted suicide, cancer, losses due to injury on the job, and pregnancy.

In general, *major medical* contracts help to offset large medical expenses caused by serious injuries or chronic illnesses. These types of policies cover hospitalization, physician visits, lab tests, and various procedures. Under these plans, the insured patient is known as a *subscriber, member, policyholder,* or *recipient.* The *dependents* of the insured individual include the spouse, children, and sometimes parents, other family members, and domestic partners. The insured may also be an organization instead of an individual. Major group insurance considers the employer to be the insured party, with the employees considered to be *risks.* Supplemental major medical insurance, which is purchased in addition to major medical when a comprehensive major medical plan does not exist, covers extended care and skilled nursing facilities.

Patients without insurance must pay full prescription prices, which vary widely. Costs can be reduced by the use of coupons or substituting generic drugs for name brand drugs. The amount of coverage per drug is determined by the insurance coverage, and it is based on two primary factors:

- Average wholesale price, as found in the *Drug Topics Red Book* or the pharmacy database.

- Copay, which is determined by whether the patient uses a government-sponsored program, HMO, or PPO. Approval of drug coverage, claim processing and collection, and payments are handled by processors, which are companies that work for insurance companies.

WHAT WOULD YOU DO?

A 25-year-old man enters your pharmacy with one prescription for an antibiotic and another for Lortab®. He hands you his insurance card, which is covered by his parents' policy until he turns 26. You enter the prescriptions into the computer when a note from the pharmacist appears on the screen. It says that the "parents of this patient have requested us not to fill pain medications for their son, reason unspecified." What do you do?

Patient Profiles

The patient profile is set up in the pharmacy computer system. An example of a computerized patient profile is shown in Figure 16-1. The patient profile must be kept up to date in order to ensure correct billing. The pharmacy computer system will allow the following information to be viewed:

- Patient information—name, date of birth, address, phone number, gender, allergies

- Insurance provider information—phone number, insurance number (per the policies of the institution or hospital)

An insurance claim may be rejected if the information is incorrect.

Prior Authorization

Insurance companies often will pay for medications only if prior authorization has been received. Reasons for prior authorization include nonformulary drugs and availability of less costly types of treatment. Two types of forms are used for prior authorization:

- Prior authorization forms—the most common type. When a third-party claim is rejected as "prior authorization required," the pharmacy will contact the patient's physician or the pharmacy will directly notify the physician's office, who then requests prior authorization from the insurance company.

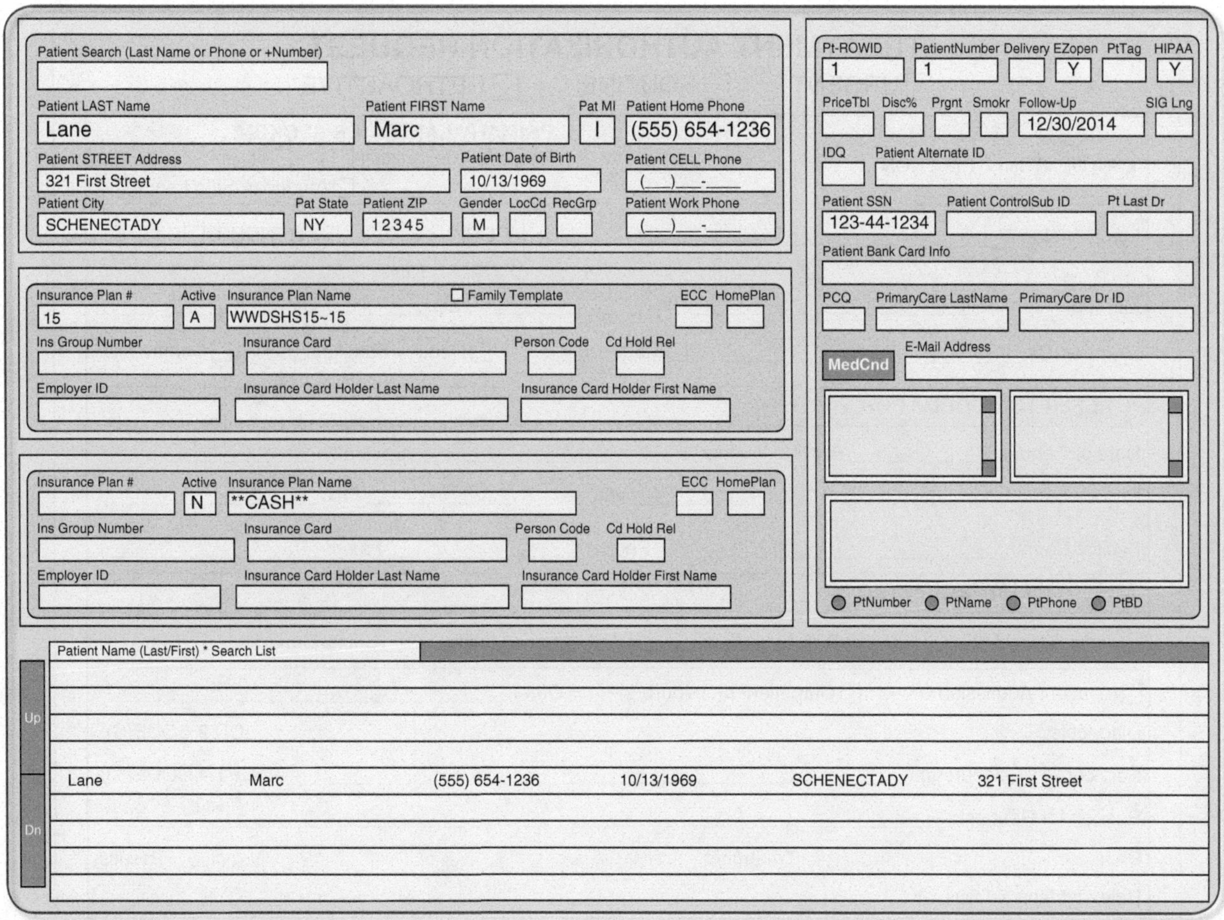

Figure 16-1 Computerized patient profile.

- Treatment authorization request (TAR) forms—used for Medicare and Medicaid. Figure 16-2 shows an example of a TAR form. The physician will most likely need to explain why a certain type of therapy is needed, usually based on previous ineffective therapies, patient allergies to certain therapies, or the requirement of diagnostic tests requiring the requested therapy. Approval then usually occurs within 24 to 48 hours. The pharmacy is seldom alerted when authorization is approved, so it should attempt to rebill the claim within 48 to 72 hours. If still denied, the pharmacy may need to contact the insurance company or the physician's office. A special override code may be needed to bill the claim. The patient must be contacted within three days regardless of the situation so that he or she will not have to wait for a denied medication without any explanation.

Claims Processing

At the time of service, pharmacy claims are processed and coverage is determined. *Adjudication* is the process of comparing submitted claims to each patient's benefits, and paying or denying them. Patient information and data about the dispensed medication are sent to the insurer or pharmacy benefits manager. To allow for real-time communications between pharmacies and payers, the National Council for Prescription Drug Programs Telecommunication Standard was developed in 1988. The current version in use is called the NCPDP D.0. Third-party claims go through a hub or *switch* so that every pharmacy does not need to establish individual connections with payers. Required claim information includes the patient's name, his or her date of birth and ID number, the payer's 6-digit NCPDP processor ID number (known as a *BIN*), the payer's processor control number (PCN), the medication name and NDC number, the quantity dispensed, the directions for use (SIG), and the days supply.

TREATMENT AUTHORIZATION REQUEST

☐ URGENT   ☐ ROUTINE   ☐ RETROACTIVE

I. PATIENT INFORMATION	PRIMARY LANGUAGE SPOKEN:
	Require Interpreter: ☐ Y ☐ N
	☐ American Sign Language

Member Name:_____   DOB:_____   GENDER: ☐ F ☐ M

Member Address:_____ City: _____ Zip: _____ Phone:_____

Member ID#:_____ ☐ Medicare   ☐ Healthy Families   ☐ Commercial

II. REFER TO INFORMATION

Date of Request:_____ Provider Name:_____ Specialty:_____

Provider Address:_____ Phone: _____ Fax:_____

Facility Name:_____ Phone:_____ Fax:_____

III. SERVICE(S) REQUESTED

☐ Initial Consult   ☐ FU visit(s)_____   ☐ Home Health   ☐ Social Services   ☐ DME

☐ Inpatient Admission   ☐ Outpatient procedure(s)   Other:_____

Diagnosis:_____   ICD 9 CODE(S):

Service(s)/Procedure(s):_____   CPT 4 CODE(S):

Reason for Request:_____

Prior   Treatment   &   Results:

Relevant labs/X-Rays, etc:_____

☐ Health Education (Specify):_____

Requesting Physicians Name

(PLEASE PRINT)   _____   PCP Phone: (_____)

Physician's Signature _____ FAX: (_____)_____

Accident: ☐ YES ☐ NO   **Where Occurred:** ☐ Home ☐ Work ☐ Auto ☐ Other

UM Decision Status: ☐ **APPROVED**   ☐ **MODIFIED**   ☐ **DEFERRED**   ☐ **DENIAL**

AUTH #:_____ Date Approved:_____ Date Auth. Expire:_____

Comments:_____

_____

_____

Reviewer's Name:_____ Signature:_____ Date:_____

INTERNAL USE ONLY: Member Eligibility as of:_____ PCP Provider ID #:_____
☐ IPA RESPONSIBILITY, Date faxed to IPA:_____

THIS REFERRAL DOES NOT GUARANTEE ELIGIBILITY. CHECK ELIGIBILITY PRIOR TO RENDERING SERVICE.
Payment will NOT be made for unauthorized services. All lab and x-rays must be ordered/performed
by contracting providers. Specialist reports must be sent to PCP promptly.

Figure 16-2 Treatment authorization request.

The NCPDP number or the National Provider Identifier (NPI) number helps identify the pharmacy that submits the claim. The switch to identify the payer and to route the claim correctly uses the BIN. The PCN and patient's *group number* provide additional identification about which program in the PBM the patient is part of, since the PBM may handle many claims, for multiple insurers, and multiple plans for each insurer. Not all payers use the group number, and it is therefore considered to be optional information in a claim. After being routed to the correct PBM and insurance plan, the individual patient must be identified to make final determination of coverage for the claim. His or her insurer assigns each covered member a **patient identification number**. The patient ID number is also called a *member ID number*, *beneficiary ID number*, *recipient ID number*, and various other names. Often, patients besides the covered member are also eligible for benefits. Examples include children or spouses of employees given insurance through their employers.

Some insurers assign every covered patient unique identification numbers. Others utilize *person codes* that indicate the patient is someone besides the member. The person codes are usually 2- or 3-digit extensions to patient identification numbers. Each patient's insurance card lists required BIN, PCN, patient identification, and group numbers (when these are used). There is no standard layout for this information, making it sometimes hard to locate. Pharmacies often are part of an eligibility service. This allows pharmacy staff members to search for patient coverages should the patient arrive at the pharmacy without an insurance card or if the card is out of date.

Third-party payers sometimes require more information to determine coverage for a claim, such as when Medicare Part B claims require a diagnosis for covered supplies and medications. This diagnosis must be submitted with the claim using an ICD-10 code (International Classification of Diseases, 10th Revision). The World Health Organization classifies medical conditions using this method. The ICD-10 creates a standardized method of documenting the diagnoses of patients.

Claims may be submitted either electronically or by using actual paper claim forms. Many third-party payers still accept paper transactions, though no longer from a pharmacy. All claims processing involving pharmacies is now done electronically, from the point of sale. Many payers require retrospective billing to be done electronically if there is a problem with the patient's insurance. In rare instances, and in the case of Medicare Part B coverage, pharmacies may bill payers using paper claim forms.

When entering data electronically, make sure to do the following:

- Use all capital letters.
- Avoid prefixes such as "Dr.," "Mr.," or "Mrs."
- Avoid special characters such as apostrophes, commas, or hyphens (unless the insurance carrier allows these).
- Use valid data in each field—avoid using words such as "same" to indicate repeated data in a new field.

Paper claims involve use of the "universal claim" form known as CMS 1500 (see Figure 16-3). Paper claims can only be used by offices that do not handle any other HIPAA-related (Health Insurance Portability and Accountability Act) transactions. Eventually, all offices will be required to use electronic claims processing, and paper forms will be done away with. When using a paper claim form, the technician must do the following:

- Proofread the claim form for errors.
- Photocopy the form and place a copy in the patient's medical record.
- Enter the date the form was sent, the patient's name, and his or her insurance carrier.
- Enter the date and the words *Insurance filed* in the patient's ledger.
- Transmit the form.

Most insurance policies have specific time limits that must be adhered to for the insured party to be able to collect from the insurance company. A **time limit** is the amount of time from the date of service to the date (deadline) a claim can be filed with the insurer. In order for a person to become eligible for insurance coverage, a **waiting period** (elimination period) may be required. A waiting period is the amount of time that an individual must wait to become eligible (usually 30 days) before coverage begins, or for a specific benefit. For example, many plans require employees to wait nine months before they can claim maternity benefits.

HEALTH INSURANCE CLAIM FORM

APPROVED BY NATIONAL UNIFORM CLAIM COMMITTEE (NUCC) 02/12

CARRIER

| | PICA | | | | | | | | PICA | |

1. MEDICARE (Medicare#) MEDICAID (Medicaid#) TRICARE (ID#/DoD#) CHAMPVA (Member ID#) GROUP HEALTH PLAN (ID#) FECA BLK LUNG (ID#) OTHER (ID#)

1a. INSURED'S I.D. NUMBER   (For Program in Item 1)

2. PATIENT'S NAME (Last Name, First Name, Middle Initial)

3. PATIENT'S BIRTH DATE   SEX
MM   DD   YY   M   F

4. INSURED'S NAME (Last Name, First Name, Middle Initial)

5. PATIENT'S ADDRESS (No., Street)

6. PATIENT RELATIONSHIP TO INSURED
Self   Spouse   Child   Other

7. INSURED'S ADDRESS (No., Street)

CITY   STATE

8. RESERVED FOR NUCC USE

CITY   STATE

ZIP CODE   TELEPHONE (Include Area Code)
(   )

ZIP CODE   TELEPHONE (Include Area Code)
(   )

9. OTHER INSURED'S NAME (Last Name, First Name, Middle Initial)

10. IS PATIENT'S CONDITION RELATED TO:

11. INSURED'S POLICY GROUP OR FECA NUMBER

a. OTHER INSURED'S POLICY OR GROUP NUMBER

a. EMPLOYMENT? (Current or Previous)
YES   NO

a. INSURED'S DATE OF BIRTH   SEX
MM   DD   YY   M   F

b. RESERVED FOR NUCC USE

b. AUTO ACCIDENT?   PLACE (State)
YES   NO

b. OTHER CLAIM ID (Designated by NUCC)

c. RESERVED FOR NUCC USE

c. OTHER ACCIDENT?
YES   NO

c. INSURANCE PLAN NAME OR PROGRAM NAME

d. INSURANCE PLAN NAME OR PROGRAM NAME

10d. CLAIM CODES (Designated by NUCC)

d. IS THERE ANOTHER HEALTH BENEFIT PLAN?
YES   NO   If yes, complete items 9, 9a, and 9d.

READ BACK OF FORM BEFORE COMPLETING & SIGNING THIS FORM.

12. PATIENT'S OR AUTHORIZED PERSON'S SIGNATURE I authorize the release of any medical or other information necessary to process this claim. I also request payment of government benefits either to myself or to the party who accepts assignment below.

SIGNED   DATE

13. INSURED'S OR AUTHORIZED PERSON'S SIGNATURE I authorize payment of medical benefits to the undersigned physician or supplier for services described below.

SIGNED

PATIENT AND INSURED INFORMATION

14. DATE OF CURRENT ILLNESS, INJURY, or PREGNANCY (LMP)
MM   DD   YY   QUAL.

15. OTHER DATE
QUAL.   MM   DD   YY

16. DATES PATIENT UNABLE TO WORK IN CURRENT OCCUPATION
FROM   MM   DD   YY   TO   MM   DD   YY

17. NAME OF REFERRING PROVIDER OR OTHER SOURCE

17a.
17b.   NPI

18. HOSPITALIZATION DATES RELATED TO CURRENT SERVICES
FROM   MM   DD   YY   TO   MM   DD   YY

19. ADDITIONAL CLAIM INFORMATION (Designated by NUCC)

20. OUTSIDE LAB? $ CHARGES
YES   NO

21. DIAGNOSIS OR NATURE OF ILLNESS OR INJURY Relate A-L to service line below (24E)   ICD Ind.
A. ___   B. ___   C. ___   D. ___
E. ___   F. ___   G. ___   H. ___
I. ___   J. ___   K. ___   L. ___

22. RESUBMISSION CODE   ORIGINAL REF. NO.

23. PRIOR AUTHORIZATION NUMBER

24. A. DATE(S) OF SERVICE		B. PLACE OF SERVICE	C. EMG	D. PROCEDURES, SERVICES, OR SUPPLIES (Explain Unusual Circumstances)		E. DIAGNOSIS POINTER	F. $ CHARGES	G. DAYS OR UNITS	H. EPSDT Family Plan	I. ID. QUAL.	J. RENDERING PROVIDER ID. #
From MM DD YY	To MM DD YY			CPT/HCPCS	MODIFIER						
1											NPI
2											NPI
3											NPI
4											NPI
5											NPI
6											NPI

25. FEDERAL TAX I.D. NUMBER   SSN   EIN

26. PATIENT'S ACCOUNT NO.

27. ACCEPT ASSIGNMENT? (For govt. claims, see back)
YES   NO

28. TOTAL CHARGE
$

29. AMOUNT PAID
$

30. Rsvd for NUCC Use

31. SIGNATURE OF PHYSICIAN OR SUPPLIER INCLUDING DEGREES OR CREDENTIALS (I certify that the statements on the reverse apply to this bill and are made a part thereof.)

SIGNED   DATE

32. SERVICE FACILITY LOCATION INFORMATION

a. NPI   b.

33. BILLING PROVIDER INFO & PH # (   )

a. NPI   b.

PHYSICIAN OR SUPPLIER INFORMATION

NUCC Instruction Manual available at: www.nucc.org   PLEASE PRINT OR TYPE   APPROVED OMB-0938-1197 FORM 1500 (02-12)

Centers for Medicare and Medicaid Services

Figure 16-3 CMS 1500 claim form.

BILLING SECONDARY PAYERS

Pharmacy patients sometimes have several insurance plans covering their prescriptions. The *primary payer* is the one billed first, and the *secondary payer* is billed once the primary payer has paid his or her share of the bill. Billing more than one insurer for the same claim is called a **coordination of benefits** (COB). Codes are used to send information from primary payers to secondary payers. These are called *Other Coverage Codes* (OCC). They inform the secondary payer about what was covered by the primary payer and for which items the secondary payer is being billed. The majority of pharmacy management systems use special fields into which this information is entered as part of a transmission to the payer.

Once a patient's primary insurance payer has posted an RA/EOB (remittance advice/explanation of benefits), it may be necessary to bill the second insurance payer (if this situation applies). The secondary payer should already have been informed of the initial insurance payment, and usually no additional claim needs to be filed. An example of this situation is Medicare as the first payer, followed by Medicaid as the second.

PROBLEMS WITH CLAIMS

Many potential problems with claims can lead to situations in which a prescription is not covered for an insured patient. Examples include noncoverage of the NDC, even though all medications have an NDC number; expired coverage; exceeding coverage limits; attempting to refill a prescription too early; nonmatching information between the processor and the cardholder; a prescription written by a physician who is not the PCP of the patient; and requesting an invalid amount of medication (usually only 30-day supplies are covered).

CLAIM REJECTIONS

Almost every day in the pharmacy claims are rejected because of many different reasons. Often, third-party payers include messages within online responses that explain the cause for a claim rejection. However, these responses often need some investigation to be performed to ascertain the actual cause of the rejection. Some rejections are because of incomplete or incorrect information within a claim. They can be easily corrected in the pharmacy. Others require more documentation in order to reach a successful adjudication. Some are called *hard stops*, which means that the claim will not be adjudicated at any time.

Days Supply Exceeded Rejection

The **days supply exceeded** *rejection* occurs often in the pharmacy because of a prescription being written for a longer time frame than is covered by the insurance plan. An example is when a prescription for 60 tablets, to be taken once per day (a 60-day supply), is written but the payer covers only up to a 30-day supply for each refill. In order to resolve this rejection and have successful claim adjudication, the quantity dispensed must be changed to the accepted days supply, and then the claim is resubmitted. A notation should be made on the prescription itself or in the pharmacy computer system detailing the reason for the change in dispense quantity. When the dispense quantity is changed, the number of refills must also be correctly updated so that the patient receives what was prescribed eventually.

Refill Too Soon Rejection

Another common rejection is called **refill too soon**, in which the pharmacy tries to bill a claim for the same medication that is too close to the last time the medication was filled. This type of rejection is also called a *carryover days supply rejection*. Some insurance plans give a date by which a prescription can be filled in the rejection message but some do not. Every plan determines what is considered "too soon." In most cases, the prescription can be billed again once the patient has used about 85% of the previous supply. For a 60-day supply, 85% usage would mean it could be refilled on day 50 after the last fill. A payer can reject the claim if the cumulative days supply makes the refill too soon. When the patient or pharmacy fills a prescription five days early every month, the total days supply over multiple refillings may cause a refill too soon rejection. Resolution options for this rejection are to wait until the payer's specific fill date is reached or to call the payer and ask if there is a possible override. In certain cases, the payer will allow the patient's request for an early refill. For example, if the patient is going to travel away from home and requests and early refill, or if the patient needs to change the dose from one to two tablets per day, the payer may allow the early refill.

Plan Limitations Exceeded Rejection

A payer may set limits about how many doses of a medication can be received by a patient within a certain time frame. A common example is the limitation of certain drugs, such as proton pump inhibitors, to only 90 days per year. The rejected claim will read **plan limitations exceeded**. The pharmacy can obtain an override for this with a prior authorization. However, there is often no way to receive a paid claim if the patient has met the maximum allowable quantity or days supply for the medication. In 2017, a new rule was created by the CMS about Milligram Morphine Equivalents (MME) limits. This new rule causes this type of rejection, when a claim for opioids is submitted for a Medicare Part D beneficiary when the daily dose or the cumulative dose exceeds the allowed limits.

Patient Not Covered Rejection

A *patient not covered rejection* may result from a change in a patient's coverage status or from a submission of information that is incorrect. The claim will be rejected if the date of birth submitted by the pharmacy is not the same as what is on file with the payer. Also, some payers do not recognize nicknames, such as Greg for Gregory or Pat for Patricia. The full name may be required on the request in order for the claim to be covered. If a patient's last name has a hyphen in it, the hyphenated name must match exactly. An example is a married woman who is registered with the payer as Mary Johnson-Thomas but whose prescription uses only her married name Mary Thomas. It is important to verify that all patient information in the claim is correct before a rejection is issued. This includes the first and last names of the patient spelled correctly, date of birth, gender, group number, identification number, and person code. A payer may provide more specific rejection information, such as Missing or Invalid Cardholder ID, Missing or Invalid Date of Birth, or Patient or Card Holder ID Name Mismatch.

Provider Not Covered Rejection

A *provider not covered rejection* involves a payer limiting eligible prescribers or even pharmacies for an insurance plan. More commonly, an identifier for the prescriber or pharmacy is submitted incorrectly. It is important to verify that the prescriber's NPI and DEA numbers, if applicable, are correct. The rule about hyphenated names also applies to prescribers if the prescriber uses such a last name. Many community pharmacies subscribe to online providers that offer search tools, allowing staff members to find prescriber state license numbers, DEA numbers, and NPI numbers. For example, provider NPI numbers can be searched at npiregistry.cms.hhs.gov. Another option is to call the prescriber to verify that the correct numbers are being submitted. Sometimes a patient is limited to a particular pharmacy, such as for specialty medications, or the payer has a limited pharmacy network. Usually, these are related to contracting factors and cannot be resolved in the pharmacy at the actual time of service.

Coverage-Terminated Rejection

A *coverage-terminated rejection* occurs when a claim is submitted to a payer after the patient's coverage period has ended. This is true for most commercial insurance plans.

Prior Authorization Required Rejection

A *prior authorization required rejection* is more commonly seen in today's pharmacy. A prior authorization is abbreviated as a "PA" and is an extra step used when determining coverage. The payer will be asked for more information prior to a decision being made whether the medication is covered for the beneficiary. In most cases, prior authorizations occur with new or expensive mediations but can also occur with older or inexpensive medications when there are preferred courses of treatments available. These rejections are common when a patient or prescriber prefers a brand name medication, but there is a generic version available. Prior authorizations were designed to ensure the most cost-effectiveness, but because of the complex process of obtaining authorization, prescriptions are often abandoned. Up to 40% of patients prescribed medications that require a prior authorization do not receive any treatment. The process of PAs should be understood and communicated to patients and prescribers, which can greatly impact patient drug therapy. The length of time from the start of the process to the approval or denial of a claim varies between payers and methods. Sometimes it takes only one day but at times may take more than one week.

In general, the PA process begins when the patient is informed that a PA is required. In the pharmacy, there must be an explanation of the amount of time to expect for the approval or denial. Since a PA means that the payer is asking for more information, if this is explained to the patient, it can help reduce frustration and decreases risks of the patient abandoning the prescription. A prior authorization usually requires information that is not in the pharmacy, not easily obtained by the pharmacy, or the prescriber's signature—meaning that the pharmacy usually must contact the prescriber about the PA. This can be done via phone, fax, or electronically. Though not required, pharmacies often find that it is helpful to complete as much of the PA form as possible before it is sent to the prescriber.

Online sites, some of which are free, allow pharmacies to find most available PA forms. When completed or nearly completed, the form can be faxed or delivered electronically for the prescriber to finish completing. Some pharmacy management systems include this type of Internet service, allowing information to be exchanged with much less interaction from the pharmacy staff. In the absence of such a service, pharmacy staff or prescriber staff members must contact individual payers to get the needed PA forms. Once they are completed, the forms are returned to the payer for a final decision about medication coverage. When all steps are done electronically, these forms can be completed in one day or less. The more the manual steps undertaken, the longer the process. Often, prior authorization approval or denial is not sent to the pharmacy, and the pharmacy staff must then contact the payer to find out the final PA outcome.

Special Billing

Pharmacies must sometimes bill a third-party payer for special items that are not medications. These include immunizations and durable medical supplies, and may also involve clinic and inpatient billing, medication therapy management (MTM), and the Healthcare Common Procedure Coding System (HCPCS).

IMMUNIZATIONS

Today, more pharmacies than ever before are recognized by third-party payers as providers of immunizations. Claims for immunizations are submitted similarly to medication claims. Payers may require additional information in order to reimburse for the administration of a vaccine. Usually, immunization claims require diagnosis codes, drug utilization review (DUR) codes, and administration fees, which are sometimes known as *incentive fees*. The administration of vaccines is coded within the ICD-10 as *Z23*. The DUR codes utilized to indicate needed administration of medications include Professional Service Code MA (Medication Administration), Reason for Service Code PH (preventive Health Care), and Result of Service Code 3N (Medication Administered). An administration fee is charged by the pharmacy for the immunization, along with the cost of the medication being injected and its associated dispensing fee. The information that is entered into this field, within the pharmacy software, may be accepted by certain payers but can cause the claim to be rejected by others. The payer's help desk or the actual insurance contract can provide details about the fields that are required and the values that are acceptable for those required fields when a pharmacy provides billing for immunizations.

Vaccination claims to major medical plans and Medicare Part B require a Current Procedural Terminology (CPT) code along with the ICD-10 code. Every vaccine, and often its manufacturer, has a unique CPT code. This is another example in which information may be added by the pharmacy management system or the clearinghouse. If this information is not added, the pharmacy staff handling vaccination billing must ensure it is included on the claim in order to get the reimbursement.

DURABLE MEDICAL SUPPLIES

Durable medical equipment, including prosthetics, orthotics, and various supplies, is abbreviated as DMEPOS. DMEPOS includes canes, walkers, diabetic blood glucose test strips and lancets, wound care supplies, and ostomy supplies. For eligible beneficiaries, Medicare Part B covers these supplies. They may also be covered as pharmacy benefits via state Medicaid programs and some commercial plans. Medicare Part B requires an ICD-10 code and an HCPCS code for items that do not have the NDC number. The NDC is actually used instead of the HCPCS code for any supplies containing one. When an ICD-10 diagnosis code and HCPCS, if required, is added, these claims are processed similar to drug claims. Individual commercial plans and state Medicaid programs may require more information. Pharmacies regularly contract with a *clearinghouse* to complete billing, making the process as simple as possible. If a clearinghouse is not used, there may be more steps needed for the billing process. The payer's *help desk* should be contacted for information and questions regarding supply claims.

CLINIC AND INPATIENT BILLING

Medications administered within hospitals and clinical are often also billed to a patient's insurance. This type of billing is extremely different from outpatient or retail billing, and it is usually not done by the pharmacy staff. In a hospital setting, administered medications are not billed individually. Costs for medications are part of a diagnosis-related group (DRG) used by health insurers. They determine payments made to the hospital based on the type of patient, the diagnosis, and the expected factors required for treatment. However, most drugs administered in outpatient clinics are billed individually. The needed information in a clinic is different from what is required on a community pharmacy claim. For a clinic-administered medication, the required information includes the patient's name and ID number; the date of services; the HCPCS, CPT, and ICD-10 codes; the NDC; the quantity; and the place of service.

MEDICATION THERAPY MANAGEMENT

MTM involves many services provided by pharmacists. These include the following:

- Comprehensive Medication Review (CMR)
- Patient Adherence Consultations
- Prescriber Consultations
- Targeted Medication Review (TMR)

   Pharmacy MTM claims are increasing since payers are starting to use the CMR completion rate as a way to measure pharmacy performance. Medicare has created standards for providing MTM services to its beneficiaries. Additionally, certain state Medicaid programs and commercial plans reimburse for clinical pharmacy services. Documentation and billing is usually done outside of the standard pharmacy filling system, varying by payer. Most documentation and billing for these services is completed via online portals. These have different formats, but much of the information they require for billing is identical. All MTM claims, for example, require the reason for service, the actual service rendered, and the outcome of the service. All online documentation and billing portals offer training about how to document each type of service provided.

Healthcare Common Procedure Coding System

The HCPCS codes for drugs that often begin with the letter "J." Therefore, they are often called "J-codes." The quantity that is submitted in a clinic-administered drug claim is not exactly the same as the quantity submitted in a community pharmacy claim. In a clinic-administered claim, quantity is expressed in billing units or service units. These units are often not related to package size. There is no standard unit between drugs. Some medications are billed in increments of 10 mg, meaning that a billing unit of "2" would indicate 20 mg in this example. Others are billed in 1 mg increments or in milliliters.

Payments

In the pharmacy, insurance specialists track claims, process payments, verify accuracy of payments, and file secondary payer claims. Following up on claims effectively and timely payment processing are important health insurance activities. An **overpayment** is a payment made by either an insurer or a patient that is greater than the actual amount due.

CLAIM ADJUDICATION

Electronic responses are sent to the pharmacy after it sends a claim to an insurer. The insurer then *adjudicates* the claim, which involves the claim's initial processing, followed by automated and manual reviews. As a result of this process, the insurer determines whether the claim is correct and should be paid, and if so, makes the payment. During initial processing, the claim is checked for problems; these include problems with the patient's name, insurance plan number, and other items. Diagnosis codes are not used in prescription processing. In the pharmacy, coding systems such as ICD-9 CM or CPT are not used. Automated review is then conducted, applying edits reflecting payment policies to the claim. If an automated review identifies problems with the claim, it is reviewed manually. Many claims examiners are knowledgeable about insurance payment policies but have no actual medical background—hence, the discrepancies that often occur between insurance companies and service providers. The insurance payer then makes a *determination* about whether to pay the claim, deny the claim, or pay a reduced amount.

If the claim has been determined payable, the insurance payer sends it to the service provider along with a remittance advice (RA), which explains the payment decisions, or an electronic remittance advice (ERA), which does the same thing, but in an electronic (rather than paper) format. A paper RA was formerly known as an explanation of benefits (EOB). Therefore, the term RA/EOB signifies both formats of the document.

MONITORING CLAIM STATUS

Each pharmacy's practice management program (PMP) is used to closely track its accounts receivable (A/R). When claims are monitored while being adjudicated, the most important information needed is the amount of time the payer has to respond and how long the claim has been in the process. Payers usually have 30 to 60 days after claim submission to adjudicate the claim. Insurance aging reports are used to document how long a payer has had a claim in process.

HIPAA has standard claim status category codes that are used to indicate various claim conditions:

A—acknowledging that the claim has been received

E—indicating a transmission error, usually requiring the claim to be resent

F—indicating that a claim has been finalized

P—indicating that a claim is pending; that the payer needs information before making a payment decision

R—indicating that a request for more information has been sent; requests for information must be answered quickly, courteously, and completely

Third-Party Audits

Third-party payers conduct **audits** on a periodic basis. They ensure that pharmacies are following terms of contracts between them and payers. They also identify overpayments by the PBM and help prevent abuse from occurring. **Desk audits** involve electronic claims data being reviewed by the PBM. The pharmacy is usually sent a communication with a list of prescriptions included in the audit. The requested information is detailed, and it usually includes copies of original prescriptions, proof of delivery (with patient signature or courier information if it was shipped to the patient), notations of changes to the prescription, and notes from the prescriber. The audit request will detail how responses must be made and give a deadline for the responses.

Field audits involve an auditor actually visiting the pharmacy. These audits are more complicated and take more time than desk audits. The pharmacy will be notified and given a time frame or list of prescriptions that the auditor will be reviewing. It is suggested that a staff member should be assigned to the auditor for the actual audit, since the information that will be requested is extensive. Extra items that may be reviewed include the pharmacy and staff licenses, drug purchasing invoices, refill procedures, compounding logs, return-to-stock procedures, expired medication processes, HIPAA compliance, and many other operational items. The auditor may take photographs of the pharmacy. These will be submitted to the PBM along with the results of the audit. Today, audits are more common. If the payer finds a pharmacy not to be compliant, significant financial losses can occur.

DISPENSED QUANTITY EXCEEDS AUTHORIZED QUANTITY

Extended days supply prescription claims are requested and covered often. Previously, payers limited patients to a one-month supply at each refill. However, three-month supply prescriptions are paid at an increasing rate. The pharmacy must be aware that, to fill the extended days supply, the prescription must be written with a higher quantity included. In some states, filling for more than the originally written quantity is allowed, but there must be sufficient refills available to cover the quantity dispensed. Payers usually do not accept this practice, however. Pharmacies must obtain a new prescription for the increased quantity. Discrepancies, while legal per a state board of pharmacy, are usually discovered during an audit. When a prescriber is contacted for authorization of a three-moth supply, he or she should note, on the face of the prescription, exactly who approved the change and the date the authorization was made. Another option is to have the prescriber send a new prescription, such as in the case of e-prescribing. Some payers may accept electronic notes in the pharmacy filling system but others may not.

HIGHER THAN EXPECTED USAGE

An audit may also result because of *higher than expected usage*. The payer usually will question an excessively large amount of medication submitted as a seven-day supply. If the amount of medication is actually needed by the patient, this must be documented well so that the days supply can be justified during an audit. Audit findings will result from prescriptions billed to the third party but not delivered to the patient. Prescriptions filled and placed into a will-call area must be regularly reviewed. Prescriptions filled more than a week prior must be considered for return to stock and claim reversal. When the pharmacy does not have the entire quantity to be dispensed in stock, the claim should not be billed to the payer until the entire quantity is available. Audits consider billing for a total amount of dosages, but only dispensing a lower quantity, even when the pharmacy intends to dispense the remainder, a major finding.

Third-party payer audits are a regular part of today's pharmacy. When findings result, the costs can be extreme. Many other issues also cause recovery of payments. Therefore, all pharmacies must keep complete documentation, careful days supply calculations, and focus on correct quantities when dispensing. This helps avoid audit findings and allows pharmacies to keep the payments they receive from the payers.

INCONSISTENT DAYS SUPPLY

When a day's supply is not shown to be appropriate for the amount dispensed, the third party can take back some or all of the reimbursement for the prescription, as a result of an audit. Though an automated system that approves claims could at first send a paid claim response to the pharmacy, an auditor may later calculate that the day's supply was incorrect. Any prescriptions with incomplete or vague instructions that do not allow a correct calculation of the days supply are usually discovered during audits. Claims that have an SIG with the words "as directed" or "insulin per sliding scale" are examples of those that do not allow for calculation of the total quantity that should be taken per day. In order to submit acceptable instructions to the payer, it may be necessary to contact the prescriber and obtain clarification of these prescriptions. When the prescriber is contracted and instructions are changed, the discussion must be documented so that if an audit occurs, the situation can be understood.

WRONG PACKAGE SIZE

Wrong package sizes are also commonly found in audits. Besides various forms of pills, most other items are dispensed and billed in grams or milliliters. Some items are dispensed as *packages*. If the incorrect quantity is used, this can cause overpayment or underpayment of a claim. Quantities may be very difficult to determine for inhalers, nebulizer solutions, and prefilled syringes for injection. Most inhalers are billed in grams or number of doses. However, some are billed as *one unit*. For example, if the billing for a certain inhaler should be "1," but since it contains 30 actual doses, a billing of "30" would cause an extreme overpayment. This would be subject to payment recovery if discovered in an audit. To determine if an item is billed in milliliters or in number of dispensed packages, it is important to review the pack size that is listed in the pharmacy filling system item file.

INAPPROPRIATE DISPENSE-AS-WRITTEN CODE

Sometimes, a patient or prescriber prefers a brand name product over an available generic product. In these cases, a Dispense-as-Written (DAW) code allows the pharmacy to indicate the individual making the product selection. When the prescriber indicates upon the prescription that the brand name product must be used, the DAW-1 code is selected, which informs the payer. If the patient indicates that he or she wants the brand name product, the DAW-2 code is selected. Note that the third party can charge the patient a higher copay, require a prior authorization, or reject the claim completely, based on the limitations of the insurance plan. Auditors can search for the appropriate use of DAW codes when reviewing prescriptions. Payers may recover payment when an incorrect DAW code has been submitted.

MISSING OR INCOMPLETE ORIGINAL PRESCRIPTION

The most common item that is requested during an audit is a copy of an original prescription. If this cannot be found, or is incomplete, it will be considered an audit finding. Incomplete prescription findings may be due to lack of a written date, a missing prescriber signature, a missing dispense quantity that cannot be otherwise calculated based on the SIG, an incomplete or unclear SIG, and other factors. Incomplete or missing documentation of prescription changes are often found. Whenever a prescription is altered, this must be correctly documented. Audit findings for unapproved refills are often discovered. These can be due to data entry errors or incomplete documentation of refills that were authorized by the prescriber. When a prescriber authorizes refills of a medication, it is important to create a new prescription instead of adding refills to a current prescription.

Role of the Insurance Billing Pharmacy Technician

Pharmacy technicians must be familiar with many different aspects of health insurance billing and transactions. In the community pharmacy, they will use software to bill insurance companies, including Medicare and Medicaid. Hospital pharmacies and other types of pharmacy have departments that handle insurance billing, so pharmacy technicians in these settings will have little interaction with insurance companies—billing is directed automatically to the billing department.

When a prescription is filled, information must be sent to the insurance company for a payment decision. This is the *pharmacy claim*. It identifies the patient or policyholder, the prescriber, the pharmacy, and the medications involved. The patient is asked for his or her prescription drug card prior to the claim being submitted. This card contains information about the patient's insurance. See Figure 16-4 for an example of a prescription drug card. Most claims are sent electronically by the electronic data interchange (EDI). Once the insurer decides the amount that it will pay, it sends this information back to the pharmacy. This often occurs very quickly but sometimes takes more time due to the level of information involved in the claim. The pharmacy technician may then collect payment from the patient according to the amount that the insurer will pay.

The *accounts receivable* portion of the pharmacy is then responsible for collecting the outstanding amount from the insurance carrier. Most of these outstanding amounts are paid within 30 to 60 days after the date of service. The pharmacy technician who works with insurance claims should follow up on all uncollected sums and solve any problems to ensure that payment is received.

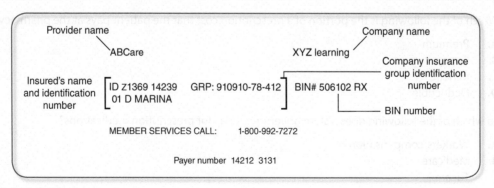

Figure 16-4 Prescription drug card.

WHAT WOULD YOU DO?

A disheveled looking young man presents two prescriptions from two different physicians. One is for a stimulant and one is for a depressant. Because prescribing these two types of drugs at the same time is not something that is done in general, you suspect that at least one or both of these prescriptions may be fraudulent. The filling of these prescriptions could result in a later audit finding, potentially costing the pharmacy extreme financial penalties. What would you do?

POINTS TO REMEMBER

An important role of the pharmacy technician handling insurance billing is to follow up on any balances that are still outstanding and make sure that the responsible payer sends payment.

Summary

Understanding various types of insurance coverage is essential for pharmacists and pharmacy technicians. The practice of pharmacy is a business, with the costs of medical care and drug prescriptions continually increasing. Customers and patients without medical insurance may not be able to afford to purchase their prescriptions and durable medical equipment. Thus, a pharmacy technician must understand the challenges involved in medical insurance as it applies to the management of the pharmacy. Health care professionals must be able to explain insurance procedures to patients and be able to contact appropriate representatives in order to determine eligibility and answer questions about coverage.

Pharmacy technicians must be familiar with the health insurance claim form (CMS 1500) and common reasons why claim forms are delayed or rejected. They must learn the skills required for electronic data interchange and computer confidentiality. It is also important to understand the different reasons for claims being rejected by payers. Today's pharmacy includes areas of special billing, such as immunizations, durable medical supplies, and the use of clinic and inpatient billing, medication therapy management, and the Healthcare Common Procedure Coding System. Third-party payers also regularly conduct audits to ensure that pharmacies are following the terms of their contracts. The pharmacy technician must participate in accurate documentation of all activities to help prevent extreme financial penalties to the pharmacy.

REVIEW QUESTIONS

1. Which of the following is the portion of a prescription cost that the patient pays at the pharmacy?

    A. Premium
    B. Copay
    C. Benefit
    D. Deductible

2. To which of the following does a state government pay for prescription medications?

    A. Workers' compensation
    B. Medicare
    C. Tricare
    D. Medicaid

3. What is the definition of adjudication?

    A. The transmission of claims
    B. The coordination of benefits
    C. Comparing claims to patient benefits and paying or denying them
    D. The management of medication therapy

4. Which of the following statements is true about Medicare Part C plans?

    A. The patient will not need coverage under Part A and Part B.
    B. These plans do not receive a fixed amount of money from Medicare to spend on their Medicare members.
    C. These plans are designed for low-income and disabled people.
    D. These plans cover the expenses of the families of veterans with total and service-connected disabilities.

5. Which of the following is optional for inclusion on a prescription insurance claim?

    A. Patient date of birth
    B. Patient identification number
    C. Patient group number
    D. Payer BIN

6. For which of the following is an ICD-10 code submitted to a payer?

    A. Description of the medication
    B. Patient diagnosis
    C. Benefit coordination
    D. Prescriber's type of practice

7. A specific amount of money that must be paid yearly, before the policy benefits begin, is called a:

    A. premium.
    B. time limit.
    C. deductible.
    D. beneficiary.

8. An example of private health insurance is:

    A. Blue Cross®–Blue Shield®.
    B. Medicaid.
    C. Medicare.
    D. CHAMPVA.

9. The cost of the coverage that the insurance policy contains is known as the:

    A. deductible.
    B. premium.
    C. preauthorization.
    D. discount.

10. Which of the following is the most common reason for a "patient not covered rejection"?

    A. Incorrect diagnosis
    B. Incorrect race of the patient
    C. Incorrect patient address
    D. Incorrect patient date of birth

11. Which of the following describes a prior authorization?

    A. The payer determines that the drug is covered but for a different patient
    B. The payer determines that the medication is not indicated for the patient's condition
    C. The payer finds that the patient is not covered
    D. The payer asks for additional information before determining coverage

12. Which of the following Medicare programs covers hospital charges?

    A. Part A
    B. Part B
    C. Part C
    D. Part D

13. How are most pharmacy bills for MTM services processed?

    A. By using a clearinghouse
    B. Through a contract with an outside provider
    C. Via online portals
    D. As part of the pharmacy's management software

14. A plan in which a member may seek care outside the network, or directly from preferred providers, is known as:

    A. fee-for-service.
    B. capitation.
    C. independent practice association.
    D. point-of-service.

15. Which of the following is the best way to reduce the chances of a large payment recovery because of an audit?

    A. Using DAW codes on every prescription
    B. Request a prior authorization for each claim
    C. Including "take as directed" on prescriptions
    D. Complete and accurate documentation

CRITICAL THINKING

A 72-year-old man comes to your pharmacy with two different types of insurance: Medicare and Blue Cross®–Blue Shield®. He wants to get a vaccine for shingles.

    1. Compare private health insurance with government plans.

    2. Identify the items that are required as part of a pharmacy immunization claim.

WEB LINKS

Affordable Health Insurance: www.healthinsurance.org

Health Information Privacy: www.hhs.gov/hipaa/index.html

Medicare: www.medicare.gov

Medicare Learning Network: www.cms.gov/outreach-and-education/medicare-learning-network-MLN/MLNproducts/downloads/msp_fact_sheet.pdf

National Provider Identifier Registry: npiregistry.cms.hhs.gov

Overview of Pharmacy Billing: www.verywellhealth.com/how-to-do-pharmacy-billing-2663842

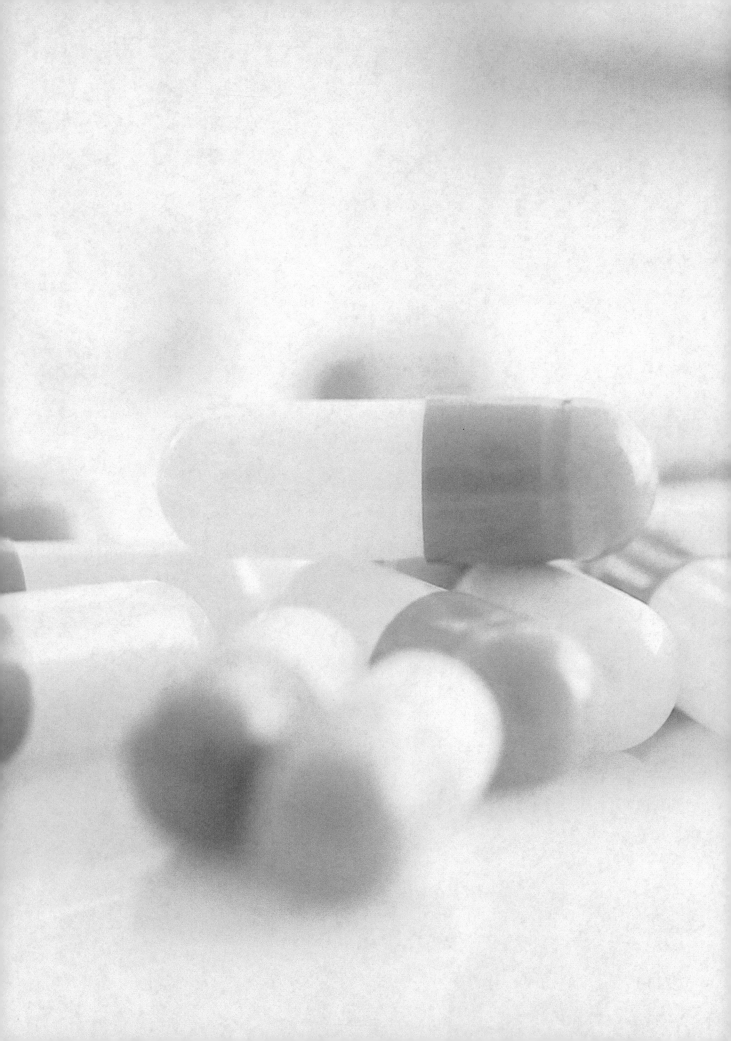

Inventory Control and Management

OBJECTIVES

Upon completion of this chapter, the reader should be able to:

1. Describe the specific storage requirements for inventory stock.
2. Explain inventory management.
3. Define the term *want book*.
4. Describe the importance of computerized inventory systems.
5. Explain the system that is the most flexible for pharmacy inventory control.
6. Explain the duties of pharmacy technicians in inventory control.
7. Describe the use of bar coding in the pharmacy.
8. Discuss waste control in relation to well-managed inventory programs.
9. Explain the use of perceptual inventory in the pharmacy.
10. Discuss special purchasing of controlled substances.

KEY TERMS

bar coding	inventory control	posting	want book
inventory	point-of-sale (POS) master	prime supplier	

Overview

Proper inventory control systems help to streamline the hectic activities of the pharmacies of today. They ensure that the correct products are stocked to serve the needs of patients and minimize the total inventory investment. Computerized inventory systems have become central to efficient pharmacy practice, reducing errors and improving patient service. Point-of-sale (POS) masters aid in inventory control by accurately controlling pharmacy stock and increasing the numbers of customers and transactions that can be handled, enhancing the pharmacy's operational abilities.

Inventory Control

Inventory control is of vital importance to pharmacies of all types. Inventory is typically a pharmacy's largest asset. Because so much is invested in inventory, proper inventory control has a strong and direct effect on a pharmacy's return on investment.

Inventory control is also important because a pharmacy must have the correct inventory to properly serve its patients. It must have those products that patients need in the quantities in which they need them. This aspect of inventory control is much harder to quantify and control but equally important. If a community pharmacy does not have the products that its patients need, at the time they need them, sales will be lost. If this happens often, the pharmacy will lose patients.

The two goals of effective inventory control are minimizing total inventory investment and carrying the right mix of products to satisfy patient demand. **Inventory** is a list of articles in stock, with the description and quantity of each. In other words, inventory is the entire stock of products on hand at a given time in the pharmacy. Inventory control is closely associated with the function of purchasing. Inventory control is important to the pharmacist because it is the means by which he or she ensures that all medications and products are accounted for and used legitimately, that adequate stocks are available when needed, and that the costs of too large an inventory are avoided. Several important issues relating to inventory must be addressed, among them are the following:

- How much inventory should be maintained?
- When should inventory levels be adjusted?
- Where should inventory be stored?

In an ideal system, pharmaceutical products would arrive shortly before they are needed.

Example

To better understand how important inventory is in relation to overhead expenses, consider the following scenario. The *total overhead* of the R.X. Drugstore is broken down as follows:

Supplies and Drug Purchases	$1,700,000
Pharmacist's Salary	$70,000
Pharmacy Technician's Salary	$24,000
Rent	$16,000
Utilities	$7400
Business Insurance	$4000
Liability Insurance	$3500
TOTAL OVERHEAD	**$1,824,900**

Therefore, if the R.X. Drugstore has an annual income of $2,100,000, it will be making a 15% profit. If a 15% profit is desired, what amount of income has to be received to meet this goal?

$$\text{Overhead} \times 0.15 = \text{Profit}$$
$$\$1,824,900 \times 0.15 = \$273,735$$

Because profit is equal to incoming receipts minus overhead:

$$\text{Overhead} + \text{Profit} = \text{Income}$$
$$\$1,824,900 + \$273,735 = \$2,098,635$$

Because net profit is usually reported annually or semiannually, the retail pharmacy department may frequently measure the cost of goods as compared to the revenue generated by the sale of those goods. This reported margin of profit is known as *gross profit*. It is the marginal difference between actual cost and total reimbursement and is also known as *gross margin*. The insurance reimbursement or private pay customer's service charge most dramatically influences the *gross profit* margin.

Example

Another example involves sales and acquisition cost to calculated gross profit:

$$\text{Sales} - \text{Acquisition cost} = \text{Gross profit}$$

If the pharmacy has sales that total $2,000,000 and the cost of the items sold is $1,500,000, then the gross profit is $500,000.

A well-managed inventory program includes waste control. In institutional settings, the amount and size of parenteral pharmaceuticals is often analyzed to reduce costs by minimizing waste. In the community pharmacy, timely return for credit of a near-expired product may be considered a controllable cost-effective tool for inventory management. Pharmacy technicians should be familiar with pharmacy policies and procedures on inventory management in an effort to prevent product depreciation and improve turnover.

Inventory Management

The pharmacy department must select a method of inventory management. There are various types of inventory management systems. The following common management systems will be discussed in this chapter:

- Computerized inventory system
- Inventory of controlled substances
- Perpetual inventory system
- Point-of-sale system

Inventory management is vital for efficiency in the pharmacy. Management activities focus on ordering stock, storing medications and supplies correctly, repackaging, disposing of used or unused pharmaceutical production, and various distribution systems. Colored or dated price stickers are simple, effective techniques used for ordering and inventory management. Colored price stickers can be used to indicate the time period during which a product was received. For example, a pharmacy might use blue stickers for products received during the first six months of a year, red stickers for products received during the next six months, yellow stickers for the first six months of the next year, and so on. Because the colors change every six months, the manager can readily estimate how long an item has been in inventory by simply glancing at the sticker. The length of time an item has been in inventory gives a rough indication of the quantity of the item needed and whether the item should be discontinued.

A system of colored or dated price stickers and a **want book** are sufficient for control of specific types of items. In practice, this control amounts to having minimal amounts of each specific item on hand and eliminating items that do not sell within some predetermined length of time, for example, within 6 to 12 months. A specific person in each pharmacy does the ordering of stock, but every pharmacy employee should understand how to order stock when it is needed. Usually, these skills are taught on-the-job because each pharmacy has its own ways of ordering.

Common inventory management errors may occur for the following reasons: miscounting the final inventory, creating labels that are not easily read, poorly marked or unmarked locations for storage, improper storage due to poor lighting, data input errors, not documenting when a drug product is used, illegible handwriting, computer malfunctions, and insufficient space.

INVENTORY STOCK

Most drug products are received in bulk "stock bottles," while some are received in "unit-dose" packaging. Unit-dose products should be stored in a separate area from bulk products. It is important to stock items according to their specific storage requirements. This means that room temperature, humidity, ventilation, and light must all be taken into consideration for each drug product. Some drugs require refrigeration or freezing for storage. Both refrigerators and freezers must be calibrated and checked for temperature accuracy on a regular basis, according to the pharmacy's policy. Many retail pharmacies stock their drug products by manufacturer name. Other methods of stocking involve alphabetic organization by each drug's generic name or, less commonly, its trade name. Each drug product should be stocked in such a way that the oldest items are taken from stock first. Expiration dates must always be verified so that no expired drugs are dispensed. A locator system should be in place so that each drug product's location is numbered and stored in the pharmacy computer system. Space should be ample so that products can be stored with enough room to avoid breakage or confusion with other drugs placed close to them. Hospital pharmacies often stock medications in dispensing units known as *supply stations* or *med-stations*. All withdrawals from stock must be thoroughly and completely documented in the computer system.

Everyone who works in the pharmacy helps to maintain inventory stock and keep the individual who handles ordering aware of what is needed. Every pharmacy orders both *formulary drugs* and a smaller amount of *non-formulary drugs*. Established stock medication levels are referred to as *periodic automatic replenishment* (PAR) levels. They are minimum amounts of medications that should be kept in the pharmacy at any given time. Pharmacy technicians regularly play a role in ordering medications. Maintenance of pharmacy stock may be with POS, order card, or handheld inventory computer systems. Pharmacy technicians often handle all the steps of ordering, restocking, and returning products.

COMPUTERIZED INVENTORY SYSTEM

The traditional purchasing and inventory control system does not involve computers and is considered old-fashioned. It is more expensive and difficult to maintain all information accurately, in addition to being more time-consuming. For these reasons, most pharmacists have attempted to implement more sophisticated purchasing and inventory control systems. Computers and computerized inventory systems increase accuracy, generate more data, and require less time compared with traditional systems. Computerized systems have the capability of making it possible for pharmacies to maintain *perpetual* control of inventories. This means that inventories and sales figures for individual products are updated constantly as purchases and sales are made. However, to maintain perpetual control, the pharmacy must update inventory records whenever inventory is purchased and whenever it is sold. Thus, all purchases and sales must be entered into the computer.

Computer systems use sales and inventory information to calculate and record points, to identify low turnover items that should be dropped from inventory, and to generate orders to be sent to wholesalers or manufacturers. The basis of the computerized purchasing and control system is the medication database.

POINTS TO REMEMBER

The medication master file contains all of the information needed for ordering, inventory, pricing, and distribution of pharmaceuticals.

Most computerized systems provide all of the information needed to write a purchase requisition and a few systems actually produce the final purchase order. The real advantage of computerized inventory control systems is the time that is saved.

INVENTORY OF CONTROLLED SUBSTANCES

The Controlled Substances Act requires pharmacies to perform biennial inventories of all controlled substances that they stock. An exact count must be performed for Schedule II medications, and an estimated count must be done for Schedule III, IV, and V medications. As required by either state law or their own organizational policy, a hospital pharmacy may perform inventories more frequently. The Controlled Substances Act requires that a pharmacy must complete an inventory of controlled substances every two years.

WHAT WOULD YOU DO?

A drug wholesaler drops by your pharmacy and offers many medications at prices well below those the pharmacy is currently paying. Eventually, you find out that the man's company is based out of Canada and that there are many discrepancies concerning the legality of selling some of these medications to pharmacies in the United States. What would you do?

POINT-OF-SALE SYSTEM

The **point-of-sale (POS) master** is an inventory control system that allows inventory to be tracked as it is used. It is the most flexible system for inventory control and can be installed in all the computers at a main pharmacy. POS systems can control stock in the pharmacy accurately, increasing overall profitability. The system is open-ended and can handle a significant volume of customers and transactions, as well as all orders, credits, inter-store transfers, and returns. A major benefit of the POS master is that it is driven by practical requests of the users themselves. The system is easy to use and is the most suitable inventory control system in the pharmacy setting. Also, POS billing allows pharmacies to send claims electronically to insurance companies. Cure data network is used so that patients can trust that their private information will be protected. The insurer verifies eligibility, identifies drugs that are covered, handles pricing of claims, and returns the response to the pharmacy in less than a minute to assist with fast prescription processing.

Duties of Pharmacy Technicians

The duties of pharmacy technicians in relation to inventory control and management are many. Often, the technician is required to place daily orders for drug products in order to keep the supply of stock adequate. Pharmaceutical sales representatives may ask pharmacy technicians to assist in their delivery of new and alternative medication information to the person in the pharmacy who makes final purchasing decisions. Technicians are regularly involved in documentation for returns, product wasting, and recalls. They use bar code scanners, work with National Drug Code numbers, verify all types of information, and update computer files concerning medications, supplies, patients, prescribers, and insurers. Pharmacy technicians record and maintain controlled substance information, investigational medication data, and distributor records.

Ordering Process

The process of pharmacy ordering is usually done by computer, either manually or automatically. Automatic ordering occurs when stock levels and reorder points are reached that trigger the computer to reorder drug products. Pharmacy staff members should verify these automatic orders. The next step is to send the order form electronically to the supplier(s) via the computer or, in fewer situations, by fax. When using computers for ordering, the supplier's computer system interacts directly with the pharmacy's computer system to communicate quickly. The order is analyzed item-by-item, inventory of the supplier is verified, and the pharmacy is sent a confirmation of whether the order will be complete or partial. Confirmations should be printed so that the pharmacy has a hard copy of the supplier's information about the order. Sometimes, items are omitted from an order. This is most commonly because items are temporarily out of stock, are on back-order, or have been discontinued by the supplier. Once the items have shipped, the supplier will communicate to the pharmacy about the type of shipping, cost, amount of packages, and future dates of shipments of back-ordered items.

The periodic automatic replenishment level is important because a manufacturer may not fill an order on a holiday or weekend. If the pharmacy uses its stock up during one of these instances, there may be a delay until the next delivery date before products can be received. A patient should never have to wait for an essential medication because the pharmacy has depleted its stock. This is especially true in a hospital pharmacy. If such a depletion of stock does occur, the pharmacy may have to use an express delivery service or borrow medication from another pharmacy. To avoid depletion of stock, it is essential that all pharmacy employees work together to ensure proper medication ordering occurs as necessary, before stock levels get critically low.

Bar Coding

Bar codes enable easy identification of items and their associated information and can be used to verify correctness when reconciling received items with invoices and purchase orders. For this reason, **bar coding** is becoming increasingly popular in the pharmacy setting, although its implementation was delayed because of the lack of a universal bar code standard for all medications. The use of bar coding also may result in a reduction in medication errors, providing assurance that the identity and dose of the drug are as prescribed for the correct patient, along with improved timeliness and accuracy. The advent of bar coding of pharmaceuticals has required changes in label designs, production processes, and size of packages, but these are all minor setbacks when viewed alongside the overall benefits of the process. By insisting that unit-dose packaging remain the norm for the pharmaceutical industry, the U.S. Food and Drug Administration (FDA) has helped to direct the implementation of bar coding so that patient safety is kept in mind. Most pharmaceuticals have been brought into the bar coding system. Bar coding of all pharmaceuticals in a uniform, consistent manner helps to offer the following:

- Product-specific manufacturer-generated bar codes
- Product-specific pharmacy-generated bar codes
- Pharmacy information system–generated bar codes (that identify a patient and an order number but not a specific medication)

Consequently, the switch to standardized bar coding has resulted in savings of dollars, time, and, most importantly, lives. A quick pass of the bar code scanner identifies drugs, strengths, dosage forms, quantities, costs, package sizes, and other important information. When a medication is scanned at the cash register (or POS), the stock of that mediation is automatically decreased from the computerized inventory list by one unit. Then, when the in-stock quantity drops below the PAR level, it is automatically reordered. There are also other scanning devices used to identify necessary medication information, with the pharmacy technician only entering the quantity to be ordered. This information is then transferred to the primary computerized ordering system.

Manual Ordering

Manual ordering is very fast being replaced in the pharmacies everywhere, but is still used to continually monitor stock levels. Some pharmacies use visual inspection of stock or ordering cards kept inside medication boxes as part of manual ordering. The cards list drug information, ordering number, and necessary PAR levels. Just-in-time ordering allows a pharmacy to order just enough stock to reduce any excess inventory. When a bottled medication is exhausted, a single bottle is ordered just in time, replacing it on the shelf. In most pharmacies today, computerized ordering dominates.

Automated Dispensing System

Automated dispensing systems are becoming the normal way of dispensing in many pharmacy settings. These systems offer the benefits of small space requirements, fast and accurate counting, minimal renovations to existing pharmacy surroundings, unit-dose packaging, bar coding, and finished packaging procedures for pills, solids, vials, cups, injectables, ampules, and blister packs. Automated pneumatic tubing systems are also offered by some manufacturers. Alternate care settings and supply logistics are aided by these systems as well, because many of them organize, secure, and track medications for increased customer interaction, medication control, and more efficient use of pharmacy staff members.

Automated dispensing systems use technology that reduces labor, increases patient safety, stores medications, and controls electronic dispensing activities. As medications are dispensed into a drug vial from a bulk bin, ADSs monitor inventory. As each dosage form passes a beam of light, it is automatically removed from inventory. Pharmacy technicians are responsible for filling, cleaning, and troubleshooting ADS systems. In hospitals, pharmacy technicians regularly stock various clinics and nursing units. Automated dispensing systems linking these sites to pharmacy computer systems allow stock levels to be checked at any time. When a nurse indicates how much of a medication has been taken from a drug cabinet, it is deducted from current stock levels in the cabinet and transmitted electronically to the pharmacy. Different reports can be generated, providing an overall stock inventory for each drug. Controlled substance use and inventory is also monitored. Any drugs added or removed by any person from the unit are identified. A log is kept of all medication users, helping to ensure that controlled substances are not misused or stolen. Pharmacy technicians perform the same activities with hospital ADSs as community pharmacy ADSs. In hospitals, technicians also run reports required for filing medication drawers and other medication reconciliation activities.

POINTS TO REMEMBER

Most automated dispensing systems comply with the regulations of both the Health Insurance Portability and Accountability Act (HIPAA) and the Joint Commission.

Receiving New Stock

Receiving is one of the most important parts of the pharmacy operation. New stock usually arrives every day at a pharmacy, except for holidays or weekends. It comes from many different sources. In hospital pharmacies, new stock arrives from a central supply source that functions every day of the week. When items are received by the pharmacy, the items should be checked and verified individually, with a printed copy of the items actually received kept on hand. Generally, the individual who ordered the products should not be the individual receiving the products. If there are any errors, the pharmacy should contact the supplier immediately. If too many items have been received compared to the order, the supplier will have an established policy for returning items and receiving credit if any overbilling occurred. When opening a received package, pharmacy staff members must be extremely accurate in verifying the items received with the packing list. They should look for incorrect, damaged, outdated, or missing items. Items should be reconciled with invoices and purchase orders. The amount of each item and correct drug strengths must be verified. Any price changes must be identified, and it must be determined if they are correct. If controlled substances have been ordered, they will be shipped separately from other drug products and should be received into the pharmacy by a pharmacist. Any material safety data sheets (SDS) must be stored in the pharmacy's approved location for these items.

Posting

Posting is the updating of inventory in pharmacy computer software databases along with reconciling differences between current stock and new stock. When an inventory order is checked and approved, it is important that accurate posting occurs. The pharmacy technician will check newly received drug inventories for NDC numbers, expiration dates, and updates to the cost of the drugs. Large price increases should be discussed with the pharmacist so that they can be verified. Stickers are sometimes affixed to unit stock bottles when they are received. These stickers document the wholesaler item number and pricing information but should not be placed anywhere on the container that could result in harm to the original label. A wholesaler can choose to not accept any returned medication containers that appear worn or tampered with. Also, medication labels should not be affixed to original manufacturer's packages for drugs of high cost, in the event that the patient cannot afford them, and they then must be returned. After posting, new drug stock must be immediately stored in the correct area based on the requirements listed in the package inserts.

Storage

When new products are added to storage shelves, expiration dates of stock are checked. The containers are then rearranged so that the oldest (with the shortest expiration dates) are in front, for fastest access and sale. This is known as *rotating the stock*. All products near to their expiration dates must be removed from storage. Every pharmacy has its only policy for acceptable ranges of expiration dates. Commonly, expiration dates of one year or more from the date of receipt from the wholesaler are required. Products stored on shelves must usually have at least four to six months of *shelf life*.

Medication Returns

There are four primary reasons why a medication will be returned to its manufacturer or the warehouse from which it was shipped:

- Drug recalls
- Damaged stock
- Expired stock
- Nearly expired stock

In the latter case, the pharmacy can return the medication for credit or full price to the wholesaler if there is at least a nine-month expiration date.

Various types of documentation are required, depending on the reason for the return. The pharmacy's policies and procedures manual should list steps to be taken to return medications. Most medications, except for scheduled drugs, can be returned by pharmacy technicians without the signature of the pharmacist.

WHAT WOULD YOU DO?

In your training as a pharmacy technician, you learned that certain medications cannot be returned. These include expired medications, adulterated or contaminated medications, and those that cannot be donated for future use. One day, when clearing out expired medications from the pharmacy inventory, you notice that a few bottles of expired muscle relaxants are missing from the area where you placed them just a few minutes before. When you ask another employee about the bottles, he or she says that he or she packaged them up to return to the manufacturer. What would you do?

RETURN OF DECLINED DRUGS

A *declined* drug is one that has not been picked up by a customer within seven days. Often, pharmacy staff makes many attempts to alert the customer that his or her prescription is awaiting pickup, but something prevents it from being picked up. Pharmacy technicians regularly cancel or "reverse" online insurance billing, store the prescription order in the patient's profile, and return the drug product to storage. If the drug is expensive, the technician may then return it to the wholesaler for credit, as long as its box is unopened, and the prescription label can be removed without altering the packaging label.

A *return-for-credit-form* must be completed, listing the drug products and quantities being returned for credit. The pharmacy technician and wholesale driver are required to verify the contents of the return packages and sign for the credit. The signature guarantees that the drug product was purchased directly from the wholesaler. It also proves under penalty of perjury that the drugs have been properly stored and handled, following the manufacturer's guidelines and all laws—local, state, or federal. The containers are then sealed and returned to the wholesaler for credit. The signed form is filed in case it needs to be accessed in the future.

DRUG RECALLS

Under the federal Food, Drug, and Cosmetic Act, the FDA can request a recall if a drug manufacturer is not willing to remove dangerous drugs from the market without the FDA's written request. The FDA then monitors company recalls and assesses the adequacy of the firm's action. If the firm does not comply with a recall request, the FDA can seek legal action and force the recall to occur. Products that may be recalled by the FDA without requesting the manufacturer to do so include medical devices, human tissue products, and infant formulas that pose a risk to human health. After a recall is completed, the FDA makes sure that the product is destroyed or reconditioned and investigates why it was defective in the first place. Many times, however, the manufacturers themselves recall drugs when they find them to be defective. Class I recalls are for dangerous or defective products that could cause serious health problems or death. Class II recalls are for products that may cause temporary health problems or pose a slight threat of a serious nature. Class III recalls are for products unlikely to cause any adverse health reactions but which violate FDA labeling or manufacturing regulations.

Drug recall notices may reach the pharmacy by e-mail, fax, or mail. They contain all information about the drug or device being recalled and include instructions as to how to follow recall procedures. The *lot number* of the drug is included. The lot numbers are assigned by each drug manufacturer, and they identify specific batches of medication from other batches that are not affected by the recall. Pharmacy staff, when receiving a recall request, must immediately inspect and remove all of the recalled stock from shelves, freezers, and refrigerators. If some of the recalled medication is found, a report is generated of all customers who received the medication in the past 30 days. These customers are then notified of the recall. The prescriber of the medication is also notified.

Recalled medications are placed into a designated area or container for return to the manufacturer, or for disposal, following the instructions in the recall notice. Pharmacy technicians are required to check the entire drug stock to ensure that the recalled drug is not in stock. If none is found, the recall form is initialed to indicate that the time is not in stock. If recalled stock is found, the pharmacist must be notified. Manufacturers and the DNA notify prescribers of recalls in the same way. All prescribers are responsible for notifying any patient using a recalled medication or device whether treatment is to be changed or discontinued. Pharmacies can assist patients with returning or disposing of recalled medications. Manufacturers, not the FDA, issue the majority of recalls. All FDA-monitored recalls are included in a weekly Enforcement Report, with the proper recall class listed. These reports are shown on the FDA website and visitors to the site can request reports via e-mail.

DAMAGED STOCK

When a pharmacy technician finds a stock to be damaged, even if this did not occur when a new stock delivery package was opened, the damaged stock can still be returned to the manufacturer. Some manufacturers require that pharmacies contact them first and obtain a return authorization before the damaged products can be returned. If a patient comes back to the pharmacy with a drug product that he or she has found to be damaged, the pharmacy will replace the item and then undertake its return to the manufacturer.

EXPIRED STOCK

Expired, deteriorated, contaminated, or other nonusable drug products should be removed immediately from usable pharmacy stock and disposed of. Expired drugs should be placed into containers labeled with "Expired Drugs—DO NOT USE" or a similar, clearly understood warning. Disposal requirements for most drugs that have an expiration date are listed in the package inserts or on a SDS. Expired drugs and their disposal methods should be documented regardless of whether they are put into biohazard bags for collection by approved biohazard disposal companies, returned to pharmaceutical representatives, or disposed of in any other way.

Some pharmacies regularly remove any medications that will expire within three months. This way, there is a greatly reduced chance that a nearly expired medication will be dispensed. Some manufacturers allow nearly expired items to be returned if they are bundled into minim package sizes and not sent as partial returns. An example is when a medication that is three months away from expiration is returned, for full or partial credit, as long as a box of 100 units of the medication are returned in one package. It is important to always follow the manufacturer's return guidelines. Hazardous chemicals, which include cytotoxic agents, must be repackaged very carefully to avoid any breakage while being transported.

Pharmacy staff can also return slow-moving (selling) stock that still has 9 to 12 months before expiration, receiving credit from the wholesaler, who may then resell the drug to another pharmacy. Only unopened bottles can be returned in these cases. Wholesalers and manufacturers have various regulations about this practice. Many pharmacies utilize a company to process returns to drug companies, which are paid a percentage of credits that are obtained. These companies will visit the pharmacy every three months or once per year, completing all paperwork and documentation for the return of expired inventory.

Purchasing Procedures

The complexity of services offered by the pharmacy department will dictate the frequency of its involvement with the purchasing department. Among various types of pharmacies, this complexity will also differ depending on the size and type of the pharmacy. In pharmacies with intravenous programs, central supply services, or other services such as orthopedic assistance, necessitating frequent buying of equipment and supplies, there will be continual involvement with purchasing. Pharmacies with limited services may have little involvement, particularly if purchasing of medications is the pharmacy's responsibility. When the pharmacy must order and buy products for use or sale, the procedure is usually carried out in one of the following ways: independent purchasing, group purchasing, wholesale purchasing, or purchasing from prime suppliers.

WHAT WOULD YOU DO?

When assisting with an inventory of the controlled substances in the pharmacy, you find large discrepancies between what the computer inventory shows and what the actual hand-counted inventory shows. Concerned that someone might be diverting controlled substances from the pharmacy, what would you do?

INDEPENDENT PURCHASING

Independent purchasing or direct purchasing means the individual pharmacist or technician works alone and deals directly with representatives of pharmaceutical companies to negotiate price, quantity, and delivery. This type of purchasing eliminates the middleman and handling fees but requires a significant commitment of time, larger inventories, and more storage space. Many vendors must make purchases.

GROUP PURCHASING

Because larger purchases generally result in lower prices, groups of buyers who pool their buying power can usually gain lower prices than any of the individual buyers acting alone; this is group purchasing. There are costs involved in belonging to a purchasing group, however. These include the direct cost of membership, commonly called an annual fee, and a certain loss of control in product selection. The members of the group purchasing organization (GPO) must meet periodically to evaluate supplier proposals, products, and performance.

WHOLESALE PURCHASING

Purchasing from a wholesaler means that many items are purchased from one source. The wholesaler is usually located close to the institution, can provide next-day delivery, and will maintain the larger portion of the inventory. This enables the hospital to reduce inventory costs. Wholesaler purchasing also reduces the need for a large commitment of personnel to support the purchasing process. The primary disadvantage is higher costs of pharmaceuticals.

PRIME SUPPLIERS

Another approach to obtaining lower prices and better service is to establish a relationship with a single supplier for a major portion of the system's purchases; this is the **prime supplier**. A contract is established, stipulating a committed volume of purchases. In return the vendor will charge a highly competitive service fee and provide a guaranteed service level, guaranteed delivery schedule, and a guarantee that individual or group contract prices will be the base price. A contract with a prime vendor may be an independent agreement with the hospital or an agreement made through the GPO. Generally, the GPO is better able to negotiate a competitive contract. The prime vendor system has the advantages of both the direct and the wholesaler purchasing processes without the disadvantages. To reduce inventory costs, most pharmacy departments will attempt to have a just-in-time inventory system. In this system, sufficient inventory is maintained for the pharmacy to function until the next reorder period. With the prime vendor system this reorder period could be as little as 24 hours. A prime vendor agreement is made between a pharmacy and a wholesaler to purchase the majority of its products from that wholesaler.

In addition to allowing the pharmacy to maintain lower in-house inventory levels, the supplier is expected to provide the following:

- Lower prices
- Extended price protection
- Minimal occurrence of back orders
- Simplified paperwork in purchasing, receiving, and paying for items
- Other special services

Potential disadvantages of using a prime supplier include the following:

- Economic competition may be reduced over a period of time.

- Quality may be inconsistent across the supplier's complete line of products.

- The pharmacy may become overly dependent on the supplier, so that a change in supplier would be disruptive to pharmacy routines.

- Prices may creep upward if inadequate controls are placed on the relationship.

Special Purchasing Of Controlled Substances

Controlled substances require special procedures, governed by the Controlled Substances Act, concerning purchasing, receiving, and inventory records. Every pharmacy is required to register with the Drug Enforcement Administration (DEA) in order to purchase and dispense controlled substances. Also, the FDA requires all controlled-substance containers to be clearly marked with the appropriate drug schedule on the product label. The pharmacy technician must inspect containers for this schedule mark. It appears as an uppercase Roman numeral, sometimes preceded by a "C" symbol. For example, a Schedule II drug may appear as *II* or *C-II*. These indications must be at least twice as large as the other letters printed on the label. When a bottle is too small to display these numerals or symbols, they must be contained on the box and package inserts. They are not required, by law, to appear on patient containers.

SCHEDULE II PURCHASING

The DEA requires that special forms be used when ordering Schedule II controlled substances. Overall, the requirements for purchasing Schedule II agents are stricter than for other substances. For most C-II drugs, PAR levels generate automated inventory alerts in pharmacy software programs. However, purchase of these substances must be specifically begun and authorized by a pharmacist, not a pharmacy technician, and utilized DEA Form 222, either paper or electronic. To order online, every pharmacy has a DEA registration, and each pharmacist has a secure pharmacy user name and protected password. Online ordering allows for next-day delivery in most instances. When C-II drugs are borrowed from another pharmacy, the pharmacist must complete and sign a paper copy of the DEA Form 222 (see Chapter 3).

When packages of Schedule II drugs are received, the pharmacy technician must make sure the seals are not broken. The pharmacist is required to break these seals and verify the contents with the invoice. Once verified, the pharmacist uses DEA Form 222 to document the date, name and amount of each Schedule II drug received, and the NDC numbers. The pharmacy technician is allowed to post the C-II drug inventory to the database. This includes the NDC numbers, prices, and expiration dates.

SCHEDULE III, IV, AND V PURCHASING

Most pharmacies allow pharmacy technicians to order C-III, C-IV, and C-V medications. The pharmacist may be required to verify and sign for them when they are received, however. Once the invoice is compared with the ordered drug's name, dosage, and quantity, the receipt can be signed by the pharmacy technician and then verified by the pharmacist. The technician can store the medications in the proper places along with the other drug stock. This is usually done alphabetically, by generic name. All C-III, C-IV, and C-V prescriptions and records, as well as purchasing invoices, are usually stored separately from other records. They must also be kept in an easily retrievable form.

CONTROLLED SUBSTANCE DISPOSAL

Schedule II controlled substances that are expired or defective must be disposed of correctly. This requires itemization, recording, witnessing, and signing by a second pharmacist. In the majority of cases, C-II drugs are not destroyed until the next time the state drug inspector visits the pharmacy, or they are returned to an authorized destruction facility after being completely documented. Community pharmacies are allowed by the DEA to offer medication take-back programs for customers, who can bring or mail in unused, unwanted, or expired prescribed controlled substances. The pharmacy often maintains a collection receptacle in a locked area of the facility where a pharmacy staff member is always present. Community pharmacies sometimes maintain take-back control substance receptacles at long-term care facilities, which also must be within locked and staffed areas.

Summary

Inventory control is vitally important to the practice of pharmacy. Receiving reports, purchase orders, and invoices all help to support the inventory control process and should be used carefully. Inventory is extremely important in relation to a pharmacy's overhead expenses and profits. A well-managed inventory program includes waste control. A "just-in-time" system, wherein products arrive shortly before they are needed, is an ideal system to strive for. The "want book" system is one of the most common types of order book systems used in the pharmacy and is usually computerized. Computer systems integrate sales and inventory information to efficiently control pharmacy inventories.

Drugs that fall under the category of "special orders" include controlled substances, cytotoxic drugs, investigational drugs, and various hazardous substances. For hazardous substances, including chemicals, pharmacy technicians must be aware of the location of their safety data sheets (SDS). Efficient management of expired stock should be a regular part of pharmacy practice and may easily be accomplished by the use of computerized inventory control. The four primary reasons why a medication will be returned are drug recalls, damaged stock, expired stock, and nearly expired stock. Further integration with computers using point-of-sale systems enables up-to-the-minute inventory control and management of the pharmacy practice. The process of bar coding allows for easy identification of information, better reconciling of invoices and purchase orders, and an overall reduction in medication errors. Automation in the pharmacy is becoming the wave of the future, with many dispensing functions being handled by robotic machinery. Improvements in pharmacy computer systems aid in all forms of purchasing and better inventory control.

REVIEW QUESTIONS

1. One of the simplest and most widely used methods of inventory control is a:

    A. notebook.
    B. want book.
    C. red book.
    D. orange book.

2. To maintain perpetual control, the pharmacy must update inventory records:

    A. whenever inventory is purchased or sold.
    B. whenever sales figures are updated.
    C. to identify low turnover.
    D. to generate orders.

3. The most suitable, flexible, and open-ended dispensing system on the market is the:

    A. want book.
    B. point-of-sale master system.
    C. manual dispensing system.
    D. supply station system.

4. Expired, deteriorated, contaminated, and other nonreusable drug products should always be:

    A. immediately removed from stock and disposed of.
    B. immediately removed from stock and mailed back to the manufacturer.
    C. immediately flushed down a toilet or drain.
    D. sold at reduced prices as soon as possible.

5. Which of the following types of agreements is made between a pharmacy and a wholesaler to purchase the majority of its products from the same wholesaler?

    A. Prime vendor agreement
    B. Velocity agreement
    C. Primer purchaser agreement
    D. Purchase order

6. All of the following are advantages of bar coding in the pharmacy, *except*:

   A. improved accuracy.
   B. tracking of medications.
   C. changes in labeling and packaging.
   D. reduction of medication errors.

7. A document that authorizes items to be purchased from vendors is a(n):

   A. invoice.
   B. purchase order.
   C. inventory.
   D. receiving report.

8. Which of the following is placed at the front of a medication shelf?

   A. Medications with the oldest expiration dates
   B. Unit doses
   C. Expired medications
   D. Medications with the newest expiration dates

9. Which of the following is not a common type of inventory management system?

   A. Perpetual inventory system
   B. Computerized inventory system
   C. E-book system
   D. Point-of-sale system

10. How often must controlled substances be inventoried?

    A. Every month
    B. Every six months
    C. Every year
    D. Every two years

11. Which of the following statements is correct regarding pharmacy technicians and inventory control?

    A. The technician must be certified to work with pharmacy inventory.
    B. The technician should take special courses concerning inventory.
    C. The technician must be licensed for these tasks.
    D. The technician should be familiar with pharmacy policies and procedures to prevent product depreciation and improve turnover.

12. Which of the following systems allows inventory to be tracked as it is used?

    A. Perpetual inventory system
    B. Locator system
    C. Point-of-sale system
    D. Inventory record card system

13. Inventory control is closely associated with the function of:

    A. purchasing.
    B. discounting.
    C. compounding.
    D. product dating.

14. Established stock medication levels are referred to as which of the following?

    A. Inventory levels
    B. Periodic automatic replenishment levels
    C. Manual levels
    D. Guaranteed service levels

15. The basis of the computerized purchasing and control system is the:

A. PDR.
B. medication database.
C. EOQ.
D. reorder point.

CRITICAL THINKING

David, a new pharmacy technician, is assigned to be responsible for inventory in his community pharmacy. He asks the pharmacist to tell him about how the pharmacy's inventory is set up.

1. Which method of pharmaceutical inventory is more practical and common in the pharmacy setting? Explain.

2. What is the role of pharmacy technicians in inventory control? Make a list of their duties.

WEB LINKS

Food & Drug Administration Drug Recalls: www.fda.gov/safety/recalls/default.htm

Inventory Management: inventorymanagement.com

National Community Pharmacists Association: www.ncpanet.org

Pharmaceutical Multichannel Marketing: www.pharmakinnex.com

Pharmacy Automation Supplies: www.pharmacyautomationsupplies.com

RX Insider: www.rxinsider.com

CHAPTER 18

Medication Errors and Safety

Liability of Medication Errors
Minimizing Liability
Negligence, Malpractice, and Penalties

OBJECTIVES

Upon completion of this chapter, the reader should be able to:

1. Define medication errors.
2. Explain the factors causing medication errors and the ways to avoid them.
3. Explain why medication errors should be reported.
4. Describe dangerous abbreviations.
5. Explain the correct use of leading zeros and trailing zeros.
6. Discuss the FDA MedWatch program.
7. Define negligence and malpractice.
8. Compare medication errors between adults and children.
9. Identify "high alert" medications.
10. Describe risk factors for medication errors in the elderly.

KEY TERMS

biologics	hematoma	pain scales	transcription
clinical	leading zeros	trailing zeros	

Overview

The use of medication involves multiple organizations and professionals from various disciplines. A medication error is any preventable event that causes or leads to inappropriate medication use or patient harm. Medication errors can occur as a result of the actions of health care professionals, patients, or consumers. They often occur in the processes of manufacturing, prescribing, transcribing, dispensing, and administering medications. Patients also commonly make medication errors at home.

Occurrence of Medication Errors

Medication errors may happen in clinics, homes, hospitals, operating rooms, pharmacies, and physician offices. Errors can also be made when prescribing medications, administering medications, and in the processes of diagnosis and testing. The Institute for Safe Medication Practices (ISMP) estimates that approximately 251,000 Americans die each year as a result of medical errors, with over 7000 of these attributable to actual medication errors. Deaths in U.S. hospitals due to medical errors are as many as 98,000 per year, which is more than deaths from motor vehicle accidents, breast cancer, and AIDS. The Food and Drug Administration (FDA) and ISMP work to analyze dangerous medication errors. Medication errors are among the most common causes of avoidable harm to patients. Most errors occur during the physician's ordering (39%) and the nurse's administration (38%), with the remaining percentage of errors divided between **transcription** and pharmacy dispensing. During manufacturing, slight deviations can occur that may affect the potency of a packaged drug product. Though these deviations are usually not significant enough to harm patients, constant computer monitoring of machinery and processes is required to ensure quality control. When a drug is manufactured incorrectly, including how it is packaged, a drug recall may be the result.

POINTS TO REMEMBER

Medication errors can occur during manufacturing, as well as in hospitals, physician offices, or pharmacies.

MEDICATION ERROR ALERT

According to the Agency for Healthcare Research and Quality, nearly one-third of adults in the United States take five or more medications. Adverse drug events account for almost 700,000 visits to emergency departments and 100,000 hospitalizations every year.

Prescribing Errors

A *prescribing error* is an error due to the incorrect selection of a drug, its dose, concentration, dosage form, quantity, administration route, infusion rate, or usage instructions. Most medication errors occur when physicians, nurse practitioners, physician assistants, dentists, and pharmacists order prescriptions. Prescribing errors may be due to human factors, illegible handwriting, inadequate monitoring, lack of drug knowledge, lack of patient information, rule violations, and the use of some dangerous abbreviations. Miscommunication or misinformation are important factors causing prescribers to make errors. These topics are discussed in detail later in this chapter.

POINTS TO REMEMBER

Highly trained people still make mistakes. Even if clinicians are well educated and follow policies, procedures, or other guidelines, errors will still happen.

WHAT WOULD YOU DO?

You are working in a community pharmacy when you receive a prescription for an elderly man with Parkinson's disease. The prescribed drug is "risperidone," which you recognize as an agent used to treat schizophrenia. It has a name that is somewhat similar to the drug "ropinirole," which *is* used for Parkinson's disease. If you were this pharmacy technician, what would you do?

Dispensing Errors

Medication errors during dispensing can be made by pharmacists or pharmacy technicians. The pharmacy technician must have a thorough knowledge of generic and trade names of various drugs. They must be skilled in performing dosage calculations and be aware of various sound-alike and look-alike drugs. Contamination can occur when aseptic technique is not utilized correctly during the preparation or compounding of various medications. Being aware of all these factors helps in preventing medication errors. A *wrong drug preparation error* occurs from incorrect preparation of a medication. Another area of concern is medications that are considered to be "high alert." When these medications are administered inappropriately, there is an increased risk of patient harm. When an error does occur, the adverse effects upon the patient may be severe. The classes of high alert medications, by classification, include the following:

- Adrenergic agonists and antagonists
- Antiarrhythmics
- Antithrombotic agents
- Cardioplegic solutions
- Epidural or intrathecal medications

- General anesthetic agents

- Hypertonic dextrose solutions (20% or more)

- Inotropic medications

- Intravenous moderate sedatives and radiocontrast agents

- Narcotics such as morphine

- Neuromuscular blocking agents

- Oral and intravenous chemotherapy medications

- Oral antidiabetic agents

- Oral moderate sedatives (for children)

- Peritoneal and hemodialysis solutions

- Total parenteral nutrition solutions

According to The Joint Commission and the ISMP, the five specific medication classes that are most often involved in serious patient-related adverse events include insulin, intravenous anticoagulants, intravenous potassium concentrates, hypertonic sodium chloride solutions, and narcotics. Human and environmental factors that affect pharmacists and pharmacy technicians, in relation to dispensing errors, are discussed later in this chapter.

POINTS TO REMEMBER

Most experts agree that medication errors result from a poor system, or some work-oriented or environmental condition, not from professional incompetence.

MEDICATION ERROR ALERT

Dispensing errors occur at a rate of four per day in a pharmacy that fills 250 prescriptions daily. This amounts to approximately 51.5 million errors, out of the 3.6 billion prescriptions filled annually in the United States.

(Source: Carroll, J. (2011). The 3.3 percent Rx dilemma. *Biotechnology Healthcare, 8*(1), 24–25.)

Administration Errors

During administration of medication, errors may occur, whether nurses or other health care personnel handle the administration. There are many causes of administration errors. Human errors and environmental factors are discussed later in this chapter. In this section, misuse of infusion pumps and other parenteral delivery systems, as well as memory lapses, faulty drug identification, and dose verification errors are mentioned. Factors that may cause administering errors, regardless of the person performing the administration, include the following:

- Misuse of infusion pumps and other parenteral delivery systems—During administration of medications with pumps or parenteral delivery systems, the patient can be harmed if equipment and technique are not sterile, resulting in an infection. Infusion pumps can be miscalibrated, causing dosing errors. When improper technique is used, parenteral delivery systems can cause tissue damage such as **hematoma**.

- Memory lapses—Sometimes a nurse who administers medications may not remember to document such an occurrence. If a medication is not documented as being administered, it is possible that the medication may be administered a second time, too closely to the first administration, causing harm to the patient.

- Faulty drug identification or dose verification—When medications are administered, the drug and dose should be read and verified at least three times. Miscalculation of dosages or giving the wrong dose to a patient can cause potentially severe patient harm. When medications are calculated, nurses should always ask another nurse to confirm their calculations.

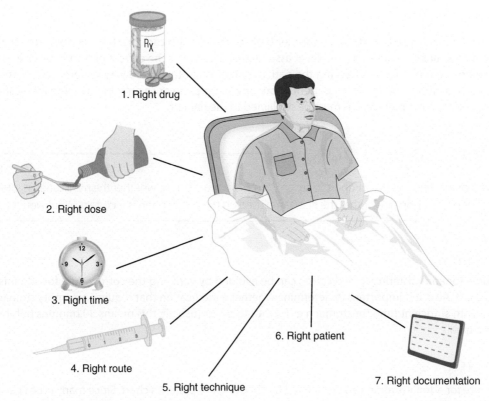

1. Right drug

2. Right dose

3. Right time

4. Right route

5. Right technique

6. Right patient

7. Right documentation

Figure 18-1 The seven rights of drug administration.

When a nurse or medical assistant is administering medications, he or she should follow the seven rights of drug administration to prevent medication errors (Figure 18-1). Not following these rights may result in giving the wrong drug, giving the wrong dosage, giving the drug to the wrong patient, giving the drug at the wrong time, giving the drug through the wrong route, giving the drug using the wrong technique, and documenting incorrect information in the patient chart. Another type of administration error is an *error of omission*, in which a needed dose is not administered to the patient.

WRONG DRUG

The physician's order must be clarified if it is unclear. Choosing the wrong drug may be avoided by verifying the label information at least three times. It should be first verified with the physician's order when it is taken out of the storage area. The next check should occur just before removing the medication from its container. The final check should occur when it is returned to storage or just before it is administered. The expiration date should also be verified so that an expired medication, or one about to expire, is not used. An *unauthorized drug error* is when a medication is administered to a patient without authorization of the prescriber. A *deteriorated drug error* is administration of a medication that is expired or obviously unstable.

WRONG DOSE

When dosage calculations are made in error, medication errors result. Another worker should always check your dosage calculations. Doses must be measured out with complete accuracy. Wrong doses can easily be avoided by using unit-dose systems because medications are already packaged in correct doses. An *improper dose error* occurs when a dose greater than, less than, or as a duplicated of a prescribed dose is administered. A *wrong dosage form error* is related to administration of a dosage form that does not correspond with the ordered dosage form.

POINTS TO REMEMBER

Dosing errors are the most common medication errors that occur in adults and children.

WRONG PATIENT

A patient may be given the medications of another patient if the health care practitioner does not ask the patient receiving the medications his or her name. Never assume that a patient is the correct person to receive a medication without verifying his or her name. Checking the patient's chart is another good way to determine that the patient is the right one. It is important to ask the patient about any allergies he or she might have. The medication's name, dosage, action, effects, and precautions must be explained to the patient.

WHAT WOULD YOU DO?

You receive a prescription for "Mrs. Robert Johnson." You are confused as to whether the medication is intended for the wife of Robert Johnson or whether the first name used on the prescription is incorrect. What would you do?

WRONG TIME

The wrong time for administering a medication can be avoided by verifying the correct time for administration on the patient's chart. Also, it is important to determine whether a medication that requires an empty stomach is being administered with sufficient time for stomach emptying to occur (usually this means 30 minutes before a meal or 2 hours after a meal).

WRONG ROUTE

The wrong route for administration can be avoided by checking the patient's chart. Since many drugs can be administered in different ways, determine the listed route for administration in the chart. The wrong route can affect the drug's absorption. If unsure about the correct route to use, verify it with the physician.

WRONG TECHNIQUE

The wrong technique of administration may cause the patient to be under- or overmedicated. The pharmacy technician must be familiar with the correct technique for every potential technique required for administration. Always ask another health care practitioner for help if there is any doubt or confusion about the technique to be used.

WRONG INFORMATION ON THE PATIENT CHART

It is important to correctly document the date and actual time of a drug's administration on the patient chart. Incorrect information on the patient chart can lead to further medication errors because additional administrations may be based on the incorrect information that was documented earlier. The patient's reactions and a notation indicating how the patient was educated about the medication should be included. Refill information should also be included.

POINTS TO REMEMBER

The health care provider who has the responsibility of administering a medication has the final opportunity to avoid a mistake.

The Patient's Role in Medication Errors

Medication errors may occur when patients self-administer drugs at home. Patients have a right to information regarding any proposed treatment, as well as the risks involved. The patient must be informed regarding his or her:

- Condition
- Treatment plan
- Prognosis

- Risks

- Benefits

- Alternative treatments

He or she must also be informed about the following:

- Complications that may occur

- Other vital pieces of information

Patients must have the answers to the following questions explained to them in order to ensure safe medication use and to avoid medication errors:

- What are the brand and generic names of the medication?

- What is the purpose of the medication?

- What is the strength and dosage?

- What are the possible adverse effects and what should be done if they occur?

- Are there medications that should be avoided while using this product?

- How long should this medication be used and what outcomes are expected?

- When is the best time to take this medication?

- How should this medication be stored?

- What should be done if a dose is missed?

- What foods should be avoided while taking this medication?

- Does this medication replace another medication currently prescribed?

- What written information is available to explain this medication?

Patients can and should play an important role in their medication therapy. Education is critical, because they can also make errors in administering medication. A *compliance error* is one that results from a patient's less-than-optimal adherence to a prescribed medication regimen.

Medication Safety for Children

According to statistics, children are highly vulnerable to medication errors. The prescription error rate per 1000 orders is highest in pediatric patients. The potential for adverse drug events in children is about three times higher than in the adult population. More than 50% of pediatric medication errors occur during prescribing, with an incorrect dose being the most common type of error. Transcribing involves interpretation and processing of the medication order, during which errors can also occur. For children, factors that increase chances for medication errors are diverse. They include the following:

- The FDA to be used for children does not approve many medications. There may be insufficient published information or FDA-approved labeling about dosing, efficacy, safety, and use in pediatric patients.

- Most medications used for children are actually formulated and packaged for adults. There may not be available dosage forms and concentrations appropriate for children. Appropriate dosage forms may require manual compounding.

- Individual doses may need calculations based on the child's age, weight, body surface area, or clinical condition.

- The overall health care system is based on adult needs.

- Younger children are unable to communicate as well as older children, teenagers, and adults.

- Neonates and other pediatric patient may have less developed organ systems to protect against medication errors.

- Children have different, changing pharmacokinetic factors at certain ages and stages of development. This may affect dosing.

- Pediatric doses may not be available in reference books.

- Many infants and children cannot swallow tablets, and prescribed doses may not fit the available tablet strengths.

- When liquid versions of a medication are not available, tablets must be manually adjusted to fit the child's needs. They can be crushed, with doses weighted, and made into powder papers. This is a time-consuming task. Therefore, tablets are usually formulated into the liquid form know as a suspension.

The steps that must be taken in order to prevent medication errors in pediatric patients include ensuring that patient information is complete, having a thorough knowledge of the types of errors that often occur, reporting errors and "near misses," remaining up to date on drug information, developing an error avoidance plan, following all procedures, and educating the child's parents on all medications.

Medication Safety for the Elderly

Since the elderly population of the United States is expected to reach 98 million by the year 2060, it is vital that medication safety for the elderly is maintained. Older people often experience *polypharmacy*—the use of multiple medications, sometimes unnecessary medications, and requirements for complicated medication regimens. The risks for medication errors are increased by the use of multiple medications. There is also a higher risk for drug interactions. Older adults often have several different chronic conditions and visit a variety of physicians and health care providers along with multiple pharmacies. Medications often related to hospitalizations for the elderly include warfarin or aspirin, which increase bleeding risks, insulin and oral diabetes medications, beta-blockers and diuretics, and anxiety medications or sleep aids.

Falling is a serious risk factor for injury in older adults, especially those who are frail. Falls are a common cause of injuries, hospitalization, and even death. Orthostatic hypotension increases with age and occurs in more than 30% of patients over the age of 75 years; in nursing home residents, this affects more than half. Falling may be linked to use of many different medications (see Table 18-1). For example, psychotropic medications, which cause sedation and alter the patient's ability to remain balanced. Medications that lower blood pressure can also be implicated in falls.

With aging, there are changes in how the body is affected by medications. Increased body fat and decreased muscle mass both affect how the body will react to various drugs. Therefore, each medication's route of administration must be correct. In older adults, there is usually decreased stomach acid, decreased gastrointestinal movements, slower stomach emptying, decreased saliva and intestinal secretions, decreased body water, alterations in blood protein in those who are frail or malnourished, decreased blood flow to the liver and kidneys, and decreased size of these organs as well. Anticholinergic medications may cause impairments of memory that cognition, delirium, drowsiness, increased dementia, fatigue, restlessness, imbalance, falling, and reduced ability to perform daily living tasks.

To increase safety for the elderly, the first step is to identify patients who are at an increased risk for adverse drugs events. Interventions include reducing polypharmacy situations, using safer alternative medications, reducing medication doses, monitoring drug levels, monitoring for sings of toxicity, and counseling patients on adherence strategies. Medication reviews should be performed by pharmacists and other qualified providers. Each medication must be assessed for appropriateness, effectiveness, safety, and assessed about whether it meets the patients' health care goals. Patients or caregivers must provide an accurate and complete list of medications being taken. Pharmacists and pharmacy technicians can ask customers to bring in all of their medications, including those that were prescribed or OTC, herbals, supplements, vitamins, inhalers, creams, ear and eye drops, suppositories, and "as-needed" medications. Pharmacists can review the correct use of all of these substances with the patient. Any newly developing symptoms must be screened for, including headache, drowsiness, dizziness, and itching. If an individual in the patient's household manages all medications, that person must be counseled as well. Important areas to assess include any unnecessary medications, conditions that are untreated or undertreated, ineffective medications, doses that are too low or too high, any adverse drug events, drug–disease interactions, and nonadherence to drug regimens. The *medication appropriateness index* is used to evaluate 10 factors about medication appropriateness. These include indication, effectiveness, dose, correct directions, practical directions, drug–drug interactions, drug–disease interactions, duplicate therapies, length of treatment, and cost.

| **Table 18-1** Medications That Cause Falls in the Elderly ||
Types of Medications	**Examples**
Anticholinergics	benztropine (Cogentin), oxybutynin (Ditropan), tolterodine (Detrol)
Anticonvulsants	gabapentin (Neurontin), pregabalin (Lyrica), valproate (Depacon)
Antidepressants (selective serotonin reuptake inhibitors)	citalopram (Celexa), fluoxetine (Prozac), sertraline (Zoloft)
Antidepressants (tricyclic)	amitriptyline (Elavil), desipramine (Norpramin), doxepin (Silenor)
Anti-Parkinson's or Restless Legs Agents	carbidopa/levodopa (Sinemet), pramipexole (Mirapex), ropinirole (Requip)
Antipsychotics	haloperidol (Haldol), olanzapine (Zyprexa), quetiapine (Seroquel)
Benzodiazepines	alprazolam (Xanax), diazepam (Valium), lorazepam (Ativan)
Blood pressure agents	amlodipine (Norvasc), lisinopril (Zestril), metoprolol (Lopressor)
Diuretics	bumetanide (Bumex), furosemide (Lasix), hydrochlorothiazide (Microzide)
Nitrates	isosorbide dinitrate (Isordil), isosorbide mononitrate (Imdur), nitroglycerin (Nitrostat)
Opioids	hydrocodone (Vicodin), morphine (Avinza), oxycodone (OxyContin)
Sleep aids	diphenhydramine (Benadryl), eszopiclone (Lunesta), zolpidem (Ambien)
Miscellaneous	digoxin (Lanoxin)

To resolve any issues that are found during counseling, a plan must be developed. This often requires collaboration between the patient, pharmacist, physician, nurses, nurse practitioners, physical therapists, social workers, pharmacy technicians, and other health care providers. Patients and caregivers must be involved in all medication decisions to ensure adherence to regimens and to understand changes that may be related to medications. Targeted patient and caregiver education is of crucial importance. Simplifying medication regimens is an important goal. This may involve the use of pill organizers, medication calendars, and assistance from family members. Lower-cost medications and prescription drug insurance options help improve adherence. All changes to a patient's medication list must be documented correctly in the electronic medical record. An updated, clearly written medication list must be provided to the patient and caregivers. It should summarize mediation names, purposes, doses, and dosing schedules, written in language understandable by nonpractitioners. Safety is ensured by regular follow-ups with patients and review of medication regimens—at least once per year.

Risk Factors for Medication Errors

Risk factors for medication errors are varied and include human factors (fatigue, noise, poor lighting, poor management, and stress), illegible handwriting, inadequate patient monitoring, lack of drug knowledge, lack of patient information, rule violations, problems with herbal remedies, problems with over-the-counter drugs, problems with medications sold over the Internet, and illegal drugs.

HUMAN FACTORS

Human factors related to medication errors include lack of attention to details, failure to recognize certain facts, choosing incorrect medications, failing to remember something concerning the medication or patient, and making incorrect choices about what actions are to be taken. A busy pharmacy setting, for example, may be distracting due to the amount of activity going on. Other human factors include consciously not following the policies and practices of work, causing required steps to be skipped. Inadequate staffing puts more stress on the existing staff members and may lead to medication errors. Poor communication between staff members can also result in errors. It is important that all health care personnel continually strive for quality work, and when errors occur, report them fully and professionally so that they can be prevented in the future.

Fatigue

Fatigue has many effects that can allow medication errors to occur. These include slowed reaction times, reduced accuracy, inability to recognize changes in the patient, lapses of attention, impaired communication ability, memory lapses, and decreased energy. Long work hours are often required in the health care setting, but the effects of these shifts can be dangerous. Lack of sleep and stress also cause fatigue. It is recommended that many health care professionals work no more than 12 hours per day and no more than 60 hours per week in order to avoid fatigue. In the workplace, fatigue can be reduced by educating workers about its effects, competent scheduling of work, taking planned naps, and providing breaks that are of adequate length in areas where work will not intrude. Higher levels of ambient lighting for night-shift workers and proven safety practices such as bar coding and "smart" infusion pumps can help in reducing fatigue.

Noise

Both internal and external noise can interrupt the concentration of health care workers and cause medication errors. Outside construction and traffic noise may contribute to lack of concentration. Interior noises such as repair work, customers' conversations, cell phones ringing, and overhead music systems may cause lack of concentration.

Poor Lighting

Adequate, bright lighting has been proven to decrease medication errors by increasing alertness and the ability to read information more accurately. Poor lighting may cause labels to be misread, including information such as drug names, dosages, and lot numbers.

Poor Management

If pharmacy technicians are not adequately supervised due to staff shortages, they may make errors that will go unchecked by pharmacists or other personnel. Another example is when a health care organization's management does not address concerns such as poor air conditioning systems, unhealthy conditions, and other distractions. When these types of situations are not managed correctly, workers are in danger of committing more medication errors due to lack of focus.

Stress

Stress is often linked to a variety of outcomes, and it certainly plays a part in medication errors. An employee who is experiencing heightened levels of stress is prone to be more distracted, often thinking about what is causing the stress when he or she should be focused on details of his or her work. Examples of stressful situations that may lead to medication errors include personal and family problems, sickness, poverty, conflicts with staff members, and dealing with upset or angry patients. Mistakes are likely to occur when focus is shifted away from the task at hand.

ILLEGIBLE HANDWRITING

Illegible handwriting has been documented as the second most prevalent cause of medication errors. It slows down the process of taking in prescriptions so that they can be processed. The order is harder to verify, and serious errors can occur if the intended drug, dosage, route, or frequency is misinterpreted. Prescribers must take the time to write their prescriptions slowly and clearly in order to protect their patients from medication errors. For example, when prescriptions are illegible, they may cause confusion among drugs with similar names. Other methods of counteracting illegible handwriting is to dictate prescriptions, type them, and review them for accuracy and clarity. Computers are a big help in maintaining legibility. Speaking to other health care professionals and patients about prescriptions ensures that everyone involved understands what medicine, dosage, route, and frequency are to be administered. This way, if the prescription itself contains an error, the chances of someone catching it are increased.

WHAT WOULD YOU DO?

A pharmacy technician received a prescription for a patient with chest pain. The prescribed medication was difficult to read, but the pharmacy technician discerned it as "Plendil," which is a calcium channel blocker. The patient died after a few days of a heart attack. The cardiologist claimed that he had written "Isordil" on the prescription, which is a nitrate used for chest pain. If you were the pharmacy technician in this example, what would you have done?

INADEQUATE PATIENT MONITORING

Health care professionals must monitor patients to ensure safe medication administration and outcomes. Vital signs and levels of consciousness can be verified to make sure that medications are acting effectively without excess. **Pain scales** are printed charts that patients can view and then respond to. They indicate various levels of pain that may be felt by the patient after a procedure or while a health condition exists. The patient is asked by the health care professional to respond about his or her level of pain by looking at the potential levels of pain on the chart. Every patient's pain tolerance level is different, and this is something that should be considered when determining the need for additional pain medication. Another area of importance is the verification of multiple pain management situations—patients should not be receiving similar medications from different prescribers because this can cause dangerous overmedication. Diagnostic tests are also important for patient monitoring. Often, these tests can reveal a potentially dangerous situation before it actually occurs. Complete blood counts, serum concentration tests, blood glucose tests, and platelet counts are commonly used to verify drug actions in the patient's system. Flow sheets are used to record each dose of each medication, allowing caregivers to track the patient's response to each drug over time. A *monitoring error* may be related to inappropriate review of a patient drug profile or the failure to use appropriate laboratory testing results to assess the patient's response to the medication.

LACK OF DRUG KNOWLEDGE

Patients who do not understand their medications and the requirements for their use may inadvertently harm themselves. Likewise, caregivers who do not understand the same information can cause harm to a patient. Patients should be encouraged to ask questions about their medications. They should understand the drug names, dosages, reasoning behind their use, how they should be administered, what they actually look like, and how they work. Health care professionals should teach patients how to protect themselves from medication errors and involve patients in drug safety programs and quality improvement measures.

POINTS TO REMEMBER

According to the ISMP, the following are medications of "highest alert" concerning medication errors:

- Insulin
- Narcotics and opiates
- Potassium chloride injections
- Heparin
- Concentrated sodium chloride (>0.9%)

MEDICATION ERROR ALERT

Recent studies have shown that 44% of hospitalized patients believed they were receiving a medication that they were not actually receiving. Also, 96% were unable to recall the name of even one medication that had been prescribed for them during their hospitalization.

(Source: *Journal of Hospital Medicine*, December 10, 2009.)

LACK OF PATIENT INFORMATION

Patient information that is essential in reducing medication errors includes age, sex, pregnancy, diagnoses, allergies, height, weight, lab test values, diagnostic study results, vital signs, patient identity, and ability to pay for prescriptions. Lack of patient information may cause serious adverse effects, drug interactions, contraindicated medications to be administered when a certain health condition exists, and incautious dosing.

RULE VIOLATIONS

All health care professionals must follow the rules of their health care practice setting. When established rules are not followed, medication errors may occur for various reasons. For example, a prescriber who does not have enough knowledge about a patient's history, including the patient's family history, may give a medication in error that he or she is allergic to. If the prescriber had followed the rules of his or her practice, the patient or family would have been asked about health and allergy histories before any drug was prescribed. Another example is when a pharmacist does not follow the rules requiring patient consultation. Without adequate consultation, a patient can misunderstand how and when to take the medication, whether it should be taken with or without meals, and so on. When the pharmacist follows the rules, the patient is adequately counseled, and these potential problems do not occur. In the cases of Medicare patients, this is an extremely important rule to follow to avoid serious legal consequences. Another instance concerns nurses when they administer medications. They must be sure to follow the "seven rights" of drug administration (see Figure 18-1); otherwise they would be in violation of the rules of their practice.

PROBLEMS WITH HERBAL REMEDIES

Herbal remedies may interact dangerously with certain medications prescribed by a physician, dispensed by a pharmacist, or administered by a nurse. Sometimes patients take herbal remedies without telling anyone. Many people incorrectly assume that herbal remedies cannot be harmful, and because they do not believe these remedies to be drugs, they omit them when asked about any medications they are taking. Therefore, the prescriber may be unaware that herbal remedies are being used by the patient. It is vital to ask what herbal remedies patients are taking—and have patients list them all—in order for medication errors to be prevented.

PROBLEMS WITH OVER-THE-COUNTER DRUGS

Over-the-counter drugs are purchased by patients to self-treat various conditions. Most people have at least one over-the-counter medication (such as aspirin) in the medicine cabinet at home to treat minor ailments. Patients are often unaware that these medications may interact poorly with prescribed medications, and they frequently fail to mention using them to their physicians. However, if a physician, for example, prescribes anticoagulants for a patient, and that patient is taking aspirin at home for pain relief, there is the potential for serious bleeding. Similarly, many patients do not realize that over-the-counter drugs can interact with other drugs, foods, or therapies (see Chapter 27). For example, a patient who takes acetaminophen while drinking alcohol is at risk for severe liver damage when these two substances are used simultaneously. Educating patients is very important to avoid medication errors. They must be told that while taking certain prescribed medications, they should not take certain over-the-counter drugs.

PROBLEMS WITH MEDICATIONS SOLD OVER THE INTERNET

Today's technology, which has provided widespread access to the Internet, has affected the pharmacy industry in both positive and negative ways. Patients often purchase medications through Internet websites in order to obtain lower prices than they can find at their local pharmacy. Some of these websites do not operate according to the law. Often, consumers who are unaware that these medications originate from other countries purchase cheaper medications. Occasionally, the FDA does not approve the formulations of these medications, and it may not even be legal to purchase them in the United States.

ILLEGAL DRUGS

Some patients use illegal drugs, which they often do not report to their physicians. If a physician prescribes a sedative for a patient who is illegally using heroin or cocaine, it is possible that a drug interaction can occur that can severely harm the patient. Ideally, the health care practitioner should be made aware of any illegal drugs that the patient is taking in order to prevent medication errors.

Dangerous Abbreviations and Numerical Terms

Medication errors frequently occur when prescribers use abbreviations. These abbreviations may cause confusion for other health care providers. As a result, The Joint Commission and the ISMP have made lists of potentially dangerous abbreviations, and established a "do not use" list. The following abbreviations must not be used because they can cause dangerous errors to occur:

- U—Write out the word "units" instead
- IU—Write out the phrase "International Units" instead
- QD or qd—Write out the word "daily" instead
- QOD or qod—Write out the phrase "every other day" instead
- µg—Write out the word "micrograms" instead
- SC or SQ—Write out the word "subcutaneous" instead
- TIW or tiw—Write out the phrase "three times a week" instead
- D/C—Write out the words "discharge" or "discontinue" instead
- HS or hs—Write out the phrases "half strength" or "hour of sleep" instead
- cc—Write out the phrase "cubic centimeters" instead, or use "milliliters" or "mL"
- AD, AS, or AU—Write out the phrases "right ear," "left ear," or "both ears" instead
- OD, OS, or OU—Write out the phrases "right eye," "left eye," or "both eyes" instead
- MS, MSO₄, or MgSO₄—Write out the phrases "morphine sulfate" or "magnesium sulfate" instead
- > or <—Write out the phrases "greater than" or "less than"
- Abbreviations for drug names—Write out drug names in full
- Apothecary nits—Use metric units
- @—Write out the word "at"

Review The Joint Commission's "Do Not Use" list (www.jointcommission.org) and the ISMP's List of Error-Prone Abbreviations (www.ismp.org/recommendations/error-prone-abbreviations-list) for rationales and other examples.

Numerical terms may also cause errors to occur. These include the use of leading zeros and trailing zeros. **Leading zeros** should be used before decimal points, for example, 0.2 mg (not ".2 mg"). **Trailing zeros** should not be used, for example, 2.0 mg should be written as "2 mg." When a leading zero is not placed before a decimal point as in the above example, the amount of ".2 mg" might be mistaken for "2 mg" if the reader does not see the decimal point. When a trailing zero is placed after a decimal point as in the second example above, the amount of "2.0 mg" might be mistaken for "20 mg" if the reader does not see the decimal point. Documented examples exist of patients inadvertently given 10 or 100 times the amount of required medication due to these types of errors. One such example involved an infant who was supposed to receive "0.4 mg" of morphine, which had been written without the leading zero, as ".4 mg." The nurse did not see the decimal point and administered "4 mg" to the infant. This overdose was 10 times the amount of morphine required. When a second dose of 4 mg of morphine was administered four hours later, the infant went into respiratory arrest and died.

MEDICATION ERROR ALERT

The most common abbreviation that has resulted in medication errors is "qd," meaning "once daily." In studies, this abbreviation has been shown to account for 43.1% of medication errors that involved abbreviations. The other most common abbreviations that resulted in medication errors were "U" for "units," "cc" in place of "mL," and "MSO₄" or "MS" for "morphine sulfate."

(Source: Brunetti, L., Santell, J. P., and Hicks, R. W. (2007). The impact of abbreviations on patient safety. *Joint Commission Journal on Quality and Patient Safety, 33*(9), 576–583.)

Avoiding Medication Errors

Prevention of medication errors must be the most important priority of all health care professionals, and they must educate patients. Pharmacists and pharmacy technicians must attempt to do everything possible to prevent medication errors. The prevention of medication errors should always be encouraged without penalties or blame. All individuals in the medication use process are responsible for ensuring prevention of medication errors. This includes the pharmacy staff as well as patients and caregivers. The following items are essentials for the technician to keep in mind:

- Confirm the patient's identity (e.g., birthdate, address, telephone number)
- Verify the original prescription
- Verify the medication calculation
- Communicate concerns to the pharmacist
- Verify the patient allergy history
- Inquire if the patient has questions for the pharmacist
- Maintain continuing education

Risk reduction strategies for preventing errors include the following:

- Consulting currently available drug reference texts
- Documenting essential patient information, including:
  - Allergies
  - Age
  - Weight
  - Current diagnoses
  - Current medication regimen
- Requiring clarification of any order that is incomplete or illegible

Human factors that increase the risk of medication errors and are preventable include the following:

- Fatigue
- Alcohol or the use of other drugs
- Illness
- Distractions
- Emotional states
- Unfamiliar situations or problems

Other factors include the following:

- Equipment design flaws
- Inadequate labeling or instructions
- Communication problems
- Hard-to-read handwriting
- Unsafe work conditions

The ISMP has set error prevention goals for physicians, nurses, pharmacists, and pharmacy technicians. Reporting and discussion of medication errors must be open and without penalties. There must be increased detection and reporting of medication errors in every facility, along with an understanding of the primary causes of these errors. Practitioners must be educated about causes of errors and ways to prevent them. Once a medication error is identified, there must be changes made to the facility's medication use process, in order to prevent similar errors in the future. Additionally, there should be continuing evaluation of biomedical literature about medication errors to improve the current methods of reducing and preventing them.

Medication Error Reporting

The reporting of medication errors and problems with products must be done whenever they occur. However, today the reporting of medication errors is a totally voluntary process. There are several medication error reporting systems:

- FDA MedWatch Program
- ISMP-MERP (formerly the United States Pharmacopeia (USP) Medication Error Reporting Program)
- ISMP-Medication Error Reporting Program
- Vaccine Adverse Event Reporting System (VAERS)

In addition to these three voluntary reporting programs and systems, many companies and institutions have developed specific reporting programs. Individuals are encouraged to report errors and other information without fear of penalties. There may be adverse drug event hotlines that allow easy reporting and interaction with pharmacists or other practitioners who are in charge of medication error tracking. In hospitals, medication errors are handled by *pharmacy and therapeutics committees*. Should an error cause patient harm, suffering, or death, some states require pharmacies to also notify the state Board of Pharmacy. Pharmacy technicians should always notify their supervising pharmacists in these cases. Information that may be required to be reported to the Board of Pharmacy includes the patient's personal data, the name and license number of each pharmacy employee involved in the error, incident date, incident description, prescriber's name, documentation of the prescriber being contacted, a description of actions taken after the event, and steps taken to prevent any recurrence.

FDA MEDWATCH PROGRAM

The FDA's MedWatch program encourages the voluntary reporting of adverse events or product problems. The official name of this program is the FDA Safety Information and Adverse Event Reporting Program. Serious adverse events, problems with product quality, product use errors, and therapeutic inequivalence or failures can be reported. MedWatch allows health care professionals and consumers to report serious suspected problems via the following:

- By telephone: (800) FDA-1088
- By fax: (800) FDA-0178
- Or through the Internet at www.fda.gov/Safety/MedWatch/

The actual MedWatch form, which contains patient information, descriptions of preventable adverse events, suspected medications and medical devices, along with reporter information, is located at

www.accessdata.fda.gov/scripts/medwatch/medwatch-online.htm.

MedWatch also provides important and timely **clinical** information about safety issues involving products, including the following:

- Prescription and over-the-counter drugs
- **Biologics** (agents that give immunity to disease or living organisms; e.g., vaccines)
- Medical and radiation-emitting devices
- Special nutritional products such as:
  - Medical foods
  - Dietary supplements
  - Infant formulas

Pharmacists and technicians can join an electronic mailing list to get up-to-date information that the FDA disseminates. They can also receive information as a result of information reported to MedWatch at the web address above.

ISMP-MEDICATION ERROR REPORTING PROGRAM

This program was originally developed and maintained by the United States Pharmacopeia (USP) but is now presented in cooperation with the ISMP. It is recognized as the official national medication error reporting program. It provides the opportunity for practitioners to voluntarily share medication error experiences through a nationwide network to help gain an understanding of why errors occur and how to prevent them. Educational information gained from the program assists health care professionals to avoid errors by recognizing circumstances and causes of actual and potential errors. Reports can be made to www.ismp.org/orderforms/reporterrortoISMP.asp. When reporting an error, there should be a description of the error, patient outcome, the type of practice site involved, generic and brand names of all involved medications, concentrations, dosage forms, other specific product information, how the error was discovered, and recommendations for future prevention of the type of error. After collection, all information is sent to the FDA, pharmaceutical manufacturers, and other interested third parties.

POINTS TO REMEMBER

Reporting is confidential and can be anonymous. Reports may be phoned to (800) FAIL-SAF(E) or 1-800-324-5723. More information can be found at *www.ismp.org/*

VACCINE ADVERSE EVENT REPORTING SYSTEM

The Vaccine Adverse Event Reporting System (VAERS) is specific for vaccine reporting. It is sponsored by the FDA as well as the CDC. The system is designed to collect post-marketing information on adverse events related to the administration of vaccines. This can occur online at vaers.hhs.gov/index.html, which features a downloadable form, by faxing the completed form to 1-877-721-0366 or by mailing in a completed form.

Liability of Medication Errors

Though pharmacy technicians work under the supervision of licensed pharmacists, the technicians themselves can be found liable for errors. If a patient of any age is affected by an error that was made by a pharmacy technician, it is possible for the family of the injured individual to file suit against both the pharmacy technician and the supervising pharmacist. Usually, the pharmacist and the facility where the technician is employed will be the focus of such lawsuits. The four elements involved in a "cause of action" related to negligence are *duty*, *breach*, *causation*, and *damages*. Pharmacists and technicians have a duty to use reasonable care to protect patients against unreasonable risks. A breach of this duty must occur. Causation means a reasonably close causal connection between the conduct that occurred and the resulting injury. There must also be an actual loss or damage that occurred. A *breach of expressed warranty* occurs when a pharmacist or technician makes express claims about a product that the product fails to meet. An example would be stating that an OTC item is just as effective as a prescription medication, though there are no clinical trial data supporting this statement.

Additional liability issues concerning the pharmacy staff and medication errors include failure to resolve possible errors, not adopting technology that could reduce medication errors that is considered a *standard of practice*, and high rates of prescription dispensing activities that result in more errors. Legal claims concerning pharmacy liability may occur at different times in different jurisdictions. In some areas, the legal claim begins when the medication error actually occurs. In other areas, it may not begin until an injury occurs, or when a patient discovers the injury and its causative factor. In most areas, when a patient does not initiate a lawsuit within two years of such events, a suit is usually then not allowed.

Minimizing Liability

Upon detecting an error in dispensing, the pharmacy technician must take all necessary steps to rectify it promptly and notify the pharmacist immediately. Failure to do so can subject the pharmacist to punitive damage liability in addition to actual damage for the injury caused. The pharmacist should inform the patient and the prescribing physician regarding the prescription error immediately upon discovery.

Negligence, Malpractice, and Penalties

Pharmacy laws are designed to protect the public by ensuring that a knowledgeable individual double-checks the results of the prescribing process and oversees the use of medications. Pharmacy technicians should be familiar with the policies and procedures manual of their workplace. Technicians must also receive training on the job. The Joint Commission requires organizations to prove that their personnel are competent.

Technicians and pharmacists need to be informed about the prevention of medication errors. In addition to the liability assumed by their employer, institution, or company, pharmacists and technicians may be held accountable for their negligence, malpractice, and penalties due to a medication error that involves the injury to, or death of, a patient.

The failure to do something that a reasonable person might do, or doing something that a reasonable person might not do, is termed negligence. A pharmacist or a supervised pharmacy technician who violates a regulation or law that establishes a standard of care, and that is designed to protect patients, may be guilty of negligence.

Negligence performed by a professional, such as a pharmacist or a pharmacist-supervised technician, is termed malpractice. A pharmacist who fails to perform a prospective drug regimen review, gives incorrect advice, or doesn't warn a patient about potential adverse effects is guilty of malpractice.

Penalties concerning negligence or malpractice may include the following:

- Restrictions on practice
- Suspension of ability to practice
- Fines
- Revocation of ability to practice
- Jail sentences

Summary

Medication errors occur during manufacturing, in hospitals, clinics, physicians' offices, pharmacies, and even at home. They can be prevented when health care professionals work together to identify potential errors and educate patients. Medication errors regularly occur during the ordering, transcribing, dispensing, and administering of medications. Illegible handwriting can cause confusion about drug names, and miscalculation may result in patients being overmedicated or under-medicated. In the pharmacy, common medication errors involve incorrect transcribing, improper preparation of products, lack of prescription monitoring, and incorrect dispensing activities. Distractions in the physician's office or the pharmacy can cause medication errors. Human factors play an important role in causing medication errors. Patients who receive proper education about their medications are less likely to experience medication errors. Labels should be checked and compared with physicians' orders at least three times to ensure accuracy. To ensure they are completely correct, health care practitioners should verify all calculations.

REVIEW QUESTIONS

1. Statistics show that the most common medication errors occur by which of the following health care professionals?

    A.   Physicians
    B.   Pharmacists
    C.   Pharmacy technicians
    D.   Transcriptionists

2. Medication error reporting is:

    A.   mandatory.
    B.   illegal.
    C.   voluntary.
    D.   required by state law.

3. Negligence performed by a professional such as a pharmacist is termed:

    A. recuperation.

    B. renumeration.

    C. diligent.

    D. malpractice.

4. Which of the following is the correct way to use a decimal point?

    A. .3

    B. 0.3

    C. 3.0

    D. .30

5. Which of the following is common in elderly patients and linked to falls?

    A. Orthostatic hypotension

    B. Hypertension

    C. Polypharmacy

    D. Polycythemia vera

6. Which of the following statements is false about medication errors in the health care setting?

    A. Medication errors can occur when ordering medications.

    B. Medication errors can occur when dispensing medications.

    C. Medication errors can occur when picking up medications from the pharmacy.

    D. Medication errors can occur when transcribing and administering medications.

7. Medication errors should be reported to which of the following agencies by using the MedWatch program?

    A. FDA

    B. CMS

    C. DEA

    D. CDC

8. Which of the following is the potential adverse event rate in pediatric patients compared to adults?

    A. Two times higher

    B. Three times higher

    C. Five times higher

    D. Ten times higher

9. Which of the following organizations has established a list of potentially dangerous abbreviations?

    A. DEA

    B. CMS

    C. ISMP

    D. CDC

10. Which of the following is false about pharmacy technicians and medication errors?

    A. They should verify the original prescription.

    B. They should verify the patient's allergy history.

    C. They should verify medication calculations.

    D. They should communicate concerns to the patient and advise him or her about taking the medications with milk.

11. Risk reduction strategies for preventing errors include all of the following, *except*:

    A. requiring clarification of any order that is incomplete or illegible.

    B. consulting with the pharmacy's attorney.

    C. documenting essential patient information.

    D. consulting currently available drug reference texts.

12. Upon detecting an error in dispensing, the pharmacy technician must take which of the following steps first?

   A. Notify the physician immediately
   B. Notify the pharmacist promptly
   C. Notify the patient immediately
   D. Notify the ISMP promptly

13. Which of the following is considered by the ISMP to be a "high alert" medication?

   A. Morphine
   B. Ampicillin
   C. Acetaminophen
   D. Atorvastatin

14. Which of the following makes it more likely for an elderly person to experience adverse drug events?

   A. Staying at home
   B. Medication usage review
   C. Multiple chronic conditions
   D. Taking a single medication

15. Which of the following must be included in a patient's medication list?

   A. Medication name, pharmacy contact, and quantity
   B. Medication name, purpose, dose, and dosing schedule
   C. Mediation name, quantity, and dose
   D. Medication name, prescriber, dose, and allowed refills

CRITICAL THINKING

A 45-year-old woman was suffering from a yeast infection. She received a prescription for metronidazole (Flagyl®). The person who transcribed the prescription into the computer typed in that the medication was to be used for *five* weeks, because he couldn't read what the physician wrote due to poor handwriting. (The physician had actually written "two weeks"). Because metronidazole has carcinogenic properties, patients should not use this drug for more than two weeks.

1. Explain the importance of preventing medication errors.

2. Briefly explain the most important risk factors for medication errors.

WEB LINKS

Agency for Healthcare Research and Quality; Patient Safety Network: www.psnet.ahrq.gov

American Pharmacists Association: www.pharmacist.com

Institute for Safe Medication Practices: www.ismp.org

ISMP Error-Prone Abbreviations List: www.ismp.org/recommendations/error-prone-abbreviations-list

ISMP Error Reporting: www.ismp.org/orderforms/reporterrortoISMP.asp

The Joint Commission: www.jointcommission.org

Medical News Today: www.medicalnewstoday.com

MedWatch Reporting Form: www.accessdata.fda.gov/scripts/medwatch/medwatch-online.htm

U.S. Food and Drug Administration: www.fda.gov

Vaccine Adverse Event Reporting System: vaers.hhs.gov/index.html

WebMD Medscape: www.medscape.com

Drug Actions and Interactions

OUTLINE

OBJECTIVES

Upon completion of this chapter, the reader should be able to:

1. Explain the processes of drug excretion.
2. Identify the organ that releases enzymes for drug metabolism.
3. Explain cytochrome P-450.
4. List factors that may cause drug interaction.
5. Describe synergism, potentiation, and antagonism.
6. Describe the term "conjugation."
7. Discuss what is meant by the term "adverse drug reaction."
8. Explain the processes of drug metabolism in newborns.
9. List foods and beverages that may interact with monoamine oxidase (MAO) inhibitors.
10. Explain the effect of smoking on the activity of drug metabolism.

KEY TERMS

absorption	biotransformation	first-pass effect	placebo
additive effect	conjugation	half-life	polypharmacy
adverse reactions (adverse effects)	cytochrome P-450	hypersensitivity reaction	potentiation
	diffusion	idiosyncratic reaction	receptor
agonist	distribution	metabolism	side effects
anaphylactic reaction	drug interaction	pharmacodynamics	specific affinity
antagonism	excretion	pharmacokinetics	synergism
bioavailability			

Overview

Some drug-related problems develop unexpectedly, without being predicted. Others are related to known drug actions and properties and can reasonably be anticipated. When patients are being treated with two or more drugs, they may interact and alter the effects of each drug. In this situation, the ability to predict specific drug actions is lessened to a great degree. This is a serious concern for elderly people, since many of them take a variety of prescription drugs. It is essential that complete and current medication records be maintained for patients. It is also important that drug therapy be closely monitored and supervised so that problems can be prevented or detected at an early stage in their development. The pharmacist is in a unique position to meet these needs. Many drug-related problems are caused by drug interactions. Pharmacy technicians must be familiar with this important matter and understand factors that may have an effect on different agents.

Pharmacokinetics

Pharmacokinetics is the study of the action of drugs within the body, including the mechanisms of absorption, distribution, metabolism, and excretion (see Figure 19-1). To fully understand how drug interactions take place, the pharmacy technician must understand the basics of pharmacokinetics. A drug's pharmacokinetics is described in terms of its concentration in the blood or plasma over time.

DRUG ABSORPTION

Absorption refers to the movement of a drug from its site of administration into the bloodstream, and thus the systemic circulation. In many cases, a drug must be transported across one or more biological membranes to reach

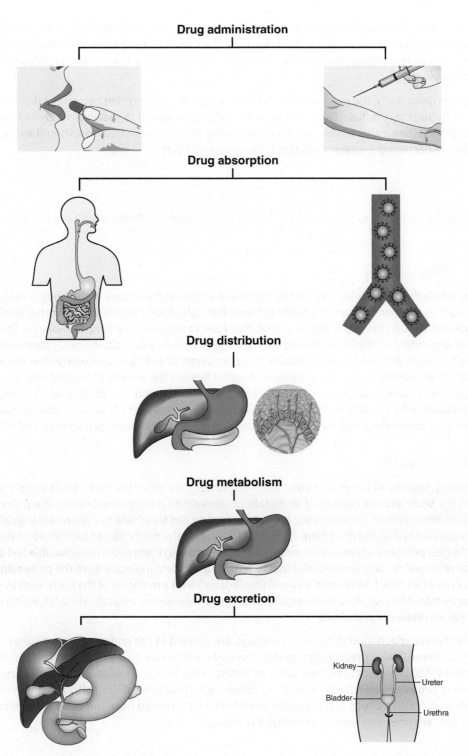

Figure 19-1 The actions of drugs in the body.

the circulation. The most common and important way in which drugs traverse membranes is through diffusion. **Diffusion** is the process by which particles in a fluid move from an area of higher concentration to an area of lower concentration, resulting in an even distribution of the particles in the fluid.

Generally, absorption takes place in the digestive system unless an agent is administered directly into the bloodstream by injection into veins, arteries, muscles, or other injection sites. Water solubility is best for drug dissolution in the stomach, while lipid solubility is best for absorption. Therefore, most drugs are weak acids or weak bases, which dissolve easily for absorption. Often, drugs are formulated as salts such as morphine sulfate or potassium penicillin, improving water solubility with no negative effects upon absorption or altering other drug characteristics. When the drug is injected directly into the bloodstream and distributes throughout the body, it acts rapidly and the process of absorption is bypassed.

When drugs are given orally, the small intestine is the primary site of absorption because of the very large surface area across which drugs may diffuse. Drugs are then immediately exposed to metabolism by enzymes in the liver before reaching the systemic circulation. This exposure, called the **first-pass effect**, results in the drug being partly metabolized before becoming available to the body for systemic effects.

POINTS TO REMEMBER

Medications that are metabolized too rapidly in the liver cannot be given orally due to the first-pass effect.

DRUG DISTRIBUTION

The process by which drug molecules leave the bloodstream and enter the tissues of the body is called **distribution**. When a drug reaches the bloodstream, it is ready to travel through blood, lymphatics, and other fluids to its site of action. To reach sites beyond the major organs, a drug may have to pass over the lipid membranes. The rate of distribution is highly dependent on the blood flow to various organs as well as lipid solubility. Organs with higher blood flow, including the heart, liver, and kidneys, receive larger amounts of a drug more quickly than organs with lower blood flow, such as fat, muscles, and peripheral tissues. Another factor is the amount of binding with plasma and tissue proteins. Drugs bind at different degrees to plasma proteins, such as albumin. Two drugs that are highly plasma protein-bound can compete for identical binding sites, causing high concentrations of unbound, pharmacologically active drugs. An example of competing drugs includes the antiseizure medications known as *phenytoin* and *valproic acid*.

DRUG METABOLISM

The overwhelming majority of drugs undergo **metabolism** after they enter the body. Most drugs are acted upon by enzymes in the body and are converted to metabolic derivatives during metabolism. The process of conversion is called **biotransformation**. In most cases, biotransformation can terminate the pharmacological action of the drug and increase removal of the drug from the body. The liver is the major site of biotransformation. In phase I metabolism, the liver produces enzymes that metabolize drugs, making them more water soluble and easier to eliminate. Chemical reactions result in a metabolite that is actually a different molecule from the parent drug. In phase II metabolism, a drug or a phase I metabolite is joined (conjugated) with a molecule of the body, such as glucuronides, glutathione, or sulfate. An example is when aspirin undergoes **conjugation** into salicylic acid, which is conjugated with glucoronide via phase II metabolism.

Numerous enzymes, which biotransform many drugs, are present in the endoplasmic reticulum. One of these enzymes is cytochrome P-450, present throughout the body, which has a very important role in drug metabolism. Cytochrome P-450 is present in highest concentrations in the liver and intestines. Several enzymes may also metabolize a drug. Drug metabolism influences drug action such as duration of drug effects, drug interactions, drug activation, and drug toxicity. Drugs that are water soluble can be removed from the body most easily, mostly via metabolism by liver enzymes and excretion through the kidneys.

DRUG EXCRETION

Excretion is the process of eliminating drugs from the body. Drugs may be excreted from the body in many forms, including urine, feces, saliva, sweat, breast milk, breath, and tears. However, the kidney is the major site of excretion for most drugs, involving three processes. These are glomerular filtration, tubular secretion, and tubular reabsorption. Glomerular filtration and tubular secretion actually remove drugs from the body, while tubular reabsorption prevents drugs from being excreted into the urine. Drugs that are lipophilic and non-ionized are reabsorbed from the glomerular filtrate back into the bloodstream. On the contrary, hydrophilic and ionized drugs are not reabsorbed but excreted. Cellular transporters and urine pH additionally affect drug reabsorption. Glomerular filtration is affected by blood pressure, dehydration, extreme blood loss, heart failure, and nonsteroidal anti-inflammatory drugs. Drugs can compete with each other for secretion, such as when probenecid competes with cellular transporters for penicillin. Changing urine pH can alter excretion. Drugs that are weakly acidic become more ionized when the urine is alkaline. Drugs that are ionized are not reabsorbed back into the bloodstream and are excreted with the urine. For example, if a patient takes too much aspirin, intravenous sodium bicarbonate is administered. This alkalinizes the urine and a larger amount of aspirin, since it is a weak acid, will remain ionized. Then it cannot be reabsorbed, and the toxic levels of aspirin will be reduced.

Pharmacodynamics

Pharmacodynamics is the study of the biochemical and physiological effects of drugs. It is also defined as the study of the mechanism of action of drugs. A basic understanding of the factors that control drug concentration at the site of action is important for the optimal use of drugs. To fully understand medication actions in the body, the pharmacy technician must understand the basics of pharmacodynamics.

DRUG ACTION

Drugs produce their effects by altering the normal function of the cells and tissues of the body. Correct cells are chosen because a particular drug has a **specific affinity** for a particular recipient site, which is usually located on the surface of the cell. This recipient site is called a **receptor**, and the drug that attaches to it and produces a functional change in the cell is known as an **agonist** (Figure 19-2). Not all drugs that bind to specific cells cause a functional change in the target cell. Some drugs act as antagonists to the natural process by binding to cells and blocking a sequence of biochemical events from occurring.

Various factors need to be considered in determining the correct drugs for a patient. These include drug half-life, diurnal body rhythms, psychological factors, drug toxicity, and possible side effects.

Drug Half-Life

The **half-life** of a drug is the time it takes for the plasma concentration to be reduced by 50%. This is one of the most common methods used to explain drug actions. The half-life of each drug given to a patient may differ; thus, a drug with a short half-life, such as 2 or 3 hours, will need to be administered more often than one with a long half-life, such as 8 hours. Another important factor when considering a drug's half-life is bioavailability. **Bioavailability** is a term that indicates measurement of both the rate of drug absorption and total amount of drug that reaches the systemic blood circulation from an administered dosage form.

POINTS TO REMEMBER

If a drug has a half-life of 4 hours, half of the drug's potency has diminished in 4 hours. In 4 more hours, half of the remaining potency has diminished, and so forth.

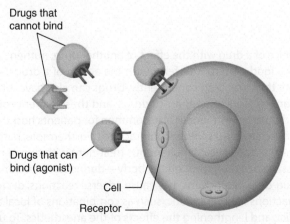

Figure 19-2 Cell receptor and agonist.

Diurnal Body Rhythms

Diurnal (during the day) body rhythms play an important role in the effects of some drugs. For example, sedatives given in the morning will not be as effective as those administered before bedtime. On the other hand, the preferred time for corticosteroid administration is in the morning, because this best mimics the body's natural pattern of corticosteroid production and elimination.

Psychological Factors

Psychological factors involve how patients feel about the drug(s) prescribed for them and the different ways they respond to them. If an individual believes in the therapy, even a **placebo**—a simulated medication that contains no active ingredients—may help to bring relief. Some patients cooperate in following the directions for a specific drug, others do not, and a patient's mental attitude can reduce or increase an expected response to a drug.

Drug Toxicity

Almost all drugs are capable of producing toxic effects. There is a range between the therapeutic dose of a drug and its toxic dose. This range is measured by the therapeutic index, which is used to explain the safety of the drug. The therapeutic index is expressed in the form of a ratio: therapeutic index (TI) = LD50/ED50, where LD50 is the lethal dose of a drug that will kill 50% of animals tested and ED50 is the effective dose that produces a specific therapeutic effect in 50% of animals tested. The greater the therapeutic index, the safer the drug.

Side Effects and Adverse Effects of Drugs

Side effects are usually defined as mild, but annoying, responses to a medication. **Adverse reactions** or **adverse effects** usually are characterized as more severe symptoms or problems that develop due to the administration of a drug. Adverse effects may require the patient to be hospitalized or may even pose a threat to the patient's life. Examples of problematic side effects are hyperactivity or inability to sleep, bleeding, nephrotoxicity, or hepatotoxicity.

Idiosyncratic Reactions   When a patient has experienced a unique, strange, or unpredicted reaction to a drug, this is termed an **idiosyncratic reaction**.

Hypersensitivity or Allergy   Allergies or **hypersensitivity reactions** are another type of unpredictable reaction caused in some patients by drugs such as aspirin, penicillin, or sulfa products. Hypersensitivity reactions generally occur when a patient has received a drug, and his or her body has developed antibodies against it. After this process of antibody production, if the patient is exposed to the drug again, the antigen-antibody reaction produces itching, hives, rash, or swelling of the skin. This is a common type of allergic reaction.

Anaphylactic Reaction   An **anaphylactic reaction** to a drug is a severe form of allergic reaction that is life-threatening. The patient develops severe shortness of breath and may even have cardiac collapse. An anaphylactic reaction is a true medical emergency because the patient may exhibit paralysis of the diaphragm, swelling of the oropharynx, and an inability to breathe.

Mechanism of Drug Interaction

A **drug interaction** is an interference of a drug with the effect of another drug, nutrient, or laboratory test. In addition, a drug interaction is possible if a food or herb interferes with the action of a drug. Drug interaction is usually the result of a patient receiving more than one drug concurrently. Drugs can also have interactions with certain disease states. Surgical patients commonly receive more than 10 drugs, and these patients often experience the effects of several drugs at once. Multiple-drug administration is also common for patients hospitalized for infections and other disorders. The aging process also increases risks for drug interactions. Furthermore, patients may have more than one unrelated disorder, which means that they need simultaneous treatment with two or more drugs. Drug interactions may occur at any step in the passage of a drug through the body—during its liberation, absorption, distribution, biotransformation, or excretion. Drug-drug interactions may cause adverse reactions, decreased therapeutic benefits, or harm to the patient. Some interactions are therapeutic, such as combinations of local anesthetics with epinephrine, causing blood vessels to constrict, and lengthening the effects of the anesthetics. To understand the mechanism of drug interaction, it is essential to look at three effects associated with it: synergism, potentiation, and antagonism.

SYNERGISM

Synergism refers to the cooperative effect of two or more drugs given together to produce a stronger effect than that of either drug given alone. When two drugs with similar actions are taken, the effect of the drugs will be double. Sometimes synergism is desirable; for example, when meperidine (Demerol®) is given for pain along with promethazine (Phenergan®), which is used as an antiemetic and sedative. Synergism is a problem when the drug combination produces undesirable effects that are dangerous to the body. An example is the combination of warfarin sodium (Coumadin®) and aspirin, which causes an excessive risk of hemorrhage because the two together can potentiate blood loss. Another example is the combination of nitrates such as nitroglycerine with erectile dysfunction drugs such as sildenafil. This combination may cause a potentially life-threatening reduction in blood pressure.

POTENTIATION

Potentiation occurs when one drug prolongs the effects of another drug. An example is the combination of acetaminophen (Tylenol®) and codeine for pain relief or fever reduction. Desirable potentiation is a wanted effect used to build up a drug level in the body or to prolong its effect; for instance, the combination of penicillin and probenecid is given to prolong the excretion time of penicillin in the body. When toxic effects occur from drug potentiation, the potentiation is undesirable. An example is the use of cimetidine (Tagamet®) for a stomach disorder and theophylline to assist in relieving asthma. Cimetidine increases serum levels of theophylline.

ANTAGONISM

Antagonism occurs when two drugs decrease each other's effects. This may occur at the receptor level or by other mechanisms of action. For example, ibuprofen and aspirin, when taken together, stop each other's action. Antagonism may be desirable to stop the effects of a medication. Another example is the use of activated charcoal to stop the effect of syrup of ipecac for a drug overdose or poisoning. Undesirable antagonism is the unwanted cancelation of drug actions. An example is in the use of tetracycline and antacids together. Because tetracycline is partially absorbed from the stomach and upper gastrointestinal (GI) tract, antacids can inhibit the gastric absorption of tetracycline.

Causes of Drug Interaction

A number of factors may be associated with drug interaction. These include multiple pharmacological effects, multiple prescribers, nonprescription drug use, patient noncompliance, and drug abuse.

MULTIPLE PHARMACOLOGICAL EFFECTS

Many drugs used currently have the capacity to influence many physiological systems. For example, combined therapy with a phenothiazine antipsychotic (such as chlorpromazine), a tricyclic antidepressant (amitriptyline), and an anti-Parkinson's agent (trihexyphenidyl) is used in some patients. Each of these agents has a different primary effect; however, all three possess anticholinergic activity. Even though the anticholinergic effect of any one of the drugs may be slight, the additive effects of the three agents may be significant. An **additive effect** is the combined effect of more than one agent, which is equal to the sum of the effects of each drug taken alone. An example is when sleep medications are taken after alcohol has been ingested, which can cause much more drowsiness than the sleep medications would have on their own—potentially to dangerous levels.

WHAT WOULD YOU DO?

During the Christmas holidays, a pharmacy technician went to see her family. Her grandmother said that she needed to take more multivitamins because she lacked energy and asked her granddaughter her opinion. If you were this pharmacy technician, what would you do?

MULTIPLE PRESCRIBERS

Sometimes an individual sees more than one physician for health care or two or more specialists in addition to a family physician. It can be difficult for any one of these physicians to be aware of all the drugs that have been prescribed by the others for this patient. For example, one prescriber may give an antihistamine to a patient and another physician may prescribe an antianxiety agent, with the possible consequence of an excessive depressant effect from the two drugs.

Many patients, especially those who are elderly, take several medicines each day. The term **polypharmacy**, which means "many drugs," refers to taking multiple medications for necessary or unnecessary reasons. The chance for individuals to develop an undesired drug interaction increases rapidly with the number of drugs used. One drug may interact with another to increase, decrease, or stop the effects of the other drug.

POINTS TO REMEMBER

Even though a patient may be seeing different physicians, he or she often has all prescriptions dispensed by the same pharmacy. Therefore, the pharmacy technician plays an important role in the detection and prevention of drug-related problems.

WHAT WOULD YOU DO?

A 76-year-old man told his grandson, who was a pharmacy technician, that he was taking four different medications. He then asked his grandson if he could take them all at once, upon going to bed, rather than throughout the day. If you were this pharmacy technician, what would you do?

NONPRESCRIPTION DRUG USE

Sometimes patients neglect to mention the nonprescription medications they have purchased when their physician questions them about medications they are taking. When patients take over-the-counter drugs such as antacids, analgesics, and laxatives for long periods in a routine manner, they may not consider them to be drugs. This increases the likelihood that interactions will occur. Because many individuals fill their prescriptions at their local pharmacy but purchase nonprescription drugs elsewhere, identification of potential problems can be extremely difficult for the pharmacist as well as for the physician. For these reasons, patients should be encouraged to obtain both their prescription and nonprescription medications at a pharmacy.

POINTS TO REMEMBER

Many reports of drug interactions involve the concurrent use of a prescription drug with nonprescription drugs such as aspirin, antacids, decongestants, and herbal supplements (such as St. John's wort).

PATIENT NONCOMPLIANCE

For a variety of reasons, many patients do not take medication in the manner intended by the prescriber. Sometimes patients receive inadequate instruction about how to take their medications. Older patients, who may be taking five or six medications, can forget to take all or some of them. Upon realizing they have forgotten to take a dose of medication, some patients double the next dose to make up for the missing one.

DRUG ABUSE

The tendencies of some individuals to abuse or deliberately misuse drugs also may lead to an increased incidence of drug interactions. Opioids, barbiturates, analgesics, and amphetamines are among the agents most often abused, and the inappropriate use of these drugs can result in many problems, including an increased potential for drug interaction.

WHAT WOULD YOU DO?

Amanda is a pharmacy technician. Her brother had chronic insomnia and had been taking diazepam for six months. He began developing tolerance to the drug over time, and then asked Amanda if he could get a stronger medication or combine the diazepam with alcohol. If you were Amanda, what would you do?

Patient Variables that Affect Drug Interaction

Many factors can influence the response to a drug in humans. These factors may predispose a patient to the development of adverse effects to a drug, and it can be anticipated that many of these considerations also apply to the development of drug interactions. Examples of these factors are discussed in the following sections.

AGE

Age is always an important factor in the risk of drug interaction. Studies indicate that there is an increased incidence of adverse drug reactions in both young and elderly patients, and, thus, the occurrence of drug interactions also is highest in these patient groups.

Drug-related problems in young patients are encountered most commonly in newborn infants. Newborn infants do not have fully developed enzyme systems. A system of enzymes called **cytochrome P-450** has been identified as the factor that contributes to many drug interactions. Cytochrome P-450 plays a key role in the oxidative biotransformation of drugs. The enzymes are involved in the metabolism of certain drugs. Newborn infants also have immature renal function, which plays a part in drug-related problems.

Most elderly patients have at least one chronic illness, for example, diabetes or hypertension. Renal disorders may also contribute to an altered drug response, and increased sensitivity to the action of certain drugs occurs with advancing age. The factor of age also has a role in the absorption, distribution, metabolism, and excretion of certain drugs, which increases the possibility of adverse drug reactions and drug interactions.

MEDICATION ERROR ALERT

Some elderly patients have cognitive deficits that put them at risk for taking incorrect dosages of prescribed medications. They may forget to take their medication on time, or they may double the doses for a single day because they forget having already taken them. The prescription drugs that are most often involved in patient deaths include opioids, benzodiazepines, antidepressants, drugs used for epilepsy, and drugs used for Parkinson's disease. In three out of four benzodiazepine deaths, patients also had opioids in their system.

GENETIC FACTORS

Genetic factors may be responsible for the development of an unexpected drug response in some patients. For example, an acetylation process, the rate of which appears to be under genetic control, metabolizes isoniazid. Some patients metabolize isoniazid rapidly, whereas others metabolize it slowly. Isoniazid may cause peripheral neuritis in some patients, and this effect has been noted most commonly in people termed slow acetylators (because their metabolism of substances derived from radicals of acetic acid is slow). Isoniazid may inhibit the metabolism of phenytoin, which can result in nystagmus, ataxia, and lethargy.

DISEASES AND CONDITIONS OF PATIENTS

Some diseases influence a patient's responses to a particular drug. Impaired renal function and hepatic function are the most important conditions that may alter drug activity and cause drug interactions.

DIET

Food often may affect the rate and extent of absorption of drugs from the GI tract. For example, many antibiotics should be taken at least 1 hour before or 2 hours after meals to achieve optimal absorption. The type of food that is eaten may have important effects on the absorption of concurrently administered drugs. For example, dietary items such as milk and other dairy products that contain calcium may decrease the absorption of tetracycline and fluoroquinolone derivatives by combining with them in the GI tract to produce a complex that is absorbed poorly. Grapefruit juice has been found to affect many different drugs—specifically those drugs that are metabolized by cytochrome P-450 in the liver and the wall of the GI tract. Based on current data, the following drugs should not be given concurrently with grapefruit juice:

- Estrogens
- Cyclosporine
- Midazolam
- Triazolam
- All calcium channel blockers
- Simvastatin

The toxicity of some drugs increases when the drugs interact with foods such as wine, cheese, or yogurt. Any patient taking a monoamine oxidase (MAO) inhibitor (an antidepressant) should avoid these foods because of the potential toxic effects. Medications that stimulate the central nervous system may cause a toxic stimulation if caffeine or caffeine-containing foods are also consumed. The combination of potassium-sparing diuretics and salt substitutes can result in dangerously high blood potassium levels. Aluminum-based antacids taken with citrus juices (such as orange juice) result in excess absorption of the aluminum. Vegetables such as broccoli, cabbage, or Brussels sprouts may inactivate anticoagulants such as warfarin sodium because they contain vitamin K. Table 19-1 shows some examples of the most common food and drug interactions that are considered to be of greatest clinical significance. For more information about common drug and food interactions, refer to the *Physician's Desk Reference* and other reference books.

Table 19.1 Clinically Significant Drug or Food Interactions

Drugs	Interactions	Nature of Interaction
Acetaminophen	Carbamazepine	Increases acetaminophen breakdown
		Increases risk of hepatotoxicity
	Oral contraceptives	Decreases acetaminophen effects
Aminoglycosides	Penicillins	Decreases aminoglycoside effects
Anticholinergics (cholinergic-blocking agents)	Antacids	Decreases absorption of anticholinergics
	Antihistamines	Increases anticholinergic side effects
	Corticosteroids	Increases intraocular pressure
Anticoagulants (oral)	Aspirin	Increases effects of anticoagulants by decreasing plasma protein binding
	Oral contraceptives	Decreases anticoagulant effects
	Thyroid preparations	Increases anticoagulant effects

(Continued)

Table 19.1 Clinically Significant Drug or Food Interactions (*Continued*)

Antidepressants	Oral contraceptives	Decreases antidepressant effects
Antidiabetic drugs	Alcohol	Possible disulfiram-like syndrome
	Anticoagulants	Increases hypoglycemic action
	Estrogens	Decreases hypoglycemic effects
Antihypertensives	Garlic	Increases antihypertensive effects
Antipsychotic agents (phenothiazines)	Alcohol	Potentiates action of phenothiazines
	Lithium	Increases extrapyramidal effects
	MAO inhibitors	Increases phenothiazine effects
Aspirin	Alcohol	Increases risk of GI bleeding associated with use of aspirin
	Antacids	Decreases salicylate levels due to increased rate of renal excretion
	Ascorbic acid (vitamin C)	Increases effects of aspirin
Atenolol	Anticholinergics	Increases effects of atenolol
Benzodiazepines	Antacids	Decreases absorption of benzodiazepines
	Opiates	Additive central nervous system effects
	Oral contraceptives	Increases benzodiazepine effects
Beta-adrenergic blocking agents	Anesthetic agents	Increases depression of myocardium
	Aspirin	Decreases action of beta-adrenergic blocking agents by inhibiting prostaglandin
	Epinephrine	Increases blood pressure
Calcium channel blockers (CCBs)	Cimetidine	Increases effects of CCBs
	Fentanyl	Severe hypotensive crisis
	Ranitidine	Increases effects of CCBs
Cephalosporins	Alcohol	Disulfiram-type responses
	Aminoglycosides	Increases risk of nephrotoxicity
	Antacids	Decreases effects of cefaclor, cefdinir, and cefpodoxime
Ciprofloxacin	Aluminum and magnesium hydroxides	Reduces ciprofloxacin absorption
	Iron supplements	Reduces ciprofloxacin absorption
Clonidine	Propranolol	Rapid discontinuation can cause hypertensive crisis
Digoxin	Antacids	Decreases digoxin levels; administer at least 1.5 hours before antacids
	Ibuprofen	Increases risk of digoxin toxicity
	Insulin	Use with caution because of effects on potassium levels
Diuretics	Anticholinergics	Increases thiazide effects
	Corticosteroids	Enhances potassium loss

(Continued)

Table 19.1 Clinically Significant Drug or Food Interactions (*Continued*)

Drugs	Interactions	Nature of Interaction
Potassium-sparing	Indomethacin	Decreases diuretic effects
	Potassium supplements	Hyperkalemia
Doxycycline	Carbamazepine	Decreases doxycycline effect
	Phenobarbital	Decreases doxycycline effect
	Phenytoin	Decreases doxycycline effect
Estrogen	Barbiturates	Decreases estrogen effects
	Rifampin	Decreases estrogen effects
Heparin	Aspirin	Because of increased platelet aggregation by aspirin, concomitant use may increase risk of bleeding
	Garlic	Increases antiplatelet effects
	Nonsteroidal anti-inflammatory drugs	Increases risk of bleeding
Hypoglycemics (oral)	Aspirin	Increases hypoglycemic action
Insulin	Alcohol	Increases hypoglycemic effect and risk of insulin shock
	Propranolol	Inhibits rebound of serum glucose after insulin-induced hypoglycemia
	Tetracyclines	Increases hypoglycemic effects
Isoniazid	Corticosteroids	Decreases isoniazid effects
Nifedipine	Cimetidine	May cause up to an 80% increase in nifedipine blood levels, which can result in hypotensive crisis
Nitroglycerin	Aspirin	May cause hypotension
Nonsteroidal anti-inflammatory drugs (NSAIDs)	Aspirin	May decrease serum levels of NSAIDs
	Loop diuretics	Decreases NSAID effects
	Phenobarbital	Decreases NSAID effects
Oral contraceptives	Penicillins	Decreases contraceptive effects
	Phenobarbital	Decreases contraceptive effects
	Tetracyclines	Decreases contraceptive effects
Penicillins	Antacids	Decreases penicillin effects
	Aspirin	Increases penicillin effects
	Tetracyclines	Decreases penicillin effects
Propranolol	Indomethacin	Decreases propranolol effects
	Nicotine	Decreases propranolol serum levels
Spironolactone	Aspirin	Decreases diuretic effect
Sulfonamides	Anticoagulants	Increases sulfonamide effects
	Aspirin	Increases sulfonamide effects
	Diuretics, thiazide	Increases risk of thrombocytopenia

(Continued)

Table 19.1 Clinically Significant Drug or Food Interactions (*Continued*)

Drugs	Interactions	Nature of Interaction
Tetracyclines	Antacids	Decreases tetracycline effects
	Iron preparations	Decreases tetracycline effects
	Lithium	May increase or decrease tetracycline effects
Theophylline	Barbiturates	Decreases theophylline levels
	Caffeine	Increases theophylline levels
	Nicotine	Decreases theophylline levels
Thyroid hormones	Estrogens	Decreases thyroid effects
	Salicylates	Decreases thyroid effects by competing with thyroid-binding sites on proteins
	Soy	Decreases absorption of thyroid hormones, so space at least 2 hours apart
Warfarin	Amiodarone	Increases warfarin effect
	Carbamazepine	Decreases warfarin effect
	Erythromycin	Increases warfarin effect
	Phenobarbital	Increases warfarin effect

ALCOHOL CONSUMPTION

Chronic use of alcoholic beverages may increase the rate of metabolism of drugs such as warfarin, phenytoin, and tolbutamide, probably by increasing the activity of liver enzymes. Conversely, acute use of alcohol by individuals who are not chronic drinkers may cause inhibition of hepatic enzymes.

Concurrent use of alcoholic beverages with sedatives and other depressant drugs can result in an excessive depressant response. The use of such combinations on a regular basis cannot be a reason for failing to exercise the caution that must be observed if problems are to be averted.

POINTS TO REMEMBER

Individuals who consume alcoholic beverages should avoid taking acetaminophen at least 3 hours before or after drinking, because this drug can cause severe liver damage when alcohol is used.

MEDICATION ERROR ALERT

The combination of alcohol with prescription medications is never a good idea. Many prescription drug users who are not addicted to their medications, or are dependent upon them, consume alcohol concurrently. Mixtures of anesthetics, antianxiety agents, and analgesics are particularly dangerous with alcohol. The combined effects of these agents with alcohol can cause respiratory failure, paralysis, and death. This interaction is a growing concern in the field of pharmacy and an important area for both pharmacists and pharmacy technicians to educate patients.

SMOKING

A number of investigations have suggested that smoking increases the activity of drug-metabolizing enzymes in the liver. As a result, certain therapeutic agents such as diazepam, theophylline, chlorpromazine, and amitriptyline are metabolized more rapidly, and their effect is decreased. This response may be more pronounced in young and middle-aged individuals than in older patients.

Reducing the Risk of Drug Interaction

Reducing the risk of drug interactions is a challenge for both health care providers and pharmacy staff. Although they could be applied to drug therapy in general, the following guidelines are offered to assist health professionals who have the responsibility of selecting and monitoring therapeutic regimens.

IDENTIFY PATIENT RISK FACTORS

Factors such as age, the nature of the patient's medical problems (e.g., impaired renal function), dietary habits, smoking, and problems such as alcoholism will influence the effects of certain drugs. These factors should be considered during the initial patient interview.

OBTAIN A DRUG HISTORY

An accurate and complete record of the prescription and nonprescription medications as well as herbal products and dietary supplements a patient is taking must be obtained. Numerous interactions have resulted from a lack of awareness of prescription medications prescribed by another physician or nonprescription medications the patient did not consider important enough to mention.

BE KNOWLEDGEABLE ABOUT THE ACTIONS OF DRUGS

Knowledge of the properties, including the primary and secondary pharmacological actions of each of the agents used or being considered for use, is essential if the interaction potential is to be assessed accurately.

CONSIDER THERAPEUTIC ALTERNATIVES

In the majority of cases, two drugs that are known to interact can be administered concurrently as long as adequate precautions are taken, for example, closer monitoring of therapy or dosage adjustments to compensate for the altered response. However, if another agent with similar therapeutic properties and a lesser risk of interacting is available, it should be used.

REFRAIN FROM ADMINISTERING COMPLEX THERAPEUTIC REGIMENS

The number of medications used should be kept to a minimum. In addition, the use of medications or dosage regimens that require less frequent administration may help avoid interactions that result from an alteration of absorption, for example, when a drug is administered close to mealtime.

EDUCATE THE PATIENT

Most patients know little about their illnesses and the benefits or problems that could result from drug therapy. Individuals who are aware of and understand this information can be expected to comply better with the instructions for administering medications and be more attentive to the development of symptoms that could be early indicators of drug-related problems. Patients should be encouraged to ask questions about their therapy and to report any excessive or unexpected responses. There should be no uncertainty on the part of patients about how to use their medications in the most effective and safest way.

MEDICATION ERROR ALERT

To prevent medication errors, patient education is highly encouraged. Patients must be encouraged to actively participate in their own health outcomes, learn about their conditions, put questions to health care professionals for more information, maintain strong and trusting relationships with their physicians, find out why a new medication is required, and always ask to read their own test results. All of these methods are suggested to reduce medication errors by making patients take a more active and informed role in their treatments.

Summary

Some drug-related problems develop unexpectedly and cannot be predicted; many others are related to known pharmaceutical actions of the drugs and can be reasonably anticipated. However, as drug therapy becomes more complex and because many patients are being treated with two or more drugs, the ability to predict the magnitude of a specific action of any given drug diminishes. Maintaining complete and current medication records for patients is essential. The pharmacist is in a unique position to meet these needs to supervise drug therapy and prevent problems. Many drug-related problems are caused by drug interactions. A number of factors may be associated with drug interactions. Multiple prescribers, consumption of nonprescription drugs, patient noncompliance, drug abuse, and patient variables (such as age, genetic factors, diseases, diet, alcohol consumption, and smoking) are factors that are known to cause drug interactions.

Pharmacists, physicians, and other health care workers can prevent some of these problems by being knowledgeable about the actions of drugs, considering therapeutic alternatives, refraining from administering complex therapeutic regimens, and educating the patient. Pharmacists and pharmacy technicians have a valuable opportunity to make significant contributions to further enhance the efficacy and safety of drug therapy.

REVIEW QUESTIONS

1. The cooperative effect of two or more drugs given together to produce a stronger effect than that of the drugs given alone is known as:

   A. potentiation.
   B. synergism.
   C. antagonism.
   D. noncompliance.

2. Drug-related problems in young patients are encountered most commonly in which of the following age groups?

   A. Newborns
   B. School age
   C. Toddlers
   D. Teenagers

3. Which of the following explains the movement of drugs throughout the body and includes absorption, distribution, metabolism, and excretion?

   A. Pharmacodynamics
   B. Pharmacokinetics
   C. Pharmacotherapy
   D. Pharmacology

4. In which of the following forms is a drug most easily excreted?

   A. Nonionized form
   B. Protein-bound form
   C. Fat-soluble form
   D. Water-soluble form

5. How does a drug cause a pharmacologic effect to occur?

   A. It must be absorbed in the stomach.
   B. It must be given intravenously.
   C. It must bind to a cell receptor.
   D. It must stimulate the heart.

6. What is the term used to describe the phase II metabolic process of a drug being jointed to a molecule that was produced by the body?

    A. Catabolism
    B. Conjugation
    C. Integration
    D. Anabolism

7. Any patient taking a MAO inhibitor should avoid which of the following foods?

    A. Seafood
    B. Yogurt
    C. Tea
    D. Broccoli

8. Which of the following processes keep drugs from being excreted with the urine?

    A. Tubular reabsorption
    B. Tubular secretion
    C. Creatinine clearance
    D. Glomerular filtration

9. Which of the following enzymes has been identified as the factor that may contribute to many drug interactions?

    A. Lipase
    B. Pepsin
    C. Enterokinase
    D. Cytochrome P-450

10. Which of the following organs produces the majority of enzymes that metabolize drugs?

    A. Kidneys
    B. Liver
    C. Lungs
    D. Pancreas

11. Which of the following is true about drug interactions?

    A. They require consideration of patient and drug-specific factors to determine actual risks.
    B. No two drugs should ever be taken at the same time.
    C. When an interaction occurs, it will be clinically significant.
    D. All interactions can be harmful, causing adverse effects.

12. Newborn infants are most at risk for drug interaction because of their:

    A. large skulls.
    B. large hearts.
    C. immature bone marrow function.
    D. immature renal function.

13. Which of the following means any unexpected, unintended, undesired, or excessive response to a drug?

    A. Overdose
    B. Drug-drug interaction
    C. Adverse drug reaction
    D. Drug toxicity

14. What effect does smoking have upon the activity of drug-metabolizing enzymes in the liver, resulting in a decreased effect of drugs such as diazepam and theophylline?

    A.   Smoking decreases activity

    B.   Smoking potentiates activity

    C.   Smoking increases activity

    D.   Smoking inhibits activity

15. When two drugs decrease the effects of each other, it is known as:

    A.   potentiation.

    B.   synergism.

    C.   agonism.

    D.   antagonism.

CRITICAL THINKING

A 25-year-old woman had chlamydia with vaginal discharge. Her gynecologist ordered tetracycline for 10 days. After 10 days, the patient had not improved. She returned to the gynecologist's office, complaining of the same signs and symptoms. The gynecologist asked about her daily consumption of milk, yogurt, and other dairy products. He or she explained that tetracycline was contraindicated with these foods because it interacts with calcium.

1. What interactions occur between tetracycline and other drugs such as insulin and oral contraceptives?

2. How do dairy products containing calcium interfere with tetracycline?

WEB LINKS

Food Medication Interactions: www.foodmedinteractions.com

Hansten and Horn Drug Interactions: www.hanstenandhorn.com

Healthline—Drug Interactions: www.healthline.com/health/drug-interactions

National Council on Alcoholism and Drug Dependence, Inc.: www.ncadd.org

National Institute on Drug Abuse: www.drugabuse.gov

The Good Drugs Guide: www.thegooddrugsguide.com

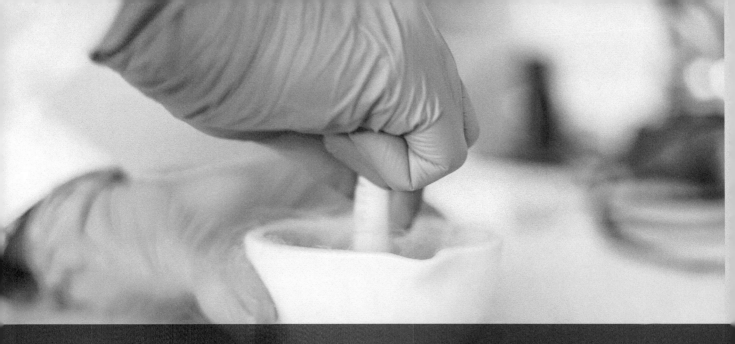

MEDICATION EFFECTS ON BODY SYSTEMS

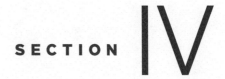

SECTION IV

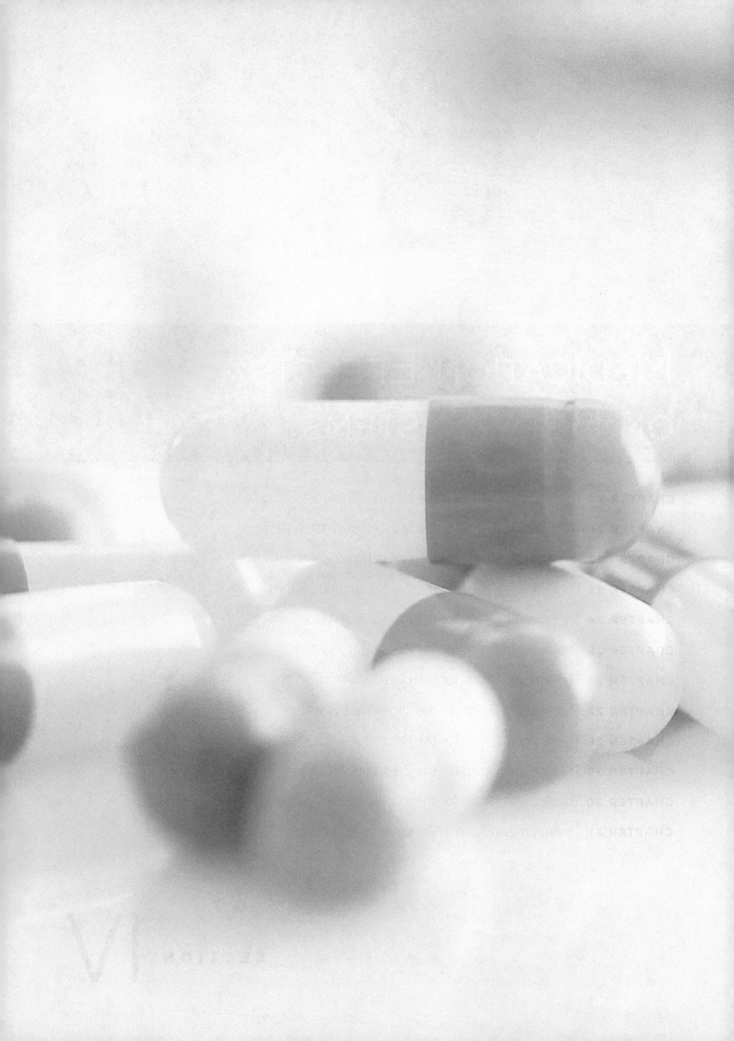

CHAPTER 20

Therapeutic Drugs for the Nervous System

OUTLINE

OBJECTIVES

Upon completion of this chapter, the reader should be able to:

1. Describe the structures and functions of the nervous system.
2. Distinguish between the sympathetic and parasympathetic divisions of the autonomic nervous system (ANS).
3. Describe neurons and their functions.
4. Describe neurotransmitters.
5. Discuss drugs used for migraine headaches.
6. Explain the main drugs used to treat epilepsy.

7. Describe the causes and major signs and symptoms of Parkinson's disease.

8. Describe the cause of Alzheimer's disease and its treatments.

9. Describe schizophrenia and the common drugs used for treatment.

10. List the trade names of the selective serotonin reuptake inhibitors (SSRIs).

KEY TERMS

acetylcholine (ACh)	homeostasis	myelin	sedation
anxiety	hyperpyrexia	neurohormone	sedatives
Bell's palsy	hypnosis	neuron	
corpus callosum	hypnotic	opiates	
headache	multiple sclerosis	opioids	

Overview

The nervous system consists of the interconnected neurons of the brain, spinal cord, and nerves. Neurons carry electrical impulses throughout the body for the control and regulation of activities.

Nervous System

The nervous system is composed of the brain, spinal cord, and nerves (see Figure 20-1). It is divided into two sections: the central nervous system (CNS) and the peripheral nervous system (PNS).

CENTRAL NERVOUS SYSTEM

The CNS is located in the dorsal cavity of the body, which consists of the cranial cavity (enclosing the brain) and the spinal cavity (containing the spinal cord). Together, the brain and spinal cord comprise the CNS. The CNS receives information from the afferent division of the PNS. It sends instructions to the rest of the body via the efferent division of the PNS.

The brain is subdivided into the cerebrum, diencephalon, brain stem, and cerebellum (see Figure 20-2). The cerebrum consists of two cerebral hemispheres, connected by the **corpus callosum**. The cerebrum is the largest portion of the brain. The diencephalon contains the thalamus (which relays incoming sensory impulses) and the hypothalamus (which maintains **homeostasis**). The brain stem consists of the midbrain, pons, and medulla oblongata. The medulla oblongata is the major center for the autonomic control of blood pressure, heart rate, breathing, and digestive activities. The cerebellum, consisting of two hemispheres, coordinates skeletal muscle movements and maintains equilibrium.

POINTS TO REMEMBER

The hypothalamus, which is a part of the diencephalon, controls the endocrine system by secreting hormones that regulate the activity of the anterior pituitary gland. It also secretes several important hormones, including oxytocin and antidiuretic hormone.

MEDICAL TERMINOLOGY REVIEW

homeostasis:

home/o = *same*

stasis = *control*

control of a stable environment

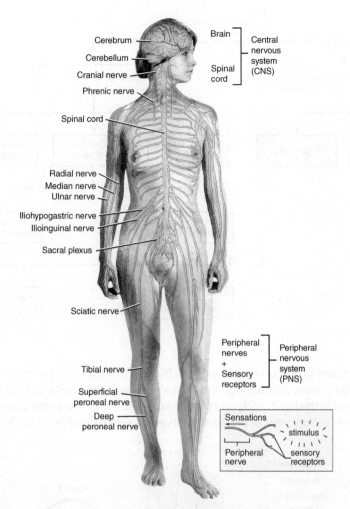

Figure 20-1 The nervous system.

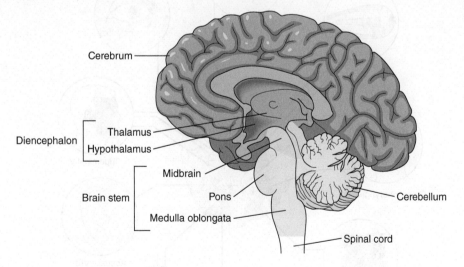

Figure 20-2 The principal parts of the brain.

PERIPHERAL NERVOUS SYSTEM

The PNS is outside the CNS and connects the CNS to the remainder of the body. The combined parts of the nervous system control sensory functions, integrative functions, and motor functions. Subdivision of these two systems is summarized in Figure 20-3.

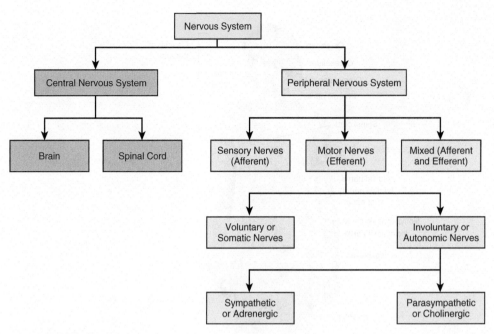

Figure 20-3 Organization of the nervous system.

The PNS consists of cranial and spinal nerves. These nerves branch from the brain and spinal cord to all body parts. The PNS is subdivided into the somatic and autonomic nervous systems (ANS). Twelve pairs of cranial nerves connect the brain to various structures in the head, neck, and trunk (see Figure 20-4). Thirty-one pairs of spinal nerves originate from the spinal cord. Primary functions of the cranial nerves are summarized in Table 20-1.

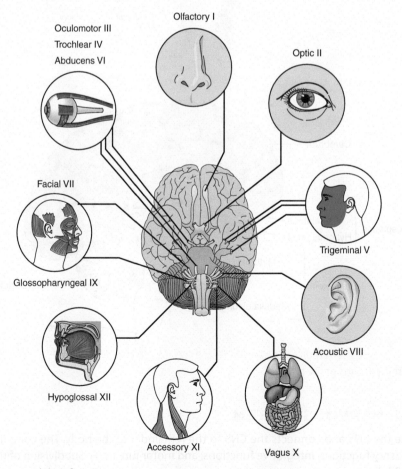

Figure 20-4 Cranial nerves and their functions.

Table 20-1 Classifications of Cranial Nerves and Their Functions

Name, Number	Functions
Olfactory (I)	Sensory (special sensory: smell). Mucous membranes in the nose send information to part of the cerebral cortex, which processes it, then sends responses resulting from the information
Optic (II)	Sensory (special sensory: vision). The optic nerves receive images captured by the retinas. They travel through the thalamus to the visual cortex for processing
Oculomotor (III)	Motor (eye movements). Related muscles are involved in movement of parts of the eyes and eyelids
Trochlear (IV)	Motor (eye movements). Control other areas of the eyes related to eye movements
Trigeminal (V)	Mixed (sensory and motor, to face). Located in the brainstem, providing sensations to the scalp, face, eyes, nasal mucous membranes, and mouth; also responsible for sensations in the skin and muscles of the jaw
Abducens (VI)	Motor (eye movements). Provides even more control of eye movements
Facial (VII)	Mixed (sensory and motor, to face). Involved in taste sensation at the front of the tongue. Connected to face and head muscles, controls facial expressions
Vestibulocochlear (VIII)	Sensory (special sensory: balance and equilibrium via vestibular nerve, and hearing via cochlear nerve). Connected to inner ear
Glossopharyngeal (IX)	Mixed (sensory and motor, to head and neck). Connected to sinuses, back of tongue, soft palate, parotid glands, and reflexive control of the heart; also involved in swallowing
Vagus (X)	Mixed (sensory and motor, widely distributed in thorax, abdomen). Extends from brainstem through the neck to reach final locations. Involved in swallowing, breathing, heartbeat, speaking, and digestion. Connected to nerves that receive messages from the ears, pharynx, chest, esophagus, and abdominal areas
Accessory (XI)	Motor (to muscles of neck and upper back). There are two divisions. Cranial branch controls pharynx, larynx, and palate muscles, helping in swallowing and digestive tract movements. Spinal branch assists in muscle movements of the head, neck, and upper shoulders
Hypoglossal (XII)	Motor (controls the movements of the muscles of the tongue)

Autonomic Nervous System

The ANS acts as a control system to maintain homeostasis in the body. It functions without any conscious effort and regulates the visceral activities that maintain homeostasis. The ANS is subdivided into the sympathetic and parasympathetic nervous systems (see Figure 20-5). The sympathetic nervous system responds to stress and emergency situations. The parasympathetic nervous system is most active under ordinary conditions.

The nervous system is able to cope with different types of stressors at different times of life, which is part of normal living or mental health. When daily stressors cause normal activities of the brain to become abnormal, a mental disorder may result. Sensory nerves gather body information and environmental information and carry it to the CNS. The brain puts this information together into a plan of action or movement, which is then carried out by the motor nerves. The body's muscles and glands respond to the CNS information brought to them by the motor nerves.

Somatic Nervous System

The somatic nervous system is associated with voluntary control of body movements and the reception of external stimuli. It is part of the efferent section of the PNS. The somatic nervous system is made up of the fibers of motor

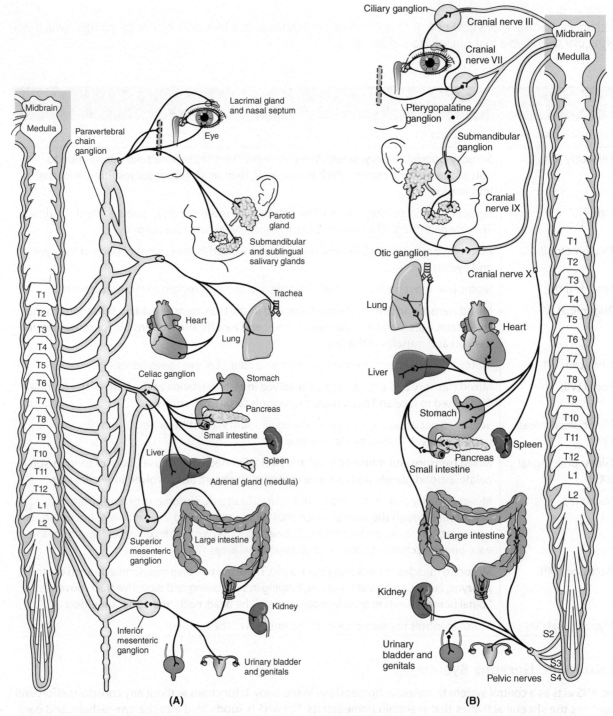

Figure 20-5 Nerve pathways of (A) the sympathetic nervous system and (B) the parasympathetic nervous system.

neurons that supply skeletal muscles. The cell bodies of nearly all the motor neurons are within the spinal cord. Though the somatic nervous system is under voluntary control, a significant amount of skeletal muscle activity used for balance, posture, and stereotypical movements is under subconscious control.

NEURONS

The **neuron** is the basic cell of the nervous system, carrying nerve impulses from one part of the body to another. It consists of three parts: dendrites, cell body, and axons (see Figure 20-6). Dendrites are the receptors that carry information to the nerve cell body, and axons carry nerve information away from the nerve cell body.

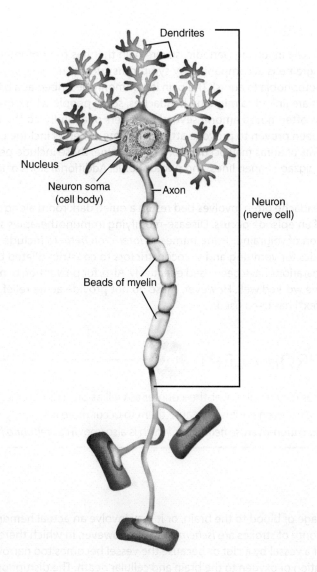

Figure 20-6 The neuron.

Neurons are closely associated with much smaller cells called neuroglia or glial cells. There are six types of neuroglia that support the neurons in the body.

NEUROTRANSMITTERS

At the junction of neurons, the continuation of messages is performed by neurotransmitters such as **acetylcholine (ACh)**, which stimulates the nerve endings, and cholinesterase, which inhibits ACh. Other neurotransmitters, called **neurohormones**, include the catecholamines (norepinephrine, epinephrine, and dopamine), serotonin, and endorphins.

Disorders of The Nervous System and Their Treatments

Disorders or conditions of the nervous system include migraine headache, stroke, epilepsy, Parkinson's disease, Bell's palsy, tic douloureux, multiple sclerosis, Alzheimer's disease, schizophrenia, bipolar disorder, major depressive disorder, anxiety disorders, and sleep disorders.

MIGRAINE HEADACHE

A migraine is a type of **headache** involving periodic, severe pain that has the potential to totally incapacitate the patient. Nearly always, a migraine is accompanied by symptoms such as nausea, vomiting, and visual signs and symptoms (ranging from photophobia to auras). The pain is commonly described as a bilateral or hemicranial throbbing. Though certain factors are linked to migraine headaches, some people who experience them have no identified cause. Susceptibility is often noted among several members of a family, so the disorder may be genetic or inherited. Foods that have been proven to provoke attacks in some sufferers include chocolate, aged cheese, and red wine. Signs and symptoms of auras may occur prior to a migraine; these include perception of flashing "lights," areas of complete darkness, zigzag-shaped lines, and photophobia. Additional signs of impending migraine include fatigue and irritability.

Treatment of migraine headache often involves bed rest in a quiet, dark room along with administration of analgesics when the first sign of an episode occurs. Disease-modifying immunotherapies such as interferon may slow and diminish the progression of migraine. Trade names of *interferon beta-1a* include Avonex® and Rebif®. Some patients also need antiemetics for vomiting and vasoconstrictors to constrict dilated blood vessels. To prevent or lessen symptoms, ergot preparations have been used effectively. Also, for prevention of migraines, beta-blockers and tricyclic antidepressants have worked well. However, these do not provide acute relief. At the onset of a migraine, sumatriptan succinate (Imitrex®) has been used.

MEDICATION ERROR ALERT

Though migraine headaches may require over-the-counter as well as prescription medications, taking them too often may actually make the headaches worse or cause them to occur more frequently. Frequent use of headache medications can cause **medication-overuse headache**, which is also known as **rebound headache**.

STROKE

A *stroke* is the arterial blockage of blood to the brain, or it may involve an actual hemorrhage, which is known as a *hemorrhagic stroke*. The majority of strokes are *ischemic strokes*, however, in which there is decreased blood flow to the brain due to blockage of a vessel by a clot or because the vessel becomes too narrow. Blockage or restriction of blood flow results in deprivation of oxygen to the brain and cellular death. The disruption occurs within the vascular system, but eventually affects the structures and functions of the nervous system. The severity of damage is based on the size of the blockage and the extent to which the brain tissue is harmed. Outcomes include weakness of the limbs, paralysis of one side of the body, and loss of speech. A stroke is usually signified by dizziness, headache, loss of balance, visual difficulties, and loss of normal movements on one side of the body. If it causes weakness of the facial muscles, the patient will have difficulty with speech.

EPILEPSY

Epilepsy is a chronic brain disorder in which sudden and abnormally intense electrical activity results in seizures. The more than 30 different seizure disorders are classified by their location in the brain and their clinical features. Epileptic seizures are classified as generalized or partial. Changes in consciousness and sensory phenomena may or may not occur.

MEDICAL TERMINOLOGY REVIEW

hyperpyrexia:

hyper- = *excessive*   abnormally high fever

-pyrexia = *fever*

Partial seizures arise from a localized area in the brain, which is often in the cerebral cortex (see Figure 20-7), and may or may not involve altered consciousness. However, partial seizures may progress to generalized seizures. The terms epilepsy, convulsions, and seizures are commonly used interchangeably, although they each have a slightly different medical meaning. Convulsions are actually involuntary muscle contractions.

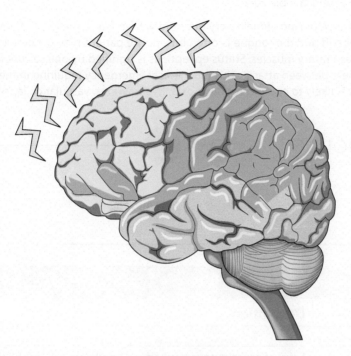

Partial seizure

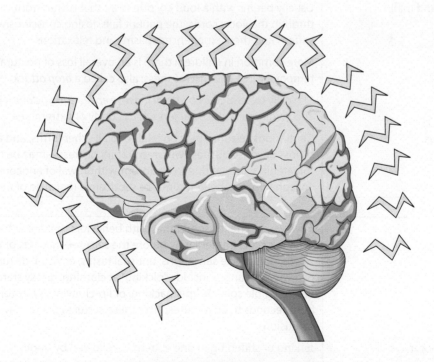

Generalized seizure

Figure 20-7 A partial seizure is characterized by chaotic firing occurring in one portion of the brain, while a generalized seizure is characterized by chaotic firing all over the brain.

Generalized seizures have multiple foci that may cause loss of consciousness. They cause diffuse electrical activity in the brain and include absence (petit mal) and tonic-clonic (grand mal) seizures. In an absence seizure, there is a brief change in the level of consciousness, resulting in blinking, blank staring, and loss of awareness of the surrounding environment. An individual may have more than one seizure disorder simultaneously. The international classification of seizures is summarized in Table 20-2.

Tonic-clonic seizures often cause the individual to cry out loudly, then fall to the ground, unconscious. In the tonic phase, the body becomes stiff and the tongue is often bitten. The patient may become cyanotic if there is prolonged contraction of the respiratory muscles. Status epilepticus is signified by one seizure following another without recovery of consciousness between attacks. This is a medical emergency requiring immediate administration of anticonvulsants, since it is likely to cause cerebral anoxia, **hyperpyrexia**, vascular collapse, and potentially, death.

MEDICAL TERMINOLOGY REVIEW

bradykinesia:

brady = *slow*   slow movement

kinesia = *movement*

Table 20-2 Classifications of Seizures	
Type	**Description**
Generalized Seizures	
Absence (petit mal)	Level of consciousness is changed briefly; there is eye blinking or rolling, a blank stare, and slight movements of the mouth. It takes about 10 seconds, and it is seen more in children
Tonic-clonic (grand mal)	Usually begins with a loud cry due to air that rushes from the lungs through the vocal cords; the patient falls, losing consciousness; the body stiffens and then experiences spasms and relaxations
Akinetic	More common in children: there is an overall loss of postural tone, and temporary loss of consciousness; also called a *drop attack*
Myoclonic	Clinically described as *bilateral massive epileptic myoclonus*; involves brief and involuntary muscular jerks of the body or extremities
Status epilepticus	Continuous seizures; may be related to all other forms, and accompanied by loss of consciousness with respiratory distress—may be life-threatening; can be due to an abrupt withdrawal of anticonvulsants, encephalopathy, head trauma, or septicemia (because of meningitis)
Partial Seizures	
Complex partial	Have varied effects, sometimes with behaviors that are without purpose; an aura occurs immediately before the seizure—nausea, pungent smells, dream-like sensations, unusual tastes, or visual disturbances; behavioral changes include "picking" at clothing, glassy stare, wandering, unintelligible speech, lip-smacking, or lip-chewing; symptoms last from seconds to 20 minutes; after these seizures, there may be mental confusion
Simple partial motor	Jerking or stiffening in one extremity, followed by tingling sensations in the same area; consciousness usually retained, but seizure may progress to a generalized seizure
Simple partial sensory	Involves hallucinations and other perceptual distortions

Anticonvulsants are the treatment of choice for epilepsy. The most commonly used anticonvulsants include phenytoin (Dilantin®), carbamazepine (Tegretol®), primidone (Mysoline®), and valproic acid (Depakene®). Patients given these medications must be closely monitored, and dosages must be carefully adjusted. Rarely, surgical intervention may be performed to remove identified brain lesions. Epileptic patients may have restricted lifestyles. Driver's licenses are commonly not obtainable unless the patient has been seizure-free for a certain period of time and has been receiving medical treatment. The patient and his or her family should also receive emotional support to aid in coping with this lifelong chronic condition. Table 20-3 gives examples of antiepileptic drugs.

PARKINSON'S DISEASE

Parkinson's disease is a slowly progressive degenerative disorder that affects motor function through the loss of extrapyramidal activity. Characteristic signs and symptoms include muscle tremor, muscle rigidity, bradykinesia, and disturbances of posture and equilibrium (see Figure 20-8). Affected individuals often exhibit a tremor of the thumb and forefinger, described as a "pill-rolling" movement.

Table 20-3 Examples of Antiepileptic Drugs (Anticonvulsants)

Generic Name	Trade Name	Route of Administration	Average Adult Dosage
carbamazepine	Tegretol®, Tegretol XR®	PO	200 mg bid, gradually increased to 800 to 1200 mg/day in three to four divided doses. Tegretol XR dosed bid
ethosuximide	Zarontin®	PO	250 mg bid, may increase q4 to 7d prn (maximum 1.5 g/day)
lamotrigine	Lamictal®	PO	25 mg/day, may increase up to 375 mg/day
levetiracetam	Keppra®	PO	Initial: 1000 mg/day, in two divided doses, may increase up to maximum 3000 mg/day
lorazepam	Ativan®	IV for status epilepticus	4 mg injected slowly at 2 mg/min, may repeat dose once if inadequate response after 10 minutes
oxcarbazepine	Trileptal®	PO	Initial: 600 mg/day, bid. May be increased by up to 600 mg/day in weekly intervals (maximum 1200 mg/day)
phenobarbital	Luminal®	PO, IM, IV	PO: 100 to 300 mg/day; IV/IM: 200 to 600 mg up to 20 mg/kg
phenytoin	Dilantin®	PO, IV	PO: 15 to 18 mg/kg or 1 g loading dose, then 300 mg/day in one to three divided doses; IV: 15 to 18 mg/kg or 1g loading dose, then 100 mg tid
tiagabine hydrochloride	Gabitril®	PO	Start with 4 mg every day, may increase dose by 4 to 8 mg/day q week
valproic acid	Depakene®	PO, IV	PO and IV: Start with 10 to 15 mg/kg/day; increase by 5 to 10 mg/kg/week to achieve optimal clinical response

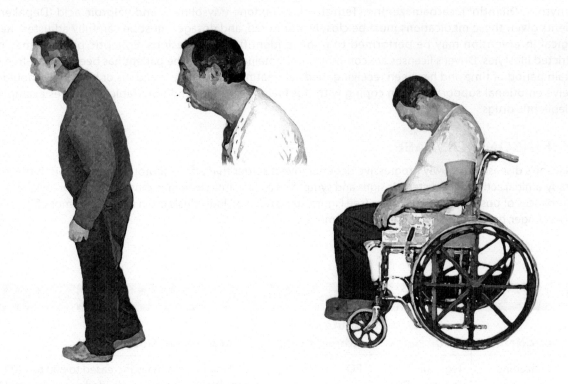

Figure 20-8 Parkinson's disease is characterized by shuffling gait and early postural changes.

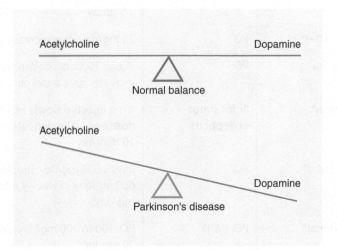

Figure 20-9 Dopamine imbalance exhibited in Parkinson's disease.

This disorder causes dysfunction and changes in the basal nuclei (clusters of nerve cells at the base of the brain), principally in the substantia nigra, which is an area of pigmented cells in the midbrain responsible for the production of the inhibitory neurotransmitter dopamine. In patients with Parkinson's disease, a decreased number of neurons in the brain secrete dopamine, leading to an imbalance between excitation and inhibition in the basal nuclei. This imbalance is seen in the altered ratio of the neurotransmitters acetylcholine and dopamine in the brain (see Figure 20-9).

As the disease progresses, the patient's posture becomes stooped, with the head bowed and body flexed forward. The walking gait is described as "shuffling." The knees remain slightly bent while walking, and falling is more likely. Swallowing becomes difficult, speech is muffled, and the face becomes relatively expressionless. Some patients experience gradual behavior and mental activity changes. Though an early-onset form of Parkinson's disease may occur in younger people, the disease usually affects adults older than 60 years. More men than women are affected, and life span after diagnosis averages 10 years.

Treatment of this incurable disease involves supportive management to control symptoms. Commonly used medications include levodopa (Larodopa®), carbidopa (Lodosyn®), antidepressants, and anticholinergics. Selegiline (Eldepryl®, Zelepar®) is another drug that has caused certain patients' symptoms to improve. Newer agents include rasagiline (Azilect®), pramipexole (Mirapex®), and ropinirole (Requip®)—see Table 20-4. It is important to initiate drug treatment as early as possible, before the disease becomes disabling, because this can prevent the disease from becoming severe. To help maximize mobility, physical therapy is often helpful. The patient is given support to encourage self-care and independence.

POINTS TO REMEMBER

Parkinson's disease affects men more often than women, occurring in all races and ethnic groups. It is not common before the age of 40, and symptoms usually begin between the ages of 45 and 65.

MEDICATION ERROR ALERT

Patients with Parkinson's disease may require assistance in correctly taking their medications. Often, patients are required to take these medications six times a day, in 3-hour intervals. If the patient is late in taking a dose, even by a few minutes, he or she may experience *leg freezing*, in which the legs slow down to the point that walking becomes impossible.

Table 20-4 Examples of Anti-Parkinson Drugs

Generic Name	Trade Name	Route of Administration	Average Adult Dosage
amantadine	Symmetrel®	PO	100 mg 1 to 2 times/day, start with 100 mg/day if patient is on other anti-Parkinsonism medications
benztropine	Cogentin®	PO	0.5 to 1 mg/day, may be gradually increased prn up to 6 mg/day
carbidopa/levodopa	Sinemet®	PO	*If not currently receiving levodopa:* 1 tablet containing 10 mg carbidopa/100 mg levodopa or 25 mg carbidopa/100 mg levodopa tid, increased by 1 tablet every day to every other day up to 6 tablets/day *If currently receiving levodopa:* 1 tablet of the 25/250 mixture tid to qid, adjusted by ½ to 1 tablet prn up to 8 tablets/day (start at 20% to 25% of initial dose of levodopa)
entacapone	Comtan®	PO	200 mg with each dose of carbidopa/levodopa to a maximum of 8 times/day (maximum 1600 mg/day)
levodopa	Larodopa®	PO	500 mg to 1 g daily in two or more equally divided doses, may increase by 100 to 750 mg q3 to 7d (maximum 8 g/day); if used in combination with carbidopa, decrease levodopa dose by 75% to 80%

(Continued)

Table 20-4 Examples of Anti-Parkinson Drugs *(Continued)*

Generic Name	Trade Name	Route of Administration	Average Adult Dosage
pramipexole	Mirapex®	PO	Initial: 0.375 mg/day in three divided doses, not to be increased more frequently than q5 to 7d Maintenance: 1.5 to 4.5 mg/day in three divided doses, with or without levodopa at 800 mg/day
rasagiline	Azilect®	PO	1 mg/day; may need to be started at 0.5 mg/day initially and then increased; may be used with or without levodopa
ropinirole	Requip®	PO	Initial: 0.25 mg tid, increased in weekly increments as follows: Week two: 0.5 mg tid Week three: 0.75 mg tid Week four: 1 mg tid Increases continue similarly up to maximum dose of 24 mg/day
selegiline	Zelapar® Eldepryl®	PO	Initial: 1.25 mg/day for at least six weeks; then may increase to 2.5 mg/day
trihexyphenidyl	Artane®	PO	Trihexy®: 1 mg on day 1, 2 mg on day 2, then increase by 2 mg q3 to 5d up to 6 to 10 mg/day in three or more divided doses (maximum 15 mg/day); Artane®: 2 to 5 mg in three divided doses taken with meals

BELL'S PALSY

Bell's palsy is paralysis of the facial nerve (seventh cranial nerve) on one side of the face, which causes the affected side to "droop." It is usually caused by compression or trauma to the facial nerve or an infection with the *Herpes simplex* virus. In some patients, pain or a pulling sensation is felt behind the ear. The patient may not be able to close the affected eye or control drooling from the affected side of the mouth. Usually temporary, the condition can also be permanent. Bell's palsy often appears early in the morning, causing a distorted facial expression and inability to smile, frown, or whistle. Patients may have diminished taste perception.

Early treatment is vital. Recommended measures include gentle massage, application of warm and moist heat, and facial exercises. To reduce inflammation of the facial nerve, prednisone is prescribed, though analgesics may also be given. If the patient cannot close the eye, it may become dried out and sore, requiring artificial tears and an eye patch for protection when outdoors. To prevent muscle atrophy, electrotherapy is used to stimulate the facial nerve.

TIC DOULOUREUX (TRIGEMINAL NEURALGIA)

Tic douloureux is pain in the area innervated by the trigeminal nerve (fifth cranial nerve). Its cause is not fully understood, but this form of neuralgia is often related to nerve root compression because of a tumor or vascular lesion. The condition is sometimes a result of herpes zoster infection or multiple sclerosis. Most cases are of unknown cause. Signs and symptoms include intense pain radiating along the trigeminal nerve, but this is transient. It may affect any of the three fifth cranial nerve branches, but predominantly affects the second or third branch. If the ophthalmic branch is affected, the patient feels pain in the eye and forehead. The nose, upper lip, and cheek become painful if the maxillary branch is involved. When the mandibular branch is involved, pain occurs in the lower lip, outer area of the tongue, and in the cheek near the ear. Pain is always unilateral, triggered by mechanical or thermal stimuli. Chewing, swallowing, or touching of the area often triggers the pain.

Analgesics are commonly used for treatment, and many people respond to carbamazepine. When medications are insufficient, surgery may be performed to dissect the nerve roots. Patients should quit smoking, since this exacerbates the condition.

MULTIPLE SCLEROSIS

Multiple sclerosis is a disease caused by progressive demyelination of nerve cells of the brain and spinal cord. Believed to be an autoimmune disease, it results in lesions that lead to sclerosis of the fatty **myelin** sheaths, reducing nerve impulse conduction. It is most commonly seen in early adulthood with stages of progression and remission. Symptoms include double vision, muscle weakness, abnormal reflexes, vertigo, and sometimes problems in urinating. Though incurable, multiple sclerosis is treated by various medications, which help patients to live relatively normal lives. In the later stages, patients often need mobility-assisting devices. For the treatment of multiple sclerosis, medications include interferon beta-1a (Avonex®, Rebif®), interferon beta-1b (Betaseron®), and glatiramer (Copaxone®).

ALZHEIMER'S DISEASE

Alzheimer's disease (senile dementia) is one of the most common causes of severe cognitive dysfunction in adults older than 65 years of age (see Figure 20-10). Its incidence is markedly increased in those older than age 85. Pathologically, the brains of people with Alzheimer's disease show progressive atrophy (shrinkage) and senile plaques. Although its exact cause is unknown, beta-amyloid deposits in neuritic plaques and arterial walls appear to play a role in pathogenesis of the disease. Alzheimer's disease may be genetically linked in some families, with affected members having an abnormality on chromosome 21, but most investigators consider the disease to be multifactorial. One theory has focused on the loss of neurotransmitter stimulation by choline acetyltransferase as having a role in causation. Other causes that have been put forward include biochemical changes, autoimmune reactions, slowly developing viral infections, chemical deficiencies, toxic chemical excess, defects of blood vessels, and deficient neurochemical factors in the brain. Head trauma has also been implicated in some cases.

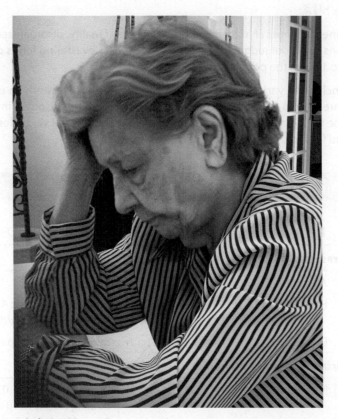

Figure 20-10 A patient with Alzheimer's disease.

Alzheimer's disease is a devastating illness characterized by progressive short-term memory failure, impaired thinking and concentration, inability to learn new information or reason normally, confusion, disorientation, personality changes, restlessness, speech disturbances, and the inability to perform routine tasks. As the disease progresses, patients may no longer be able to speak to others, walk without assistance, or sit without some form of support. Deterioration of brain function occurs over 5 to 10 years and requires increasing levels of care. Patients with advanced disease seem emotionally detached, restless, and disoriented, and may be hostile and combative. Sleep disturbances are common. Eventually most patients are bedridden, and death often occurs from an infection or complication.

Alzheimer's disease is incurable, and it has been difficult to accurately diagnose until after death. Pathologic brain examination shows characteristic neuronal loss and senile plaques, including microscopic deposits of amyloid materials. Treatment is supportive, using medications that help alleviate cognitive symptoms such as cholinesterase inhibitors. The primary drug used is donepezil hydrochloride (Aricept®). Other medications include galantamine (Reminyl®) and rivastigmine (Exelon®). Table 20-5 summarizes medications used for Alzheimer's disease.

It is believed that persistent activation of N-methyl-D-aspartate (NMDA) receptors by the excitatory amino acid glutamate contributes to Alzheimer's symptoms. Therefore, memantine (Namenda®), an NMDA inhibitor, may be used. Additional medications include tacrine (Cognex®), antipsychotics or neuroleptics such as haloperidol (Haldol®), antianxiety agents (alprazolam [Xanax®], lorazepam [Ativan®], and buspirone [Buspar®]), and selective serotonin reuptake inhibitors (SSRIs, including paroxetine hydrochloride). Lorazepam works for longer periods of time than alprazolam. For aggression and delusional symptoms, risperdone (Risperdal®) and olanzapine (Zyprexa®) are used. Additional treatments for Alzheimer's disease include the prescription dietary supplement known as Axona®, the combination vitamin product known as Cerefolin®, and vitamin B_{12} supplementation.

SCHIZOPHRENIA

Schizophrenia is a mental illness characterized by distortion of reality, disorganized thought patterns, social withdrawal, hallucinations, and poor judgment. It is one of the most devastating forms of mental illnesses and occurs in approximately 1% to 1.5% of the population.

Schizophrenia includes a variety of syndromes, which present differently in each individual. However, characteristic changes are seen in the brains of patients suffering from the disorder, including reduction of the cortex (outer portion) of the temporal lobes, enlargement of the third and lateral ventricles, excessive dopamine secretion, and decreased blood flow to the front of the brain.

Table 20-5 Examples of Drugs Used to Treat Alzheimer's Disease

Generic Name	Trade Name	Route of Administration	Average Adult Dosage
Acetylcholinesterase Inhibitors			
donepezil	Aricept®	PO	5 to 23 mg/day
galantamine	Razadyne®	PO	Immediate release: 4 to 12 mg bid; extended release: 8 to 24 mg/day
rivastigmine	Exelon®	PO, transdermal path	PO: 3 to 6 mg bid; patch: 4.6 to 13.3 mg/day
N-Methyl-D-aspartate Receptor Antagonist			
memantine	Namenda®	PO	Immediate release: 10 mg bid (initial: 5 mg/day, titrating weekly to 10 mg bid); extended release: 14 to 28 mg/day (initial: 7 mg/day titrating up to 28 mg/day)

The cause of schizophrenia has not been fully determined but may have a genetic link. Other possible causes include brain damage to the fetus caused by perinatal complications or viral infections in the mother during pregnancy. The onset of schizophrenia is usually between 15 and 25 years of age in men and between 25 and 35 years of age in women. Stressful events appear to initiate the onset and recurrence of the disorder.

Treatment during the acute phase of schizophrenia involves antipsychotics. Dosage is determined by identifying the smallest amount of the chosen medication that causes remission of symptoms without producing significant adverse effects. Long-term multiple therapies are used; these include medications, supportive psychotherapy, and family counseling. Once the patient is stabilized, treatment focuses on reestablishing his or her sense of self, using personal, social, and vocational therapies. Atypical antipsychotics used as first-line therapy include risperidone (Risperdal®) and olanzapine (Zyprexa®). Less common drugs include ziprasidone (Geodon®) and quetiapine (Seroquel®). For patients who do not respond well to these drugs, older medications such as chlorpromazine (Thorazine®), haloperidol (Haldol®), and fluphenazine (Prolixin®) are most commonly used.

POINTS TO REMEMBER

Neuroleptic agents used for schizophrenia may cause extrapyramidal side effects (EPS). These appear as involuntary motor movements. Tardive dyskinesia is one form of EPS. It is characterized by involuntary, repetitive, movements that have no purpose.

BIPOLAR DISORDER

Bipolar disorder is a mental illness characterized by periods of extreme excitation or mania and deep depression. It is not commonly understood why it takes months to move from one of these extremes to the other. Some patients have predominantly manic episodes or predominantly depressive episodes. Few patients experience the classic swing from mania to depression and back. Bipolar disorder is also called manic-depressive illness.

Treatment for bipolar disorder may involve hospitalization (for severe conditions), medications, and, if coexisting drug or alcohol abuse is present, treatment for substance abuse. Medications for bipolar disorder include lithium, anticonvulsants, antipsychotics, antidepressants, benzodiazepines, and a combination of the antidepressant fluoxetine and the antipsychotic olanzapine, which is marketed under the name Symbyax®. Table 20-6 lists examples of antipsychotic medications.

Table 20-6 Examples of Antipsychotic Drugs

Generic Name	Trade Name	Route of Administration	Average Adult Dosage
lithium	Eskalith®	PO	900 to 1800 mg/day in three or four divided doses
haloperidol	Haldol®	PO, IM	PO: 0.2 to 5 mg bid to tid; IM: 2 to 5 mg repeated q4h prn
thiothixene	Navane®	PO, IM	PO: 2 mg tid, may increase up to 15 mg/day prn or tolerated (maximum 60 mg/day); IM: 4 mg bid to qid (maximum 30 mg/day)
trifluoperazine	Stelazine®	PO, IM	PO: 1 to 2 mg bid, may increase up to 20 mg/day in hospitalized patients; IM: 1 to 2 mg q4 to 6h (maximum 10 mg/day)
cariprazine	Vraylar®	PO	Initial dose is 1.5 mg once daily; may be increased to 3 mg once daily
loxapine	Loxitane®	PO, IM	PO: Start with 10 mg bid and rapidly increase to maintenance levels of 60 to 100 mg/day in two to four divided doses (maximum 250 mg/day); IM: 12.5 to 50 mg q4 to 6h

(Continued)

Table 20-6 Examples of Antipsychotic Drugs *(Continued)*

Generic Name	Trade Name	Route of Administration	Average Adult Dosage
perphenazine	Perphenazine®	PO, IM, IV	PO: 4 to 16 mg bid to qid; 8 to 32 mg sustained release bid (maximum 64 mg/day); IM: 5 mg q6h (maximum 15 to 30 mg/day); IV: Dilute to 0.5 mg/mL in NS, administer at not more than 1 mg q1 to 2 min or 5 mg by slow infusion
chlorpromazine	Thorazine®	PO, IM, IV	PO: 25 to 100 mg tid to qid, may need up to 1000 mg/day; IM/IV: 25 to 50 mg up to 600 mg q4 to 6h
thioridazine	Mellaril®	PO	50 to 100 mg tid, may be increased up to 800 mg/day prn or as tolerated
clozapine	Clozaril®	PO	Initial: 25 to 50 mg/day, titrate to target dose of 350 to 450 mg/day in three divided doses at 2-week intervals; increase prn (maximum 900 mg/day)
olanzapine	Zyprexa®	PO	Initial: 5 to 10 mg/day, may be increased by 2.5 to 5 mg q week until desired response (usual range: 10 to 15 mg/day, maximum 20 mg/day)
quetiapine	Seroquel®	PO	Initial: 25 mg bid, may be increased by 25 to 50 mg bid to tid on second or third day as tolerated to target a dose of 300 to 400 mg/day in divided doses bid to tid, may adjust dose by 25 to 50 mg bid every day prn (maximum 800 mg/day)

MAJOR DEPRESSIVE DISORDER

Major depressive disorder is characterized by one or more major depressive episodes. It is a mood disorder that is not linked to a history of manic or hypomanic episodes. It is one of several subgroups of depression. Major depression, or unipolar disorder, is a chemical deficit within the brain, and a precise diagnosis is based on biologic factors or personal characteristics. The causes of depression include genetic and psychosocial stressors. Depression may also occur as a reactive episode, a response to a life event, or secondarily to many systemic disorders (including cancer, diabetes, heart failure, and AIDS). Clinical depression is a common problem, and many patients with milder forms may be misdiagnosed and not receive treatment. Signs and symptoms of major depressive disorder include deep, persistent sadness, hopelessness, and despair. Symptoms generally develop over days to weeks, and patients are often anxious or brooding, describing feelings of emptiness, heaviness, or a vague sense of loss. Other signs include remorse, self-blame, guilt, or loss of self-esteem.

The most effective treatment involves combined medications and psychotherapy. Patients who respond well to antidepressants, obtaining good symptom relief, generally have good prognoses. SSRIs are usually tried first. Additional medications include serotonin-norepinephrine reuptake inhibitors (SNRIs) such as duloxetine (Cymbalta®), venlafaxine (Effexor®), and desvenlafaxine (Pristiq®), as well as atypical antidepressants such as bupropion (Wellbutrin®). Family support and education are very important for recovery. Additional treatments may include electroconvulsive therapy (ECT), if the patient is severely incapacitated, psychotic, or unresponsive to other therapies. Table 20-7 lists examples of antidepressants.

ANXIETY DISORDERS

Anxiety is a common psychological disorder that, for most people, is only a temporary stress response. It is defined as a persistent and irrational fear of a specific object, activity, or situation. When exposed to chronic stress, some people develop excessive anxiety. In others, the response may simply be inappropriate to the stressor. It is termed an illness

Table 20-7 Examples of Antidepressants

Generic Name	Trade Name	Route of Administration	Average Adult Dosage
Selective Serotonin Reuptake Inhibitors (SSRIs)			
citalopram	Celexa®	PO	20 mg/day, increased to maximum dose of 40 mg/day at an interval of no less than one week
escitalopram	Lexapro®	PO	10 mg/day
fluoxetine	Prozac®	PO	20 to 80 mg/day, in the morning
fluvoxamine	Luvox®	PO	Initial: 50 mg/day at bedtime; Maint: 100 to 300 mg/day
paroxetine	Paxil®	PO	20 mg/day, in the morning
sertraline	Zoloft®	PO	50 mg/day
Serotonin-Norepinephrine Reuptake Inhibitors (SNRIs)			
desvenlafaxine	Pristiq®	PO	50 mg/day
duloxetine	Cymbalta®	PO	40 to 60 mg/day, in two divided doses
venlafaxine	Effexor®	PO	75 mg/day, in two to three divided doses, with food
Atypical Antidepressants			
bupropion	Wellbutrin®	PO	Initial: 150 mg/day, in the morning; Maint: if tolerated, increase to 300 mg/day on day 4, in the morning
mirtazapine	Remeron®	PO	15 mg/day, at bedtime (maximum 45 mg/day, at bedtime)
trazodone	Desyrel®	PO	150 mg/day; may be increased by 75 mg/day q3d (maximum 375 mg/day)
Tricyclic and Tetracyclic Antidepressants			
amitriptyline	Elavil®	PO, IM	PO (initial): 25 to 100 mg/day in three to four divided doses, or 50 to 100 mg at bedtime; PO (maint): 25 to 150 mg/day in one dose or three to four divided doses; IM: 20 to 30 mg up to qid; switch to PO therapy as soon as possible
clomipramine	Anafranil®	PO	25 mg/day; if tolerated, increase gradually to 100 mg at end of week 2 (maximum 250 mg/day)
desipramine	Norpramin®	PO	100 to 200 mg/day (maximum 300 mg/day)
doxepin	Silenor®	PO	Initial: 25 to 150 mg/day in one to three divided doses; Maint: 25 to 300 mg/day in one to three divided doses
imipramine	Tofranil®	PO, IM	PO (initial): 30 to 100 mg/day in divided doses, gradually increase to 200 mg/day prn; IM: up to 100 mg/day in divided doses; switch to PO dosage as soon as possible
nortriptyline	Pamelor®	PO	25 mg tid to qid (maximum 150 mg/day)

(Continued)

Table 20-7 Examples of Antidepressants *(Continued)*

Generic Name	Trade Name	Route of Administration	Average Adult Dosage
protriptyline	Vivactil®	PO	15 to 40 mg/day in three to four divided doses (maximum 60 mg/day)
trimipramine	Surmontil®	PO	Initial: 75 mg/day in divided doses, increased to 150 mg/day; Maint: 50 to 150 mg/day
Monoamine Oxidase Inhibitors (MAOIs)			
isocarboxazid	Marplan®	PO	Initial: 10 mg bid, increase by 10 mg increments q2 to 4d up to 40 mg/day by end of week 1; then increase by up to 20 mg/week prn (maximum 60 mg/day); divide daily dosage into two to four doses
phenelzine	Nardil®	PO	15 mg tid, may increase prn (maximum 90 mg/day)
selegiline	Emsam®	Transdermal patch	One patch (6 mg) q24h
tranylcypromine	Parnate®	PO	30 mg/day in divided doses; increase prn in 10 mg/day increments at intervals of one to three weeks (maximum 60 mg/day)

when the affected person can no longer live a normal life. According to the Anxiety Disorders Association of America, anxiety disorders are the most common psychiatric illnesses in the United States, affecting 40 million adults, with a higher incidence in women than in men.

Anxiety is an uncomfortable state that has both psychological and physical components. The psychological component is characterized by emotions such as fear, apprehension, dread, and uneasiness. The physical components include tachycardia, palpitations, trembling, dry mouth, sweating, weakness, fatigue, and shortness of breath. Untreated, anxiety disorders often lead to severe disorders such as depression and alcoholism. Fortunately, anxiety disorders respond well to treatment such as behavior therapy, psychotherapy, or drug therapy.

In general, treatments for the various anxiety disorders include increased physical activities, relaxation exercises, and anxiolytic drugs. SSRIs are used first, often with amitriptyline/nortriptyline. Benzodiazepines are often prescribed, including lorazepam (Ativan®), clonazepam (Klonopin®), and alprazolam (Xanax®). These are used on an "as-needed" basis for only a short time due to dependence potential.

Anxiety disorders may be classified as generalized anxiety disorder, panic disorder, obsessive-compulsive disorder, social anxiety disorder, or post-traumatic stress disorder. Brief explanations of the different types of anxiety follow.

Generalized Anxiety Disorder

Generalized anxiety disorder is a chronic condition characterized by uncontrollable worrying. Most patients with generalized anxiety disorder also have another psychiatric disorder, usually depression. The hallmark of this disorder is unrealistic or excessive anxiety about several events or activities (e.g., work or school performance). Generalized anxiety disorder may last for six months or longer.

Panic Disorder

Panic disorder is characterized by recurrent, intensely uncomfortable episodes known as panic attacks. Panic attacks have a sudden onset, reaching peak intensity within 10 minutes. Symptoms may include trembling, shortness of breath, heart palpitations, chest pain (or chest tightness), sweating, nausea, dizziness (or slight vertigo), lightheadedness, hyperventilation, paresthesias (tingling sensations), and sensations of choking or smothering. These symptoms typically disappear within 30 minutes. Many patients go to an emergency department because they think they are having a heart attack. Some patients experience panic attacks daily; others have only one or two per month.

According to the *American Journal of Psychiatry*, the incidence of panic disorders in women is two to three times higher than seen in men. Onset of panic disorder usually occurs in the late teens or early 20s.

Obsessive-Compulsive Disorder

Obsessive-compulsive disorder is a potentially disabling condition characterized by persistent obsessions and compulsions that cause marked distress, consume at least 1 hour per day, and significantly interfere with daily living. An obsession is defined as a recurrent, persistent thought, impulse, or mental image that is unwanted and distressing, and comes involuntarily to mind despite attempts to ignore or suppress it. A compulsion is a ritualized behavior or mental act that a person is driven to perform in response to his or her obsessions.

Social Anxiety Disorder

Social anxiety disorder, formerly known as social phobia, is characterized by an intense, irrational fear of situations in which one might be scrutinized by others, or might do something that is embarrassing or humiliating. Exposure to the feared situation almost always elicits anxiety. As a result, the person avoids the situation, or, if it cannot be avoided, endures it with intense anxiety. Manifestations include blushing, stuttering, sweating, palpitations, dry throat, and muscle tension.

Social anxiety disorder is one of the most common psychiatric disorders and the most common anxiety disorder. This disorder typically begins during the teenage years and, if left untreated, is likely to be lifelong.

Post-Traumatic Stress Disorder

Post-traumatic stress disorder develops following a traumatic event that elicited an immediate reaction of fear, helplessness, or horror. It is more common in women than in men, and it is the fourth most common psychiatric disorder. Traumatic events that involve interpersonal violence (e.g., assault, rape, or torture) are more likely to cause post-traumatic stress disorder than are traumatic events that do not (e.g., car accidents or natural disasters).

Treatments for post-traumatic stress disorder include counseling and drug therapy. Counseling helps the patient to accept the intense memories that trigger the condition. A sense of safety is established and feelings of guilt and self-blame are addressed. Cognitive behavior training increases self-esteem and self-control. Sleep disturbances are also investigated and treated. Medications include benzodiazepines, antianxiety agents, and SSRIs. Recovery varies, and while some patients return to a normal state within a short time period, others never recover.

SLEEP DISORDERS

Insomnia is the inability to fall asleep or stay asleep. Difficulty in falling asleep or disturbed sleep patterns both result in insufficient sleep. Sleep disorders are common and may be short in duration or of long standing. They may have little or no apparent relationship to other immediate disorders. Sleep disorders can be secondary to emotional problems, pain, physical disorders, and the use or withdrawal of drugs. Excess alcohol consumed in the evening can shorten sleep and lead to withdrawal effects in the early morning.

Treatments for sleep disorders begin with identification and removal of their cause. Sleep hygiene is then improved. Patients are taught to reduce tension and stress. A regular sleep schedule is instituted, with regular bedtimes and awakening times, and anything detrimental to good sleeping patterns is removed from the bedroom. Daily activities are increased to balance against sleep times. Beginning in the late afternoon, the patient must avoid caffeine, nicotine, and stimulants. Strenuous exercise must not occur in the few hours prior to sleep. The bedroom must be darkened and quiet. If all these preparations are insufficient, hypnotic benzodiazepines are prescribed. The three newest hypnotics commonly used for sleep disorders include zolpidem (Ambien®), zaleplon (Sonata®), and eszopiclone (Lunesta®).

WHAT WOULD YOU DO?

A 21-year-old woman who seems extremely sad and depressed asks you, the pharmacy technician, which over-the-counter sleeping pills are the strongest that your pharmacy sells. You ask her if she has been having trouble sleeping, and she says yes. When you ask if she has seen a physician about her condition, she says there is no reason to do that. After finding the tablets she wants, she returns to your counter to purchase them. What would you do in this situation?

ATTENTION DEFICIT AND HYPERACTIVITY DISORDER

Attention deficit and hyperactivity disorder (ADHD) affects brain physiology, resulting in inability to focus and loss of attention, an inability to remain quiet and passive in behavior, or both. The diagnosis of ADHD affects 3% to 5% of school-aged children, with boys three times more likely than girls to have symptoms, which include explosive outbursts, impulsiveness, and irritability. The child's intelligence is not affected, but it is difficult to retain focus and be productive in school. When ADHD affects older children or adults, there are distractions because of various sights, sounds, or thoughts. The affected individual often gets "lost" in daydreams. They become unable to meet deadlines and finish projects and often lose items that they need.

SEDATIVES, HYPNOTICS, AND ANTIANXIETY DRUGS

Sedatives and **hypnotic** drugs are used to treat patients with anxiety and sleep disorders. Sedatives can reduce anxiety. **Sedation** is characterized by decreased anxiety, motor activity, and mental acuity; it induces calmness or sleep. **Hypnosis** is a trance-like state defined by an increased tendency to sleep. Hypnotic drugs are used to produce sleep or drowsiness. Some examples of antianxiety drugs are shown in Table 20-8.

Table 20-8 Examples of Antianxiety Drugs

Generic Name	Trade Name	Route of Administration	Average Adult Dosage
Benzodiazepines			
alprazolam	Xanax®	PO	0.25 to 0.5 mg tid (maximum 4 mg/day)
chlordiazepoxide	Librium®	PO, IM, IV	PO: 5 to 10 mg tid to qid; IM/IV: 50 to 100 mg 1 hour before surgery
diazepam	Valium®	PO, IM, IV	PO: 2 to 10 mg bid to qid or 15 to 30 mg/day sustained release; IV/IM: 2 to 10 mg, repeat if needed in 3 to 4 hours
estazolam	Prosom®	PO	1 mg at bedtime, may be increased up to 2 mg if necessary
lorazepam	Ativan®	PO, IM, IV	PO: 2 to 6 mg/day in divided doses; IM: 2 to 4 mg (0.05 mg/kg) at least 2 hours before surgery; IV: 0.044 mg/kg up to 2 mg 15 to 20 minutes before surgery
oxazepam	Oxazepam®	PO	10 to 30 mg tid to qid
Nonbenzodiazepines			
buspirone	BuSpar®	PO	7.5 to 15 mg/day in divided doses
secobarbital	Seconal®	PO	100 to 300 mg/day in three divided doses
zolpidem	Ambien®	PO	5 to 10 mg at bedtime, limited to 7 to 10 days

POINTS TO REMEMBER

Ambien is a hypnotic (sedative) used for short-term treatment of sleep disorders. It is an immediate-release tablet taken at bedtime that helps the user to fall asleep more easily. Another form is Ambien CR, which is extended-release. It acts not only by making it easier for the patient to fall asleep, but also—when its second layer is dissolved—by helping him or her to remain asleep. This medication must be used exactly as prescribed due to the potential for dangerous adverse effects.

MEDICATION ERROR ALERT

Sedatives are one type of "high-alert medication"; these are the drugs that are most likely to cause significant patient harm. Examples of "high-alert" drugs used for sedation include dexmedetomidine (Precedex®), midazolam (Midazolam HCl®), and chloral hydrate (Noctec®).

NARCOTIC ANALGESICS

Narcotic analgesics are also referred to as **opioids,** which is the general term for drugs with morphine-like activity that reduce pain and induce tolerance and physical dependence. Drugs made from opium (such as morphine and heroin) are referred to as **opiates.** Due to their potential for addiction and abuse, prescriptions for these agents have become more controlled. Narcotic analgesics carry many risks and have multiple label warnings, mostly the risk for serious and life-threatening respiratory depression—often linked to deaths from their use. Also, these agents are even more dangerous when used with benzodiazepines or other CNS depressants, including alcohol. It is very important to assess risk factors for each patient before these agents are prescribed. For chronic pain, narcotic analgesics should be started by using immediate-release/short-acting formulations and not the longer acting forms. The long-acting forms include methadone, fentanyl, and the extended-release forms of oxycodone, hydrocodone, hydromorphone, and morphine. Practitioners should always start opioid medications at the lowest effective dosages, and increase dosages very slowly, every one to three months. There are many adverse effects of these agents. They include nausea, vomiting, constipation, drowsiness, confusion, tolerance, physical dependence, and ultimately, respiratory depression. Adverse effects are seen more often in older patients, especially when kidney or liver abnormalities are present. Table 20-9 shows some examples of common narcotic analgesics.

POINTS TO REMEMBER

There is an epidemic of narcotic drug overuse in the United States, primarily with morphine, heroin, and similar opioid-derived drugs. To save the lives of individuals who are overdosing, naloxone is administered. This drug is not addictive, is a nonscheduled prescription medication and works only if there are opioids in the patient's system.

WHAT WOULD YOU DO?

Opioids, such as narcotic analgesics, are among the drugs that are most commonly abused by college students. You are a recent college graduate and have just started working in a community pharmacy. One day as you are stocking medications, one of your college friends enters and asks another pharmacy technician for a refill of a prescription opioid. Your friend has the same name as his father (Timothy O'Brien), and you think may be he is trying to use his father's prescription to obtain the drug for himself. What would you do in this situation?

Naloxone

Naloxone is an opioid antagonist that blocks or temporarily reverses the effects of opioids. It is used for the emergency treatment of opioid overdose, regardless of whether this is known or suspected. It acts by competing for the same receptors as opioids. Naloxone reverses opioid effects, including sedation, hypotension, and respiratory depression. The drug is available in many dosage formulations, administered intramuscularly or intranasally, both of which are equally effective. Naloxone may be prescribed along with opioids, and patients must be educated about the potential hazards of misusing opioids, as well as the effectiveness of naloxone in reversing overdose. All 50 states have passed laws increasing access to naloxone. Most states now have standing orders allowing pharmacists to provide naloxone without an actual prescription.

Table 20-9 Examples of Narcotic Analgesics

Generic Name	Trade Name	Route of Administration	Average Adult Dosage
codeine	(generic only)	PO, IM, SC	15 to 60 mg qid
fentanyl	Subsys®, Abstral®, Actiq®, Fentora®, Lazanda®, Duragesic®, Ionsys®, Sublimaze®	Sublingual, Buccal, Intranasal, Transdermal patch, IM, IV	Transmucosal products: varied dosages; transdermal patch: 25 mcg/h q72h; IM: 50 to 100 mcg q1 to 2h; IV: 25 to 50 mcg/h
hydrocodone	(oral IR only available with acetaminophen: Lorcet®, Lortab®, Norco®, Vicodin®, Verdrocet®, Xodol®); Hysingla ER®, Zohydro ER®	PO	Immediate-release: 5 to 10 mg q4 to 6h (in combination with 300 to 325 mg acetaminophen per tablet); extended-release: 10 to 20 mg q12 to 24h
hydrocodone and homatropine	Hycodan®	PO	5 to 10 mg q4 to 6h prn (maximum 15 mg/dose)
hydromorphone	Dilaudid®	PO, IM, IV, rectal, SC	PO/IM/IV/SC: 1 to 4 mg q4 to 6h prn; extended release: 12 to 32 mg q24h; rectal: 3 mg q4 to 6h
meperidine	Demerol®	PO, IM, IV, SC	50 to 150 mg q3 to 4h prn
methadone	Dolophine®, Methadone®	PO, IM, SC	2.5 to 10 mg q3 to 4h prn
morphine	MS Contin®, Kadian®, Arymo ER®, MorphaBond ER®, Infumorph®, Mitigo®	PO, IM, IV	PO: 15 to 30 mg q4h; extended- release: 15 to 30 mg q8 to 12h; IM/IV: 5 to 15 mg q4h
oxycodone	Oxaydo®, Roxicodone®, RoxyBond®, OxyContin®, Xtampza ER®	PO	Immediate-release: 5 to 15 mg q4 to 6h; extended- release: 10 to 20 mg q12h (for OxyContin), 9 to 18 mg q12h (for Xtampza ER)
oxymorphone	Opana®, generic	PO	Immediate-release: 5 to 10 mg q4 to 6h; extended-release: 5 to 10 mg q12h
pentazocine	Talwin®	PO, IM, IV, SC	PO: 50 to 100 mg q3 to 4h (maximum 600 mg/day); IM/IV/SC: 30 mg q3 to 4h (maximum 360 mg/day)
pentazocine and naloxone	Talwin NX®	PO	One tablet (50 mg pentazocine/0.5 mg naloxone q3 to 4h); dosage may be doubled when needed; maximum 12 tablets/day
tapentadol	Nucynta®, Nucynta ER®	PO	Immediate-release: 50 to 100 mg q4 to 6h prn; extended- release: 50 to 250 mg q12h
tramadol	Ultram®, ConZip®	PO	Immediate- release: 50 to 100 mg q4 to 6h prn; extended- release: 100 to 300 mg/day

ANESTHETICS

Anesthesia is the unique condition of reversible unconsciousness or a loss of sensation. It is characterized by four reversible actions: unconsciousness, analgesia, immobility, and amnesia. There are four stages of general anesthesia (see Table 20-10).

Table 20-10 The Four Stages of General Anesthesia

Stage	Characterized By
Stage I	Analgesia
	Euphoria
	Perceptual distortions
	Amnesia
Stage II	Delirium
	Hypertension
	Tachycardia
Stage III	Surgical anesthesia
Stage IV	Medullary depression begins with cessation of respiration and circulatory collapse

Table 20-11 Examples of Local Anesthetics

Generic Name	Trade Name	Route of Administration	Average Adult Dosage
Amides			
bupivacaine	Sensorcaine®	IM (local infiltration, sympathetic block, lumbar epidural, caudal block, peripheral nerve block, retrobulbar block)	0.25% to 0.75% solution, depending on how administered
lidocaine	Xylocaine®	Caudal, Epidural, Infiltration, Nerve Block, Saddle Block, Spinal, Topical (jelly, ointment, cream, or solution)	0.5% to 2% solution (infiltration, nerve block, epidural, caudal); spinal: 5% with glucose; saddle block: 1.5% with dextrose; topical: 2.5% to 5%
Esters			
benzocaine	Americaine®	Topical	Lowest effective dose
procaine	Novocain®	SC, Peripheral nerve block	SC: 10% solution diluted with NS at 1 mL/5 seconds; PNB: 0.5% solution (up to 200 mL), 1% solution (up to 100 mL), or 2% solution (up to 50 mL)

Anesthetics are agents that act generally on the nervous tissue. Local anesthetics act to produce a loss of sensation in a local area of the body by depressing the excitability of excitable tissues. General anesthetics produce a state affecting overall body function. In anesthetic concentrations, they do not produce detectable generalized effects on all nerves. Examples of local anesthetics are shown in Table 20-11, and examples of general anesthetics that are currently in use are shown in Table 20-12.

Table 20-12 Examples of Currently Used General Anesthetics

Generic Name	Trade Name	Route of Administration	Average Adult Dosage
diazepam	Valium®	IV, IM	5 to 10 mg, repeat if needed in 2 to 4 hours
propofol (a benzodiazepine)	Diprivan®	IV	Induction: 2 to 2.5 mg/kg q10s until induction onset; Maint: 100 to 200 mcg/kg/min
thiopental sodium (a barbiturate)	Pentothal®	IV	IV test dose: 25 to 75 mg, then 50 to 75 mg at 20 to 40 seconds intervals; an additional 50 mg may be given prn

Summary

The nervous system consists of the interconnected neurons of the brain, spinal cord, and nerves. Together, the brain and spinal cord comprise the central nervous system. The peripheral nervous system connects the central nervous system to the remainder of the body. It consists of the cranial and spinal nerves. The autonomic nervous system controls homeostasis in the body. The somatic nervous system is associated with voluntary control of body movements and the reception of external stimuli. The neuron is the basic cell of the nervous system, and neurotransmitters enable nerve impulses to be transmitted throughout the body.

Disorders of the nervous system include migraine headache, stroke, epilepsy, Parkinson's disease, Bell's palsy, tic douloureux, multiple sclerosis, Alzheimer's disease, schizophrenia, bipolar disorder, major depressive disorder, anxiety disorders, sleep disorders, and attention deficit and hyperactivity disorder. Medications used to treat central nervous system disorders include sedatives, hypnotics, antianxiety drugs, anticonvulsants, anti-Parkinson drugs, antidepressants, antipsychotics, narcotic analgesics, and anesthetics.

REVIEW QUESTIONS

1. All of the following are parts of the neuron, *except:*

    A. synapse.
    B. cell body.
    C. dendrite.
    D. axon.

2. The portion of the brain that coordinates skeletal muscle activity is the:

    A. pons.
    B. medulla oblongata.
    C. hypothalamus.
    D. cerebellum.

3. Which of the following connects the two cerebral hemispheres?

    A. Pons
    B. Corpus callosum
    C. Medulla oblongata
    D. Thalamus

4. Which of the following foods cannot provoke a migraine attack?

    A. Red wine
    B. Aged cheese
    C. Broccoli
    D. Chocolate

5. Which of the following types of seizures is a medical emergency requiring immediate action?

   A. Petit mal
   B. Grand mal
   C. Tonic-clonic
   D. Status epilepticus

6. Paralysis of which of the following cranial nerves may cause Bell's palsy?

   A. Third
   B. Fifth
   C. Seventh
   D. Tenth

7. Which of the following is a newer drug used for Parkinson's disease?

   A. Phenytoin
   B. Rasagiline
   C. Lithium
   D. Morphine

8. Which of the following agents is an anticonvulsant?

   A. Carbamazepine
   B. Estazolam
   C. Levodopa
   D. Perphenazine

9. Conventional antipsychotics act by blocking the action of which of the following neurotransmitters?

   A. Dopamine
   B. Serotonin
   C. Acetylcholine
   D. All of the above

10. The generic name of Demerol® is:

    A. hydrocodone.
    B. meperidine.
    C. pentazocine.
    D. propoxyphene.

11. Which of the following signifies stage III of general anesthesia?

    A. Euphoria
    B. Delirium
    C. Surgical anesthesia
    D. Cessation of respiration

12. Atypical antipsychotics are thought to act by blocking the action of which of the following neurotransmitters?

    A. Dopamine
    B. Acetylcholine
    C. Serotonin
    D. A and C

13. Which of the following is the trade name of diazepam?

    A. Prosom®
    B. Ativan®
    C. Valium®
    D. Xanax®

14. What is the trade name of alprazolam?

    A.   BuSpar®

    B.   Ativan®

    C.   Serax®

    D.   Xanax®

15. Deposition of which of the following materials may cause Alzheimer's disease?

    A.   Serotonin

    B.   Amyloid

    C.   Uric acid

    D.   Creatinine

CRITICAL THINKING

A 70-year-old man presented with nondisabling, intermittent resting tremor of his left hand that over one year had progressed to the right hand. His cognition was normal, as were his oculomotor movements. There were mild signs of asymmetrical cogwheel rigidity and bradykinesia. The patient was diagnosed with Parkinson's disease.

    1. Which treatment options should be considered to initiate treatment?

    2. Why should treatment be initiated early and not after this patient's symptoms become disabling?

WEB LINKS

Alzheimer's Association: www.alz.org/

Alzheimer's Foundation of America: alzfdn.org/

American Academy of Sleep Medicine: aasm.org/

American Headache Society: americanheadachesociety.org/

Anticonvulsants for Bipolar Disorder: www.webmd.com/bipolar-disorder/guide/anticonvulsant-medication

Anti-Parkinson Drugs: www.webmd.com/parkinsons-disease/guide/drug-treatments#1

Anxiety and Depression Association of America: adaa.org

Central Nervous System Disorders—Related Drugs by Generic Name: www.drugs.com/condition/cns-disorder.html

Epilepsy Foundation: www.epilepsy.com

National Multiple Sclerosis Society: www.nationalmssociety.org/

National Sleep Foundation: www.sleepfoundation.org

Nervous System Diseases: www.nervous-system-diseases.com

Parkinson's Disease Foundation: www.parkinson.org

Schizophrenia and Related Disorders Alliance of America: sardaa.org

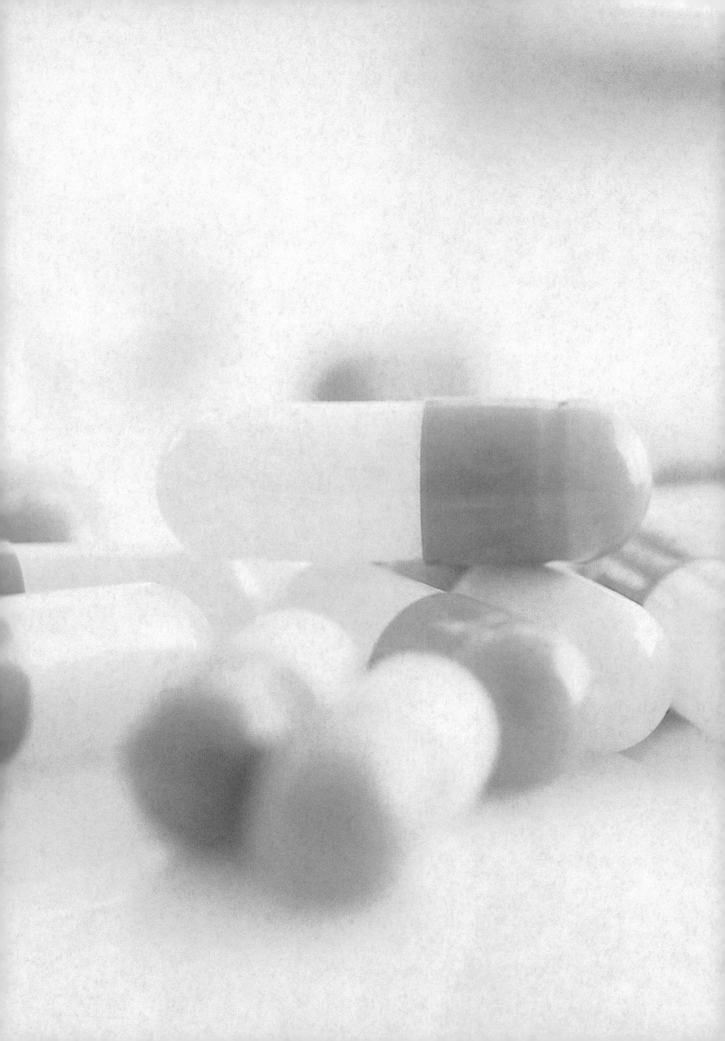

CHAPTER 21

Therapeutic Drugs for the Musculoskeletal System

OUTLINE

OBJECTIVES

Upon completion of this chapter, the reader should be able to:

1. Identify the axial and appendicular skeletons and name the major bones of each.
2. Discuss the major functions of bones.
3. Describe the various types of joints.
4. Identify the types of muscle that make up the muscular system.
5. Describe osteoarthritis and the medications used for it.
6. Define gout and explain its causes.
7. Describe the treatment of osteoporosis.
8. Compare the signs and symptoms of osteomalacia and rickets.
9. Describe fibromyalgia and its treatment.
10. Describe various types of muscle relaxants.

KEY TERMS

agonist

amphiarthroses

antagonist

arthritis

articulation

bursa

cartilage

centrally acting skeletal muscle relaxants

contusions

diarthroses

fibromyalgia

gout

lacerations

ligaments

muscular dystrophy

myasthenia gravis

neuromuscular blocking agents

osteoblasts

osteoclasts

osteocytes

osteogenic cells

osteomalacia

osteomyelitis

osteoporosis

rheumatoid arthritis

skeletal muscle

synarthroses

synergist

tendinitis

tendons

Overview

The musculoskeletal system actually consists of two different systems that work closely together: the skeletal system that provides the frame of the body and the muscular system that provides movement of the body. The musculoskeletal system includes a collection of connective tissue, muscles, bones, and joints. As the human skeleton forms, it is made up of **cartilage** and fibrous membranes. Bones soon mostly replace these. With continued growth and development, connective tissue in the skeletal muscle increases and the muscles develop stronger bonds. In later life, the process reverses, leading to decreases in skeletal muscle mass and weakening of muscular bonds.

The musculoskeletal system is affected by a large number of disorders. These disorders affect persons of all age groups and occupations. They are a major cause of pain and disability.

A broad spectrum of musculoskeletal injuries results from numerous physical forces, including blunt tissue trauma, disruption of tendons and ligaments, and fractures of bony structures. Many of the forces that cause injury to the musculoskeletal system are typical for a particular environmental setting, activity, or age group. Trauma resulting from high-speed motor vehicle accidents is a common cause of injury in adults younger than 45 years. The most common causes of childhood injuries are falls, bicycle-related injuries, and sports injuries. Falls are the most common causes of injury in people 65 years of age and older, with fractures of the hip and proximal humerus particularly common in this age group.

Anatomy and Physiology of the Musculoskeletal System

The musculoskeletal system consists of the skeletal muscles, bones, joints, tendons, and ligaments. The primary structures that influence body movements are the skeletal muscles, which are attached to the bones. Nearly half of the body's mass is made up of muscle tissues, which transform chemical energy into mechanical energy in order to cause skeletal movements.

SKELETAL SYSTEM

The skeletal system consists of bones and the joints where bones meet. Bones, which are considered the organs of the skeletal system, comprise a variety of very active, living tissues: bone tissue, cartilage, dense connective tissue, blood, and nervous tissue. They are multifunctional, providing points of attachment for muscles, protecting and supporting softer tissues, housing cells that produce blood, storing inorganic salts such as calcium and phosphorus, supporting and protecting the body's vital organs, and forming passageways for blood vessels and nerves. The 206 bones of the skeletal system differ in size and shape but are similar in structure, development, and function. Bones are classified by shape: long, short, flat, irregular, or round.

There are five major types of bone cells: **osteoblasts**, **osteocytes**, **osteoclasts**, *osteogenic cells*, and *bone lining cells*. Osteoblasts produce the bone matrix. Osteocytes are mature bone cells. Osteoclasts are large, multinucleated bone cells involved in resorption and deposition of bone. **Osteogenic cells** are also called *osteoprogenitor cells*. They are mitotically active stem cells in the periosteum and endosteum that, when stimulated, often differentiate into osteoblasts or bone lining cells. The bone lining cells are flattened and are found on bone surfaces where bone remodeling does not occur. They are believed to help maintain the bone matrix.

Divisions of the Adult Skeleton

The skeleton is divided into two major portions: an axial skeleton and an appendicular skeleton. The axial skeleton includes the skull, the vertebral column, and the thoracic cage. The appendicular skeleton includes the pectoral girdle, the upper limbs, the pelvic girdle, and the lower limbs. Table 21-1 summarizes the divisions of the adult skeleton.

Joints

The joints allow the body to be mobile and flexible. The **articulation** sites are covered with cartilage. Joints are classified based on their degree of movement and the types of material that hold them together. The three major groups of joints are called synarthroses, amphiarthroses, and diarthroses.

Synarthroses do not allow movement. There are three types of synarthroses:

- Sutures—Fibrous joints that occur only in the skull
- Syndesmoses—Bones that are connected by ligaments; for example, where the radius articulates with the ulna in the arm

Table 21-1 Divisions of the Adult Skeleton

Type of Skeleton	Type of Bones
Axial skeleton	Skull (22)
	Eight cranial bones: frontal (1), parietal (2), occipital (1), temporal (2), sphenoid (1), ethmoid (1)
	Fourteen facial bones: maxilla (2), zygomatic (2), palatine (2), inferior nasal concha (2), mandible (1), lacrimal (2), nasal (2), vomer (1)
	Middle ear (6)
	Malleus (2), incus (2), stapes (2)
	Hyoid (1)
	Hyoid bone (1)
	Vertebral column (26)
	Cervical vertebrae (7), thoracic vertebrae (12), lumbar vertebrae (5), sacrum (1), coccyx (1)
	Thoracic cage (25)
	Rib (24), sternum (1)
Appendicular skeleton	Pectoral girdle (4)
	Scapula (2), clavicle (2)
	Upper limbs (60)
	Humerus (2), radius (2), ulna (2), carpal (16), metacarpal (10), phalanx (28)
	Pelvic girdle (2)
	Hip bone (2)—includes the ilium, ischium, and pubis
	Lower limbs (60)
	Femur (2), tibia (2), fibula (2), patella (2), tarsal (14), metatarsal (10), phalanx (28)

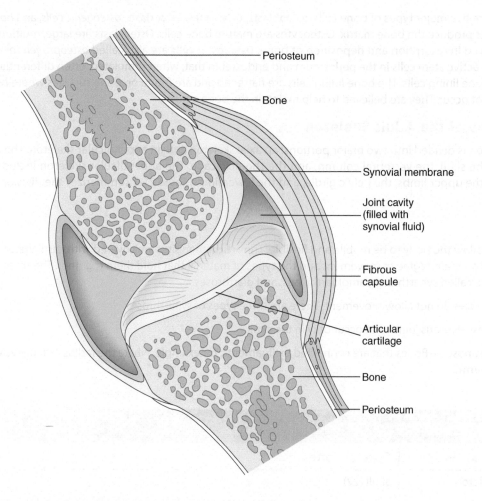

Figure 21-1 The structure of a synovial joint.

- Gomphoses—Exemplified by the way each tooth fits in its socket and is held there by a periodontal ligament

Amphiarthroses allow slight movement. An example is the symphysis pubis, which permits expansion of the lower pelvis, increasing the size of the birth canal to allow delivery of a baby.

Diarthroses allow free movement. These joints are also called synovial joints. The capsule surrounding a joint is lined with a connective membrane called the synovial membrane, with fluid inside (see Figure 21-1). The knee is an example of a synovial joint.

MUSCULAR SYSTEM

There are more than 600 muscles in the body. The muscular system consists of three types of muscles: **skeletal muscle**, which is attached to bones and joints by connective tissue (**tendons** and **ligaments**); smooth muscle; and myocardium. Skeletal muscle is also called voluntary muscle because it is the only type of muscle that can be consciously controlled. It is responsible for overall mobility of the body, and contracts rapidly. However, skeletal muscle tires easily and must be rested frequently.

Muscles require electrical impulses from motor nerves for stimulation (see Figure 21-2). When the muscles are excited, the muscle fibers respond by contracting and relaxing. A muscle that performs an actual movement is called a prime mover or an **agonist**. A muscle that opposes the actions of an agonist is called an **antagonist**. A muscle that assists an agonist is called a **synergist**. Beyond their role in enabling movement, skeletal muscles have other functions. They maintain body posture, stabilize joints, produce heat, and maintain body temperature.

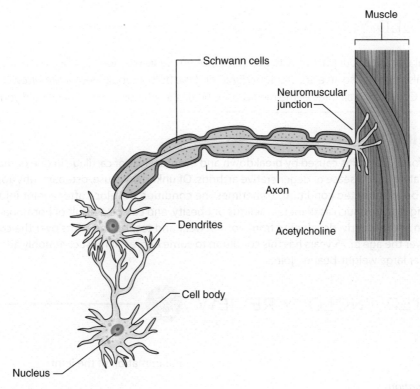

Figure 21-2 A neuron stimulating a muscle.

Musculoskeletal System Disorders

Diseases and disorders of the musculoskeletal system may occur at any age. Some conditions are the result of trauma to the affected part. They may be acute (i.e., of short duration) or chronic (requiring medications or treatments throughout an individual's life).

TRAUMATIC INJURY

Most traumatic skeletal injuries are accompanied by soft tissue (muscle, tendon, or ligament) injuries. These injuries include **contusions**, hematomas, and **lacerations**.

Sprains and strains are both musculoskeletal injuries, but they differ in terms of the tissue that is affected. A sprain involves the supporting ligaments of a joint. A strain is a stretching or a partial tear in a muscle or a muscle-tendon unit. A complete tear in a muscle or tendon is described as a rupture. Strains commonly result from the sudden stretching of a muscle that is actively contracting. They can occur at any age but are more common in middle-aged and older adults. Muscle strains are usually characterized by pain, stiffness, swelling, and local tenderness. Pain is increased with stretching of the muscle group.

ARTHRITIS

Arthritis is inflammation of an entire joint. This condition usually affects all of a joint's tissues, including its blood supply, bone, cartilage, ligaments, muscles, nerves, tendons, and other components. Approximately 10% of all humans experience arthritis, for which there is no cure, and there are over 100 different varieties of the disorder. Analgesics are commonly used for arthritis pain relief.

POINTS TO REMEMBER

Physical therapy helps to restore mobility and relieve pain in patients with back pain, arthritis, and joint and muscle injuries.

WHAT WOULD YOU DO?

An elderly patient comes to your pharmacy to get a prescription medication for his or her severe arthritis. You notice that he or she is also purchasing an extra-strength NSAID and the herbal supplement *white willow bark,* which is also used for arthritis. Considering all three of the medications he or she intends to use, what would you do?

OSTEOARTHRITIS

Osteoarthritis is a form of arthritis caused by breakdown and eventual loss of cartilage in one or more joints. It is also known as degenerative joint disease or degenerative arthritis. Of unknown cause, osteoarthritis appears to be linked to aging and may be an inherited condition. Sometimes the condition develops after a joint injury. It may also be linked to underlying diseases, such as diabetes mellitus or obesity, and can be a result of hormonal disorders. Osteoarthritis is common in the elderly, developing from normal wear and tear on the joints over the course of a lifetime. Nearly everyone over the age of 75 years has this condition to some degree. It most commonly affects the knees and hips, as well as other large weight-bearing joints.

MEDICAL TERMINOLOGY REVIEW

arthritis:

arthr = *joint*   inflammation of the joint

-itis = *inflammation*

Although there is no cure for osteoarthritis, treatment is aimed at reducing inflammation, minimizing pain, and maintaining joint function. These goals may be achieved by a combination of medications, physical therapy, nutritional management, and supportive care. Medications include analgesics, muscle relaxants, and non-steroidal anti-inflammatory drugs (NSAIDs).

Anti-inflammatory drugs include salicylates and NSAIDs. Aspirin (acetylsalicylic acid) has antipyretic, analgesic, and anti-inflammatory effects (at higher doses). Anti-inflammatory drugs reduce swelling. Along with acetaminophen and the cyclooxygenase-2 (COX-2) selective inhibitors, these drugs are also called *non-opioid analgesics.* Table 21-2 lists various non-opioid analgesics. For specific or individual joints, intra-articular steroid injections may be indicated. For example, in the knees, intra-articular hyaluronic acid helps to reduce pain.

In severe cases, opioid analgesics are used. Opioid analgesics act upon the brain's opioid receptors—primarily the *mu*, *kappa*, and *delta* receptors. Analgesia is effective via changes in pain perception at the spinal cord level of the central nervous system. The clinically effective opioid analgesics have mu-receptor agonist actions. Morphine is considered to be the prototype of the opioid analgesics. When the mu-receptors are activated, it causes analgesia, miosis, respiratory depression, euphoria, decreased gastrointestinal motility, and physical dependence. Therefore, opioid medications are controlled substances. Overdose may be life threatening. Examples of opioid antagonists, which can reverse opioid agonist effects by competing for opioid receptor sites, include naloxone and naltrexone. See Chapter 20 for detailed information on opioid analgesics.

Nondrug treatment includes alternation of moist heat and cold applications, range-of-motion exercises, elastic supportive bandages and splints, and massage therapy.

OSTEOMYELITIS

Osteomyelitis is a bacterial infection of the bones that may be acute or chronic. Approximately 90% of cases are caused by *Staphylococcus aureus*, with the next most prevalent bacterium being streptococcus. Patients may be predisposed to osteomyelitis if they have diabetes mellitus, neuropathy, and vascular insufficiency, a history of recent trauma or surgery, or foreign bodies such as prosthetic implants.

Treatment includes aggressive, long-term antibiotic therapy, usually for at least six weeks, followed by preventative care directed against reinfection. Antibiotics are often administered intravenously, but local antibiotics may

Table 21-2 Non-opioid Analgesics

Generic Name	Trade Name	Route of Administration	Average Adult Dosage
acetaminophen	Tylenol®	PO	500 mg (1 to 2 tablets q6h)
Salicylates			
aspirin (acetylsalicylic acid)	Alka-Seltzer®, Bayer®, Ecotrin®	PO, rectal	350 to 650 mg q4h (maximum 4 g/day)
choline magnesium trisalicylate	Trilisate®	PO	2 to 3 g/day in two divided doses
salsalate	Disalcid®	PO	325 to 3000 mg/day in divided doses (maximum 4 g/day)
Non-steroidal Anti-inflammatory Drugs			
diclofenac	Cataflam®, Solaraze®, Voltaren®	PO, ophthalmic, topical	PO: 150 to 200 mg/day in three to four divided doses; ophthalmic: 1 drop of 0.1% solution in affected eye qid beginning 24 hours after surgery and continuing for two weeks; topical: apply to affected area bid for 60 to 90 days
etodolac	Lodine®	PO	200 to 400 mg q6 to 8h (maximum 1000 mg/day)
ibuprofen	Advil®, Motrin®	PO	400 to 800 mg tid to qid (maximum 3200 mg/day)
indomethacin	Indocin®, Indocin SR®	PO, IV, rectal	PO: 25 to 50 mg bid to tid (maximum 200 mg/day) or 75 mg sustained release 1 to 2 times daily; IV: less than 48 hours, 0.2 mg/kg followed by two doses of 0.1 mg/kg q12 to 24h; two to seven days, 0.2 mg/kg followed by two doses of 0.2 mg/kg q12 to 24h; less than seven days, 0.2 mg/kg followed by two doses of 0.25 mg/kg q12 to 24h; rectal: 50 mg tid until pain is tolerable, then rapidly taper
ketorolac	Toradol®	PO	20 mg once, then 10 mg q4 to 6h prn (maximum 40 mg/day)
meclofenamate sodium	Meclofenamate®	PO	200 to 400 mg/day in three to four divided doses (maximum 400 mg/day)
meloxicam	Mobic®	PO	7.5 to 15 mg once daily
nabumetone	Relafen®	PO	1000 mg/day (maximum 2000 mg/day)
naproxen	Aleve®, Naprosyn®	PO	550 mg once, then 275 mg q6 to 8h or 550 mg q12h prn
oxaprozin	Daypro Alta®	PO	1200 mg/day
Cyclooxygenase-2 Selective Inhibitor			
celecoxib	Celebrex®	PO	200 mg/day or 100 mg bid

also be used. Aqueous penicillin, cephalosporin, erythromycin, ampicillin, and tetracycline are among the drugs that may be given. Dosages are based on patient age and the causative organism. The patient may require supportive measures, such as increased protein intake; supplementation with vitamins A, B, and C; bed rest; and the control of chronic conditions that may be related to osteomyelitis.

POINTS TO REMEMBER

The duration of therapy for acute osteomyelitis is four to six weeks, and for chronic osteomyelitis, it is more than eight weeks.

RHEUMATOID ARTHRITIS

Rheumatoid arthritis (RA) is a systemic inflammatory disease that attacks the connective tissue of the joints. It produces inflammation of the synovial membranes that leads to the destruction of the articular cartilage and underlying bone. Women are affected by this severely debilitating condition two to three times more frequently than men. Although the disease occurs in all age groups, its prevalence increases with age. The peak incidence among women is between the ages of 40 and 60 years, with the onset at 30 to 50 years of age.

The cause of RA has not been established. However, evidence points to a genetic predisposition and an autoimmune component. Joint involvement is usually bilateral, involving the same joints on both sides of the body, and systemic, involving more than one joint. The patient may complain of joint pain and stiffness that lasts for 30 minutes or longer after arising in the morning, and frequently for several hours. The most commonly affected joints initially are those of the fingers, hands, wrists, knees, and feet.

Treatment of RA includes medications to reduce inflammation, relieve pain, and prevent or slow joint damage. These medications include NSAIDs, steroids, disease-modifying antirheumatic drugs (DMARDs), immunosuppressants, tumor necrosis factor-alpha inhibitors, and others. Injectable drugs include etancercept (Enbrel®), adalimumab (Humira®), tocilizumab (Actemra®), certolizumab (Cimzia®), anakinra (Kineret®), abatacept (Orencia®), infliximab (Remicade®), golimumab (Simponi®), and a combination of rituximab (Rituxan®) with methotrexate. If improvement is not achieved, second-line agents are used, which include gold salts such as auranofin and gold sodium thiomalate, as well as methotrexate in a singular formulation. Physical and occupational therapy are used to improve joint mobility and help teach patients how to protect their joints from damage. Severe RA may require surgical procedures such as total joint replacement, tendon repair, and joint fusion.

GOUT

Gout is a chronic, usually inherited condition in which uric acid is not metabolized normally. There is either overproduction or decreased excretion of uric acid or urate salts, which leads to an acute, episodic type of arthritis, chronic deposition of uric acid in tissues, and kidney stones or impairment. The uric acid deposits form hard nodules in tissues, causing pain. Gout usually affects the first metatarsal joint of the great toe, resulting in severe to excruciating pain. It may also affect joints in the feet, ankles, and knees, with pain peaking over several hours, then slowly subsiding. The condition usually affects people older than 30 years, with men more commonly affected than women.

Treatment of an acute attack of gout includes bed rest, to lower the pressure on the affected joints, immobilization of affected limbs, and application of ice. Oral or parenteral NSAIDs or corticosteroids are helpful. When injection is chosen, it must be given locally into the area of persistent pain. Adequate fluid intake and a diet low in purines is also recommended. When gout is chronic, antihyperuricemic medications are indicated (see Table 21-3). For overweight patients, gradual weight reduction is suggested.

MEDICATION ERROR ALERT

The use of *colchicine* (*Colcrys*®) for gout and other conditions must be carefully monitored due to its toxicity. Intravenous doses of more than 2 to 4 mg per attack of gout have resulted in life-threatening toxicities.

TABLE 21-3 Drugs for Treatment of Gout

Generic Name	Trade Name	Route of Administration	Average Adult Dosage
allopurinol	Zyloprim®	PO	200 to 300 mg/day for mild gout; 400 to 600 mg/day for moderately severe gout (maximum 800/day)
colchicine	Colcrys®	PO	0.6 mg/day or bid (maximum 1.2 mg/day)
febuxostat	Uloric®	PO	40 to 80 mg/day
probenecid and colchicine	Probecid and Colchicine®	PO	500 mg probenecid/0.5 mg colchicine daily for one week, followed by the same dosage bid thereafter
Corticosteroids			
methylprednisolone	Depo-Medrol®	IM	4 to 120 mg/day
prednisone	Deltasone®	PO	5 to 60 mg/day
triamcinolone	Kenalog®	Intra-articular	2.5 to 20 mg/day

OSTEOPOROSIS

Osteoporosis is a condition in which there is a loss of normal bone density. It is the most common metabolic bone disease and is caused by an imbalance between the breakdown and resorption of older bone tissue and the creation and deposition of new bone tissue. Its most common forms are senile osteoporosis and postmenopausal osteoporosis (related to declining estrogen levels). Many conditions and factors are linked to the development of osteoporosis, including malabsorption, radiation therapies, immobility, smoking, and chronic conditions such as RA. It can also result from the use of medications such as heparin, phenytoin, prednisolone, and prednisone. Signs and symptoms of osteoporosis include wasting or deterioration of bone mass and decreased bone density. The condition most often affects women who are postmenopausal, small boned, of Asian or northern European heritage, smokers, and those who have a family history of osteoporosis. Symptoms are usually only produced when the condition affects the vertebrae or weight-bearing bones. It progresses silently until pain is caused by a bone fracture.

MEDICAL TERMINOLOGY REVIEW

> **osteoporosis:**
>
> oste/o = *bone*   -osis = *condition*
>
> por = *porous, lessening in density*   condition of porous bones

Treatment of osteoporosis is based on the cause. If untreated, the condition may result in permanent disability. Dietary changes are important and include increased intake of calcium, calcium carbonate with or without sodium fluoride, phosphate supplements, and vitamin D or other supplements. If the patient is postmenopausal, estrogen replacement therapy may be initiated. Loss of calcium may be slowed by exercise. Other medical therapies include bisphosphonates, parathyroid hormone, a nasal spray form of calcitonin, calcitonin salmon, and monoclonal antibodies (see Table 21-4).

WHAT WOULD YOU DO?

A pharmacy technician's 56-year-old aunt told him she was taking 400 mg of calcium and 200 units of vitamin D per day to prevent osteoporosis. If you were this pharmacy technician, what else would you suggest that she do to prevent osteoporosis?

OSTEOMALACIA AND RICKETS

Osteomalacia is a metabolic bone disease characterized by defective mineralization of the bones. When it occurs in children, the condition is called rickets, and occasionally the term *adult rickets* is applied to the adult form of the disease. Deficiency or ineffective usage of Vitamin D causes osteomalacia, the body cannot absorb calcium or phosphorus, and therefore, bone building is insufficient. The disease may result from inadequate exposure to sunlight (which is required for the natural synthesis of vitamin D), as well as chronic renal conditions and intestinal malabsorption of vitamin D.

Table 21-4 Examples of Medications for Osteoporosis

Generic Name	Trade Name	Route of Administration	Average Adult Dosage
Bisphosphonates			
alendronate	Fosamax®	PO	5 to 10 mg/day or 35 to 70 mg/week
ibandronate	Boniva®	PO, IV	PO: 150 mg/month; IV: 3 mg bolus q3 months
risedronate	Actonel®	PO	5 mg/day, or 35 mg/week, or 150 mg/month
zoledronic acid	Reclast®	IV	5 mg q1 to 2 years
Calcitonin Hormone Analogue			
calcitonin salmon	Fortical®	Nasal spray, IM/SC	Nasal spray: 200 units (1 spray) in one nostril/day, switching nostrils daily; IM/SC: 100 units/day
Selective Estrogen Receptor Modulator (SERM)			
raloxifene	Evista®	PO	60 mg/day
Parathyroid Hormone Analogue			
teriparatide	Forteo®	SC	20 mcg/day for up to two years
Monoclonal Antibody			
denosumab	Prolia®	SC	60 mg once q6 months
Supplements			
vitamin D and calcium	Citracal®, Caltrate®	PO	1000 to 1200 mg in two to three divided doses of calcium, and 400 to 800 international units of vitamin D

MEDICAL TERMINOLOGY REVIEW

osteomalacia:

oste/o = *bone*   softening of the bones

malacia = *softening*

Treatment of osteomalacia includes increased dietary intake of calcium, vitamin D (in the diet and via supplements), and calcitonin. In elderly persons more than any other group, it is important to increase sunlight exposure, which helps increase vitamin D metabolism and absorption to levels approaching normal. Any underlying condition must also be treated in order to reverse the deficiency. The treatments for rickets are the same as for osteomalacia, but may also include surgical intervention to correct a slipped femoral epiphysis in infants and young children. For deformities, bracing may be required.

POINTS TO REMEMBER

Studies suggest that osteomalacia caused by vitamin D deficiency is relatively common in elderly people who are acutely ill, and often is undiagnosed.

MEDICATION ERROR ALERT

The American Academy of Pediatrics recommends a daily dose of 400 units of vitamin D for infants. However, infants who drink less than 1 L of formula per day may need a lower dose of vitamin D supplements. Too much vitamin D can cause nausea, vomiting, loss of appetite, abdominal pain, muscle weakness, joint pain, confusion, fatigue, and kidney damage.

TENDINITIS

Tendinitis is inflammation of a tendon. It is also sometimes spelled *tendonitis*. A common example of this condition is tennis elbow, in which the elbow tendons become inflamed due to repetitive motion injury to the area. There may be associated calcium deposits and involvement of the **bursa**.

Treatment involves resting the injured area, administration of oral anti-inflammatory medications, and ice packs. Steroids may be injected into the affected joint space. Tendinitis sometimes affects the shoulder, causing it to become fixed (or "frozen") because of adhesions that form. Surgery may be required to release the tissues and return the joint to full range of motion.

MEDICATION ERROR ALERT

The risk of developing tendinitis increases when certain fluoroquinolones are administered. These include ciprofloxacin, levofloxacin, and similar drugs. Fluoroquinolones are also linked to tendon rupture. Therefore, dosages of these agents must be controlled carefully.

FIBROMYALGIA

Fibromyalgia is a common chronic condition affecting muscles, tendons, and joints in the entire body. The cause is unknown, but onset may be linked to infections, psychological distress, or trauma. Patients with fibromyalgia experience pain in response to normal stimuli that would otherwise be perceived as benign. The condition may be worsened by inappropriate exercise, poor posture, and smoking.

Fibromyalgia has no cure, but treatment can lessen the symptoms and help to restore normal function. Treatment involves a combination of patient education, physical activity, stress reduction, and medications. The focus of treatment is on reducing pain and improving sleep patterns. Medications designed to help improve sleep may be used, including the antidepressant amitriptyline (Elavil®), in low doses. To help with muscle and joint soreness, additional medications such as NSAIDs and muscle relaxants may be given.

POINTS TO REMEMBER

Fibromyalgia is more common in women, people of lower socioeconomic status, those with poor functional status, and people experiencing stressful life events.

WHAT WOULD YOU DO?

A pharmacy technician was diverting anabolic steroids from the hospital pharmacy in which he or she worked, so that his or her brother could use them to improve his physical performance in the hopes of obtaining a college athletic scholarship. If you discovered that your co-worker in the pharmacy was doing this, what would you do?

MUSCULAR DYSTROPHY

Muscular dystrophy is a rare, inherited condition that usually affects males. It causes degeneration of muscle tissue over time, eventually resulting in total incapacitation. There is no effective treatment for muscular dystrophy. However, patients may benefit from exercise, physical therapy, orthopedic appliances, and surgery. Corticosteroids help to slow degeneration of muscles. Additional medications that may be given, depending on symptoms, include anticonvulsants, immunosuppressants, and antibiotics.

MYASTHENIA GRAVIS

Myasthenia gravis is a condition of muscle weakness that causes affected individuals to become tired easily. The condition usually begins in the muscles of the face and is caused by abnormal destruction of acetylcholine receptors at neuromuscular junctions. Myasthenia gravis is an autoimmune disorder that primarily affects women between the ages of 20 and 40 years and men older than age 60. In most patients (80% to 90%), autoantibodies against the acetylcholine receptor are found. There is often drooping of one or both eyelids, diplopia, and difficulty in chewing, swallowing, and speaking. Signs and symptoms may differ over hours, days, weeks, and years and may worsen upon exposure to cold, sunlight, emotional stress, and infections. Muscular weakness often occurs after strenuous exercise or late in the day, and short rest periods may restore normal function. Eventually, however, paralysis of the muscles occurs. *Myasthenic crisis* is a severe manifestation in which the patient cannot swallow or breathe normally. This life-threatening complication may develop in response to a stressor or as part of the disease progression; it is a medical emergency that requires immediate care.

Treatment for myasthenia gravis is supportive and based on symptoms, patient age, and pregnancy status. Restricted activity, a soft or liquid diet, and, in severely affected patients, complete bed rest may be indicated. Medications include anticholinesterases, but their effect lessens over time. The drug of choice is pyridostigmine bromide (Mestinon®). A thymectomy is indicated if there is a thymus gland tumor. If the patient does not improve after surgery, corticosteroids may be required. Patients who experience a myasthenic crisis require immediate care, including intubation and mechanical ventilation. The patient's anticholinesterase medications are stopped and then reintroduced, along with plasmapheresis, as his or her condition improves.

POINTS TO REMEMBER

Myasthenic crisis causes respiratory muscle weakness, which produces respiratory insufficiency and can lead to respiratory failure.

Other Medications Used to Treat Musculoskeletal System Disorders

Skeletal muscle pain is very common. Chronic pain or severe injury needs special care. Treatments include analgesics, muscle relaxers, and sometimes physical therapy.

MUSCLE RELAXANTS

Muscle relaxants work by affecting skeletal muscle function and decreasing muscle tone. They are used to relieve muscle spasms, pain, and hyperreflexia. There are two major types of muscle relaxants, with different actions: *neuromuscular blocking agents* and *spasmolytics*.

Neuromuscular Blocking Agents

Neuromuscular blocking agents prevent muscles from moving. They interfere with transmission at the neuromuscular end plate and lack central nervous system activity. These drugs have no effect on pain or level of consciousness. Another group of skeletal muscle relaxants is used orally for painful muscle conditions. Examples of neuromuscular blocking agents are listed in Table 21-5.

Table 21-5 Examples of Neuromuscular Blocking Agents

Generic Name	Trade Name	Route of Administration	Average Adult Dosage
Short Duration			
succinylcholine	Anectine®	IM, IV	IM: 2.5 to 4 mg/kg up to 150 mg; IV: 0.3 to 1.1 mg/kg administered over 10 to 30 seconds, may give additional doses prn
Intermediate Duration			
atracurium	Tracrium®	IV	0.4 to 0.5 mg/kg initial dose, then 0.08 to 0.1 mg/kg 20 to 45 minutes after the first dose prn; reduce doses if used with general anesthetics
cisatracurium	Nimbex®	IV	Intubation: 0.15 or 0.20 mg/kg; Maint: 0.03 mg/kg q20min prn or 1 to 2 mcg/kg/min
pancuronium	Pavulon®	IV	Initial: 0.04 to 0.1 mg/kg (later incremental doses starting at 0.01 mg/kg may be used)
rocuronium	Zemuron®	IV	Initial: 0.6 mg/kg, though a lower dose of 0.45 mg/kg may be sufficient
vecuronium	Vecuronium Bromide®	IV	Initial: 0.08 to 0.1 mg/kg as a bolus; maintenance: 0.01 to 0.015 mg/kg
Extended Duration			
doxacurium	Nuromax®	IV	0.05 mg/kg administered as rapid bolus injection over 5 to 10 seconds; use lower doses in older adults or patients with renal or hepatic dysfunction
mivacurium	Mivacron®	IV	Loading: 0.15 mg/kg given over 5 to 15 seconds (over 60 seconds in patients with cardiovascular disease); Maint: 0.1 mg/kg generally q15min

Spasmolytics

Spasmolytics are also called **centrally acting skeletal muscle relaxants**. They are used to relieve musculoskeletal pain and spasms and to reduce spasticity for many conditions. Some examples of these drugs are listed in Table 21-6.

POINTS TO REMEMBER

Neuromuscular blocking agents prevent muscles from moving. These drugs have no effect on pain or the level of consciousness.

Table 21-6 Examples of Centrally Acting Skeletal Muscle Relaxants (Spasmolytics)

Generic Name	Trade Name	Route of Administration	Average Adult Dosage
baclofen	Lioresal®	PO, intrathecal	PO: 5 mg tid, may increase by 5 mg/dose q3d prn (maximum 80 mg/day); intrathecal: prior to infusion pump implantation, initiate trial dose of 50 mcg/mL bolus administered by barbotage up to 1 minute
carisoprodol	Soma®	PO	350 mg tid
chlorzoxazone	Parafon Forte®	PO	500 mg tid to qid (maximum 3 g/day)
cyclobenzaprine	Flexeril®	PO	5 to 10 mg tid (maximum 60 mg/day)
diazepam	Valium®	PO, IM, IV	PO: 2 to 10 mg bid to qid or 15 to 30 mg/day sustained release; IM/IV: 2 to 10 mg, repeat prn in 3 to 4 hours
metaxalone	Skelaxin®	PO	800 mg tid to qid
methocarbamol	Robaxin®	PO	Initial: 1500 mg qid; maintenance: 1000 mg qid

Summary

The musculoskeletal system is made up of connective tissue, muscles, bones, and joints. Bones provide points of attachment for muscles. Bone cells include osteoblasts, osteocytes, and osteoclasts. The skeleton is divided into two major portions: an axial skeleton and an appendicular skeleton. The joints allow the body to be mobile and flexible. The muscular system consists of three types of muscles: skeletal, smooth, and cardiac muscle. Skeletal muscles are voluntary, meaning they are consciously controlled.

Musculoskeletal disorders affect persons of all age groups and occupations. Injury and trauma result from numerous physical forces, including falls and high-speed motor vehicle accidents. Disorders of this system affect the bones, joints, muscles, and tendons. There are many different types of arthritis. Osteoarthritis is very common in elderly adults. Rheumatoid arthritis is a systemic inflammatory disease that attacks joints. Gouty arthritis is caused by the accumulation of crystalline deposits of uric acid in joint surfaces, bones, soft tissue, and cartilage. Osteoporosis is the most common metabolic bone disease, involving a loss of normal bone density, primarily in postmenopausal women. Fibromyalgia is an extremely common chronic condition affecting muscles, tendons, and joints in the entire body. Medications used to treat musculoskeletal system disorders include muscle relaxants, analgesics, antipyretics, and anti-inflammatory drugs.

REVIEW QUESTIONS

1. Which of the following types of bone cells are involved in resorption and deposition of bone?

   A. Osteoblasts
   B. Osteoclasts
   C. Osteocytes
   D. Osteogens

2. Which of the following is not a route of administration for indomethacin?

   A. Rectal
   B. Oral
   C. Topical
   D. Intravenous

3. Which of the following is not a type of synarthroses?

   A. Amphiarthroses
   B. Gomphoses
   C. Sutures
   D. Syndesmoses

4. Which of the following is a neuromuscular blocker?

   A. Baclofen
   B. Mivacurium
   C. Ibuprofen
   D. Fentanyl

5. Which of the following is the trade name of probenecid?

   A. Deltasone
   B. Benadryl
   C. Zyloprim
   D. Colcrys

6. Which of the following is not used to treat rheumatoid arthritis?

   A. Humira
   B. Enbrel
   C. Boniva
   D. Actemra

7. Which of the following is a degenerative joint disease?

   A. Rheumatoid arthritis
   B. Gouty arthritis
   C. Osteomyelitis
   D. Osteoarthritis

8. The trade name of meloxicam is:

   A. Meclomen.
   B. Meclofen.
   C. Mobic.
   D. Motrin.

9. Osteoarthritis most commonly affects the:

   A. neck and shoulders.
   B. knees and hips.
   C. wrists and fingers.
   D. elbows and hips.

10. To treat osteomyelitis, antibiotics are usually administered:

    A. orally.
    B. topically.
    C. intravenously.
    D. locally.

11. Deposition of which chemical substance in the tissues of the toes may cause gout?

    A. Uric acid
    B. Alpha protein
    C. Phosphoric acid
    D. Beta amyloid

12. Treatment of postmenopausal women with osteoporosis includes all of the following, *except*:

    A. Fosamax®.
    B. Actonel®.
    C. Mivacron®.
    D. Boniva®.

13. Which of the following is a muscle relaxant?

    A. cisatracurium (Nimbex)
    B. cyclobenzaprine (Flexeril)
    C. teriparatide (Forteo)
    D. vecuronium (Norcuron)

14. The trade name of diclofenac is:

    A. Voltaren®.
    B. Indocin®.
    C. Indameth®.
    D. Meclomen®.

15. All of the following are trade names of methotrexate, *except*:

    A. Mexate®.
    B. Rheumatrex®.
    C. Myochrysine®.
    D. Amethopterin®.

CRITICAL THINKING

A 34-year-old woman went to her physician complaining about muscle weakness and becoming easily tired. She was diagnosed with myasthenia gravis.

1. What are the most common signs and symptoms of this condition?

2. What factors can worsen the signs and symptoms of myasthenia gravis?

3. What is the purpose of using a neuromuscular agent such as pyridostigmine?

WEB LINKS

American Academy of Orthopaedic Surgeons: aaos.org

American Orthopaedic Association: www.aoassn.org

Arthritis Foundation: www.arthritis.org

Bone, Joint, and Muscle Disorders: bone-muscle.health-cares.net/

Health Information, including Musculoskeletal: www.healthpages.org

Muscular Dystrophy Association: www.mda.org

National Fibromyalgia Association: www.fmaware.org

National Osteoporosis Foundation: www.nof.org

Skeletal System: www.getbodysmart.com

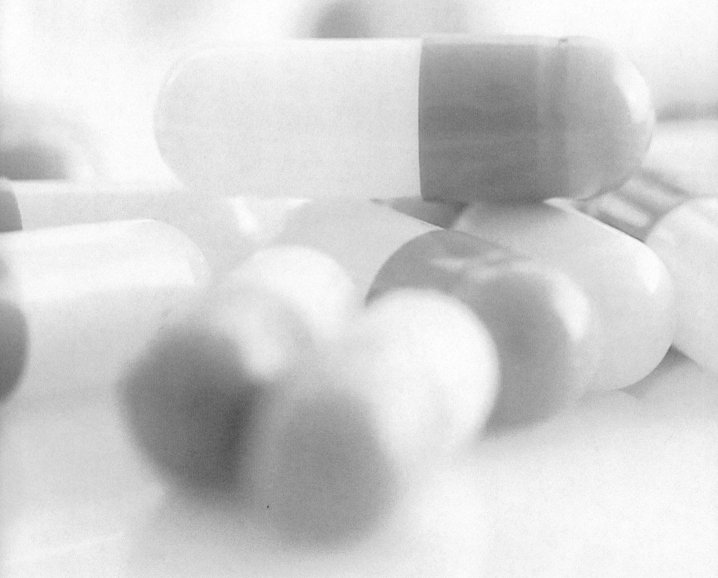

Therapeutic Drugs for the Endocrine System

OBJECTIVES

Upon completion of this chapter, the reader should be able to:

1. Define the term *hormone* and name some of the functions of the anterior pituitary gland.
2. Describe the locations of the major endocrine glands and the hormones they secrete.
3. Define thymosin, oxytocin, prolactin, and melatonin.
4. Describe the causes of Cushing's syndrome.
5. Compare Hashimoto's disease with simple goiter.
6. Compare the characteristics of myxedema and cretinism.
7. Describe type 2 diabetes mellitus.
8. List drugs for the treatment of hypothyroidism.
9. Describe different types of insulin.
10. List five generic and trade names of oral hypoglycemics.

KEY TERMS

acromegaly	dwarfism	hyperglycemia	pituitary gland
calcitonin	gigantism	insulin	prolactin
catecholamines	glucagon	islets of Langerhans	thymosin
corticosteroids	Graves' disease	melatonin	thyroxine
cretinism	growth hormone	myxedema	vasopressin
diabetes mellitus	hormones	neurohypophysis	

Overview

The endocrine system consists of specialized cell clusters, glands, hormones, and target tissues. The glands and cell clusters secrete hormones and chemical transmitters in response to stimulation from the nervous system and other sites. Together with the nervous system, the endocrine system regulates and integrates the body's metabolic activities and maintains internal homeostasis. Each target tissue has receptors for specific hormones. Hormones connect with the receptors, and the resulting hormone-receptor complex triggers the target cell's response.

Anatomy and Physiology of the Endocrine System

The endocrine system is composed of endocrine glands, which are distributed throughout the body. Endocrine glands secrete hormones, or chemical messengers, directly into the bloodstream. The major organs of the endocrine system are the hypothalamus, pituitary gland, thyroid gland, parathyroid glands, adrenal glands, pancreas, testes, and ovaries (see Figure 22-1).

Hormones are natural chemical substances secreted into the bloodstream from the endocrine glands that regulate and control the activity of an organ or tissues in another part of the body. A list of major hormones and endocrine glands is provided in Table 22-1. Hormones from the various endocrine glands work together to regulate vital processes of the body such as the following:

- Secretions in the digestive tract
- Energy production
- Composition and volume of extracellular fluid

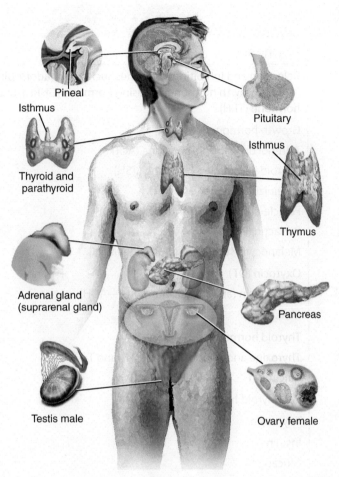

Figure 22-1 The endocrine glands.

- Adaptation and immunity
- Growth and development
- Reproduction and lactation

The body is conservative and secretes hormones only as needed. For example, **insulin** is secreted when the blood glucose level rises. **Glucagon**, another hormone, works antagonistically to insulin and is released when the blood glucose level falls below normal. Hormones are potent chemicals, thus, their circulating levels must be carefully controlled. When the level of a hormone is adequate, its further release is stopped. This type of control is called a negative feedback mechanism. Overactivity or underactivity of a gland is the most common cause of endocrine diseases. If a gland secretes an excessive amount of its hormone, it is hyperactive. When a gland fails to secrete its hormone or secretes an inadequate amount, it is hypoactive.

Inactivation of hormones occurs enzymatically in the blood, liver, kidneys, or target tissues. Hormones are secreted primarily via the urine and, to a lesser extent, the bile. In medicine, hormones generally are used in three ways: (1) for replacement therapy; (2) for pharmacological effects beyond replacement; and (3) for endocrine system diagnostic testing.

HYPOTHALAMUS

The hypothalamus is the main integrative center for the endocrine and autonomic nervous systems. The hypothalamus helps control some endocrine glands by neural and hormonal pathways. Neural pathways connect the hypothalamus to the posterior pituitary gland. The hypothalamus releases two effector hormones: antidiuretic hormone (ADH, also known as vasopressin) and oxytocin. These hormones are stored in the posterior pituitary gland.

Table 22-1 Endocrine Glands and Their Hormones

Gland	Hormones
hypothalamus	Releasing and inhibiting hormones such as gonadotropin-releasing hormone (GnRH), growth hormone-releasing hormone (GHRH), and thyrotropin-releasing hormone (TRH)
anterior pituitary	Growth hormone (GH; hGH)
	Adrenocorticotropic hormone (ACTH)
	Thyroid-stimulating hormone (TSH)
	Luteinizing hormone (LH)
	Follicle-stimulating hormone (FSH)
	Prolactin (PRL)
	Melanocyte-stimulating hormone (MSH)
posterior pituitary	Oxytocin (OT)
(hormone storage site)	Vasopressin (antidiuretic hormone—ADH)
pineal	Melatonin
thyroid	Thyroid hormones
	Thyroxine and triiodothyronine (T_4 and T_3)
	Calcitonin
parathyroid	Parathyroid hormone
thymus	Thymosin
pancreas (islets of Langerhans)	Insulin
	Glucagon
adrenal cortex	Cortisol (a glucocorticoid)
	Aldosterone (a mineralocorticoid)
	Androgens
adrenal medulla	Epinephrine
	Norepinephrine
testes	Testosterone
ovaries	Estrogen
	Progesterone

The hypothalamus also exerts hormonal control at the anterior pituitary gland, by releasing and inhibiting hormones, which arrive by a portal system. Hypothalamic hormones stimulate the pituitary gland to synthesize and release tropic hormones. These hormones include corticotropin (also called adrenocorticotropic hormone), thyroid-stimulating hormone, and gonadotropins, such as luteinizing hormone and follicle-stimulating hormone. Secretion of tropic hormones stimulates the adrenal cortex, thyroid gland, and gonads. Hypothalamic hormones also stimulate the pituitary gland to release or inhibit the release of effector hormones, such as growth hormone and prolactin.

MEDICAL TERMINOLOGY REVIEW

hypothalamus:

hypo- = *under*

-thalamus = *mass of gray matter with relay functions*

gray matter in the brain that relays nerve impulses

PITUITARY GLAND

The small, marble-shaped **pituitary gland** is under the control of the hypothalamus in the brain. The pituitary gland is small and is situated at the base of the brain. It is also called the "master gland." It secretes hormones directly into the bloodstream to control and regulate the other endocrine glands. The pituitary gland consists of two lobes: an *anterior lobe* (adenohypophysis) and a *posterior lobe* (neurohypophysis), which are under the influence of hypothalamic hormones. These hormones control the secretion of specific tropic hormones that regulate peripheral endocrine gland secretions and target tissues.

Anterior Pituitary Gland

The anterior lobe of the pituitary gland is particularly important in sustaining life. The anterior pituitary gland secretes at least six hormones: **growth hormone** (GH, hGH somatotropin), adrenocorticotropic hormone (ACTH), thyroid-stimulating hormone (TSH, thyrotropin), follicle-stimulating hormone (FSH), luteinizing hormone (LH), and **prolactin** (PRL). Since FSH and LH both affect the male and female gonads, they are collectively referred to as *gonadotropins*. Another hormone, melanocyte-stimulating hormone (MSH), stimulates melanocytes in the skin to produce more melanin, which darkens the skin pigment. Figure 22-2 illustrates the major hormones of the pituitary gland and their principal target organs.

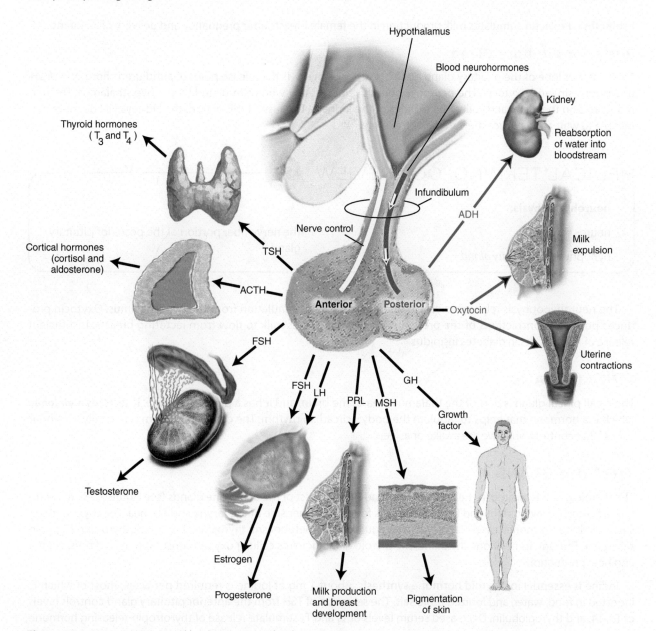

Figure 22-2 Hormones secreted by the pituitary gland.

Growth Hormone   Growth hormone (somatotropin) promotes body growth by stimulating cells to increase in size and divide rapidly.

Adrenocorticotropic Hormone   ACTH stimulates the growth of the adrenal gland cortex and the secretion of corticosteroids. Under normal conditions, a diurnal rhythm occurs in ACTH secretion, with an increase beginning after the first few hours of sleep and reaching a peak at the time a person awakens.

Thyroid-Stimulating Hormone   Thyroid-stimulating hormone controls the release of thyroid hormone and is necessary for the growth and function of the thyroid gland. TSH stimulates the thyroid gland to increase the uptake of iodine and increase the synthesis and release of thyroid hormones. It is prescribed for hypothyroidism and diagnostic tests.

Follicle-Stimulating Hormone   Follicle-stimulating hormone controls development of the ova in the ovaries and sperm in the testes. It also stimulates the ovaries to secrete estrogen.

Luteinizing Hormone   Luteinizing hormone stimulates sex hormone secretion in both genders (progesterone in the female and testosterone in the male), as well as plays a role in release of the ova from the ovaries in females.

Prolactin   Prolactin stimulates milk production in the female breasts after pregnancy and delivery of an infant.

Posterior Pituitary Gland

The posterior lobe of the pituitary gland, or the **neurohypophysis**, is the release point of antidiuretic hormone (ADH, or vasopressin) and oxytocin. The neurohypophysis releases ADH when stimulated by the hypothalamus. The hormone acts on the distal and collecting tubules of the kidneys. Because of this action, the kidneys will be more permeable to water and reduce the volume of the urine.

MEDICAL TERMINOLOGY REVIEW

neurohypophysis:

neuro- = *nerve*

hypophysis = *pituitary gland*

the nerve fiber portion of the posterior pituitary gland

The neurohypophysis releases oxytocin under appropriate stimulation from the hypothalamus. Oxytocin produces powerful contractions of the pregnant uterus and causes milk to flow from lactating breasts. Insufficient release of ADH results in diabetes insipidus.

PINEAL GLAND

The small pineal gland is part of the thalamus area of the brain, and it has a pinecone shape. It secretes **melatonin**, which is a hormone that helps to regulate the body's circadian rhythm. The circadian rhythm is basically a 24-hour "clock" that controls when we are awake or asleep.

THYROID GLAND

The thyroid gland is located in the anterior neck and is the largest of the endocrine glands (see Figure 22-3). It resembles a butterfly, having right and left lobes, and is found on either side of the larynx and trachea. The thyroid gland secretes three hormones essential for proper regulation of metabolism: **thyroxine** (T_4), triiodothyronine (T_3), and **calcitonin**. Through its hormone thyroxine, the thyroid gland governs cellular oxygen consumption, and thus, energy and heat production.

Iodine is essential for thyroid hormone synthesis. About 1 mg of iodine is required per week, most of which is ingested in food, water, and iodized table salt. The secretion of TSH from the anterior pituitary gland controls levels of T3, T4, and thyroglobulin. Decreased serum levels of T_3 and T_4 stimulate release of thyrotropin-releasing hormone

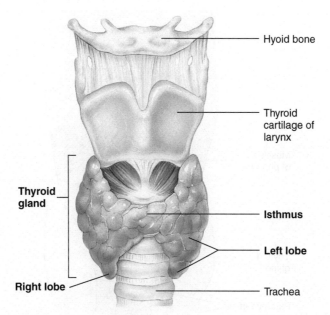

Figure 22-3 Thyroid gland.

(TRH) from the hypothalamus, which stimulates the pituitary gland to secrete TSH. Then, TSH stimulates the thyroid gland to release T_4 and thyroglobulin. The hormone calcitonin has a very important role in calcium metabolism. Normally, calcitonin decreases the level of blood calcium; therefore, this hormone is used to treat hypercalcemia, osteoporosis, and Paget's disease.

POINTS TO REMEMBER

Up to 80% of the iodine in the body is in the thyroid gland. In this gland, the concentration of iodine is 25 times that of the iodine concentration in the bloodstream.

PARATHYROID GLANDS

Four tiny parathyroid glands lie along the posterior (dorsal) surface of the thyroid gland (see Figure 22-4). The parathyroid glands secrete parathyroid hormone (PTH, parathormone). The stimulus for the release of PTH is a low plasma level of calcium. PTH has three target organs: bones, digestive tract (intestines), and kidneys. The overall effect of PTH is to increase plasma calcium levels. This stimulates bone breakdown, resulting in the release of more calcium into the blood.

Spontaneous atrophy or injury that results in removal of the parathyroid glands is followed by a decrease in the concentration of serum calcium and an increase in the concentration of serum phosphorus. The biological function of calcitonin is to prevent excessive hypercalcemia from PTH activity. When plasma calcium levels are elevated, thyrocalcitonin is released in increased quantities. Thus, it tends to oppose PTH but at different cell targets.

THYMUS GLAND

The thymus gland is located in the mediastinal cavity, and is both superior and anterior to the heart. It plays an important role in "kick-starting" the immune system following birth. Its endocrine function involves secretion of the hormone **thymosin**, which is important for proper development of the immune system. Though present at birth, the thymus grows to its greatest size during puberty. It then begins to shrink continually through life, and is replaced by adipose and connective tissues.

The primary function of the thymus is to develop the immune system in newborns. The thymus is critical for the growth and development of the thymic lymphocytes, also called T lymphocytes or T cells. These lymphocytes are vital for the immune system to be able to protect the body.

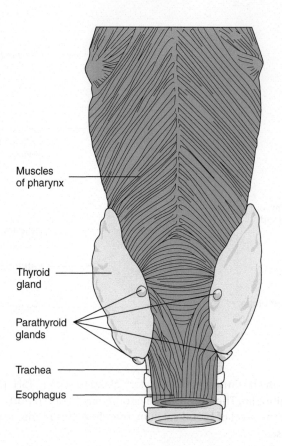

Muscles
of pharynx

Thyroid
gland

Parathyroid
glands

Trachea

Esophagus

Figure 22-4 Parathyroid glands.

MEDICAL TERMINOLOGY REVIEW

corticosteroids:

cortico- = *cortex*

-steroids = *hormones affecting sex organs*

steroids formed in the cortex of the adrenal gland that affect the sex organs

ADRENAL GLANDS

The adrenal glands are located at the top of each kidney. They consist of two parts: the outer *adrenal cortex* and the inner *adrenal medulla* (see Figure 22-5). The adrenal cortex synthesizes three important classes of hormones: glucocorticoids or adrenocorticosteroids (cortisol), mineralocorticoids (primarily aldosterone), and androgens, which are steroid sex hormones. All these three classes are referred to as **corticosteroids** because they are produced by the adrenal cortex, which is one of the endocrine structures most vital for normal metabolic function. Aldosterone regulates sodium and potassium levels, while cortisol regulates carbohydrates in the body. In both genders, the adrenal cortex secretes androgens, which can be converted to estrogen following release into the bloodstream. Androgens regulate secondary sex characteristics. All of the hormones from the adrenal cortex are steroid hormones.

The adrenal medulla secretes two **catecholamines**: epinephrine (adrenaline) and norepinephrine (noradrenaline). Both of these hormones are vital for emergency situations since they increase heart rate, blood pressure, and respiration levels, allowing the body to perform better when under stress.

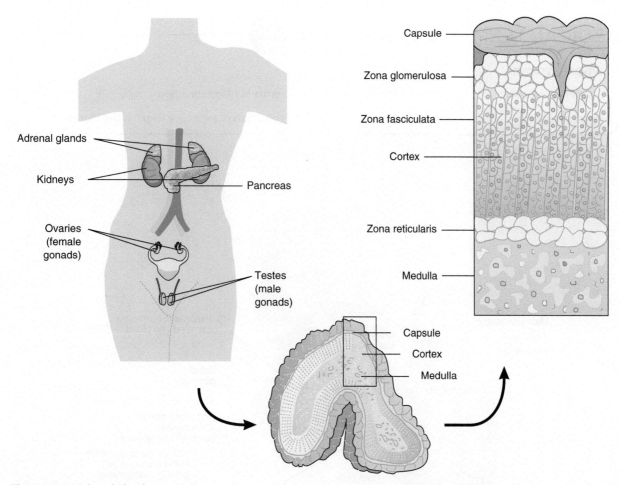

Figure 22-5 Adrenal glands.

Tumors in the adrenal medulla can increase hormonal secretion. Release of norepinephrine usually predominates and causes high blood pressure, increased heart rate, and elevated blood glucose.

PANCREAS

The pancreas is one of the accessory organs of the digestive system, located beneath the great curvature of the stomach (see Figure 22-6). It is the only body organ with both endocrine and exocrine functions. The pancreas produces digestive enzymes that are deposited in the duodenum of the small intestine. Throughout the pancreas, there are clusters of specialized cells (**islets of Langerhans**). The alpha cells produce glucagon to raise blood glucose levels and the beta cells release insulin, which lowers blood glucose levels. This occurs after eating, when carbohydrates have been absorbed as sugar (glucose) into the bloodstream. The body's cells can then obtain the required amounts of glucose needed for cellular respiration.

When serum blood glucose levels decline, glucagon facilitates the breakdown of glycogen in the liver to glucose. The conversion of glycogen to glucose results in an increase in blood glucose. Several hours after a meal has been digested, or when the body begins strenuous physical activity, glucagon is released to supply glucose to the cells. The release of glucagon stimulates insulin secretion, which then inhibits the release of glucagon. The most important disease involving the endocrine pancreas is diabetes mellitus, a disorder of carbohydrate metabolism that involves insulin deficiency, insulin resistance, or both. Diabetes, if untreated or uncontrolled, leads to **hyperglycemia**. Severe hyperglycemia and ketoacidosis may produce diabetic coma or unconsciousness, which requires much higher doses of insulin.

MEDICAL TERMINOLOGY REVIEW

hyperglycemia:

hyper- = *excessive*

glyc = *sugar*

-emia = *blood condition*

condition of excessive sugar in the blood

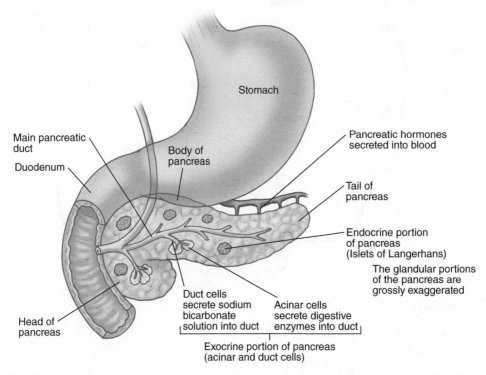

Figure 22-6 The pancreas.

OVARIES

The ovaries are the two female gonads; they are located in the lower abdominopelvic cavity. They produce the female sex hormones, which include estrogens and progesterone. The ovaries are discussed in greater detail in Chapter 28.

TESTES

In males, the testes are the two oval glands inside the scrotum. They are the male gonads, producing the male sex hormone (testosterone) and gametes (sperm). The testes are discussed in greater detail in Chapter 28.

Disorders of the Endocrine System and their Treatments

Diseases and conditions of the endocrine system include pituitary diseases, diabetes, and thyroid diseases. Common dysfunctions of the endocrine system are classified as hypofunction, hyperfunction, inflammation, and tumor. The most common endocrine disorders are explained here.

HYPOPITUITARISM

Hypopituitarism is a condition caused by a deficiency or absence of any of the pituitary hormones, especially those produced by the anterior pituitary lobe. Hypopituitarism leads to growth retardation in children. Causes include a pituitary or hypothalamic tumor, though congenital deficiencies may also be involved. Another cause is damage to the pituitary gland because of radiation, surgical removal, or ischemia due to basilar skull fracture, infarct, or a tumor. When ischemia is severe and ongoing, glandular tissue begins to be permanently destroyed. If panhypopituitarism occurs, which is destruction of the entire anterior lobe, no important anterior pituitary hormones can be secreted. This is most common in females, and its cause is unknown. Signs and symptoms of hypopituitarism include metabolic dysfunction, growth retardation, or sexual immaturity. The specific hormone deficiency affects the physical findings.

If there is deficiency of pituitary hormones that stimulate other endocrine glands, the glands may atrophy. If TSH secretion is reduced, the thyroid gland's function is affected, and hypothyroidism symptoms develop. If ACTH secretion is reduced, nutrient metabolism and sodium balance are affected. If gonadotropins are deficient, sexual functions are impaired, including libido, menstruation, and sexual development. In children, hypopituitarism causes growth retardation. Because of tumor infringement on the optic nerve, there may be headache and even blindness.

Treatment of hypopituitarism is based on the patient's age, severity of the condition, type of deficiency, and underlying cause. Tumor removal usually reverses the condition if neoplasia was the cause. After this surgery, radiation is indicated. If needed, replacement therapy may involve hormones such as cortisone, thyroxine, human growth hormones, or sex hormones. Continual monitoring of hormone levels is required during therapy.

Dwarfism is the abnormal underdevelopment of the body that occurs in children. Hyposecretion of growth hormone results in growth retardation. Dwarfism may be congenital, or it may be caused by a cranial hemorrhage after birth. It may also be of an unidentified cause. Secondary hypopituitarism results from head trauma, infection, or a tumor, causing deficiency of the growth hormone-releasing hormone (GHRH). Signs and symptoms of dwarfism include extremely short height, with a body that is small in proportion. Prepubescent children do not develop secondary sex characteristics. Dwarfism may be linked to other abnormalities, and mental disability may be present in varying degrees.

Treatments for dwarfism involve administration of somatotropin until a height of 5 feet is reached. The patient may also require thyroid and adrenal hormone replacements. If required, sex hormones may be administered as puberty approaches.

HYPERPITUITARISM

Hyperpituitarism is a chronic and progressive disease that is caused by excessive production and secretion of pituitary hormones (particularly human growth hormone [hGH]). Excessive hGH produces one of two distinct conditions, **gigantism** or **acromegaly**, depending on the time of life at which the dysfunction begins.

Gigantism describes an abnormal pattern of growth and stature. It occurs before puberty, resulting in a proportional overgrowth of all body tissue. Growth is accelerated, especially affecting the long bones. There may be delay of sexual and mental development. Gigantism is often caused by an anterior pituitary adenoma. It may affect several members of the same family. Also, by delaying puberty and the closure of the epiphyses of bones, hypogonadism may lead to taller than normal stature but not actual gigantism.

The goal of treatment for gigantism is to reduced amounts of growth hormone that are secreted. This is best achieved by transsphenoidal surgery, with or without the use of radiation to the pituitary gland in order to reduce its size. In children or adolescents, gonadal hormone treatments may be required if hypogonadism is present. The patient should have yearly follow-up examinations.

Acromegaly is a chronic metabolic condition in adults caused by hypersecretion of hGH. It occurs after puberty, when epiphyseal closure has already occurred, thereby resulting in an overgrowth of just the bones of the face, hands, and feet (as well as an excessive overgrowth of soft tissue). The cause is also often a pituitary tumor or adenoma. This condition affects both genders equally. Signs and symptoms usually appear after the age of 30 or 40 years. The patient experiences the need for larger shoes and gloves, and continuing jaw growth results in larger spaces between teeth. The overproduction of hGH can reduce mortality, so life may be extended. However, a variety of clinical symptoms may occur throughout the body, including joint pain because of osteoarthritis. Treatment for acromegaly is designed to reduce hGH secretion and prevent mass effects from an existing tumor. If successful, treatment may prevent additional disfigurement. Ideal treatment is the same surgery used for gigantism, with or without radiation therapy to the pituitary gland. Success depends on how tumor cells respond to the treatments. In some cases of acromegaly, octreotide (Sandostatin®) is indicated.

DIABETES INSIPIDUS

Diabetes insipidus is a disturbance of water metabolism. It is a deficiency in the release of **vasopressin** (antidiuretic hormone [ADH]) by the posterior pituitary gland and causes the excretion of larger than normal amounts of colorless, dilute urine by the kidney. Diabetes insipidus may be hereditary or caused by damage to the hypothalamus or pituitary gland from cerebral edema, head trauma, or an intracranial lesion. Nephrogenic diabetes insipidus occurs because of renal tubular resistance to vasopressin. Diabetes insipidus is more common in males and may occur in childhood or early adulthood. Often its cause is unknown. Insufficient vasopressin levels result in distal nephron tubules of the kidney being unable to reabsorb water from filtrate back into the bloodstream, resulting in excessive urine volume.

Signs and symptoms of diabetes insipidus include polyuria, polydipsia, fatigue, and symptoms of dehydration. These include drying of mucous membranes, dizziness, hypotension, and poor skin turgor (cellular tension), all of which may develop rapidly.

Treatment of diabetes insipidus involves injection or nasal sprays of vasopressin or oral desmopressin acetate (DDAVP). Some drugs prescribed to stimulate secretion of ADH include chlorpropamide, carbamazepine, and clofibrate. For nephrogenic diabetes insipidus, thiazide diuretics are administered to block the kidneys' excretion of free water. They work by inhibiting sodium and chloride reabsorption and by increasing sodium, chloride, and water excretion. Underlying causes must be identified and treated. If pituitary gland trauma was the cause, symptoms subside as the lesions resolve.

SIMPLE GOITER

The term goiter refers to any enlargement of the thyroid gland. Simple (nontoxic) goiter results from a shortage of iodine in the diet. Iodine is necessary for the synthesis of thyroxine (T_4), which is the major form of thyroid hormone in the blood. When thyroid hormone levels in the blood are less than needed, the anterior pituitary gland increases secretion of thyrotropin (TSH). This hormone continually tries to stimulate production of thyroid hormone from the thyroid gland, and the gland then increases in size. Though deficiency of iodine is no longer prevalent because of improved diets that include iodized salt, fresh vegetables, and seafood, simple goiter still occurs in people who eat large amounts of goitrogenic foods. Examples of these foods include cabbage and turnips. Drugs such as lithium are also goitrogenic.

Simple goiter, which is also known as hyperplasia of the thyroid gland, produces conspicuous swelling of the anterior neck (see Figure 22-7). Over time, the hyperplasia causes pressure upon the esophagus, making swallowing difficult. If further enlargement occurs, compression of the trachea causes dyspnea. However, the condition can be asymptomatic in its early stages. Females are more often affected than males.

Treatment in the early stages of simple goiter includes one drop of saturated solution of potassium iodide per week. Thyroid hormones such as thyroxine may also be beneficial. To prevent simple goiter, iodine must be added to the diet in iodine-deficient areas of the world. When goiter occurs sporadically, prevention involves avoiding goitrogenic foods or drugs. Table 22-2 summarizes various medications used to treat thyroid gland conditions.

HASHIMOTO'S DISEASE

Hashimoto's disease, also known as Hashimoto's thyroiditis or chronic thyroiditis, is a chronic disease of the immune system that attacks the thyroid gland. This condition occurs more in women than in men, is most common between ages 45 and 65, and is the leading cause of non-simple goiter and hypothyroidism. It is of unknown cause but believed to be genetically linked. In Hashimoto's disease, antibodies appear to destroy the thyroid instead of simulating it, making this disorder autoimmune-related. Enlargement of the thyroid occurs due to extensive infiltration by plasma cells and lymphocytes. Over time, the glandular tissue is replaced by fibrous tissue.

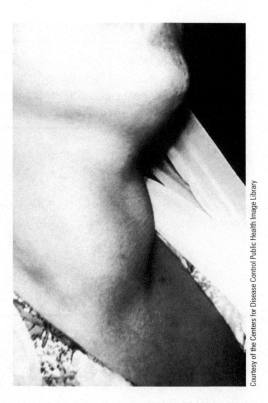

Courtesy of the Centers for Disease Control Public Health Image Library

Figure 22-7 Simple goiter.

Signs of Hashimoto's disease include gradual, painless enlargement of the thyroid gland. The patient feels pressure in the neck and experiences difficulty in swallowing. With disease progression, symptoms of hypothyroidism develop, including sensitivity to cold, mental apathy, and weight gain. Treatment requires replacement of thyroid hormones throughout the patient's lifetime, which also prevents additional goiter growth.

HYPERTHYROIDISM

Hyperthyroidism is the overproduction of thyroid hormone, causing increased metabolism and changes in multiple body systems. **Graves' disease** is a condition of primary hyperthyroidism. It occurs when the entire thyroid gland is enlarged, resulting in a diffuse goiter. The cause of Graves' disease is not certain but is believed to be autoimmune-related. Antibodies to thyroid antigens stimulate hyperactivity of the thyroid gland. The condition is seen in families, implying a genetic link.

Signs and symptoms relate to increased metabolic activity and numerous multisystem changes and include palpitations, rapid heartbeat, excitability, nervousness, insomnia, weight loss, increased perspiration, warm and moist skin, muscular weakness, and onycholysis of the nails. The patient is hyperactive, often loses hair, and may experience tremors. One of the distinguishing manifestations of hyperthyroidism is exophthalmos, which is abnormal protrusion of the eyeballs due to edema in the tissues behind the eyes (see Figure 22-8). Also, the skin may change from its normal condition. Sudden worsening of symptoms may signal a life-threatening condition known as *thyrotoxicosis* or *thyroid storm*, which occurs because of greatly raised thyroid hormone levels.

Treatment is aimed at reducing formation and secretion of thyroid hormone. This begins with administration of antithyroid medications, including methimazole (Tapazole®), propylthiouracil and *Lugol's solution. Lugol's solution is a medication containing iodine and potassium iodide*. For hypertension and tachycardia, beta-blockers are used, including atenolol (Tenormin®) and propranolol hydrochloride (Inderal®). Additional treatments include radioactive iodine therapy and surgical thyroidectomy, though this surgery is very uncommon in the United States. The patient must be continually supervised, with thyroid hormone levels monitored. He or she may need assistance coping with physical symptoms or anxiety caused by Graves' disease.

WHAT WOULD YOU DO?

You are aware that your pharmacy manager has been treated for hyperthyroidism. One day, he or she comes to work feeling feverish and says he or she feels like his or her heart is pounding. He or she soon becomes nauseated and weak and seems confused. Bearing in mind his or her hyperthyroidism, what would you do?

POINTS TO REMEMBER

Propylthiouracil is currently the drug of choice to treat hyperthyroidism during pregnancy because methimazole causes the congenital defect of esophageal atresia.

MEDICATION ERROR ALERT

Dosing errors involving Lugol's solution for Graves' disease are relatively common. While often only 5 drops of the solution are intended for administration, errors that have occurred include administering 5 mL instead of 5 drops, causing a potentially fatal outcome. One contributing factor may be that unfamiliarity with the solution may cause some health care professionals to assume that milliliters would be given, and not drops.

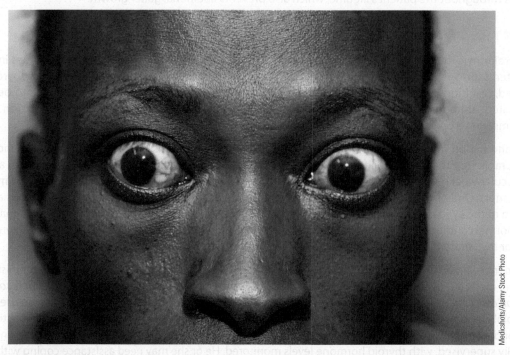

Figure 22-8 Graves' disease.

HYPOTHYROIDISM

Hypothyroidism can affect males and females of any age. Many people across the world are at high risk for hypothyroidism due to iodine-deficient diets. This can result in congenital hypothyroidism, which can lead to mental deficiency. Hypothyroidism is very common and may occur in families. **Cretinism** is a form of congenital hypothyroidism that manifests in infancy or early childhood. It is typified by the absence of the thyroid gland or the lack of thyroid hormone synthesis by the thyroid gland. In most cases, abnormal fetal development results in failure of the thyroid gland to develop or function. An enzyme required for thyroid hormone synthesis may also be lacking. The lack of thyroid hormones causes mental and physical retardation in infants and young children. Antithyroid drugs taken during pregnancy, or a maternal thyroid deficiency may also cause this condition.

Signs and symptoms of hypothyroidism may not develop for weeks to years. Initial symptoms include cold intolerance, fatigue, constipation, and dry skin that flakes easily. The condition is diagnosed by blood testing to obtain levels of TSH, T_3, and T_4. Increased TSH levels and decreased T_3 and T_4 levels indicate hypothyroidism. In cretinism, the child will have stunted growth, with an extended abdomen, stocky build, broad nose, short forehead, small and wide-set eyes, puffy eyelids, expressionless face, dry skin, wide-open mouth, and a thickened and protruding tongue. The sex organs do not develop, and there is retardation of growth, mental ability, and physical strength. The child may be unable to stand or walk due to poor muscle tone.

Treatment of hypothyroidism includes hormone replacement throughout the patient's lifetime. Popular medications include Levoxyl® and Synthroid®. Careful monitoring of hormone levels in the blood is required. Without treatment, the condition causes more intense symptoms and may become very severe. For cretinism, early thyroid hormone replacement can promote normal physical development but cannot prevent mental retardation. The hormone replacement therapy must continue throughout the patient's life.

MEDICATION ERROR ALERT

Patients must be educated to avoid compounded hormones for treating thyroid conditions. One patient, who had been receiving Synthroid® for 10 years with no problems, changed physicians and was switched to a compounded T_4/T_3 combination. After six weeks, his thyroid levels were dangerously high. The compounded pills had been made in error and contained 11 times the dose per pill. After recovering, he was switched back to Synthroid®, and his condition returned to normal.

MYXEDEMA

Myxedema is severe, prolonged hypothyroidism. It develops in older children or adults due to impairment of the thyroid gland's ability to form thyroxine. This may be linked to lowered amounts of thyrotropin, failure of the gland to function, damage due to radiation, a tumor, or surgical removal of the gland with T_4 replacement therapy. Also, myxedema may be secondary to inability of the pituitary gland to produce thyrotropin. In children and teens, Hashimoto's thyroiditis often causes hypothyroidism.

Signs and symptoms of myxedema vary with age of onset but include skin thickening and other changes; lack of sweating; excessive tiredness or fatigue; muscular weakness; bloating of the face; thickening of the tongue; puffy eyelids; weight gain; thin, brittle hair; loss of hair; constipation; and cold intolerance. Most patients are female, and in these patients menorrhagia occurs. Physical abilities are impaired, the speech becomes slower and slurred, and the patient experiences mental apathy. Rarely, severe myxedema may result in a coma, which is considered life threatening and requires intensive care.

Treatment of myxedema involves the use of levothyroxine sodium (T_4), in the lowest possible doses, to achieve normal function of the thyroid. Therapy should continue throughout the patient's lifetime.

HYPERPARATHYROIDISM

Hyperparathyroidism is caused by increased parathyroid hormone secretion in the bloodstream. It can originate from one or several of the four parathyroid glands, usually because of a benign tumor. A related condition, *secondary*

Table 22-2 Examples of Medications for Thyroid Gland Conditions

Generic Name	Trade Name	Route of Administration	Average Adult Dosage
Antithyroid Preparations			
methimazoleole	Tapazole®	PO	5 to 15 mg q8h
potassium iodide	Pima®, SSKI®	PO	50 to 250 mg tid for 10 to 14 days before surgery
Calcitonin			
calcitonin (salmon)	Calcimar®, Miacalcin®	IM, SC	100 IU/day, may be increased to 50 to 100 IU/day or every other day
Natural Thyroid Replacement			
thyroid (T_3 and T_4) (desiccated)	Armour Thyroid®, Thyrar®	PO	60 mg/day, may be increased to q30d to 60 to 180 mg/day
Synthetic Thyroid Replacement			
levothyroxine sodium (thyroxine, T_4)	Levothroid®, Synthroid®	PO, IV	PO: 25 to 50 mcg/day, gradually increase by 50 to 100 mcg q1 to 4 weeks to usual dose of 100 to 400 mcg/day; IV: half of usual PO dose
liothyronine sodium (triiodothyronine, T_3)	Cytomel®, Triostat	PO	25 to 75 mcg/day
liotrix (T_3, T_4)	Euthroid®, Thyrolar®	PO	12.5 to 30 mcg/day, gradually increase to desired response

hyperparathyroidism involves the parathyroid glands compensating for chronic hypocalcemia caused by renal failure or poor calcium absorption. Both of these forms of hyperparathyroidism involve increased calcium levels. Increased parathyroid hormone levels promote calcium release from the bones into the bloodstream. This causes weakening of the bones and a higher incidence of fractures. Increased blood calcium levels cause calcium salts to build up in the kidneys, which sometimes causes kidney stones. Other effects of hypercalcemia include lethargy, muscle weakness, and changes in heart conduction. Treatment is based on the cause. Surgical removal of a tumor may be required. Several parathyroid glands may also require surgical removal. Kidney dialysis or transplantation may be required. Other treatments include reduction of calcium levels by increasing fluid intake or by limiting calcium dietary intake. Osteoporosis medications have been used to treat hyperparathyroidism, including bisphosphonates, raloxifene, and estrogen/progestin therapy. Additional medications include calcimimetics and vitamin D analogues.

HYPOPARATHYROIDISM

Hypoparathyroidism is caused by malfunction of the parathyroid glands. It is often due to damage of these glands that occurs during thyroid surgery. Hypocalcemia develops, which then reduces levels of vitamin D. Symptoms include irregular heart contractions, muscle spasms, and altered nerve conduction. Hypoparathyroidism can be treated with supplemental calcium and vitamin D. Other treatments to correct hypocalcemia include parenteral injections of calcium.

CUSHING'S SYNDROME

Cushing's syndrome is a condition of chronic hypersecretion of cortisol from the adrenal cortex. It results in excessive circulating levels of cortisol. Cushing's syndrome may be caused by hyperplasia or tumors of the pituitary gland or adrenal gland, resulting in excessive corticotropin (ACTH) secretion by the pituitary gland or by the production of corticotropin in other organs, such as the lungs when they are cancerous. The syndrome can also be brought on by large doses or prolonged administration of corticosteroids when they are used to treat other diseases.

Signs and symptoms of Cushing's syndrome include fatigue, muscular weakness, and changes in body appearance. The abdomen protrudes because of fat deposits, and there are additional deposits in the shoulder area, commonly described as *buffalo humps*. The face assumes a characteristic "moon" shape, and retention of salt and water cause edema and hypertension. Additional signs include hyperlipidemia, atherosclerosis, osteoporosis, and psychiatric problems. The skin thins, may bruise easily, and develops striae (stretch marks) that are red or purple in color. Since Cushing's syndrome suppresses the immune response, the patient may develop infections more easily. Additional related manifestations include amenorrhea, excessive hair growth, impotence, and development of diabetes mellitus. Characteristic signs of Cushing's syndrome are shown in Figure 22-9A, while resolution of the condition after treatment is shown in Figure 22-9B.

Treatment of Cushing's syndrome depends on the cause. Hormone-secreting pituitary or adrenal tumors are surgically removed or treated with radiation therapy. Along with radiation, or separately, medication therapies may be used to suppress secretion of ACTH, for example, metyrapone or mitotane, which decrease cortisol levels.

POINTS TO REMEMBER

Cushing's disease is defined as an excess of glucocorticoid because of excessive ACTH secretion, most often from a pituitary tumor. It is the most common cause of primary Cushing's syndrome.

HYPERALDOSTERONISM

Hyperaldosteronism is caused by excessive aldosterone secretion from the cortices of the adrenal glands. The condition can be primary or secondary. Primary hyperaldosteronism is caused by an abnormality of the adrenal cortex. Secondary hyperaldosteronism is caused by some stimulus that is outside of the adrenal glands. Aldosterone promotes the retention of sodium and water, as well as the excretion of potassium. The primary signs and symptoms of hyperaldosteronism are hypertension and hypokalemia. If an aldosterone-secreting tumor exists, it must be surgically removed. Treatments of hyperaldosteronism include medications to manage hypertension and potassium supplements to reverse hypokalemia. Once the disorder is identified and treated, the prognosis is good.

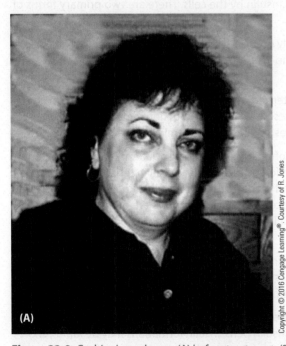 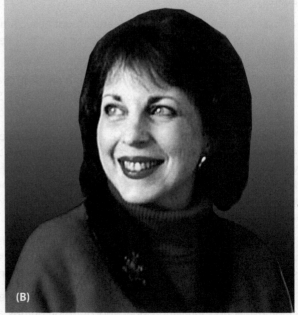

Figure 22-9 Cushing's syndrome: (A) before treatment; (B) after treatment.

ADDISON'S DISEASE

Addison's disease is partial or total failure of adrenocortical function. Its onset is usually gradual, with progressive destruction of the adrenal glands and the resulting reduction of many important hormones that they secrete. It may be linked to an autoimmune condition, hemorrhage, tuberculosis, fungal infection, neoplasms, or surgical removal of the adrenal glands. Some rare genetic defects may cause Addison's disease, and the disorder may also occur secondary to hypopituitarism.

Signs and symptoms of Addison's disease include fatigue, weakness, decreased appetite, weight loss, and gastrointestinal disturbances. The skin may appear "bronze," and cardiovascular problems may occur. These include irregular pulse, orthostatic (postural) hypotension, and reduced cardiac output. Other common symptoms are hypoglycemia, anxiety, depression, and emotional distress. When aldosterone levels are reduced, the patient may be unable to retain salt or water. The condition can become life threatening when dehydration, electrolyte imbalance, or hyperkalemia occur.

Treatment of Addison's disease includes administration of glucocorticoids such as hydrocortisone (Cortef®), methylprednisone (Medrol®), prednisolone, and prednisone; and mineralocorticoids such as fludrocortisone acetate, to replace natural hormones. This must occur over the patient's entire life, with close supervision. Potassium and sodium levels must be corrected. Patient education is important so that he or she may understand signs of overdosage or underdosage, as well as how infection and stress are related to the condition. If there is a sudden decrease or insufficiency in adrenocortical hormone levels, a life-threatening emergency known as *addisonian crisis* may develop. Patients experiencing addisonian crisis require immediate treatment with hydrocortisone.

WHAT WOULD YOU DO?

A patient in your pharmacy complains of a sudden, severe pain in the lower back, then vomits and passes out. You run around the pharmacy counter and upon checking the patient, notice a medical ID bracelet on his or her arm that says he or she has Addison's disease. If you were this pharmacy technician, what would you do?

DIABETES MELLITUS

Diabetes mellitus is a chronic disorder of carbohydrate, fat, and protein metabolism. It is caused by inadequate production of insulin by the pancreas, or ineffective utilization of insulin by the cells. There are two primary forms of diabetes mellitus:

- Type 1 diabetes mellitus has an early, abrupt onset. It usually occurs before 30 years of age and most often manifests in late childhood. The pancreas secretes little or no insulin, and this condition can be difficult to control.

- Type 2 diabetes mellitus is the more common form, characterized by a gradual onset in adults older than age 30. It occurs more often in people older than 55 years. Since some pancreatic function remains, control of symptoms by dietary management is possible. In some cases, an oral hypoglycemic medication is required.

Although diabetes mellitus may be acquired, type 1 disease often has a genetic association. Patients have abnormalities of metabolism that are linked to abnormal insulin secretion by the pancreas, insulin resistance, or abnormal levels of glucose production by the liver. The exact cause of type 1 diabetes mellitus is still unknown; however, it may follow an infection early in life that initiates an autoimmune process, in which antibodies are produced that destroy pancreatic beta cells. Type 2 diabetes mellitus is more prevalent in older adults who are overweight and is thought to be lifestyle related.

Diabetes mellitus may be induced when the pancreas is destroyed by a tumor, pituitary gland trauma, or other endocrine disorders. Insulin production by the body can also be suppressed by certain medications. Various genetic disorders are able to cause insensitivity of the body's insulin receptors to insulin.

Type 1 diabetes mellitus may require insulin replacement therapy. Insulin may be injected in a variety of ways, including injection, inhalation, open-loop infusion pumps, and insulin pens. Insulin formations may be rapid-, short-, intermediate-, or long-acting, as well as premixed formulations containing both long- and short-acting insulins.

Type 2 diabetes mellitus usually does not require insulin administration and is commonly controlled through a restricted diet, exercise, and oral hypoglycemics. The major risk factors for type 2 diabetes include age, family history, ethnicity, obesity, and prediabetes. Family history combines a genetic predisposition with environmental, cultural, and behavioral factors. Family history is a major predictor of developing this form of diabetes. Risk is twice as high when a parent or sibling has diabetes and four times higher when two or more first-degree relatives have diabetes. Environmental factors are believed to play a role in the etiology of the disease, but these are not fully understood. The most important environmental risk factor is obesity, especially central or visceral obesity. Medical conditions that may increase the risks for type 2 diabetes include *acanthrosis nigricans*, which involves skin discolorations in patchy areas due to overproduction of insulin, hypertension (blood pressure 130/80 mm Hg or higher), high LDL cholesterol (70 mg/dL or higher), high triglycerides (250 or higher), polycystic ovary syndrome (which carries risks for type 2 diabetes that are three to five times higher), and *prediabetes*.

MEDICATION ERROR ALERT

Medication errors involving insulin are very common. Patients have self-administered large doses of glulisine (Apidra®), thinking they were administering a basal dose of glargine (Lantus®), since the packaging for these products is very similar. Glulisine is a rapid-acting insulin with a more rapid onset and shorter duration of action, while glargine is the 24-hour basal insulin indicated for once-daily subcutaneous administration.

GESTATIONAL DIABETES

Gestational diabetes mellitus, also known as type 3 diabetes, is a condition that develops in many women during pregnancy. Elevated levels of estrogen and progesterone during pregnancy appear to play a role by blocking the effects of insulin. Maternal insulin thus has reduced effectiveness, leading to elevations in glucose levels. The cycle of elevated glucose and resulting increased insulin production triggers increased placental production of human placental *lactogen* (which facilitates the energy supply of the fetus). The fetus receives its glucose from the mother, hence the importance of the balance of glucose production and glucose utilization.

Risk factors for gestational diabetes include a family history of diabetes, obesity, and maternal age over 25 years. The condition is most often detected between 24 and 28 weeks of gestation when excessive glucose levels are noted during routine prenatal blood and urine screening. Though some patients are asymptomatic, common manifestations include polydipsia, polyuria, and polyphagia.

Treatment of gestational diabetes requires close supervision of both mother and fetus and dietary control, which includes limiting intake of simple sugars. Walking and other moderate exercise is indicated. Medications may include oral hypoglycemics or insulin. The patient must monitor blood glucose levels regularly using home testing devices. Usually, delivery of the baby and placenta resolves the condition, but if not, treatment must continue.

WHAT WOULD YOU DO?

Your co-worker is a female pharmacy technician who is pregnant. One day, she complains of nausea, abdominal pain, headache, and double vision while at work. She tries to focus on her work and not think about her symptoms, but when she begins to tremble, become uncoordinated, and feel faint, she asks you what you think she should do. You help her to sit on the floor carefully first. If found yourself in this scenario, what would you do next?

SELECTED DRUGS FOR DIABETES MELLITUS

Type 1 diabetes is characterized by a lack of insulin production from the pancreas, or an inability of glucose to enter the cells, and must be treated with insulin. Type 2 diabetes may be characterized by either decreased production of insulin or normal amounts of insulin with abnormal sensitivity of the tissues to the insulin that is present. Common differences between type 1 and type 2 diabetes are summarized in Table 22-3. There are several serious

Table 22-3 Characteristics of Type 1 and Type 2 Diabetes

Characteristics	Type 1 Diabetes	Type 2 Diabetes
Onset age	Usually under 30 years	Usually over 30 years
Obesity association	No	Extremely common
Ketoacidosis that requires insulin treatment	Yes	No
Endogenous insulin in the plasma	Very low to undetectable	Varied; low, normal, or elevated based on degree of insulin resistance, defects in insulin secretion
Occurrence in twins	Up to 50%	More than 90%
Related to certain HLA-D antigens	Yes	No
Islet cell antibodies present at diagnosis	Yes	No
Islet pathology	Insulitis; selective loss of most beta cells	Smaller, normal-looking islets; amyloid (amylin) deposits common
Development of complications such as retinopathy, nephropathy, neuropathy, atherosclerotic cardiovascular disease	Yes	Yes
Hyperglycemia response to oral antihyperglycemics	No	Yes, initially for many patients

complications of diabetes, including retinopathy, neuropathy, nephropathy, stroke, and diabetic ketoacidosis. Insulin can be given only by injection, either subcutaneously or intravenously. Only regular insulin can be administered intravenously. Insulin doses are measured in units. Table 22-4 shows a list of different types of insulin. There are also older, intermediate-acting insulins. These include the following:

- *Humulin N and Novolin N*: Onset of 1 to 2 hours, duration of 16 to 24 hours, concentration of 100 units per mL, expiration varies (Humulin N Kwikpen—14 days; Humulin N vial—31 days; Novolin N vial—42 days), dosage form either vial or Kwikpen, pen dial of one unit, can be taken without regard to meals, usually dosed once or twice per day alone or mixed with a rapid- or short-acting insulin

- *Humulin R, U-500*: Onset of 30 minutes, duration of 12 to 24 hours, concentration of 500 units per mL, expiration of pens 28 days, expiration of vials 40 days, dosage form: pen or vial, pen dial of five units, taken 30 minutes before meals, usually dosed three to four times per day before meals or snacks

Insulin pumps were first developed in 1963, and today they have evolved to become extremely small. They now are about the size of a cell phone and are powered by a battery. They can easily be clipped onto a belt or clothing. As many as 1 million people globally use insulin pumps to deliver insulin in extremely small doses, subcutaneously, similar to how the pancreas normally releases insulin. They offer flexible dosing and eliminate the need for multiple injections of insulin per day. Most pumps are attached via plastic tubing to the patient via a subcutaneous cannula or steel needle. Infusion sets are changed every two to three days, ensuring that the insulin is potent, and to minimize any chance of infection. Candidates for insulin pumps are individuals who have to check blood glucose four or more times per day, and then take three or more insulin injections. Each patient must be thoroughly instructed in the proper use of these devices in order to avoid ketoacidosis.

Inhaled insulin was first developed in 2005; it is used to help reduce the amount of daily insulin injections that are needed. For type 1 diabetes, inhaled insulin is administered along with a basal insulin. A patient using inhaled insulin must have sufficient lung capacity to be able to inhale the entire prescribed dose. Before starting inhaled insulin, there must be a detailed medical history, physical examination, and spirometry performed. There must also be additional spirometry testing. Inhalers are replaced every 15 days, and the same inhaler can be used for different cartridge dose sizes.

Table 22-4 Various Insulins Used to Treat Diabetes Mellitus

Long-Acting Insulins

Properties	Degludec U-100 (Tresiba)	Degludec U-200 (Tresiba)	Detemir U-100 (Levemir)	Glargine U-100 (Lantus)	Glargine U-300 (Toujeo)
Onset	30 to 90 minutes	30 to 90 minutes	1.1 to 2 hours	1.1 hours	6 hours
Duration of action	42 hours	42 hours	7.6 to 24 hours	10.8 to 24 hours	24 to 36 hours
Formulation	Pen	Pen	Pen or vial	Pen or vial	Pen
Concentration	100 units per mL	200 units per mL	100 units per mL	100 units per mL	300 units per mL
Expiration	56 days	56 days	42 days	28 days	42 days
Maximum units injected per dose	80 units	160 units	80 units	80 units	80 units
Pen dial	One unit	Two units	One unit	One unit	One unit
Units per pen	300 units in 3 mL	600 units in 3 mL	300 units in 3 mL	300 units in 3 mL	450 units in 1.5 mL

Rapid-Acting, Ultra-Rapid-Acting, and Short-Acting Insulins

Insulin Aspart (Fiasp)	Insulin Aspart (Novolog)	Insulin Glulisine (Apidra)	Insulin Lispro (Humalog) U-100, U-200	Human Insulin Regular (Novolin R, Humulin R)	Inhaled Insulin (Afrezza)
Onset: 2.5 minutes	10 to 20 minutes	25 minutes	15 to 30 minutes	30 minutes	15 to 30 minutes
Duration: 3 to 5 hours	3 to 5 hours	4 to 5.3 hours	3 to 6.5 hours	8 hours	160 minutes
Expiration: 28 days	28 days	28 days	28 days	Humulin R: 31 days; Novolin R: 42 days	Open strips: three days; unopened foil package: 10 days; inhaler: 15 days
Maximum per dose: 60 units	60 units	80 units	60 units	60 units	4, 8, or 12 unit cartridges
Units per pen: 300 units in 3 mL	300 units in 3 mL	300 units in 3 mL	U-100: 300 units in 3 mL; U-200: 600 units in 3 mL	300 units in 3 mL	Not applicable
Dosage form: Vial or pen	Vial or pen	Vial or pen	U-100: Vial or pen; U-200: pen only	Vial	Inhaled
Meal timing: Subcutaneous (SC): at start of meal, 20 minutes after meal	SC: 5 to 10 minutes before meals	SC: within 15 minutes before or 20 minutes after starting meal	SC: up to 15 minutes before or immediately after a meal	SC: 30 minutes before meal	Inhaled at start of meal

Oral hypoglycemics are used to lower blood glucose level in type 2 diabetes. Table 22-5 shows some examples of oral hypoglycemics. Also, since many people with type 2 diabetes need multiple medications, there are combination oral agents available. These are summarized in Table 22-6. Two newly approved medications are insulin glargine (Toujeo®) and inhaled insulin (Afrezza®). Toujeo has the same active ingredient as Lantus but is three times more concentrated at 300 units per mL. It is also more effective at controlling blood sugar while the patient is sleeping. Only small dosage adjustments are usually needed when a patient is converted from Lantus to Toujeo. The new medication Afrezza is the same as Humulin but is inhaled instead of being injected. This medication has not gained wide acceptance because the patient must be able to breathe in a complete dose, and regular lung testing is required. People who smoke and those who have COPD usually cannot take this dosage form. An injectable, long-acting insulin must also be injected along with this inhaled product.

Table 22-5 Examples of Oral Hypoglycemic Drugs

Generic Name	Trade Name	Average Adult Dose	Comments
Sulfonylureas			
First Generation			
chlorpropamide	Diabinese®	Initial: 100 to 250 mg/day with breakfast; adjust by 50 to 125 mg/day q3 to 5d until glycemic control is achieved, up to 750 mg/day	Long-acting agents
Second Generation			
glimepiride	Amaryl®	Initial: 1 to 2 mg/day with breakfast or first main meal; may increase to usual maintenance dose of 1 to 4 mg/day (maximum 8 mg/day)	May cause GI upset, hypoglycemia, weight gain
glipizide	Glucotrol®, Glucotrol XL®	Initial: 2.5 to 5 mg/day 30 minutes before breakfast; may be increased by 2.5 to 5 mg q1 to 2 weeks; >15 mg/day in divided doses 30 minutes before a.m. and p.m. meal (maximum 40 mg/day); 5 to 10 mg sustained release tablets once daily	
glyburide	DiaBeta®	1.25 to 20 mg once or twice/day with first meal (maximum 20 mg/day)	
micronized glyburide	Glynase®	0.75 to 12 mg once or twice/day with first meal (maximum 12 mg/day)	
Meglitinides (secretogogues)			
acarbose	Precose®	25 to 100 mg tid with meals (maximum 150 mg/day if weighing 60 kg or less; maximum 300 mg/day if weighing more than 60 kg)	May cause flatulence, GI upset, weight loss
miglitol	Glyset®	25 to 100 mg tid with meals (maximum 300 mg/day)	

(Continued)

Table 22-5 Examples of Oral Hypoglycemic Drugs (*Continued*)

Generic Name	Trade Name	Average Adult Dose	Comments
nateglinide	Starlix®	60 to 120 mg tid 1 to 30 minutes before meals	May be used as monotherapy or with metformin; may cause hypoglycemia and weight gain
repaglinide	Prandin®	Initial: 0.5 mg 15 to 30 minutes before meals; initial dose for patients previously using glucose-lowering agents: 1 to 2 mg 15 to 30 minutes before meals (2 to 4 doses/day depending on meal pattern; maximum 16 mg/day); dosage range: 0.5 to 4 mg 15 to 30 minutes before meals	
Biguanides			
metformin	Fortamet®, Glucophage®, Glucophage XR®, Glumetza®, Riomet®	Initial: 500 mg every day–tid or 850 mg every day–bid with meals; may be increased by 500 to 850 mg/day q1 to 3 weeks (maximum 2550 mg/day); or start with 500 mg sustained release with p.m. meal; may increase by 500 mg/day at p.m. meal q week (maximum 2000 mg/day)	One-a-day formulation that helps with gastrointestinal discomfort
Thiazolidinediones (Glitazones)			
pioglitazone	Actos®	15 to 30 mg once daily (maximum 45 mg every day)	Monitoring of liver enzymes
rosiglitazone	Avandia®	Initial: 4 mg every day or 2 mg bid; may increase after 12 weeks (maximum 8 mg/day in 1 to 2 divided doses)	
Dipeptidyl Peptidase-4 (DPP-4) Inhibitors			
alogliptin	Nesina®	25 mg/day	
linagliptin	Tradjenta®	5 mg/day	
saxagliptin	Onglyza®	2.5 to 5 mg/day (maximum 5 mg/day)	
sitagliptin	Januvia®	50 to 100 mg/day (maximum 100 mg/day)	May cause GI upset, headache, sinusitis
Sodium-Glucose Co-Transporter 2 (SGLT2) Inhibitors (used with caution in kidney disease)			
canagliflozin	Invokana®	100 to 300 mg/day (maximum 300 mg/day)	May cause genital fungal infections
dapagliflozin	Farxiga®	5 to 10 mg/day (maximum 10 mg/day)	May cause increased urination
empagliflozin	Jardiance®	10 to 25 mg/day (maximum 25 mg/day)	May cause orthostasis
Glucagon-like Peptide-1 (GLP-1) Receptor Agonists			
albiglutide	Tanzeum®	30 to 50 mg subcutaneous once/week	May cause GI upset, hypoglycemia, nausea/vomiting, weight loss

(*Continued*)

Table 22-5 Examples of Oral Hypoglycemic Drugs (*Continued*)

Generic Name	Trade Name	Average Adult Dose	Comments
exenatide	Byetta®	5 to 10 mcg subcutaneous twice/day	May cause GI upset, hypoglycemia, nausea/vomiting, weight loss
exenatide suspension	Bydureon®	2 mg subcutaneous once/week	
liraglutide	Victoza®	0.6 to 1.8 mg subcutaneous/day	
Synthetic Amylin Analog			
pramlintide	Symlin®	15 to 120 mcg subcutaneous immediately before large meals (maximum 120 mcg/dose)	May cause GI upset, hypoglycemia

Table 22-6 Combination Oral Agents for Type 2 Diabetes Mellitus

Generic Name	Trade Name	Average Adult Dose
alogliptin-metformin	Kazano®	Two forms: 12.5 mg alogliptin/500 mg metformin per day, or 12.5 alogliptin/1000 mg metformin per day (maximum 25 mg alogliptin/2000 mg metformin per day)
alogliptin-pioglitazone	Oseni®	Various forms: 25 mg alogliptin/15 mg pioglitazone per day, up to 25 mg alogliptin/45 mg pioglitazone per day
glipizide-metformin	Metaglip®	Various forms: 2.5 mg glipizide/250 mg metformin once per day, up to 10 mg glipizide/2000 mg metformin per day
glyburide-metformin	Glucovance®	Various forms: 1.25 mg glyburide/250 mg metformin once or twice per day, up to 20 mg glyburide/2000 mg metformin once per day
linagliptin-metformin	Jentadueto®	Various forms: 5 mg linagliptin/1000 mg metformin once per day, up to 5 mg linagliptin/2000 mg metformin once per day
pioglitazone-glimepiride	Duetact®	30 mg pioglitazone/2 mg glimepiride or 30 mg pioglitazone/4 mg glimepiride once per day, gradually titrated prn (maximum 15 mg/30 mg)
pioglitazone-metformin	ActoPlus Met®, ActoPlus Met XR®	Various forms: 15 mg pioglitazone/500 mg metformin bid or 15 mg pioglitazone/850 mg metformin once per day, titrated prn to a maximum of 45 mg/2550 mg
repaglinide-metformin	PrandiMet®	4 mg repaglinide/1000 mg metformin bid or tid, up to a maximum of 10 mg/2500 mg per day
saxagliptin-metformin	Kombiglyze XR®	Various forms: 5 mg saxagliptin/500 mg metformin once per day, up to 2.5 mg/1000 once per day
sitagliptin-metformin	Janumet®	Initial: 100 mg sitagliptin/1000 mg metformin once per day, titrated up to a maximum of 100 mg sitagliptin/2000 mg metformin once per day

OBESITY

Obesity is extremely common in the United States as well as in many other countries. The Centers for Disease Control and Prevention (CDC) reports that 39.8% of adults and 18.5% of children are obese. Obesity increases the risks for serious chronic health conditions, including heart disease, atherosclerosis, hypertension, stroke, diabetes, sleep apnea, asthma, blood clots, fatty liver, cirrhosis, gallstones, cancer, pancreatitis, abnormal menstruation, infertility, arthritis, and gout. Diagnosis of obesity is based on body mass index (BMI), with a BMI of 30 or more considered obese.

To prevent obesity, physical activity and a good diet are essential. Foods that are high in added sodium, sugar, and saturated fats should be avoided. Dietitians or nutritionists are great resources to support a healthy diet. Moderate physical activity every day should be gradually increased over time, with the involvement of a health care professional. For extreme obesity, surgery may be performed to reduce the size of the stomach or install a gastric band to reduce stomach volume. Medication options are available for patients who exercise and are on a healthy diet. They work by reducing fat absorption in the intestines or by reducing hunger sensations from the hypothalamus.

Summary

The endocrine system consists of many glands and other organs, and its master gland is the pituitary gland. Hormones are natural chemical substances secreted from endocrine glands that control many different functions. The hypothalamus is the main integrative center for the endocrine and autonomic nervous systems. The anterior pituitary gland secretes growth, adrenocorticotropic, thyroid stimulating, follicle stimulating, and luteinizing hormones, as well as prolactin and melanocyte-stimulating hormone. The posterior pituitary gland releases antidiuretic hormone and oxytocin.

The pineal gland secretes melatonin, which regulates the circadian rhythms. The thyroid gland secretes three hormones essential for proper regulation of metabolism. Parathyroid hormone targets the bones, intestines, and kidneys to increase plasma calcium levels. The thymus gland plays an important role in kick-starting the immune system following birth. The adrenal glands synthesize glucocorticoids, mineralocorticoids, corticosteroids, epinephrine, and norepinephrine. The pancreas has both endocrine and exocrine functions and produces glucagon and insulin.

Common disorders of the endocrine system include diabetes insipidus, hypopituitarism, hyperpituitarism, simple goiter, Hashimoto's disease, hyperthyroidism, hypothyroidism, myxedema, Cushing's syndrome, Addison's disease, diabetes mellitus, and gestational diabetes. Medications used to treat endocrine system disorders are used for hormonal deficiencies or excesses, or non-endocrine diseases. Thyroid hormones and insulins are among the most commonly used medications for endocrine system disorders. The most important disease involving the endocrine pancreas is diabetes mellitus, a disorder of carbohydrate metabolism that involves insulin deficiency, insulin resistance, or both. Type 2 diabetes mellitus is a common complication of obesity, which affects more than one of every three adults in the United States, and more than one of every six children.

REVIEW QUESTIONS

1. Which of the following glands releases glucagon and calcitonin?

   A. Posterior pituitary and pancreas
   B. Anterior pituitary and thymus
   C. Pancreas and thyroid
   D. Adrenal cortex and parathyroid

2. Antidiuretic hormone is also known as:

   A. oxytocin.
   B. vasopressin.
   C. glucocorticoid.
   D. thymosin.

3. Which of the endocrine glands releases the hormone *aldosterone*?

    A.   The pituitary gland
    B.   The thyroid gland
    C.   The thymus gland
    D.   The adrenal gland

4. Which of the following is the generic name of Tapazole?

    A.   Levothyroxine
    B.   Liotrix
    C.   Metformin
    D.   Methimazole

5. What is the name of the condition caused by hypersecretion of growth hormone before puberty?

    A.   Myxedema
    B.   Dwarfism
    C.   Gigantism
    D.   Acromegaly

6. Which of the following agents is used in the treatment of thyroid gland disorders?

    A.   Glipizide
    B.   Metformin
    C.   Norgestrel
    D.   Potassium iodide

7. Cretinism is a congenital disorder developing in early childhood that results from deficiency of hormone(s) released by which endocrine gland?

    A.   Thymus
    B.   Thyroid
    C.   Adrenal (cortex)
    D.   Anterior pituitary

8. Treatment of hypopituitarism is based on the patient's:

    A.   gender.
    B.   family history.
    C.   race.
    D.   age.

9. Which of the following is the primary function of the thymus gland?

    A.   Secreting calcitonin
    B.   Synthesizing growth hormone
    C.   Developing the immune system
    D.   Releasing melatonin

10. The goal of treatment for gigantism is to reduce amounts of:

    A.   prolactin.
    B.   aldosterone.
    C.   growth hormone.
    D.   thyroid hormone.

11. Hyperplasia or a tumor of the adrenal cortex may cause:

    A.   Cushing's syndrome.
    B.   Addison's disease.
    C.   diabetes mellitus.
    D.   Hashimoto's disease.

12. Starlix® is the trade name of:

   A. glyburide.
   B. nateglinide.
   C. glipizide.
   D. repaglinide.

13. Which of the following is the trade name of a natural thyroid replacement?

   A. Tapazole®
   B. Levothroid®
   C. Armour Thyroid®
   D. Calcimar®

14. Overgrowth of just the bones of the face, hands, and feet, with an excessive overgrowth of soft tissue, is called:

   A. myxedema.
   B. acromegaly.
   C. gigantism.
   D. cretinism.

15. Which of the following is considered to be long-acting insulin?

   A. Insulin aspart (Novolog)
   B. Insulin glulisine (Apidra)
   C. Insulin NPH
   D. Insulin glargine U-300 (Toujeo)

CRITICAL THINKING

A 13-year-old boy had a car accident and was brought to the emergency room with a fractured tibia. His physician noticed that he was much taller than normal for his age. He suspected that the boy might have gigantism.

   1. Make a list of anterior and posterior pituitary hormones.

   2. Compare gigantism and acromegaly.

WEB LINKS

Adrenal Fatigue: adrenalfatigue.org

American Diabetes Association: www.diabetes.org

American Thyroid Association: www.thyroid.org

Cushing's Syndrome: www.cushings-help.com

Endocrine Diseases: www.endocrineweb.com

Hormone Health Network: www.hormone.org

Parathyroid Diseases: www.parathyroid.com

Pituitary Network Association: pituitary.org

Thyroid Disease: www.thyroid-info.com

CHAPTER 23

Therapeutic Drugs for the Cardiovascular System

OUTLINE

OBJECTIVES

Upon completion of this chapter, the reader should be able to:

1. Name the structures of the heart layers and chambers.
2. Describe the metabolism of cholesterol.
3. Compare arteriosclerosis with atherosclerosis.
4. Describe the classifications of hypertension and antihypertensives.
5. Explain the difference between myocardial infarction and angina pectoris.
6. Define the terms cardiac output and ejection fraction.
7. Describe the risk factors for heart failure.
8. Differentiate between anticoagulants and thrombolytics.
9. List generic and trade names of statin drugs.
10. Give three examples each of ACE inhibitors and angiotensin receptor blockers.

KEY TERMS

agranulocytes	diastole	lumen	pulmonary valve
angina pectoris	ejection fraction	mediastinum	stent
angioplasty	erythropoiesis	mitral valve	systole
aortic valve	formed elements	myocardial infarction (MI)	tachypnea
arrhythmias	granulocytes	pacemaker	tricuspid valve
coronary artery bypass graft	hyperlipidemia	pernicious anemia	vacuole
cyanosis	hypertension	phagocytosis	venae cavae
	lipoproteins	plasma	

Overview

Cardiovascular disorders are the most common causes of death in the United States. These disorders include hyperlipidemia, hypertension, chest pain (angina), heart attack (myocardial infarction), cardiac arrhythmias, heart failure, stroke, and various blood disorders. Approximately 85.6 million American adults have one or more types of cardiovascular disease (CVD), with about half of these people being aged 60 or older. About one of every three deaths is from CVD. Fortunately, in the past decade, death rates from CVD have declined by almost 29%. Today, prevention of CVD has become a focus of the American Heart Association (AHA), along with treatment. The seven areas of prevention defined by the AHA include a heart healthy diet, adequate physical exercise, avoiding smoking, and control of body weight, blood pressure, and cholesterol and glucose levels. Risks for CVD death are lowered when more of these risk factors are controlled.

Anatomy and Physiology of the Cardiovascular System

The cardiovascular system is also known as the circulatory system; it consists of the heart and blood vessels. Two parts make up the cardiovascular system: the pulmonary circulation and the systemic circulation. The pulmonary circulation involves movement of blood between the heart and the lungs through the pulmonary trunk. Deoxygenated blood is transported to the lungs to pick up oxygen and is then pumped back to the heart. In the systemic circulation, oxygenated blood is carried from the heart to the body tissues and cells and is then transported back to the heart. The systemic circulation supplies all body cells with blood, oxygen, and other nutrients. The cardiovascular system also collects waste products such as carbon dioxide from the cells. These waste products are products of metabolic reactions. They are eliminated from the body through the lungs, liver, and kidneys.

MEDICAL TERMINOLOGY REVIEW

epicardium:	**myocardium:**	**endocardium:**
epi- = *upon, over*	my/o- = *muscle*	endo- = *within*
cardi- = *heart*	cardi- = *heart*	cardi- = *heart*
-ium = *mass*	-ium = *mass*	-ium = *mass*
upon the heart mass	muscle of the heart	within the heart

THE HEART

The heart is a hollow muscular organ located within the **mediastinum**, resting on the diaphragm. It is slightly left of the centerline of the chest cavity. It is approximately the size of an adult's fist, with a shape like an inverted pear. It lies directly behind the sternum, and the tip of its lower edge is called the apex.

Layers of the Heart

The wall of the heart has three layers (the epicardium, myocardium, and endocardium) as shown in Figure 23-1. The endocardium is its inner layer, which lines the heart chambers. The myocardium is the thicker and muscular middle heart layer. When this layer contracts, it establishes sufficient pressure to pump blood through the blood vessels. The epicardium is the outer heart layer. Enclosing the heart is a two-layered pleural sac known as the pericardium. The inner layer of this sac is composed of the epicardium, also known as the visceral pericardium. The sac's outer layer is called the parietal pericardium. While the heart beats, friction is reduced by fluid found between these two layers.

POINTS TO REMEMBER

Pericarditis is an inflammation of the pericardium that roughens the serous membrane surfaces. As a result, the beating heart rubs against its pericardial sac.

Chambers of the Heart

The heart is divided into two atria and two ventricles. The atria are the upper chambers, and the ventricles are the lower chambers. A wall of tissue known as the interatrial septum separates the left and right atria. The right atrium receives blood from the **venae cavae**. The left atrium receives blood from the pulmonary veins. Another wall of tissue, the interventricular septum, separates the left and right ventricles. These are the pumping chambers of the heart; consequently, their myocardium is much thicker. When they contract, they eject blood out of the heart and into the larger arteries.

Valves of the Heart

The right atrium is separated from the right ventricle by the **tricuspid valve** (see Figure 23-2). It controls the opening between the right atrium and the ventricle. The **pulmonary valve** is located between the right ventricle and the pulmonary trunk. The left atrium is separated from the left ventricle by the **mitral valve**. The **aortic valve** is between the left ventricle and the aorta.

POINTS TO REMEMBER

An incompetent or insufficient valve forces the heart to re-pump the same blood over and over since the valve does not close properly and blood backflows.

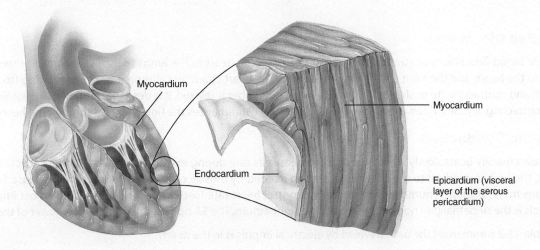

Figure 23-1 Walls of the heart.

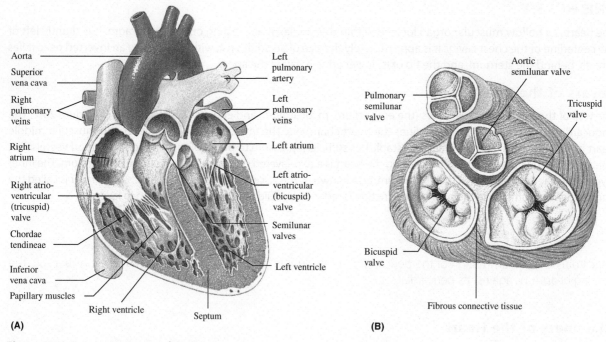

Figure 23-2 Interior structures of the heart.

Table 23-1 Cardiac Blood Flow

- Deoxygenated blood from the body tissues enters the relaxed right atrium, through two large veins: the superior vena cava and the inferior vena cava.
- The right atrium contracts, pushing blood through the tricuspid valve into the relaxed right ventricle.
- The right ventricle contracts, pushing blood through the pulmonary valve, into the pulmonary artery. This artery carries blood to the lungs, where it is oxygenated.
- The left atrium receives blood after it has been oxygenated by the lungs. The blood enters the relaxed left atrium through the four pulmonary veins.
- The left atrium contracts. Blood is pushed through the mitral valve, into the relaxed left ventricle.
- The left ventricle contracts, pushing blood through the aortic valve into the aorta, which is the body's largest artery. The aorta carries the blood to the rest of the body.

Cardiac Blood Flow

Cardiac blood flow is very controlled, progressing through the heart to the lungs to receive oxygen. It then moves back to the heart, and then out to the rest of the body. The heart chambers alternate between relaxing (to fill with blood) and contracting (to push blood forward). When a chamber is relaxed, it is described as being in **diastole**. When it is contracting, it is described as being in **systole**. Table 23-1 summarizes the flow of blood through the heart.

Cardiac Conduction

The heart usually beats slowly while at rest but increases its rate during exercise or increased physical activity. As a result, the body can adjust to the changes in oxygen needed by muscle cell activity or inactivity. Increased activity requires more oxygen. A number of mechanisms control heart rate (see Figure 23-3). One of the most important controls is the sinoatrial (SA) node in the wall of the right atrium. The SA node is the primary **pacemaker** of the heart.

Table 23-2 summarizes the path traveled by electrical impulses in the heart.

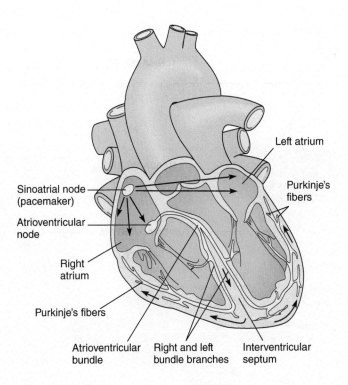

Figure 23-3 Conduction system of the heart.

Table 23-2 Cardiac Conduction
• The heart's pacemaker is the sinoatrial (SA) node. Electrical impulses begin in this node, with an electrical wave traveling through the atria, causing them to contract (systole).
• The atrioventricular node is stimulated. It transfers the stimulation wave to the atrioventricular bundle (or bundle of His).
• The electrical impulse then travels down the bundle branches in the interventricular septum.
• The Purkinje fibers in the ventricular myocardium are then stimulated. This causes ventricular systole.

BLOOD VESSELS

The blood vessels include the arteries, the capillaries, and the veins (see Figure 23-4). Arteries have thicker walls than veins. The capillaries are the sites of nutrient, electrolyte, gas, and waste exchange. Networks of capillaries are called capillary beds. The walls of capillaries are extremely thin.

Capillaries converge into venules, which in turn converge into veins that return blood to the heart, completing the closed system of blood circulation. Veins have valves that allow blood to move in only one direction—toward the heart. The movement of blood through the veins is also aided by muscular action against them and skeletal muscle contractions.

A functional cardiovascular system is vital for survival because, without circulation, tissues lack a supply of oxygen and nutrients and wastes accumulate. Under such conditions, the cells soon begin irreversible changes that quickly lead to cell death. Figure 23-5 shows the general pattern of blood transport in the cardiovascular system (pulmonary and systemic circulation).

POINTS TO REMEMBER

Arteries have narrow central tubes (lumens), while the lumens of veins are larger. This is related to the fact that the walls of arteries are thicker than those of veins. The vasomotor fibers control the smooth muscles and, in response to the body's needs, can cause vasoconstriction (reducing lumen diameter) or vasodilation (increasing lumen diameter).

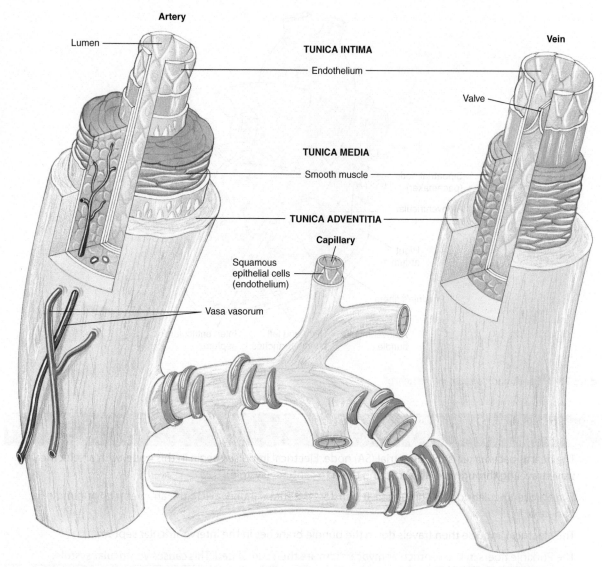

Figure 23-4 Arteries, capillaries, and veins.

BLOOD

Blood transports substances between body cells and the external environment, helping to maintain a stable internal environment. It can be separated into **formed elements** and a liquid portion called **plasma**. The formed elements in the blood consist of red blood cells, white blood cells, and platelets. The liquid plasma includes water, gases, hormones, plasma proteins, nutrients, electrolytes, and cellular wastes. Blood volume varies with body size, fluid and electrolyte balance, and the content of the adipose tissue. The process of red blood cell production is called **erythropoiesis**. This process increases when oxygen levels in the blood decrease. Red blood cells contain hemoglobin, which combines with oxygen. Mature red blood cells do not have a nucleus. White blood cells are either **granulocytes** (neutrophils, eosinophils, and basophils) or **agranulocytes** (which include monocytes and lymphocytes), as shown in Figure 23-6.

Neutrophils and monocytes ingest foreign particles in a process known as **phagocytosis**. They do so by engulfing solid particles within a cell membrane to form an internal membrane-bound compartment known as **vacuole**. Neutrophils are the most numerous white blood cells in the peripheral circulation. Eosinophils kill parasites and help to control inflammation and allergic reactions. Basophils release heparin, which inhibits blood clotting, and histamine, which increases blood flow to injured tissues. Lymphocytes produce antibodies that attack specific foreign substances. Platelets help to close breaks in blood vessels. They are formed from megakaryocytes in the bone marrow.

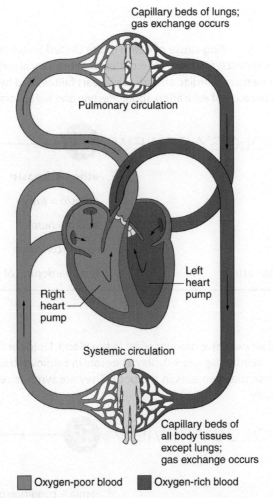

Figure 23-5 Pulmonary and systemic circulation.

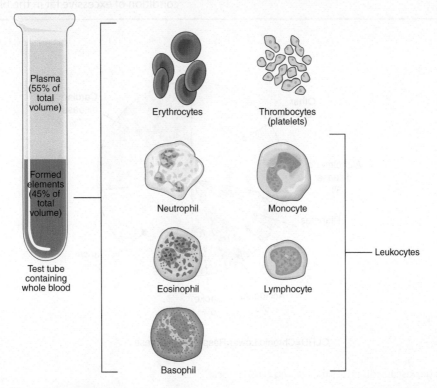

Figure 23-6 Major components of blood.

Disorders of the Cardiovascular System

Cardiovascular disease (CVD) is the leading cause of death in the United States today (see Figure 23-7). These disorders and conditions include arteriosclerosis and atherosclerosis, coronary artery disease (CAD) (angina pectoris), myocardial infarction (MI), hypertension, cardiac arrhythmias, heart failure, and hyperlipidemia. The risk of CVD has decreased for some individuals because of education about lifestyle and behavioral changes.

MEDICAL TERMINOLOGY REVIEW

arteriosclerosis:

ateri/o = *artery*

sclero = *hard*

-osis = *condition*

condition of hardening of the artery

atherosclerosis:

ather/o = *fatty*

sclero = *hard*

-osis = *condition*

fatty hardening of the artery

HYPERLIPIDEMIA

Hyperlipidemia is a condition of an excessive amount of fat in the blood. Lipids or fats, which are usually transported in various combinations with proteins (**lipoproteins**), play a key role in cardiovascular disorders. Lipids, including cholesterol and triglycerides, are essential elements in the body. They are synthesized in the liver; therefore, they can never be eliminated from the body.

MEDICAL TERMINOLOGY REVIEW

hyperlipidemia:

hyper = *excessive*

lipid = *fat*

-emia = *condition of blood*

condition of excessive fat in the blood

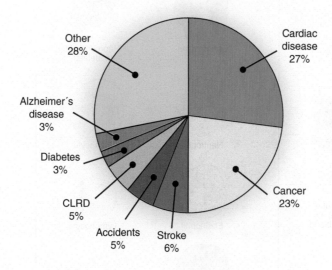

CLRD=Chronic Lower Respiratory Disease

Figure 23-7 Cardiovascular disease is the leading cause of death.

Dietary or drug therapy of elevated plasma cholesterol levels can reduce the risk of atherosclerosis, and subsequent CVD. Lipoproteins consist of four different types: chylomicrons, very-low-density lipoproteins (VLDL), low-density lipoproteins (LDL), and high-density lipoproteins (HDL). A patient with high serum cholesterol and increased LDL is at risk of atherosclerotic coronary disease and myocardial infarction. Atherosclerosis is a disorder in which lipid subgroups (total cholesterol, triglycerides, LDL, and HDL) in various proportions indicate risk factors for the individual. Particles of LDL contain 60% to 70% of all blood cholesterol. Table 23-3 shows normal values of cholesterol and triglyceride levels.

Diseases associated with plasma lipids can manifest as an elevation in triglyceride levels (hyperlipidemia) or as an elevation in the cholesterol level. Medications are not the first line of treatment for hyperlipidemia. Antihyperlipidemic drugs are used only if diet modification and exercise programs fail to lower LDL, or "bad cholesterol" levels, to normal. Table 23-4 shows examples of lipid-lowering drugs.

ARTERIOSCLEROSIS AND ATHEROSCLEROSIS

Arteriosclerosis is the term used to describe degenerative changes in small arteries, which commonly occur in older adults and individuals with diabetes. Elasticity is lost, and the walls become thick and hard. The **lumen** gradually narrows and may become obscured. This leads to diffuse ischemia and death in various tissues, such as those of the heart, kidneys, or brain. Hypertension, hyperlipidemia, diabetes mellitus, and aging add to the progression of arteriosclerosis.

Atherosclerosis is a syndrome differentiated by the presence of atheromas (plaques consisting of lipids, cells, and cell debris, often with attached thrombi, which form inside the walls of large arteries). Atheromas form primarily in

Table 23-3 Normal Values of Cholesterol and Triglyceride Levels

Cholesterol Level	Cholesterol Category
<200 mg/dL	Desirable
200 to 239 mg/dL	Borderline
≥240 mg/dL	High
HDL Cholesterol Level	**HDL Cholesterol Category**
<40 mg/dL (for men) <50 mg/dL (for women)	Low HDL cholesterol; a major risk factor for heart disease
≥60 mg/dL	High HDL cholesterol; an HDL of 60 mg/dL and higher is considered protective against heart disease
LDL Cholesterol Level	**LDL Cholesterol Category**
<100 mg/dL	Optimal
100 to 129 mg/dL	Above optimal
130 to 159 mg/dL	Borderline high
160 to 189 mg/dL	High
≥190 mg/dL	Very high
Triglyceride Level	**Triglyceride Category**
<150 mg/dL	Normal
150 to 199 mg/dL	Borderline high
200 to 499 mg/dL	High
≥500 mg/dL	Very high

Table 23-4 Examples of Antihyperlipidemic Drugs

Generic Name	Trade Name	Route of Administration	Average Adult Dosage
Bile Acid Sequestrants			
cholestyramine	Questran®	PO	One packet or one level scoopful once/day; maint: two to four packets or scoopfuls/day, always mixed with water or other fluids
colesevelam	Welchol®	PO	3 tablets bid with meals or 6 tablets every day with a meal, may be increased to 7 tablets/day
colestipol	Colestid®	PO	15 to 30 g/day in two to four doses with meals and at bedtime or 1 to 2 tablets 1 to 2 times/day
Fibrates			
fenofibrate	Tricor®	PO	54 mg every day (maximum 160 mg/day)
gemfibrozil	Lopid®	PO	600 mg bid 30 minutes before a.m. and p.m. meal, may be increased up to 1500 mg/day
Nicotinic Acid			
niacin	Niacor®, Niaspan®	PO	PO: 500 mg to 2 g at bedtime
HMG-CoA Reductase Inhibitors (Statins)			
atorvastatin	Lipitor®	PO	Initial: 10 to 40 mg every day, may be increased up to 80 mg/day
fluvastatin	Lescol®	PO	20 mg at bedtime, may be increased up to 80 mg/day in one to two doses
lovastatin	Altoprev®, Mevacor®	PO	20 to 40 mg 1 to 2 times/day
pitavastatin	Livalo®	PO	Initial: 2 mg once per day; (maximum 4 mg once per day)
pravastatin	Pravachol®	PO	10 to 80 mg every day
rosuvastatin	Crestor®	PO	5 to 40 mg once/day, usually starting at 10 to 20 mg once/day
simvastatin	Zocor®	PO	5 to 40 mg every day (maximum 80 mg/day) Patients taking danazol or cyclosporine should not exceed 10 mg every day
Omega-3 Fatty Acids (fish oil)			
omega-3-acid ethyl esters	Lovaza®	PO	4 g per day, taken in a single dose or as two 2-g divided doses
Cholesterol-Absorption Inhibitors			
ezetimibe	Zetia®	PO	10 mg once per day
Proprotein Convertase Subtilisin-Kexin Type 9 (PCSK9) Inhibitors			
alirocumab	Praluent®	Subcutaneous	75 mg once every two weeks; or 300 mg once per month
evolocumab	Repatha®	Subcutaneous	140 mg every two weeks; or 420 mg once per month

large arteries such as the aorta and the coronary arteries. Inflammation occurs because of life-long buildup of these plaques, along with small injuries in the vessel walls. The body responds to this damage by sending T lymphocytes and macrophages to combat the atheromas, and these white blood cells actually increase the blockage. The cycle continues and can result in a total blockage of a vessel—leading to heart attack or stroke. Atherosclerosis leads to CAD, in which the cardiac arteries do not receive proper oxygenation. This type of disease is a leading cause of death of both genders. Proper lifestyle and medication changes can allow for a longer lifetime, with decreased risks for heart attack and stroke. Patients with atherosclerosis also have arteriosclerosis. Figure 23-8 illustrates atherosclerosis and the narrowing of the arterial lumen.

HYPERTENSION

Hypertension is defined as an abnormal increase in arterial blood pressure. It occurs as two major types: essential (primary) hypertension, the most common, and secondary hypertension, which results from renal disease or another identifiable cause. Hypertension is a major cause of cardiac disease, renal failure, and stroke.

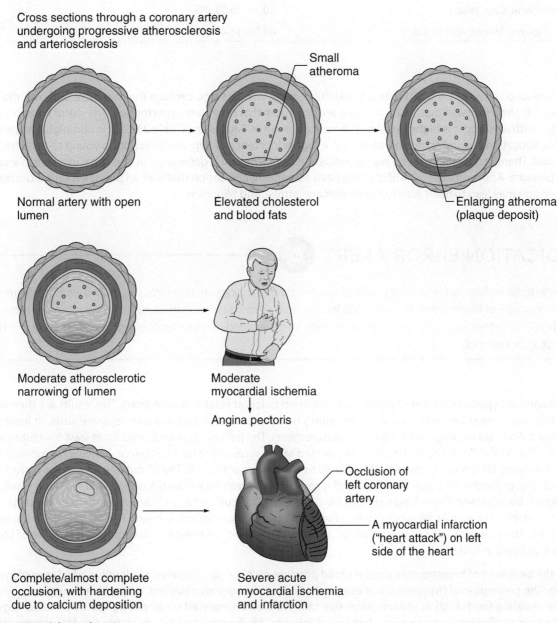

Cross sections through a coronary artery undergoing progressive atherosclerosis and arteriosclerosis

Small atheroma

Normal artery with open lumen

Elevated cholesterol and blood fats

Enlarging atheroma (plaque deposit)

Moderate atherosclerotic narrowing of lumen

Moderate myocardial ischemia

Angina pectoris

Complete/almost complete occlusion, with hardening due to calcium deposition

Severe acute myocardial ischemia and infarction

Occlusion of left coronary artery

A myocardial infarction ("heart attack") on left side of the heart

Figure 23-8 Atherosclerosis.

Table 23-5 Hypertension Prevalence in Various Ages, Genders, and Races

Age	Prevalence
18 to 39 years	7.3%
40 to 59 years	32.4%
60 years or more	65%
Age and Gender	**Prevalence**
Less than 45 years	More males than females
45 to 64 years	Males and females equivalent
65 years or more	More females than males
Race	**Prevalence**
Hispanics	29.6% to 29.9%
Non-Hispanic Caucasians	30.1% to 32.9%
Non-Hispanic African Americans	44.9% to 46.1%

Hypertension affects 32.6% of adults in the United States, which is a percentage that has increased over the last 25 years. It is also estimated that 17.3% of adults are not aware that they have hypertension. The risk of hypertension increases with age, and it is higher in African Americans than in Caucasians (Table 23-5). It is also higher in people with less education and lower income. Men have a higher incidence of hypertension during young to early-middle adulthood. Thereafter, women have a higher incidence. Hypertension is defined as an abnormal increase in arterial blood pressure. Approximately 90% of patients have essential hypertension that is of an unknown cause. Untreated hypertension may lead to heart attack, kidney damage, stroke, and blindness.

MEDICATION ERROR ALERT

In hypertensive obese patients, noninvasive blood pressure recordings are often inaccurate. This leads to incorrect interpretations of blood pressure, potentially leading to treatment errors with vasopressors or antihypertensive medications. Therefore, for critically ill obese patients, invasive blood pressure monitoring should be done quickly in critical care settings.

To diagnose hypertension, blood pressure is measured twice, at least 1 minute apart. The results are then averaged. The values must be confirmed after measuring blood pressure on two or more separate visits, at least one week apart. Accurate readings require proper measurements. The patient must be seated for at least 5 minutes, with both feet flat on the floor. The arm must be supported at the level of the heart. Tobacco, caffeine, or medications that can increase BP cannot be consumed within 30 to 60 minutes of the test. The BP cuff must be of the correct size and placed over the patient's bare arm. If the cuff is too large, the reading will be decreased, and if it is too small, the reading will be increased. The tubing must not have any leaks. The cuff remains fastened; the devices are calibrated every six months. The systolic BP is noted when the first of two or more sounds is heard. The diastolic BP is the value just prior to the disappearance of these sounds. The values are then classified into one of four categories of blood pressure, as listed in Table 23-6.

For the treatment of hypertension, regular blood pressure monitoring is required to identify early stages of hypertension. The prevention of hypertension is essential. Lifestyle changes are required, which include regular physical activity; avoiding foods high in sodium, excessive table salt, and processed meat; eating more fruits and vegetables; limiting alcohol intake to no more than two drinks per day for men and one drink per day for women; stress reduction via relaxation techniques; and cessation of smoking. When these modifications fail, medications are pre-scribed. Many classes of drugs are used to treat hypertension, including the following:

- Diuretics
- Beta-blockers
- Angiotensin-converting enzyme (ACE) inhibitors
- Angiotensin II receptor blockers (ARBs)
- Calcium channel blockers
- Alpha-blockers

Diuretics are most often used to treat hypertension and heart failure. Initially, a thiazide diuretic is usually used. Most of them work by causing the kidneys to eliminate more sodium than they normally would. Three types of diuretics are used to treat hypertension. The other drugs mentioned above may be used individually or in combina-tions with each other. Table 23-7 shows antihypertensive agents.

Table 23-6 Blood Pressure Classifications

Classification	Systolic mm Hg		Diastolic mm Hg
Normal	Less than 120	And	Less than 80
Prehypertension	120 to 139	Or	80 to 89
Stage 1 hypertension	140 to 159	Or	90 to 99
Stage 2 hypertension	160 or higher	Or	100 or higher

Table 23-7 Antihypertensive Agents

Generic Name	Trade Name	Route of Administration	Average Adult Dosage
Beta-Blockers			
atenolol	Tenormin®	PO, IV	PO: 25 to 50 mg/day, may be increased to 100 mg/day; IV: 5 mg over 5 minutes for two doses with 10 minutes in between, then switch to PO
bisoprolol fumarate	Zebeta®	PO	2.5 mg once daily, may increase to 5 to 10 mg prn (maximum 10 mg/day)
carvedilol	Coreg®	PO	Initial: 3.125 mg bid for two weeks, may be doubled, dose q2 weeks as tolerated up to 25 mg bid if less than 85 kg or 50 mg bid if more than 85 kg
labetalol	Trandate®	PO	Initial: 100 mg bid; may be titrated after two to three days in increments of 100 mg bid q2 to 3d
metoprolol	Lopressor®	IV, PO	Initial IV: 3 bolus injections of 5 mg each at 2-minute intervals; then 50 mg PO q6h, 15 minutes after last IV dose, continuing for 48 hours; maint: 100 mg PO bid
nadolol	Corgard®	PO	40 mg once daily, may be increased up to 240 to 320 mg/day in one to two divided doses
propranolol	Inderal®	PO	40 mg bid, may be increased gradually; maint: 120 to 240 mg per day (maximum 640 mg/day)

(Continued)

Table 23-7 Antihypertensive Agents (*Continued*)

Generic Name	Trade Name	Route of Administration	Average Adult Dosage
Angiotensin-Converting Enzyme (ACE) Inhibitors			
benazepril	Lotensin®	PO	10 to 40 mg/day in one to two divided doses
captopril	Capoten®	PO	6.25 to 25 mg tid, may be increased to 50 mg tid (maximum 450 mg/day)
enalapril	Vasotec®	PO, IV	PO: 5 mg/day, may be increased to 10 to 40 mg/day in one to two divided doses; IV: 1.25 q6h, may be given up to 5 mg q6h in hypertensive emergencies
fosinopril	Monopril®	PO	5 to 40 mg once daily (maximum 80 mg/day)
lisinopril	Zestril®	PO	10 mg once daily, may be increased up to 20 to 40 mg 1 to 2 times/day (maximum 80 mg/day)
moexipril	Univasc®	PO	7.5 mg, 1 hour before meals, once/day (maximum 30 mg per day)
perindopril	Aceon®	PO	4 mg once daily (maximum 16 mg/day)
quinapril	Accupril®	PO	10 or 20 mg once daily (maximum 80 mg/day)
ramipril	Altace®	PO	Initial: 2.5 mg once/day; maint: 2.5 to 20 mg/day as single dose or two equal doses
trandolapril	Mavik®	PO	1 or 2 mg once daily, with dosage adjustments once per week prn (maximum 8 mg/day)
Angiotensin II Receptor Blockers (ARBs)			
azlisartan	Edarbi®	PO	40 to 80 mg once daily
candesartan	Atacand®	PO	Start at 16 mg every day (range 8 to 32 mg divided 1 to 2 times/day)
eprosartan	Teveten®	PO	400 to 800 mg once daily
irbesartan	Avapro®	PO	Initial: 150 mg once daily, may be increased to 300 mg/day
losartan	Cozaar®	PO	25 to 50 mg in one to two divided doses (maximum 100 mg/day); start with 25 mg/day if volume depleted
olmesartan	Benicar®	PO	20 mg every day, may be increased to 40 mg every day, start with 5 to 10 mg every day if volume depleted
telmisartan	Micardis®	PO	40 mg every day, may be increased to 80 mg/day
valsartan	Diovan®	PO	80 mg every day (maximum 320 mg every day)
Calcium Channel Blockers: Dihydropyridines			
amlodipine	Norvasc®	PO	5 to 10 mg once daily
felodipine	Plendil®	PO	5 to 10 mg once daily (maximum 20 mg/day)
isradipine	DynaCirc CR®	PO	5 mg once daily (maximum 20 mg/day)
nicardipine	Cardene IV®	IV	50 mL/hr (maximum 150 mL/hr)

(Continued)

Table 23-7 Antihypertensive Agents (*Continued*)

Generic Name	Trade Name	Route of Administration	Average Adult Dosage
nifedipine	Procardia®, Procardia XL®, Adalat CC®	PO	10 to 20 mg tid up to 180 mg/day
nisoldipine	Sular®	PO	10 to 20 mg/day in two divided doses (maximum 40 mg/day), may need to reduce dose in patients with liver disease
Thiazide Diuretics			
chlorothiazide	Diuril®	PO, IV	PO: 500 to 1000 mg (10 to 20 mL oral suspension) 1 to 2 times daily; IV: 0.5 to 1 g, 1 to 2 times daily
chlorthalidone	Thalitone®	PO	Initial: 15 mg once daily, may be increased to 30 mg/day (maximum 45 to 50 mg/day)
hydrochlorothiazide	Microzide®	PO	12.5 mg once daily (maximum 50 mg daily)
indapamide	Lozol®	PO	1.25 mg in the morning; may be increased after four weeks to 2.5 mg/day, then after four weeks to 5 mg/day
metolazone	Zaroxolyn®	PO	2.5 to 10 mg once daily (maximum 20 mg daily)
Loop Diuretics			
bumetanide	Bumex®	PO, IM, IV	PO: 0.5 to 2 mg usually as a single dose; may be given IM/IV when PO is not an option but should be switched to PO as soon as possible
ethacrynic acid	Edecrin®	PO, IV	PO: 50 to 100 mg 1 to 2 times daily, increase by 25 to 50 mg prn to 400 mg/day; IV: 0.5 to 1 mg/kg or 50 mg up to 100 mg, may repeat prn
furosemide	Lasix®	PO, IM, IV	PO: 20 to 80 mg in one or more divided doses up to 600 mg/day prn; IM/IV: 20 to 40 mg in one or more divided doses up to 600 mg/day
torsemide	Demadex®	PO	5 mg once daily; in four to six weeks, may be increased to 10 mg/day
Potassium-Sparing Diuretics			
amiloride	Midamor®	PO	5 mg once daily; may be increased to 10 mg/day prn; (maximum 20 mg/day)
triamterene	Dyrenium®	PO	100 mg bid (maximum 300 mg/day), may be decreased to 100 mg/day or every other day
Aldosterone Antagonists			
eplerenone	Inspra®	PO	Initial: 50 mg/day; (maximum 100 mg/day)
spironolactone	Aldactone®	PO	25 to 200 mg/day in divided doses for at least five days prn; if no response, a thiazide or loop diuretic may be added

ANGINA PECTORIS

Angina pectoris is an episodic, reversible oxygen insufficiency in the heart muscle that causes varying forms of transient chest pain. The pain is usually felt in the chest or left arm. Anginal pain most commonly follows exertion. Atherosclerotic lesions that produce a narrowing of the coronary arteries are the major cause of angina. However, tachycardia (increased heart rate), anemia, hyperthyroidism, and hypotension can also cause an oxygen imbalance that results in insufficient myocardial oxygen.

There are several types of angina: stable (classic), unstable, decubitus (nocturnal), and silent. The most common form is classic angina, which may occur, with predictable frequency, from exertion (often from exercising), emotional stress, or a heavy meal. In stable angina, pain is predictable in frequency and duration. Rest and nitroglycerin relieve the pain.

Unstable angina is a medical emergency, and the patient must be treated in a hospital. It typically has a sudden onset and sudden worsening, which may progress to myocardial infarction. Unstable angina occurs during periods of rest.

Decubitus angina is a condition characterized by periodic attacks of cardiac pain that occur when a person is lying down. It is also known as vasospastic angina. Decubitus angina occurs when the decreased myocardial blood flow is caused by spasms of the coronary arteries. Silent angina is an impairment of vasodilator reserve that causes angina-like chest pain in a person with normal coronary arteries.

To prevent angina pectoris, cessation of smoking, stress reduction, weight loss, lowering cholesterol and blood pressure, and controlling underlying conditions such as hypertension are essential. If there is an occlusion, surgery is indicated, utilizing **angioplasty** or **coronary artery bypass graft**. The placement of a **stent** may be performed to widen arteries and improve coronary blood flow.

For the treatment of angina pectoris, there are three groups of medications that are prescribed to treat and prevent symptoms.

1. Nitroglycerin—a nitrate that dilates arteries to allow increased blood flow to the heart muscle
2. Beta-adrenergic blockers—bind to beta-adrenoreceptors, preventing sympathetic stimulation of the heart; sudden discontinuation of beta-blockers can lead to abrupt increases in blood pressure
3. Calcium channel blockers—block calcium entry, reducing electrical conduction in the heart, decreasing force of contraction, and dilating arteries

Examples of commonly used antianginal drugs are listed in Table 23-8.

POINTS TO REMEMBER

According to the American Heart Association, angina occurs more commonly in women than men.

WHAT WOULD YOU DO?

A patient in your pharmacy has just received his or her prescription for an antianginal medication when he or she exclaims that he or she is having chest pain at that moment, and he or she collapses. If you were the pharmacy technician who served him or her, what would you do?

MYOCARDIAL INFARCTION

Myocardial infarction (MI) is also known as heart attack. It results in the reduction of blood flow through one of the coronary arteries. This causes ischemia (restriction in blood supply resulting in reduced supply of oxygen) in the muscle of the heart (the myocardium), and necrosis (see Figure 23-9). It is the leading cause of death in the United States and Western Europe. Each year, about 790,000 people in the United States experience MI (Centers for Disease Control and Prevention). Predisposing risk factors for MI include the following:

- Family history of MI
- Gender (men and postmenopausal women are more susceptible to MI than premenopausal women)
- Hypertension
- Elevated triglyceride, total cholesterol, and low-density lipoprotein ("bad cholesterol") levels
- Obesity
- Sedentary lifestyle

Table 23-8 Examples of Antianginal Drugs			
Generic Name	**Trade Name**	**Route of Administration**	**Average Adult Dosage**
Nitrates			
isosorbide	Imdur®	PO	30 to 60 mg q a.m., may be increased up to 120 mg once daily after several days if needed (maximum dose 240 mg)
nitroglycerin	Nitro-Bid®, Nitrol®	PO, Topical	PO: 1.3 to 9 mg q8 to 12h; Topical: 1.5 to 5 cm (1/2 to 2 inches) of ointment q4 to 6h
	Nitrodisc®, Nitro-Dur®	Transdermal patch	Wear patch for q24h, or leave on for 10 to 12 hours, then remove and have a 10 to 12 hours nitrate-free interval
	Nitrostat®; Nitrolingual®	PO, Sublingual (SL) tablets; SL pump spray	PO: 1.3 to 9 mg q8 to 12h; SL: one to two sprays (0.4 to 0.8 mg) or a 0.3 to 0.6 mg tablet q3 to 5min prn (maximum three doses in 15 minutes)
Beta-Adrenergic Blockers			
acebutolol	Sectral®	PO	300 to 400 mg tid
atenolol	Tenormin®	PO, IV	25 to 50 mg/day, may be increased to 100 mg/day; IV: 5 mg over 5 minutes, followed by another 5 mg IV injection 10 minutes later, then switch to PO
nadolol	Corgard®	PO	40 mg once daily, may be increased up to 240 to 320 mg/day in one to two divided doses
propranolol	Inderal®	PO	10 to 20 mg bid to tid, may need 160 to 320 mg/day in divided doses
Calcium Channel Blockers			
bepridil	Vascor®	PO	Initial: 200 mg once daily, may be adjusted q7d (maximum 400 mg/day)
diltiazem	Cardizem®	PO	30 mg qid, may be increased q1 to 2d as required (usual range: 180 to 360 mg/day in divided doses)
nifedipine	Adalat®, Procardia®	PO	10 to 20 mg tid up to 180 mg/day
verapamil	Calan®, Verelan PM®	PO	80 mg q6 to 8h, may be increased up to 320 to 480 mg/day in divided doses

- Aging
- Smoking
- Drug use, especially cocaine and amphetamines
- Stress

During an acute heart attack, treatment is based on how stable the patient is, and his or her immediate risk of death. Aspirin is given as soon as possible, and often other medications that will help prevent blood clotting in the coronary arteries are also given. Oxygen is given to aid breathing, a pain medication (usually morphine) is administered for the chest pain, beta-blockers are given to reduce the heart's need for oxygen, nitroglycerin is given to help blood flow into heart muscle cells, and finally, a cholesterol-lowering statin drug is administered. Heparin may be needed along with aspirin to achieve a stronger anticlotting effect.

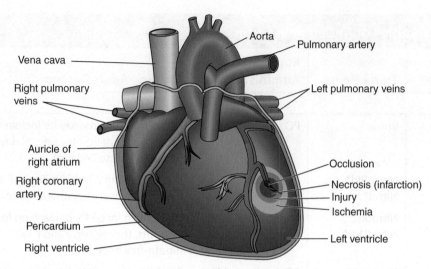

Figure 23-9 Myocardial infarction.

Reperfusion therapy is considered to restore blood flow to the injured heart muscle as quickly as possible to prevent permanent damage. This is performed mechanically in a cardiac catheterization department, with a catheter threaded through a large blood vessel toward the heart. A colored dye is injected to locate the blockage within the coronary artery. Then, percutaneous transluminal coronary angioplasty can be performed, crushing the clot and plaque. A stent may be placed to keep the artery open. Additional antiplatelet agents may be needed. Reperfusion can also be achieved with thrombolytic agents such as tissue plasminogen activator (tPA).

After a myocardial infarction occurs, cardiac rehabilitation, dietary changes, and cessation of smoking are essential. If any complications develop after the MI, there may be a need for antiarrhythmic, antihypertensive, and heart failure medications. When hospitalized, daily medications include aspirin, a beta-blocker, an ACE inhibitor, a statin, and a second anticoagulant.

CARDIAC ARRHYTHMIAS

Arrhythmias (dysrhythmias) are deviations from the normal cardiac rate or rhythm. They may result from damage to the heart's conduction system or from systemic causes such as electrolyte abnormalities, fever, hypoxia, stress, and drug toxicity.

Arrhythmias reduce the efficiency of the heart's pumping cycle. A slight increase in heart rate increases cardiac output, but a very rapid heart rate prevents adequate filling during diastole, reducing cardiac output. A very slow heart rate also reduces output to the tissues, including the brain and the heart itself. Irregular contractions are inefficient because they interfere with the normal filling and emptying cycle. Table 23-9 summarizes various cardiac arrhythmias.

WHAT WOULD YOU DO?

There are "five A's" referring to acute therapy for cardiac arrhythmias, which include *adenosine, adrenaline, ajmaline, amiodarone,* and *atropine.* There are also "B," "C," and "D" strategies that signify *beta-blockers, cardioversion,* and *defibrillation.* If you were asked to come up with a chart for the pharmacy reminding employees of these strategies in cases of emergency, what would you do to help simplify the components on it?

Antiarrhythmic drugs are classified according to their effects on the conduction of impulses through the heart and their mechanism of action. Table 23-10 shows examples of antiarrhythmic drugs.

Table 23-9 Various Cardiac Arrhythmias

Type of Arrhythmia	Beats per Minute
Bradycardia	<60
Tachycardia	150 to 250
Atrial flutter	200 to 350
Atrial fibrillation	>350
Ventricular fibrillation	Variable
Premature atrial contraction	Variable
Premature ventricular contraction	Variable

Table 23-10 Examples of Antiarrhythmic Drugs

Generic Name	Trade Name	Route of Administration	Average Adult Dosage
Class I			
disopyramide	Norpace®	PO	400 to 800 mg/day in divided doses
flecainide	Tambocor®	PO	100 mg q12h, may be increased by 50 mg bid q4d (maximum 400 mg/day)
lidocaine	Xylocaine®	IM, IV, SC	IM/SC: 200 to 300 mg, may be repeated once after 60 to 90 minutes; IV: 50 to 100 mg bolus at a rate of 20 to 50 mg/min, may repeat in 5 minutes, then start infusion of 1 to 4 mg/min immediately after first bolus
mexiletine	Mexitil®	PO	200 to 300 mg q8h (maximum 1200 mg/day)
procainamide	Pronestyl®, Procan SR®	PO, IM, IV	PO: 1 g followed by 250 to 500 mg q3h or 500 mg to 1 g q6h sustained release; IM: 0.5 to 1 g q4 to 6h until able to take PO; IV: 100 mg q5min at a rate of 25 to 50 mg/min until arrhythmia is controlled or 1 g given, then 2 to 6 mg/min
propafenone	Rythmol®	PO	Initial: 150 mg q8h (450 mg/day); may be increased over three to four day intervals, to 225 mg q8h; (maximum 900 mg/day)
quinidine	Quinidex®	PO	Initial: 300 mg q8 to 12h; dose may be cautiously increased with close monitoring
Class II (beta-adrenergic blockers)			
acebutolol	Sectral®	PO	200 mg bid increased to 600 to 1200 mg/day
esmolol	Brevibloc®	IV	500 mcg/kg loading dose followed by 50 mcg/kg/min, may be increased dose q5 to 10min prn (maximum 200 mcg/kg/min)
propranolol hydrochloride	Inderal®, InnoPran XL®	PO, IV	PO: 10 to 30 mg tid to qid, IV: 0.5 to 3 mg q4h prn
sotalol	Betapace®	PO	80 mg bid; may be increased by 80 mg/day q3d with close monitoring; (note: this drug also has Class III properties)

(Continued)

Table 23-10 Examples of Antiarrhythmic Drugs (*Continued*)			
Generic Name	**Trade Name**	**Route of Administration**	**Average Adult Dosage**
Class III (drugs that interfere with potassium outflow)			
amiodarone	Cordarone®, Nexterone®, Amiodarone HCl Injection®	PO, IV	PO (loading): 800 to 1600 mg/day in one to two doses for one to three weeks; PO (maint): 400 to 600 mg/day in one to two doses; IV (loading): 150 mg over 10 minutes followed by 360 mg over next 6 hours; IV (maint): 540 mg over 18 hours (0.5 mg/min), may be continued at 0.5 mg/min)
bretylium	Bretylium Tosylate Injection®	IM, IV	IM: 5 to 10 mg/kg, may be repeated in 1 to 2 hours if arrhythmia persists, then 5 to 10 mg/kg q6 to 8 h for maintenance; IV: 5 mg/kg rapid injection, may increase to 10 mg/kg and repeat q15 to 30min (maximum 30 mg/kg/day): may also be given by continuous infusion at 1 to 2 mg/min
dofetilide	Tikosyn®	PO	125 to 500 mcg bid with close monitoring
dronedarone	Multaq®	PO	400 mg bid
Class IV (calcium channel blockers)			
diltiazem	Cardizem®, Cartia XT®	IV	0.25 mg/kg bolus over 2 minutes, if inadequate response, may be repeated in 15 minutes with 0.35 mg/kg, followed by a continuous infusion of 5 to 10 mg/hr (maximum 15 mg/hr for 24 hours)
verapamil	Calan®, Isoptin®	PO, IV	PO: 240 to 480 mg/day in divided doses; IV: 5 to 10 mg direct, may be repeated in 15 to 30 minutes prn
Other Drugs			
atropine sulfate	Atropine®	IM, IV	IM/IV: 0.5 to 1 mg q1 to 2h prn (maximum 2 mg)
digoxin	Lanoxin®	PO, IV	*Digitalizing dose—* PO: 10 to 15 mcg/kg (1 mg) in divided doses over 24 to 48 hours; IV: 10 to 15 mcg/kg (1 mg) in divided doses over 24 hours *Maintenance dose—* PO/IV: 0.1 to 0.375 mg/day

HEART FAILURE

Heart failure is one of the most common cardiovascular disorders, affecting more than 5.7 million Americans over age 21. The prevalence of heart disease is increasing, with an estimated 8 million Americans being affected by the year 2030. Currently, about 870,000 new patients are diagnosed annually. By the age of 40, men and women have a one in five risk of developing heart failure. Risks increase with age, and the condition is more common after age 65. Heart failure is the cause of death in one of nine individuals. Risk factors include advanced age, the male gender, and the African American race. Uniquely, African American males have a much higher rate of heart failure at ages younger than 75. Other risk factors include CAD, hypertension, diabetes, and a family history of heart failure. Treating hypertension can reduce risks of developing heart failure by up to 50%.

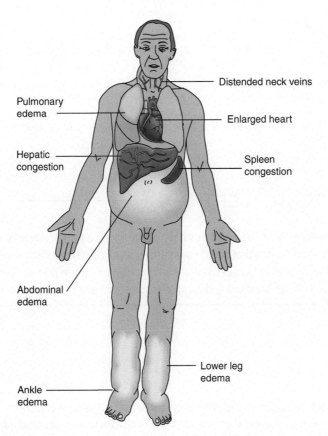

Distended neck veins

Pulmonary edema

Enlarged heart

Hepatic congestion

Spleen congestion

Abdominal edema

Lower leg edema

Ankle edema

Figure 23-10 Congestive heart failure.

Heart failure occurs when the heart is not able to pump enough blood to meet the body's metabolic demands. As a result of this failure, gradual congestion of the cardiopulmonary and general vascular system develops. The amount of blood that the heart is able to pump is measured in liters per minute, and called *cardiac output*. Common symptoms include shortness of breath, **tachypnea**, tachycardia, and enlargement of the heart. Shortness of breath is called *dyspnea on exertion* when it occurs with exercise, and is called *orthopnea* when is occurs while lying down. As CHF progresses, fluid builds up in the vascular system, leading to neck vein distention and edema in the ankles and lower legs. Right-sided heart failure leads to congestion of the liver and spleen. Left-sided heart failure leads to congestion and edema of the lungs (see Figure 23-10). There is a low **ejection fraction** from the heart, of less than 40%. Crackles or rales heard during examination reveal fluid building in the lungs, which is confirmed by chest x-rays. Related to this fluid, there is a constant, nonproductive cough. The patient often complains of fatigue and exercise intolerance.

Because there is no cure for heart failure, the treatment goals are to prevent, treat, or remove the underlying causes when possible. Drugs can relieve the symptoms of heart failure by a number of different mechanisms, including slowing the heart rate, increasing contractility, and reducing its workload.

Heart failure may be treated with a variety of drugs and methods, including cardiac glycosides, diuretics, ACE inhibitors, angiotensin receptor blockers (ARBs), beta-blockers, aldosterone antagonists, fluid restriction, and a low-sodium diet. The only currently available cardiac glycoside is digoxin (Lanoxin®). These drugs are also used for hypertension; they are listed in Table 23-7.

POINTS TO REMEMBER

The role of cardiac glycosides is not well defined, but they have been shown to increase the force of heart muscle contraction in some patients.

MEDICATION ERROR ALERT

Studies have found that nearly 50% of heart patients have experienced a potentially avoidable adverse drug event or other problem with their medications that could have caused significant harm if not discovered early. A significant component of these errors is that elderly patients with heart conditions often do not understand their health care information fully and make mistakes in dosages, dosing schedules, and assessing the effects of prescribed drugs.

Disorders of the Hematological System

Specific causes of hematological disorders include chronic disease, surgery, malnutrition, drugs, exposure to toxins or radiation, genetic or congenital defects that disrupt blood cell function or production, and trauma. Examples of some disorders and conditions include folic acid deficiency anemia, iron deficiency anemia, pernicious anemia, and thrombocytopenia.

FOLIC ACID DEFICIENCY ANEMIA

Folic acid deficiency anemia is a common, slowly progressive condition. It usually occurs in infants, adolescents, pregnant and lactating women, alcoholics, elderly people, and those with cancer. Folic acid deficiency anemia may result from alcohol abuse, poor diet, impaired absorption, overcooking of food, prolonged drug therapy, and increased folic acid requirements during pregnancy. It may also be caused by the rapid growth that occurs during infancy, childhood, and adolescence. Treatment of folic acid deficiency involves folic acid supplements, dietary changes to increase the amount of folic acid, and treating the underlying condition. Sometimes, injections of folic acid are required.

IRON DEFICIENCY ANEMIA

Iron deficiency anemia is a disorder of oxygen transport in which hemoglobin synthesis is deficient. It is a common disease worldwide and occurs most commonly in premenopausal women, infants (particularly premature babies), children, and adolescents (especially females). Possible causes of iron deficiency anemia include inadequate dietary intake of iron, iron malabsorption, blood loss caused by drug-induced gastrointestinal bleeding (from aspirin, anticoagulants, and steroids), and heavy menses. Bleeding from trauma, peptic ulcers, and cancer may also cause it. Pregnancy that diverts maternal iron to the fetus for production of red blood cells may cause iron deficiency anemia in the mother. Treatment of this condition requires iron supplements, syrups (for children), and injections. The underlying cause must be identified and treated. Iron supplements must be taken with meals since they can cause stomach upset. They should not be taken with antacids but should be taken with vitamin C.

PERNICIOUS ANEMIA

Pernicious anemia is a disorder of red blood cells that causes them to develop into an enlarged, misshapen form. It is caused by the inability to absorb vitamin B_{12} from the diet. Pernicious anemia is characterized by decreased production of hydrochloric acid in the stomach and a deficiency of intrinsic factor, which is normally secreted by the inner layer of the stomach. This factor is essential for vitamin B_{12} absorption in the ileum. The resulting deficiency of this vitamin inhibits red blood cell growth, which leads to the production of fewer and deformed cells that have poor oxygen-carrying capacity. This also causes neurological damage by impairing myelin formation. Treatment of pernicious anemia begins with treating the underlying cause, followed by daily or weekly vitamin B_{12} injections that are decreased over time. Once B_{12} levels are normalized, injections are often only required monthly. After this, oral supplements are used, along with nasal gels and sprays.

THROMBOCYTOPENIA

Thrombocytopenia is a deficiency of platelets in circulating blood. Severe thrombocytopenia can involve spontaneous bleeding. The most common cause of thrombocytopenia is cancer chemotherapy, but it may be drug induced by heparin or carbamazepine (Tegretol®). For severe cases of thrombocytopenia, medications include corticosteroids, intravenous immunoglobulins, immune blockers (such as rituximab), and platelet growth factors (such as eltrombopag). In some cases, a splenectomy is required.

MEDICATION ERROR ALERT

Documented medication errors have occurred between the drugs carbamazepine (Tegretol®) and metoprolol succinate (Toprol-XL®). Tegretol® is indicated for seizures or trigeminal neuralgia, while Toprol-XL® is indicated for hypertension, angina pectoris, and heart failure. Carbamazepine also carries warnings regarding aplastic anemia, agranulocytosis, and the fact that gradual withdrawal is required.

THROMBOPHLEBITIS

Thrombophlebitis is defined as an inflammation inside a vein along with the formation of a blood clot at the site. It is a dangerous situation because the thrombus may break away and lodge in a vital organ. Aching or cramping pain, especially in the calf when the patient is walking, characterizes deep vein thrombophlebitis. Medications for thrombophlebitis include anticoagulants and thrombolytics.

MEDICAL TERMINOLOGY REVIEW

thrombophlebitis:

thromb/o = *clot*

phleb = *vein*

-itis = *inflammation*

inflammation caused by clotting in the veins

PULMONARY EMBOLISM

Pulmonary embolism is defined as the blockage of a pulmonary artery by fat, air, tumor tissue, or a thrombus that usually arises from a peripheral vein. Most commonly, a thrombus moves from one of the deep veins of the legs. Regardless of the type, the mass moves through the veins to be pumped via the right side of the heart to the pulmonary circulation. It then lodges in a lung vessel, usually where an artery narrows and divides. The risk of pulmonary embolism is increased by immobility, injury to a blood vessel, any predisposition to clot formation, CVD, thrombophlebitis, or pulmonary disease. A variety of factors during pregnancy also predispose women to this condition. Other factors may include use of oral contraceptives that are high in estrogen, diabetes mellitus, and myocardial infarction.

Table 23-11 Examples of Anticoagulants Used for Cardiovascular Disorders

Generic Name	Trade Name	Route of Administration	Average Adult Dosage
heparin sodium	Hepalean®, Hep-Lock®	IV, SC	IV: 5000-unit bolus dose, then 20,000 to 40,000 units infused over 24 hours, dose adjusted to maintain desired activated partial thromboplastin time (APTT) or 5000 to 10,000 units piggyback q4 to 6h; SC: 10,000 to 20,000 units followed by 8000 to 20,000 units q8 to 12h
lepirudin	Refludan®	IV	0.4 mg/kg initial bolus (maximum 44 mg) followed by 0.15 mg/kg/hr (maximum 16.5 mg/hr) for 2 to 10 days, adjust rate to maintain APTT of 1.5 to 2.5
warfarin sodium	Coumadin Sodium®, Panwarfin®	PO, IV	10 to 15 mg/day for two to five days, then 2 to 10 mg once daily with dose adjusted to maintain PT 1.2 to 2 times control or international normalized ratio (INR) of 2 to 3
Low-Molecular-Weight Heparin			
dalteparin	Fragmin®	SC	120 IU/kg bid for at least five days
enoxaparin	Lovenox®	SC	1 mg/kg q12h or 1.5 mg/kg/day; monitor anti-Xa activity to determine appropriate dose
tinzaparin	Innohep®	SC	175 anti-Xa IU/kg every day for at least six days and until patient is adequately anticoagulated (INR at least 2.0 for two consecutive days)

Signs and symptoms of pulmonary embolism appear after the embolism has interrupted blood flow. They include apprehension, chest pain, cough, fever, and in more serious cases, dyspnea, tachypnea, and, sometimes, hemoptysis. If the embolism is extremely large, **cyanosis** and shock develop, often leading to death. Treatment focuses on maintaining cardiopulmonary integrity, adequate ventilation, and adequate perfusion. Oxygen therapy and anticoagulants are used. Often heparin and similar agents will be used first, followed by warfarin, which may be maintained for weeks to months. Thrombolytic drugs may be administered to dissolve a clot, often when there is low blood pressure or cardiac arrest. It is important to prevent this condition from developing in hospitalized patients, so various prophylactic therapies are used, including early ambulation, low doses of anticoagulants, thromboembolism-deterrent (TED) stockings, and sequential compression devices that pump the legs intermittently. Anticoagulants are agents that prevent formation of blood clots (thrombi). Table 23-11 shows examples of anticoagulants.

WHAT WOULD YOU DO?

A patient who previously was diagnosed with deep vein thrombosis is taking his blood pressure on a free machine in your pharmacy. He becomes short of breath and says that his chest hurts and his heart feels irregular. As a pharmacy technician, you call 911 on his behalf and assist in keeping him calm and safe until the EMTs arrive. When they arrive and assess the man, they ask if you know anything about his medication history. In this scenario, what would you do?

POINTS TO REMEMBER

Recent studies have shown that nicotinic acid, for lowering LDL cholesterol and increasing HDL cholesterol, does not have significant effects.

Summary

The cardiovascular (circulatory) system consists of the heart and the blood vessels. It is divided into pulmonary and systemic circulations. The pulmonary circulation involves movement of blood between the heart and the lungs. Deoxygenated blood is transported to the lungs to pick up oxygen and is then pumped back to the heart. In the systemic circulation, oxygenated blood is carried from the heart to the body tissues and is then transported back to the heart. The wall of the heart has three layers: epicardium, myocardium, and endocardium. The heart is divided into two atria and two ventricles. The right atrium is separated from the right ventricle by a tricuspid (atrioventricular) valve. The pulmonary (semilunar) valve is located between the right ventricle and the pulmonary artery. The left atrium is separated from the left ventricle by the mitral (bicuspid) valve. The aortic (semilunar) valve is found between the left ventricle and the aorta.

Contraction of heart chambers is known as systole, while relaxation is known as diastole. The sinoatrial (SA) node is the primary pacemaker of the heart, controlling heart rate. The blood vessels include the arteries, capillaries, and veins, along with connecting vessels known as arterioles and venules. Blood consists of red blood cells, white blood cells, platelets, and liquid plasma. The amount of force exerted by the blood against the blood vessel walls is known as blood pressure.

Cardiovascular disorders are the most common causes of death in the United States. Examples of these disorders are hyperlipidemia, arteriosclerosis, atherosclerosis, hypertension, angina pectoris, myocardial infarction, cardiac arrhythmias, and heart failure. Blood disorders are common and varied. Examples of these disorders include various anemias, thrombocytopenia, thrombophlebitis, and pulmonary embolism. Medications used to treat cardiovascular system disorders include antihyperlipidemic drugs, antihypertensive drugs, antianginal drugs, antiarrhythmics, cardiac glycosides, diuretics, ACE inhibitors, beta-blockers, and anticoagulants.

REVIEW QUESTIONS

1. Which chamber of the heart pumps deoxygenated blood through the pulmonary valve into the lungs?

   A. Right atrium
   B. Left ventricle
   C. Right ventricle
   D. Left atrium

2. Which of the following organs is mostly responsible for controlling cholesterol levels in the body?

   A. Brain
   B. Pancreas
   C. Heart
   D. Liver

3. A disease in which plaque builds up in the walls of large arteries is:

   A. atherosclerosis.
   B. coronary artery disease.
   C. arteriosclerosis.
   D. hyperlipidemia.

4. Which of the following contains 60% to 70% of all blood cholesterol?

   A. LDL
   B. HDL
   C. VLDL
   D. Chylomicrons

5. Which of the following defines hypertension?

    A.   140 mm Hg systolic or 90 mm Hg diastolic
    B.   150 mm Hg systolic or 95 mm Hg diastolic
    C.   130 mm Hg systolic or 85 mm Hg diastolic
    D.   120 mm Hg systolic or 80 mm Hg diastolic

6. Sudden discontinuation of which of the following can lead to abrupt increases in blood pressure?

    A.   ACE inhibitors
    B.   Angiotensin receptor blockers
    C.   Beta-blockers
    D.   Calcium channel blockers

7. Regarding heart failure, which of the following is not a risk factor?

    A.   Family history
    B.   Age less than 65 years
    C.   Hypertension
    D.   African American race

8. All of the following medications are used for angina pectoris, *except:*

    A.   beta-adrenergic blockers.
    B.   calcium channel blockers.
    C.   sulfates.
    D.   nitrates.

9. Which of the following agents is *not* a beta-adrenergic blocker?

    A.   Nadolol
    B.   Nitroglycerin
    C.   Atenolol
    D.   Propranolol

10. The trade name of verapamil is:

    A.   Edecrin®.
    B.   Diachlor®.
    C.   Calan®.
    D.   Hygroton®.

11. Which of the following terms describes the amount of blood pumped by the heart, in liters per minute?

    A.   Heart rate
    B.   Cardiac output
    C.   Contractility
    D.   Ejection fraction

12. Which of the following agents are able to dissolve blood clots?

    A.   Coagulants
    B.   Thrombolytics
    C.   Anticoagulants
    D.   Hemostatics

13. Which of the following is not a statin drug?

    A.   Crestor
    B.   Lopressor
    C.   Lipitor
    D.   Zocor

14. Avapro® is the trade name of:

   A. irbesartan.
   B. olmesartan.
   C. lisinopril.
   D. enalapril.

15. Which of the following is an example of a lipid-lowering drug?

   A. Bishydroxy®
   B. Lescol®
   C. Refludan®
   D. Cozaar®

CRITICAL THINKING

A 56-year-old man was playing tennis with a friend. He began feeling pain in his chest, which radiated to his chin and left arm. His friend called 911, and he was taken to the emergency department.

1. How many types of angina pectoris exist? Explain each type.

2. What is the treatment of choice for angina pectoris?

3. What are the complications of angina pectoris if it continues?

WEB LINKS

American Association of Cardiovascular and Pulmonary Rehabilitation: www.aacvpr.org

American Heart Association: www.heart.org

American Red Cross: www.redcross.org

American Society of Hematology: www.hematology.org/patients/anemia/

Heart Attack Statistics: www.cdc.gov/heartdisease/heart_attack.htm

CHAPTER 24

Therapeutic Drugs for the Immune System

OUTLINE

OBJECTIVES

Upon completion of this chapter, the reader should be able to:

1. Describe the cells and organs of the immune system.
2. Define non-Hodgkin's lymphoma and its treatment plan.
3. List the nonspecific defenses of the human body.
4. Define antigen, antibody, and immunoglobulin.
5. Describe common autoimmune disorders.
6. Discuss immunizations and their adverse effects.

7. Differentiate between active and passive immunity.

8. Describe the immune response.

9. List three ways in which vaccines are prepared.

10. Differentiate between immediate and delayed hypersensitivity.

KEY TERMS

active acquired immunity	autism	immunology	passive acquired immunity
allergen	B lymphocytes	inactivated vaccines	plasma cells
allergy	contraindication	innate immunity	precaution
anthrax	hepatitis	killer cells	spleen
antibodies	hilum	live attenuated vaccines	T lymphocytes
antigens	immunogen	lymph nodes	toxoid
antitoxins	immunogenicity	lymphatic sinuses	trabeculae
attenuation	immunoglobulins	natural active acquired immunity	vaccination

Overview

The immune system protects the body by monitoring for antigens that may be dangerous and must be destroyed. The lymphatic organs are critical in the control and destruction of many pathogenic microorganisms. These organs and tissues provide the structural basis of the immune system. They contain phagocytic cells and lymphocytes, which play vital roles in the body's defense mechanisms and resistance to disease. Autoimmune disorders involve the immune system becoming unable to identify "self" antigens, and then they attack the body's cells, tissues, and organs.

Our environment contains a great variety of infectious microbes such as viruses, bacteria, fungi, protozoa, and multicellular parasites. These can cause various infections. Most infections in normal individuals are short-lived and leave little permanent damage. This is due to the immune system, which combats infectious agents. The principal components of the immune system include the bone marrow, thymus, lymph nodes, spleen, and lymphatic vessels.

Microorganisms come in many different forms; therefore, a wide variety of immune responses are required to deal with each type of infection. For example, the skin acts as an effective barrier to most organisms; very few infectious agents can penetrate intact skin. However, many agents gain access across the epithelia of the gastrointestinal or urogenital tracts. Others can infect the nasopharynx and lungs. A small number, such as malaria and hepatitis B, can infect the body only if they enter it directly.

The site of the infection and the type of pathogen largely determine which immune responses will be effective. The most important distinction is between pathogens that invade the host's cells and those that do not. It is also important to stress that the primary function of the immune system is to eliminate infectious agents and to minimize the damage they cause.

Anatomy and Physiology of the Immune System

The immune system, which includes the lymphatic system, is made up of a vast collection of cells and biochemicals that travel through lymphatic vessels, as well as the organs and glands that produce them. The lymphatic vessels and organs are shown in Figure 24-1.

The lymphatic and immune systems have a second major function. They enable human beings to live alongside different types of organisms that can take up residence inside or on the human body and cause infectious diseases.

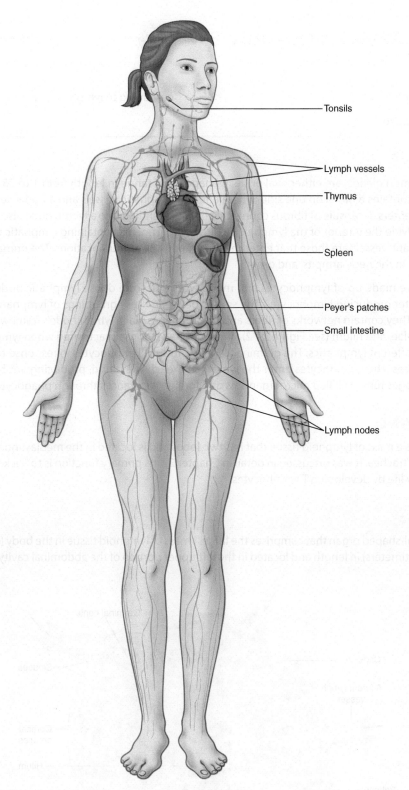

Tonsils

Lymph vessels

Thymus

Spleen

Peyer's patches

Small intestine

Lymph nodes

Figure 24-1 Lymphatic vessels and organs.

Cells and biochemicals of the lymphatic system launch both generalized and targeted attacks against "foreign" particles. As a result, the body is able to destroy infectious microorganisms and viruses. Immunity against disease also protects against toxins and cancer. When the body's immune response is not normal, many conditions may result. These include persistent infections, cancers, autoimmune disorders, and allergies. The lymphoid organs proliferate and differentiate from T and B lymphocytes (T and B cells) and monocytes (macrophages).

MEDICAL TERMINOLOGY REVIEW

lymphatic:

lymph/o = *lymph*   pertaining to lymph

-atic = *pertaining to*

LYMPH NODES

Lymph nodes, or lymph glands, are either oval or bean-shaped and range in length from 1 to 25 mm (millimeters). Each lymph node contains a **hilum** on one side, where efferent lymphatic vessels and a nodal vein leave the node, and a nodal artery enters. A capsule of fibrous connective tissue extending into a lymph node also covers its exterior. These **trabeculae** divide the interior of the lymph node into compartments containing lymphatic tissue and sinuses. The afferent lymphatic vessels are those that enter the lymph node in various locations. The primary concentrations of lymph nodes are in the neck, armpits, and groin.

Lymph nodes are made up of lymphocytes and monocytes that form dense lymphatic nodules. Each nodule has a germinal center producing lymphocytes. The spaces between these groupings of lymphatic tissue are called **lymphatic sinuses**. They contain networks of fibers and macrophages. Each lymph node's framework is made up by its capsule, trabeculae, and hilum (see Figure 24-2). The immune response is activated when lymph enters a lymph node through the afferent lymphatics. The germinal centers produce lymphocytes in response to microorganisms or foreign substances. The lymphocytes enter the lymph and reach the blood, producing antibodies against the invaders. Macrophages remove killed microorganisms and foreign substances through phagocytosis.

THYMUS GLAND

The thymus gland is a mass of lymphoid tissue that has two lobes and is located in the mediastinum, behind the sternum and along the trachea. It was discussed in detail in Chapter 22. Its primary function is to "kick-start" the immune system during early life by developing T lymphocytes.

SPLEEN

The **spleen** is an oval-shaped organ that comprises the largest mass of lymphoid tissue in the body (see Figure 24-3). It is about 12 cm (centimeters) in length and located in the left upper portion of the abdominal cavity. The spleen filters

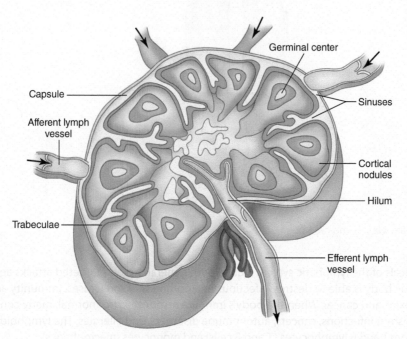

Figure 24-2 Lymph node.

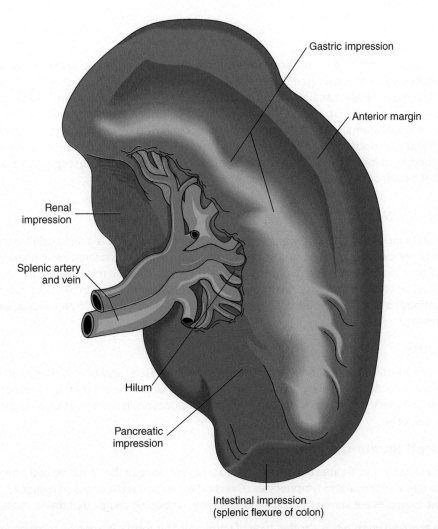

Figure 24-3 The spleen.

blood that enters its hilum via the splenic artery and leaves via the splenic vein. It functions to phagocytize bacteria and worn-out red blood cells and platelets. Hemoglobin can then be released and recycled. The spleen also produces plasma cells and lymphocytes, and it acts as a blood reservoir. If the body is hemorrhaging, the spleen releases stored blood into the blood circulation. When seriously injured, the spleen may need to be surgically removed.

POINTS TO REMEMBER

Splenomegaly is abnormal enlargement of the spleen, which may be linked to diseases such as scarlet fever, syphilis, typhoid fever, typhus, or infection with a microscopic blood fluke worm from the genus *Schistosoma*.

MEDICAL TERMINOLOGY REVIEW

splenomegaly:

splen/o = *spleen*

-megaly = *enlarged*

an enlarged spleen

Immunity

Immunity may be broadly defined as "inborn or acquired resistance to disease" and involves all of what may collectively be called the *host defenses* (see Figure 24-4). Immunity is the condition of being immune or resistant to a particular infectious disease, usually as a result of the presence of protective **antibodies** that are directed against the etiological agent of that disease. The innate or native resistance to disease found in certain individuals, races, and species of animals is not a type of immunity conferred by antibodies but rather is a resistance resulting from natural nonspecific factors. A person who is susceptible to a disease usually has inadequate levels of protective antibodies or insufficient nonspecific defenses. In some cases, this susceptibility may simply reflect a very poor state of health or the presence of an immunodeficiency disease.

TYPES OF IMMUNITY

The types of immunity include innate and acquired immunity. **Innate immunity** is a rapid cellular response to infection, and through phagocytosis, cytokines, and antigen processing, begins the *adaptive immune response*. Acquired immunity results from the active production of antibodies. If the antibodies are released within a person's body, the immunity is called **active acquired immunity**. Such protection is usually long-lasting. In **passive acquired immunity**, the person receives antibodies that were produced by another person or, in some cases, by an animal; such protection is usually only temporary.

Innate Immunity

Innate immunity occurs quickly in response to an infection. Macrophages and neutrophils phagocytize bacteria and other antigens in infection sites. They then release *cytokines* to begin the inflammatory response to infection. *Antigen-presenting cells* process antigens for presentation to lymphocytes in lymph nodes, aiding in beginning the adaptive immune response.

Active Acquired Immunity

Individuals who have had a specific infection usually have some resistance to the causative pathogen because of the presence of antibodies and stimulated lymphocytes. This is called **natural active acquired immunity**. Such resistance may be permanent. Examples are immunity against poliomyelitis, whooping cough, diphtheria, mumps, and measles.

Artificial active acquired immunity is another type of immunity. This results if a person receives a vaccination (the administration of a vaccine that stimulates the production of antibodies). The vaccine contains sufficient **antigens** of a pathogen to enable the individual to form antibodies against that pathogen. Vaccines are made from living or

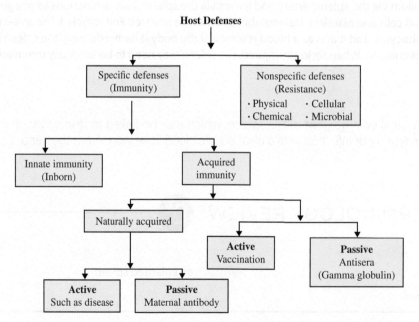

Figure 24-4 Host defenses.

dead (inactivated) pathogens or from certain toxins they excrete. Vaccines made from living organisms are the most effective, but they must be prepared from harmless organisms that are antigenically related to the pathogens or from weakened pathogens that have been genetically changed, so they are no longer pathogenic. The process of weakening pathogens is called **attenuation**, and the vaccines produced in this way are referred to as attenuated vaccines. A **toxoid** vaccine is prepared from endotoxins that have been inactivated or made nontoxic by heat or chemicals. Toxoids are protein toxins that have been modified to reduce their toxicity without significantly altering their **immunogenicity**. They can be injected safely to stimulate the production of antibodies that are capable of neutralizing the endotoxins of pathogens such as those that cause diphtheria and tetanus. A subgroup of antisera usually prepared from the serum of horses immunized against a particular toxin-producing organism are called **antitoxins**.

POINTS TO REMEMBER

Two of the oldest and best known active immunizing agents are diphtheria toxoid and tetanus toxoid, which protect against the bacterial endotoxins.

POINTS TO REMEMBER

A vaccine that stimulates the immune system to produce antibodies to a specific illness-causing toxin is called a toxoid vaccine.

Passive Acquired Immunity

Passive immunity is a form of acquired immunity resulting from antibodies that are transmitted naturally through the placenta to a fetus, or through the colostrum to an infant, or artificially by injection of antiserum (a serum containing antitoxins) for treatment or prophylaxis. Passive immunity is not permanent. It does not last as long as active immunity.

POINTS TO REMEMBER

Antibodies in colostrum protect against certain digestive and respiratory infections.

Immunology

Immunology is the study of immune responses. This area of study includes the topics of active and passive immunity to infectious agents and processes involved in antibody production, discussed earlier. Other topics, including antigens, immune responses, antibodies, hypersensitivity, and the allergic response, are explained here.

ANTIGENS

An antigen is any foreign organic substance that stimulates the production of antibodies. An antigen is also called an **immunogen**. Foreign proteins are the best antigens.

POINTS TO REMEMBER

Immunoglobulins (except for human immunoglobulins) must be kept refrigerated similarly to vaccines. Human immunoglobulins should be kept at room temperature.

ANTIBODIES

The terms *antibody* and **immunoglobulin** are often used interchangeably, but *immunoglobulin* also is used more broadly to refer to an administered blood product containing antibodies. Antibodies are produced by lymphocytes in response to bacteria, viruses, or other antigenic substances. An antibody is specific to an antigen. The antibody-producing cells are a specific type of lymphocyte called B lymphocytes (or B cells), which often work in coordination

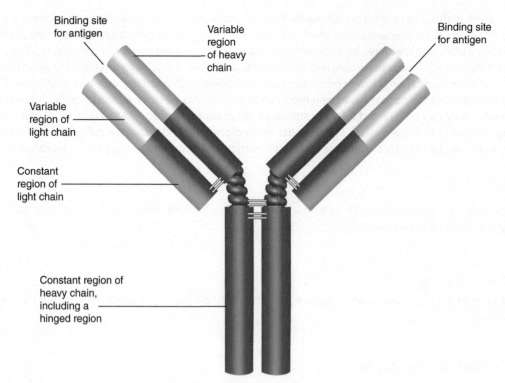

Figure 24-5 Antibody structure.

with T lymphocytes (T cells) and macrophages. The antibody is a type of protein called an immunoglobulin (Ig). Antibodies form in response to many antigens. Antibodies have a simple structure of four amino acid chains that are linked by disulfide bonds. Two of the chains are identical in structure, with approximately 400 amino acid chains, known as *heavy chains*. The other two chains are half of their length, identical to each other, and known as *light chains*. Once united, an antibody molecule has two identical halves, each with a heavy chain and a light chain. The molecule is "Y"-shaped. The "tips" of the "Y" are where antigens bind. Binding sites are varied, allowing the antibody to bind with a large number of antigens. The "stem" of the Y is always constantly the same (Figure 24-5). Each class of antibody is named for its action. There are five classes of antibodies: IgG, IgA, IgM, IgD, and IgE.

Immunoglobulin G

IgG protects against disease and is found in blood and lymphocytes. The normal concentration of IgG in the blood is about 70% to 80% of the total antibodies. IgG is the only immunoglobulin that crosses the placental barrier and protects against red cell antigens and white cell antigens.

POINTS TO REMEMBER

A newborn does not yet have its own antibodies but does retain IgG that has passed through the placenta from its mother.

Immunoglobulin A

IgA protects the mucous membranes and internal cavities against infection. The serum concentration of IgA is 15% to 20%. IgA is found in all secretions of the body and is the major antibody in the mucous membranes, in the intestines, and in the bronchi, colostrum, saliva, and tears. IgA combines with a protein in the mucosa and defends body surfaces against invading microorganisms.

POINTS TO REMEMBER

The newborn also receives IgA from colostrum, a substance secreted from the mother's breasts for the first few days after birth.

Immunoglobulin M

IgM is the largest immunoglobulin in molecular structure. It is the first immunoglobulin the body produces when challenged by antigens and is found in circulating blood. IgM activates complement and can destroy antigens during the initial antigen exposure. The serum concentration of IgM is approximately 10%.

Immunoglobulin D

IgD is a specialized protein found in small amounts in serum. The precise function of IgD is not known, but its quantity increases during allergic reactions to milk, insulin, penicillin, and various toxins. The serum concentration of IgD is less than 1%.

Immunoglobulin E

IgE is found on the surface of basophils and mast cells; it causes allergy, drug sensitivity, anaphylaxis, and immediate hypersensitivity. It also combats parasitic diseases. IgE is available in the serum in amounts of less than 1%. IgE is concentrated in the lungs, skin, and the cells of mucous membranes. It provides the primary defense against environmental antigens and is believed to be responsive to IgA. IgE reacts with some antigens to release certain chemical mediators (such as histamine) that cause type I hypersensitivity reactions characterized by wheals and flare. It can mediate the release of histamine in the immune response to parasites. Serum concentrations of IgE are low in the serum because the antibody is firmly fixed to the tissue surface.

Immune Responses

The immune system as a whole can specifically recognize many thousands of antigens. The specific cells of the immune system, the lymphocytes, undergo differentiation. Some of these cells migrate to and mature in the thymus and are referred to as thymus-derived or **T lymphocytes**. T lymphocytes manifest cellular immunity but also, when activated, play a "helper" role in humoral immunity (an immune response that leads to the production of antibodies). Another class of lymphocytes called killer cells also confers cell-mediated immunity. Most immune responses to pathogenic microorganisms include both a humeral and a cell-mediated component.

Other lymphoid stem cells influenced by fetal liver, bone marrow, or lymphoid tissue differentiate to become **B lymphocytes**. The B lymphocytes mature during immune responses and become the antibody-producing **plasma cells**. The immune response also involves three other types of immunocompetent cells: macrophages, **killer cells**, and natural killer cells. The macrophages (monocytes), neutrophils, and mast cells make up the inflammatory component of the immune response. Macrophages are nonspecific, phagocytic cells, engulfing and destroying their targets. Macrophages do not bind their targets specifically. In other words, the macrophage does not determine whether it is engulfing a virus or a fungal particle, or a sliver of wood. In fact, it can phagocytize all three at once.

When nonself (foreign) antigens are recognized, there is a cascade of T-cell and B-cell events that cause tissue inflammation and the death of the foreign cells. Cytokines are chemicals involved in activating this immune response. The most important cytokine that is involved is called interleukin-2 (IL-2). T-cell activation triggers three signals that result in cytokine production and cell proliferation. These signals are as follows:

1. An antigen presenting cell connects with a T-cell receptor—this weak signal needs assistance to amplify its strength to the cell nucleus
2. Co-stimulation occurs to amplify the signal; once it is received, production of cytokines starts
3. As interleukin-2 binds to the cytokine receptor on the T-cell surface, there are various steps that include activation of the target, leading to starting of the cell cycle and T-cell replication

POINTS TO REMEMBER

Rho(D) immune globulin is given to pregnant women who are Rh negative and have been exposed to blood that is Rh positive.

Disorders of the Immune System

Immune disorders may be temporary or permanent. When immune cells are targeted by infections, severe immune suppression may occur. Primary immune deficiency diseases are inherited genetic disorders. This chapter focuses on lymphoma, autoimmune disorders, and hypersensitivity.

LYMPHOMA

Lymphoma is a type of cancer that affects lymphocytes or other blood cells. It is often malignant and causes lymphatic tissue tumors that begin as enlarged lymph nodes, most commonly without pain. Immune response is depressed and the patient is susceptible to opportunistic infections. After leukemias and brain tumors, malignant lymphomas are the third most common type of cancers in children and young adults. Two groups of lymphomas exist: Hodgkin's disease and non-Hodgkin's lymphomas. The non-Hodgkin's lymphomas comprise nearly two-thirds of all childhood lymphomas.

MEDICAL TERMINOLOGY REVIEW

lymphoma:

lymph/o = *lymph*   a tumor in lymphatic tissue

-oma = *tumor*

MEDICATION ERROR ALERT

Chemotherapy has a narrow therapeutic window. Patients with lymphoma and other cancers often cannot physically tolerate a medication error. To prevent mistakes in chemotherapy, health care professionals must first recognize that they do occur, and then create steps and methods that emphasize medication error prevention. Chemotherapy orders must be accurate and completely clear in their wording. Staff members must be continually trained and have instantaneous access to information. Patient identification systems must be accurate, and pharmacy concerns about medications must be addressed.

Hodgkin's Disease

Hodgkin's disease (also called Hodgkin's lymphoma) has two peak ages of onset, occurring in younger people between the ages of 15 and 35 years, and then in adults aged 55 years or older. It is more common in men and usually involves the reticulum cells of the lymph nodes. This type of lymphoma represents only about 15% of all lymphomas. Risk factors include previous malignancies, prior treatment with radiation therapy or chemotherapy, family history of the condition or other lymphomas, exposure to the Epstein–Barr virus, and immunosuppression. Survival rates vary, based on stage at time of discovery, between 65% and 90%.

An abnormal cell called the Reed–Sternberg cell characterizes Hodgkin's disease. Initial symptoms include painless lymph node enlargement in the neck or mediastinum, fatigue, pruritus, and pain after consuming alcohol. These symptoms are followed by fever, night sweats, fatigue, and weight loss. Hodgkin's disease is treated with chemotherapy, radiation, and bone marrow or stem cell transplantation, based on staging. Patients with stage I or II disease and a favorable prognosis are treated with radiation therapy. For the remainder of stage I and II patients, and some in stage III, combined chemotherapy is preferred. Chemotherapy alone is often used for stage IIIB and IV patients. The preferred treatment is called ABVD therapy, and it uses the following medications:

- **A**: doxorubicin (**A**driamycin®)
- **B**: **b**leomycin (Blenoxane®)
- **V**: **v**inblastine (Velban®)
- **D**: **d**acarbazine (DTIC-Dome®)

Chemotherapy is usually used for patients who have relapses, with bone marrow or stem cell transplantation reserved for those with multiple relapses.

POINTS TO REMEMBER

Prognosis following treatment of Hodgkin's lymphoma is excellent, with at least 80% of children expected to be cured of their disease. Relapses of this disease are not common.

MEDICATION ERROR ALERT

One medication used for Hodgkin's disease, called procarbazine (Matulane®), was involved in medication errors that occurred in connection with a prenatal vitamin sold as Materna®. The errors resulted when pharmacy technicians searched for the first three letters of the vitamin name, "M-A-T," which prompted the computer systems to pull up "Matulane®." The errors were not discovered by pharmacy personnel until after at least one pregnant woman received the Hodgkin's disease drug instead of the prenatal vitamin, and miscarried her baby.

Non-Hodgkin's Lymphoma

Non-Hodgkin's lymphoma comprises a group of lymphoid cell neoplasms that vary in severity and rate of progression. Distinguishing between non-Hodgkin's and Hodgkin's lymphoma is important because their treatments and outcomes are very different. Survival rates for the various types of non-Hodgkin's lymphoma also vary, ranging from 36% to 91%. Incidence of non-Hodgkin's lymphoma peaks in preadolescents, with a second peak in older people. Risk factors include previous history of malignancies, previous radiation therapies (as well as chemotherapy and immunotherapy), certain viral infections (with HIV, human T-cell lymphotropic virus, Epstein–Barr virus, or hepatitis C virus), immunosuppression, and connective tissue disorders such as lupus erythematosus or rheumatoid arthritis. Gastrointestinal lymphoma may develop as a result of celiac disease, Crohn's disease, and chronic gastritis related to *Helicobacter pylori*.

There are various types of non-Hodgkin's lymphoma. The most common (35% to 40%) are indolent lymphomas, with subtypes that include follicular lymphoma, small lymphocytic lymphoma, mantle cell lymphoma, and marginal zone lymphoma. Grade I and II follicular lymphomas have indolent features, while grade III is aggressive. Non-Hodgkin's lymphomas may arise from B cells, T cells, or natural killer (NK) cells. Unfortunately, the aggressive forms of all the various types of non-Hodgkin's lymphoma make up 50% of cases. The most common are diffuse large B-cell lymphoma and peripheral T-cell lymphoma. The highly aggressive lymphomas are rare, comprising 5% of all the non-Hodgkin's lymphomas, and include Burkitt's lymphoma and adult T-cell lymphoma.

Signs and symptoms of non-Hodgkin's lymphomas include fatigue, painless lymphadenopathy, bone pain, and gastrointestinal symptoms. The adenoids or tonsils may become enlarged, and fever, night sweats, and weight loss may eventually occur.

Treatment for non-Hodgkin's lymphoma includes the procedures used for Hodgkin's disease but may additionally require the use of monoclonal antibodies, either with or without radioactive isotopes. Chemotherapy or local radiation is often started only after symptoms develop that might respond to such treatment, since indolent lymphomas are usually not curable using these methods. Though the aggressive lymphomas progress rapidly, they are more likely to be cured with appropriate treatment, which includes CHOP chemotherapy. This utilizes the following medications:

- **C**: cyclophosphamide (**C**ytoxan®)
- **H: h**ydroxy doxorubicin (Adriamycin®)
- **O**: vincristine (**O**ncovin®)
- **P: p**rednisone

Additionally, rituximab and radiation therapy may be used. For relapses, high-dose chemotherapy may be used, followed by bone marrow transplantation in some cases. Periodic follow-up is conducted since patients are at increased risk for developing secondary malignancies.

WHAT WOULD YOU DO?

Since hydroxy doxorubicin (Adriamycin®) can be toxic to the heart, chemotherapy for heart patients who also have non-Hodgkin's lymphoma usually uses CVP (**c**yclophosphamide, **v**incristine, and **p**rednisone), that is, CHOP without the drug Adriamycin® included. If a family member had heart disease along with non-Hodgkin's lymphoma, what would you do if he asked you about his treatment options?

Cancer and the Lymph Nodes

Cancer cells from a primary tumor may metastasize and enter the lymphatic vessels, eventually reaching the lymph nodes, where they may be trapped and reproduce. The cells may then be transported through the lymphatic and circulatory systems to other sites in the body. To combat cancer metastasis, surgical removal of lymph nodes may be indicated. For example, if a mastectomy is performed for advanced breast cancer, the axillary lymph nodes are usually removed as well, in order to stop the spread of cancer cells.

WHAT WOULD YOU DO?

You are a pharmacy technician who has been diagnosed with metastatic cancer. With your training, you understand how metastasis may be treated. Along with your medical treatments, what would you do to improve your chances of survival?

AUTOIMMUNE DISORDERS

The human immune system has natural immunity against foreign antigens, from birth. Each fetus receives this immunity from the mother. Throughout life and with exposure to certain antigens, additional immunity must be acquired. Vaccines have made it possible, working with certain infectious sources, to eradicate many diseases from the United States. Sometimes, however, the immune system does not or is unable to fight antigens. It instead becomes hyper-reactive, targeting the "self" antigens. An autoimmune disorder is any disease or condition in which the immune system cannot identify normal, healthy antigens. It then attacks the cells, tissues, and organs of the body. There are about 80 different autoimmune disorders caused by genetics, environmental factors, hormones, and infections. The American Autoimmune Related Diseases Association estimates that about 50 million Americans have autoimmune disorders, with 75% of these being females.

The symptoms of autoimmune disorders vary, but most involve fatigue, weakness, and pain. They occur because there is immune system activation. Autoimmune disorders are also chronic disease states. Patients with these disorders require nonpharmacologic and pharmacologic treatment throughout life. Remission is difficult to obtain. Treatments are aimed at slowing the immune system's attack upon healthy tissues and organs. Medications include immunosuppressants, which slow down the immune system and its responses. However, these agents may cause re-infection with diseases such as hepatitis B (Chapter 27) or tuberculosis (Chapter 25). Live vaccines that are administered to prevent a disease can actually cause an infection. Immunosuppressants can also cause skin and other cancers. They must be monitored regularly, using blood counts and liver tests. Autoimmune disorders include type 1 diabetes mellitus (Chapter 22), rheumatoid arthritis (Chapter 21), Hashimoto's thyroiditis (Chapter 22), and multiple sclerosis (Chapter 20).

HYPERSENSITIVITY

Allergy (hypersensitivity) may be defined as "an *inappropriate immunological reaction*" to an environmental immunogen called the **allergen**. Hypersensitivity is not manifested on first contact with the antigen, but it usually appears on subsequent contact. There are four types of hypersensitivity reactions (types I, II, III, and IV), but in practice these types do not necessarily occur in isolation from each other. The first three are antibody-mediated; mainly T cells and macrophages mediate the fourth.

Type I (immediate) hypersensitivity occurs when an IgE antibody response is directed against innocuous environmental antigens such as pollen, house-dust mites, or animal dander. The resulting release of pharmacological mediators by IgE-sensitized mast cells produces an acute inflammatory reaction with symptoms such as asthma or rhinitis (hay fever).

Type II, or antibody-dependent cytotoxic hypersensitivity, occurs when an antibody, usually IgG, binds to either a self-antigen or a foreign antigen on cells, which leads to phagocytosis, killer cell activity, or complement-mediated lysis (such as anaphylactic shock caused by allergy to penicillin).

Type III hypersensitivity develops when immune complexes are formed in large quantities or cannot be cleared adequately from the body, leading to serum sickness–type reactions.

Type IV, or delayed type hypersensitivity (DTH), is most seriously manifested when antigens (e.g., those on tubercle bacilli) are trapped in a macrophage and cannot be cleared. Other aspects of DTH reactions are seen in graft rejection and allergic contact dermatitis.

Vaccination

A **vaccination** is the act of giving an injection or other form of antibody to protect an individual from an infectious disease. Vaccines are classified as live attenuated or inactivated. **Live attenuated vaccines** are produced from viruses or bacteria in a laboratory. Live attenuated vaccines available in the United States include live viruses and live bacteria. Examples are polio (Sabin and oral), measles/mumps/rubella (MMR), yellow fever, varicella-zoster (human herpes virus 3), typhoid (oral), and BCG (for tuberculosis). **Inactivated vaccines** can be composed of whole viruses, bacteria, or fractions of either, which have been rendered noninfectious. The more similar a vaccine is to the natural disease, the better the response to the vaccine will be. Examples are vaccines for polio (Salk), rabies, influenza, hepatitis A, typhus, pertussis, typhoid (injectable), cholera, and plague. Live attenuated vaccines are usually effective with one dose. They may cause severe reactions and may interfere with circulating antibodies. Recommended vaccinations and immunization schedules for both adults and children are presented in Figures 24-6A, 24-6B, and 24-6C.

POINTS TO REMEMBER

In some states, pharmacists are allowed to administer selected immunizations, such as flu vaccines, in retail (community) pharmacies.

POINTS TO REMEMBER

Severely immunocompromised individuals can safely be administered inactivated vaccines but should generally not receive live vaccines because they have the potential to cause serious disease in these individuals.

POINTS TO REMEMBER

Mild toxic or allergic reactions are more common with inactivated vaccines than with live vaccines since the inactivated products usually contain more antigen and require booster doses.

ADVERSE REACTIONS

The vaccines that are routinely used today are generally very safe and highly effective. As with any drugs, there are some risks caused by vaccinations that range from common, minor, and inconvenient to rare, serious, and life threatening. An adverse reaction is an undesirable effect caused by a vaccine that is extraneous to the vaccine's primary purpose of production of immunity. Adverse reactions to vaccines fall into three general categories: local, systemic, and allergic. Local reactions are generally the least severe and most frequent. Allergic reactions are the most severe and least frequent. Recently, there have been concerns among the public that **autism** in children may be linked to certain vaccinations. Studies have proven that vaccines received during the first two years of life have no

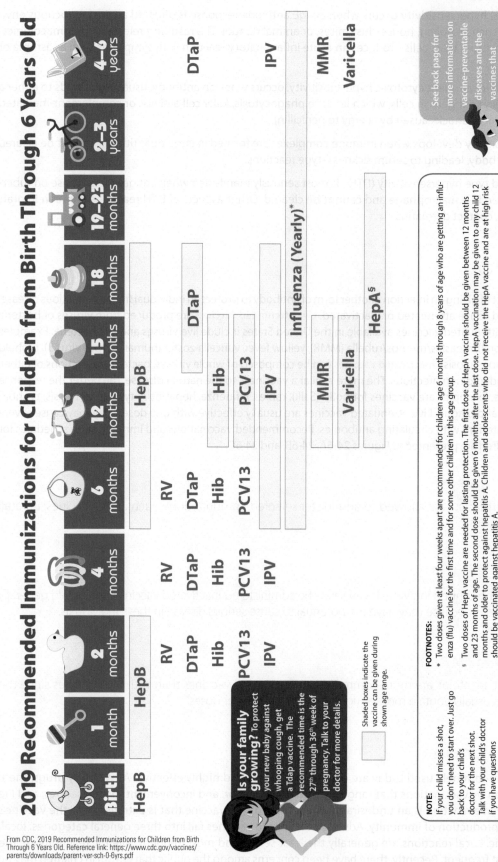

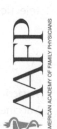
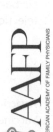

Figure 24-6A Childhood immunization schedules, ages 0 to 6 years.

Vaccine-Preventable Diseases and the Vaccines that Prevent Them

Disease	Vaccine	Disease spread by	Disease symptoms	Disease complications
Chickenpox	Varicella vaccine protects against chickenpox.	Air, direct contact	Rash, tiredness, headache, fever	Infected blisters, bleeding disorders, encephalitis (brain swelling), pneumonia (infection in the lungs)
Diphtheria	DTaP* vaccine protects against diphtheria.	Air, direct contact	Sore throat, mild fever, weakness, swollen glands in neck	Swelling of the heart muscle, heart failure, coma, paralysis, death
Hib	Hib vaccine protects against *Haemophilus influenzae* type b.	Air, direct contact	May be no symptoms unless bacteria enter the blood	Meningitis (infection of the covering around the brain and spinal cord), intellectual disability, epiglottitis (life-threatening infection that can block the windpipe and lead to serious breathing problems), pneumonia (infection in the lungs), death
Hepatitis A	HepA vaccine protects against hepatitis A.	Direct contact, contaminated food or water	May be no symptoms, fever, stomach pain, loss of appetite, fatigue, vomiting, jaundice (yellowing of skin and eyes), dark urine	Liver failure, arthralgia (joint pain), kidney, pancreatic and blood disorders
Hepatitis B	HepB vaccine protects against hepatitis B.	Contact with blood or body fluids	May be no symptoms, fever, headache, weakness, vomiting, jaundice (yellowing of skin and eyes), joint pain	Chronic liver infection, liver failure, liver cancer
Influenza (Flu)	Flu vaccine protects against influenza.	Air, direct contact	Fever, muscle pain, sore throat, cough, extreme fatigue	Pneumonia (infection in the lungs)
Measles	MMR** vaccine protects against measles.	Air, direct contact	Rash, fever, cough, runny nose, pink eye	Encephalitis (brain swelling), pneumonia (infection in the lungs), death
Mumps	MMR**vaccine protects against mumps.	Air, direct contact	Swollen salivary glands (under the jaw), fever, headache, tiredness, muscle pain	Meningitis (infection of the covering around the brain and spinal cord), encephalitis (brain swelling), inflammation of testicles or ovaries, deafness
Pertussis	DTaP* vaccine protects against pertussis (whooping cough).	Air, direct contact	Severe cough, runny nose, apnea (a pause in breathing in infants)	Pneumonia (infection in the lungs), death
Polio	IPV vaccine protects against polio.	Air, direct contact, through the mouth	May be no symptoms, sore throat, fever, nausea, headache	Paralysis, death
Pneumococcal	PCV13 vaccine protects against pneumococcus.	Air, direct contact	May be no symptoms, pneumonia (infection in the lungs)	Bacteremia (blood infection), meningitis (infection of the covering around the brain and spinal cord), death
Rotavirus	RV vaccine protects against rotavirus.	Through the mouth	Diarrhea, fever, vomiting	Severe diarrhea, dehydration
Rubella	MMR** vaccine protects against rubella.	Air, direct contact	Sometimes rash, fever, swollen lymph nodes	Very serious in pregnant women—can lead to miscarriage, stillbirth, premature delivery, birth defects
Tetanus	DTaP* vaccine protects against tetanus.	Exposure through cuts in skin	Stiffness in neck and abdominal muscles, difficulty swallowing, muscle spasms, fever	Broken bones, breathing difficulty, death

Last updated January 2019 • CS300526-A

* DTaP combines protection against diphtheria, tetanus, and pertussis.
** MMR combines protection against measles, mumps, and rubella.

Figure 24-6A Childhood immunization schedules, ages 0 to 6 years.

(*Continued*)

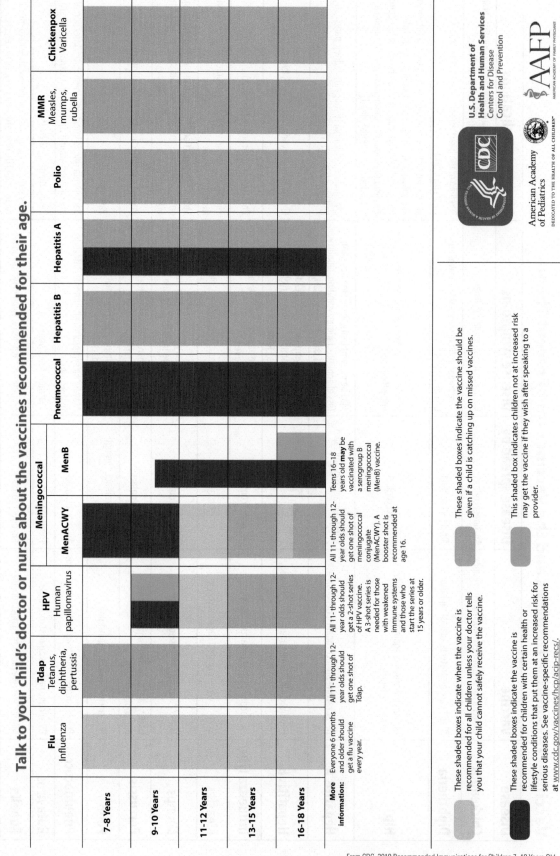

Figure 24-6B Childhood immunization schedules, ages 7 to 18 years.

Vaccine-Preventable Diseases and the Vaccines that Prevent Them

Diphtheria (Can be prevented by Tdap vaccination)

Diphtheria is a very contagious bacterial disease that affects the respiratory system, including the lungs. Diphtheria bacteria can be spread from person to person by direct contact with droplets from an infected person's cough or sneeze. When people are infected, the bacteria can produce a toxin (poison) in the body that can cause a thick coating in the back of the nose or throat that makes it hard to breathe or swallow. Effects from this toxin can also lead to swelling of the heart muscle and, in some cases, heart failure. In serious cases, the illness can cause coma, paralysis, or even death.

Hepatitis A ((Can be prevented by HepA vaccination)

Hepatitis A is an infection in the liver caused by hepatitis A virus. The virus is spread primarily from person to person through the fecal-oral route. In other words, the virus is taken in by mouth from contact with objects, food, or drinks contaminated by the feces (stool) of an infected person. Symptoms can include fever, tiredness, poor appetite, vomiting, stomach pain, and sometimes jaundice (when skin and eyes turn yellow). An infected person may have no symptoms, may have mild illness for a week or two, may have severe illness for several months, or may rarely develop liver failure and die from the infection. In the U.S., about 100 people a year die from hepatitis A.

Hepatitis B ((Can be prevented by HepB vaccination)

Hepatitis B causes a flu-like illness with loss of appetite, nausea, vomiting, rashes, joint pain, and jaundice. Symptoms of acute hepatitis B include fever, fatigue, loss of appetite, nausea, vomiting, pain in joints and stomach, dark urine, grey-colored stools, and jaundice (when skin and eyes turn yellow).

Human Papillomavirus (Can be prevented by HPV vaccination)

Human papillomavirus is a common virus. HPV is most common in people in their teens and early 20s. About 14 million people, including teens, become infected with HPV each year. HPV infection can cause cervical, vaginal, and vulvar cancers in women and penile cancer in men. HPV can also cause anal cancer, oropharyngeal cancer (back of the throat), and genital warts in both men and women.

Influenza (Can be prevented by annual flu vaccination)

Influenza is a highly contagious viral infection of the nose, throat, and lungs. The virus spreads easily through droplets when an infected person coughs or sneezes and can cause mild to severe illness. Typical symptoms include a sudden high fever, chills, a dry cough, headache, runny nose, sore throat, and muscle and joint pain. Extreme fatigue can last from several days to weeks. Influenza may lead to hospitalization or even death, even among previously healthy children.

Measles (Can be prevented by MMR vaccination)

Measles is one of the most contagious viral diseases. Measles virus is spread by direct contact with the airborne respiratory droplets of an infected person. Measles is so contagious that just being in the same room after a person who has measles has already left can result in infection. Symptoms usually include a rash, fever, cough, and red, watery eyes. Fever can persist, rash can last for up to a week, and coughing can last about 10 days. Measles can also cause pneumonia, seizures, brain damage, or death.

Meningococcal Disease (Can be prevented by meningococcal vaccination)

Meningococcal disease has two common outcomes: meningitis (infection of the lining of the brain and spinal cord) and bloodstream infections. The bacteria that cause meningococcal disease spread through the exchange of nose and throat droplets, such as when coughing, sneezing, or kissing. Symptoms include sudden onset of fever, headache, and stiff neck. With bloodstream infection, symptoms also include a dark purple rash. About one of every 10 people who gets the disease dies from it. Survivors of meningococcal disease may lose their arms or legs, become deaf, have problems with their nervous systems, become developmentally disabled, or suffer seizures or strokes.

Mumps (Can be prevented by MMR vaccination)

Mumps is an infectious disease caused by the mumps virus, which is spread in the air by a cough or sneeze from an infected person. A child can also get infected with mumps by coming in contact with a contaminated object like a toy. The mumps virus causes swollen salivary glands under the ears or jaw, fever, muscle aches, tiredness, abdominal pain, and loss of appetite. Severe complications for children who get mumps are uncommon, but can include meningitis (infection of the lining of the brain and spinal cord), encephalitis (inflammation of the brain), permanent hearing loss, or swelling of the testes, which rarely results in decreased fertility.

Pertussis (Whooping Cough) (Can be prevented by Tdap vaccination)

Pertussis spreads very easily through coughing and sneezing. It can cause a bad cough that makes someone gasp for air after coughing fits. This cough can last for many weeks, which can make preteens and teens miss school and other activities. Pertussis can be deadly for babies who are too young to receive the vaccine. Often babies get whooping cough from their older brothers or sisters, like preteens or teens, or other people in the family. Babies with pertussis can get pneumonia, have seizures, become brain damaged, or even die. About half of children under 1 year of age who get pertussis must be hospitalized.

Pneumococcal Disease (Can be prevented by pneumococcal vaccination)

Pneumonia is an infection of the lungs that can be caused by the bacteria called "pneumococcus." These bacteria can cause other types of infections, too, such as ear infections, sinus infections, meningitis (infection of the lining of the brain and spinal cord), and bloodstream infections. Sinus and ear infections are usually mild and are much more common than the more serious forms of pneumococcal disease. However, in some cases, pneumococcal disease can be fatal or result in long-term problems like brain damage and hearing loss. The bacteria that cause pneumococcal disease spread when people cough or sneeze. Many people have the bacteria in their nose or throat at one time or another without being ill—this is known as being a carrier.

Polio (Can be prevented by IPV vaccination)

Polio is caused by a virus that lives in an infected person's throat and intestines. It spreads through contact with the stool of an infected person and through droplets from a sneeze or cough. Symptoms typically include sore throat, fever, tiredness, nausea, headache, or stomach pain. In about 1% of cases, polio can cause paralysis. Among those who are paralyzed, about 2 to 10 children out of 100 die because the virus affects the muscles that help them breathe.

Rubella (German Measles) (Can be prevented by MMR vaccination)

Rubella is caused by a virus that is spread through coughing and sneezing. In children, rubella usually causes a mild illness with fever, swollen glands, and a rash that lasts about 3 days. Rubella rarely causes serious illness or complications in children, but can be very serious to a baby in the womb. If a pregnant woman is infected, the result for the baby can be devastating, including miscarriage, serious heart defects, mental retardation, and loss of hearing and eyesight.

Tetanus (Lockjaw) (Can be prevented by Tdap vaccination)

Tetanus mainly affects the neck and belly. When people are infected, the bacteria produce a toxin (poison) that causes muscles to become tight, which is very painful. This can lead to "locking" of the jaw so a person cannot open his or her mouth, swallow, or breathe. The bacteria that cause tetanus are found in soil, dust, and manure. The bacteria enter the body through a puncture, cut, or sore on the skin. Complete recovery from tetanus can take months. One to two out of 10 people who get tetanus die from the disease.

Varicella (Chickenpox) (Can be prevented by varicella vaccination)

Chickenpox is caused by the varicella zoster virus. Chickenpox is very contagious and spreads very easily from infected people. The virus can spread from either a cough or sneeze. It can also spread from the blisters on the skin, either by touching them or by breathing in these viral particles. Typical symptoms of chickenpox include an itchy rash with blisters, tiredness, headache, and fever. Chickenpox is usually mild, but it can lead to severe skin infections, pneumonia, encephalitis (brain swelling), or even death.

Last updated on January 24, 2019 – CS300526-B

If you have any questions about your child's vaccines, talk to your child's doctor or nurse.

Figure 24-6B Childhood immunization schedules, ages 7 to 18 years.   *(Continued)*

Recommended Adult Immunization Schedule
for ages 19 years or older

UNITED STATES 2019

How to use the adult immunization schedule

1 Determine recommended vaccinations by age **(Table 1)**

2 Assess need for additional recommended vaccinations by medical condition and other indications **(Table 2)**

3 Review vaccine types, frequencies, and intervals, and considerations for special situations **(Notes)**

Recommended by the Advisory Committee on Immunization Practices (www.cdc.gov/vaccines/acip) and approved by the Centers for Disease Control and Prevention (www.cdc.gov), American College of Physicians (www.acponline.org), American Academy of Family Physicians (www.aafp.org), American College of Obstetricians and Gynecologists (www.acog.org), and American College of Nurse-Midwives (www.midwife.org).

Report

- Suspected cases of reportable vaccine-preventable diseases or outbreaks to the local or state health department
- Clinically significant postvaccination reactions to the Vaccine Adverse Event Reporting System at www.vaers.hhs.gov or 800-822-7967

Injury claims

All vaccines included in the adult immunization schedule except pneumococcal 23-valent polysaccharide and zoster vaccines are covered by the Vaccine Injury Compensation Program. Information on how to file a vaccine injury claim is available at www.hrsa.gov/vaccinecompensation or 800-338-2382.

Questions or comments

Contact www.cdc.gov/cdc-info or 800-CDC-INFO (800-232-4636), in English or Spanish, 8 a.m.–8 p.m. ET, Monday through Friday, excluding holidays.

Download the CDC Vaccine Schedules App for providers at www.cdc.gov/vaccines/schedules/hcp/schedule-app.html.

Helpful information

- Complete ACIP recommendations: www.cdc.gov/vaccines/hcp/acip-recs/index.html
- General Best Practice Guidelines for Immunization (including contraindications and precautions): www.cdc.gov/vaccines/hcp/acip-recs/general-recs/index.html
- Vaccine Information Statements: www.cdc.gov/vaccines/hcp/vis/index.html
- Manual for the Surveillance of Vaccine-Preventable Diseases (including case identification and outbreak response): www.cdc.gov/vaccines/pubs/surv-manual
- Travel vaccine recommendations: www.cdc.gov/travel
- Recommended Child and Adolescent Immunization Schedule, United States, 2019: www.cdc.gov/vaccines/schedules/hcp/child-adolescent.html

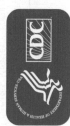

U.S. Department of Health and Human Services
Centers for Disease Control and Prevention

Vaccines in the Adult Immunization Schedule*

Vaccines	Abbreviations	Trade names
Haemophilus influenzae type b vaccine	Hib	ActHIB Hiberix
Hepatitis A vaccine	HepA	Havrix Vaqta
Hepatitis A and hepatitis B vaccine	HepA-HepB	Twinrix
Hepatitis B vaccine	HepB	Engerix-B Recombivax HB Heplisav-B
Human papillomavirus vaccine	HPV vaccine	Gardasil 9
Influenza vaccine, inactivated	IIV	Many brands
Influenza vaccine, live attenuated	LAIV	FluMist Quadrivalent
Influenza vaccine, recombinant	RIV	Flublok Quadrivalent
Measles, mumps, and rubella vaccine	MMR	M-M-R II
Meningococcal serogroups A, C, W, Y vaccine	MenACWY	Menactra Menveo
Meningococcal serogroup B vaccine	MenB-4C MenB-FHbp	Bexsero Trumenba
Pneumococcal 13-valent conjugate vaccine	PCV13	Prevnar 13
Pneumococcal 23-valent polysaccharide vaccine	PPSV23	Pneumovax
Tetanus and diphtheria toxoids	Td	Tenivac Td vaccine
Tetanus and diphtheria toxoids and acellular pertussis vaccine	Tdap	Adacel Boostrix
Varicella vaccine	VAR	Varivax
Zoster vaccine, recombinant	RZV	Shingrix
Zoster vaccine live	ZVL	Zostavax

*Administer recommended vaccines if vaccination history is incomplete or unknown. Do not restart or add doses to vaccine series for extended intervals between doses. The use of trade names is for identification purposes only and does not imply endorsement by the ACIP or CDC.

From CDC, Recommended Adult Immunization Schedule for ages 19 years or older Reference link: https://www.cdc.gov/vaccines/schedules/downloads/adult/adult-combined-schedule.pdf

Figure 24-6C Recommended adult immunization schedule.

Table 1 Recommended Adult Immunization Schedule by Age Group United States, 2019

Vaccine	19–21 years	22–26 years	27–49 years	50–64 years	≥65 years
Influenza inactivated (IIV) or Influenza recombinant (RIV) **or**	1 dose annually				
Influenza live attenuated (LAIV)	1 dose annually				
Tetanus, diphtheria, pertussis (Tdap or Td)	1 dose Tdap, then Td booster every 10 yrs				
Measles, mumps, rubella (MMR)	1 or 2 doses depending on indication (if born in 1957 or later)				
Varicella (VAR)	2 doses (if born in 1980 or later)				
Zoster recombinant (RZV) (preferred) **or**				2 doses	2 doses
Zoster live (ZVL)					1 dose
Human papillomavirus (HPV) Female	2 or 3 doses depending on age at initial vaccination				
Human papillomavirus (HPV) Male	2 or 3 doses depending on age at initial vaccination				
Pneumococcal conjugate (PCV13)				1 dose	
Pneumococcal polysaccharide (PPSV23)	1 or 2 doses depending on indication				1 dose
Hepatitis A (HepA)	2 or 3 doses depending on vaccine				
Hepatitis B (HepB)	2 or 3 doses depending on vaccine				
Meningococcal A, C, W, Y (MenACWY)	1 or 2 doses depending on indication, then booster every 5 yrs if risk remains				
Meningococcal B (MenB)	2 or 3 doses depending on vaccine and indication				
Haemophilus influenzae type b (Hib)	1 or 3 doses depending on indication				

Recommended vaccination for adults who meet age requirement, lack documentation of vaccination, or lack evidence of past infection

Recommended vaccination for adults with an additional risk factor or another indication

No recommendation

Figure 24-6C Recommended adult immunization schedule.

(Continued)

Table 2 Recommended Adult Immunization Schedule by Medical Condition and Other Indications United States, 2019

Vaccine	Pregnancy	Immuno-compromised (excluding HIV infection)	HIV infection CD4 count <200	HIV infection CD4 count ≥200	Asplenia, complement deficiencies	End-stage renal disease, on hemodialysis	Heart or lung disease, alcoholism[1]	Chronic liver disease	Diabetes	Health care personnel[2]	Men who have sex with men
IIV or RIV							1 dose annually				
LAIV		CONTRAINDICATED					PRECAUTION				1 dose annually
Tdap or Td	1 dose Tdap each pregnancy					1 dose Tdap, then Td booster every 10 yrs					
MMR	CONTRAINDICATED	CONTRAINDICATED					1 or 2 doses depending on indication				
VAR	CONTRAINDICATED	CONTRAINDICATED					2 doses				
RZV (preferred)	DELAY						2 doses at age ≥50 yrs				
ZVL	CONTRAINDICATED	CONTRAINDICATED					1 dose at age ≥60 yrs				
HPV Female	DELAY	3 doses through age 26 yrs					2 or 3 doses through age 26 yrs				
HPV Male		3 doses through age 26 yrs					2 or 3 doses through age 21 yrs			2 or 3 doses through age 26 yrs
PCV13							1 dose				
PPSV23							1, 2, or 3 doses depending on age and indication				
HepA							2 or 3 doses depending on vaccine				
HepB							2 or 3 doses depending on vaccine				
MenACWY		1 or 2 doses depending on indication, then booster every 5 yrs if risk remains									
MenB	PRECAUTION	2 or 3 doses depending on vaccine and indication									
Hib		3 doses HSCT[3] recipients only					1 dose				

Legend:
- Recommended vaccination for adults who meet age requirement, lack documentation of vaccination, or lack evidence of past infection
- Recommended vaccination for adults with an additional risk factor or another indication
- Precaution—vaccine might be indicated if benefit of protection outweighs risk of adverse reaction
- Delay vaccination until after pregnancy if vaccine is indicated
- Contraindicated—vaccine should not be administered because of risk for serious adverse reaction
- No recommendation

1. Precaution for LAIV does not apply to alcoholism. 2. See notes for influenza; hepatitis B; measles, mumps, and rubella; and varicella vaccinations. 3. Hematopoietic stem cell transplant.

Figure 24-6C Recommended adult immunization schedule.

(Continued)

Notes Recommended Adult Immunization Schedule
United States, 2019

Haemophilus influenzae type b vaccination

Special situations

○ **Anatomical or functional asplenia (including sickle cell disease):** 1 dose Hib if previously did not receive Hib; if elective splenectomy, 1 dose Hib, preferably at least 14 days before splenectomy

○ **Hematopoietic stem cell transplant (HSCT):** 3-dose series Hib 4 weeks apart starting 6–12 months after successful transplant, regardless of Hib vaccination history

Hepatitis A vaccination

Routine vaccination

○ **Not at risk but want protection from hepatitis A** (identification of risk factor not required): 2-dose series HepA (Havrix 6–12 months apart or Vaqta 6–18 months apart [minimum interval: 6 months]) or 3-dose series HepA-HepB (Twinrix at 0, 1, 6 months [minimum intervals: 4 weeks between doses 1 and 2, 5 months between doses 2 and 3])

Special situations

○ **At risk for hepatitis A virus infection:** 2-dose series HepA or 3-dose series HepA-HepB as above
- **Chronic liver disease**
- **Clotting factor disorders**
- **Men who have sex with men**
- **Injection or non-injection drug use**
- **Homelessness**
- **Work with hepatitis A virus** in research laboratory or nonhuman primates with hepatitis A virus infection
- **Travel in countries with high or intermediate endemic hepatitis A**
- **Close personal contact with international adoptee** (e.g., household, regular babysitting) in first 60 days after arrival from country with high or intermediate endemic hepatitis A (administer dose 1 as soon as adoption is planned, at least 2 weeks before adoptee's arrival)

Hepatitis B vaccination

Routine vaccination

○ **Not at risk but want protection from hepatitis B** (identification of risk factor not required): 2- or 3-dose series HepB (2-dose series Heplisav-B at least 4 weeks apart [2-dose series HepB only applies when 2 doses of Heplisav-B are used at least 4 weeks apart] or 3-dose series Engerix-B or Recombivax HB at 0, 1, 6 months [minimum intervals: 4 weeks between doses 1 and 2, 8 weeks between doses 2 and 3, 16 weeks between doses 1 and 3]) or 3-dose series HepA-HepB (Twinrix at 0, 1, 6 months [minimum intervals: 4 weeks between doses 1 and 2, 5 months between doses 2 and 3])

Special situations

○ **At risk for hepatitis B virus infection:** 2-dose (Heplisav-B) or 3-dose (Engerix-B, Recombivax HB) series HepB, or 3-dose series HepA-HepB as above
- **Hepatitis C virus infection**
- **Chronic liver disease** (e.g., cirrhosis, fatty liver disease, alcoholic liver disease, autoimmune hepatitis, alanine aminotransferase [ALT] or aspartate aminotransferase [AST] level greater than twice upper limit of normal)
- **HIV infection**
- **Sexual exposure risk** (e.g., sex partners of hepatitis B surface antigen (HBsAg)-positive persons; sexually active persons not in mutually monogamous relationships, persons seeking evaluation or treatment for a sexually transmitted infection, men who have sex with men)
- **Current or recent injection drug use**
- **Percutaneous or mucosal risk for exposure to blood** (e.g., household contacts of HBsAg-positive persons; residents and staff of facilities for developmentally disabled persons; health care and public safety personnel with reasonably anticipated risk for exposure to blood or blood-contaminated body fluids; hemodialysis, peritoneal dialysis, home dialysis, and predialysis patients; persons with diabetes mellitus age younger than 60 years and, at discretion of treating clinician, those age 60 years or older)
- **Incarcerated persons**
- **Travel in countries with high or intermediate endemic hepatitis B**

Human papillomavirus vaccination

Routine vaccination

○ **Females through age 26 years and males through age 21 years:** 2- or 3-dose series HPV vaccine depending on age at initial vaccination; males age 22 through 26 years may be vaccinated based on individual clinical decision (HPV vaccination routinely recommended at age 11–12 years)

○ **Age 15 years or older at initial vaccination:** 3-dose series HPV vaccine at 0, 1–2, 6 months (minimum intervals: 4 weeks between doses 1 and 2, 12 weeks between doses 2 and 3, 5 months between doses 1 and 3; repeat dose if administered too soon)

○ **Age 9 through 14 years at initial vaccination and received 1 dose, or 2 doses less than 5 months apart:** 1 dose HPV vaccine

○ **Age 9 through 14 years at initial vaccination and received 2 doses at least 5 months apart:** HPV vaccination complete, no additional dose needed

○ If completed valid vaccination series with any HPV vaccine, no additional doses needed

Special situations

● **Immunocompromising conditions (including HIV infection) through age 26 years:** 3-dose series HPV vaccine at 0, 1–2, 6 months as above

● **Men who have sex with men and transgender persons through age 26 years:** 2- or 3-dose series HPV vaccine depending on age at initial vaccination as above

● **Pregnancy through age 26 years:** HPV vaccination not recommended until after pregnancy; no intervention needed if vaccinated while pregnant; pregnancy testing not needed before vaccination

Figure 24-6C Recommended adult immunization schedule.

(Continued)

Notes | Recommended Adult Immunization Schedule United States, 2019

Influenza vaccination

Routine vaccination

- **Persons age 6 months or older:** 1 dose IIV, RIV, or LAIV appropriate for age and health status annually
- For additional guidance, see www.cdc.gov/flu/professionals/index.htm

Special situations

- **Egg allergy, hives only:** 1 dose IIV, RIV, or LAIV appropriate for age and health status annually
- **Egg allergy more severe than hives** (e.g., angioedema, respiratory distress): 1 dose IIV, RIV, or LAIV appropriate for age and health status annually in medical setting under supervision of health care provider who can recognize and manage severe allergic conditions
- **Immunocompromising conditions (including HIV infection), anatomical or functional asplenia, pregnant women, close contacts and caregivers of severely immunocompromised persons in protected environment, use of influenza antiviral medications in previous 48 hours, with cerebrospinal fluid leak or cochlear implant:** 1 dose IIV or RIV annually (LAIV not recommended)
- **History of Guillain-Barré syndrome within 6 weeks of previous dose of influenza vaccine:** Generally should not be vaccinated

Measles, mumps, and rubella vaccination

Routine vaccination

- **No evidence of immunity to measles, mumps, or rubella:** 1 dose MMR
  - Evidence of immunity: Born before 1957 (except health care personnel [see below]), documentation of receipt of MMR, laboratory evidence of immunity or disease (diagnosis of disease without laboratory confirmation is not evidence of immunity)

Special situations

- **Pregnancy with no evidence of immunity to rubella:** MMR contraindicated during pregnancy; after pregnancy (before discharge from health care facility), 1 dose MMR
- **Non-pregnant women of childbearing age with no evidence of immunity to rubella:** 1 dose MMR
- HIV infection with CD4 count ≥200 cells/µL for at least 6 months and no evidence of immunity to measles, mumps, or rubella: 2-dose series MMR at least 4 weeks apart; MMR contraindicated in HIV infection with CD4 count <200 cells/µL
- **Severe immunocompromising conditions:** MMR contraindicated
- **Students in postsecondary educational institutions, international travelers, and household or close personal contacts of immunocompromised persons with no evidence of immunity to measles, mumps, or rubella:** 1 dose MMR if previously received 1 dose MMR, or 2-dose series MMR at least 4 weeks apart if previously did not receive any MMR
- **Health care personnel born in 1957 or later with no evidence of immunity to measles, mumps, or rubella:** 2-dose series MMR at least 4 weeks apart for measles or mumps, or at least 1 dose MMR for rubella; if born before 1957, consider 2-dose series MMR at least 4 weeks apart for measles or mumps, or 1 dose MMR for rubella

Meningococcal vaccination

Special situations for MenACWY

- **Anatomical or functional asplenia (including sickle cell disease), HIV infection, persistent complement component deficiency, eculizumab use:** 2-dose series MenACWY (Menactra, Menveo) at least 8 weeks apart and revaccinate every 5 years if risk remains
- **Travel in countries with hyperendemic or epidemic meningococcal disease, microbiologists routinely exposed to *Neisseria meningitidis*:** 1 dose MenACWY and revaccinate every 5 years if risk remains
- **First-year college students who live in residential housing (if not previously vaccinated at age 16 years or older) and military recruits:** 1 dose MenACWY

Special situations for MenB

- **Anatomical or functional asplenia (including sickle cell disease), persistent complement component deficiency, eculizumab use, microbiologists routinely exposed to *Neisseria meningitidis*:** 2-dose series MenB-4C (Bexsero) at least 1 month apart, or 3-dose series MenB-FHbp (Trumenba) at 0, 1–2, 6 months (if dose 2 was administered at least 6 months after dose 1, dose 3 not needed); MenB-4C and MenB-FHbp are not interchangeable (use same product for all doses in series)
- **Pregnancy:** Delay MenB until after pregnancy unless at increased risk and vaccination benefit outweighs potential risks
- **Healthy adolescents and young adults age 16 through 23 years (age 16 through 18 years preferred) not at increased risk for meningococcal disease:** Based on individual clinical decision, may receive 2-dose series MenB-4C at least 1 month apart, or 2-dose series MenB-FHbp at 0, 6 months (if dose 2 was administered less than 6 months after dose 1, administer dose 3 at least 4 months after dose 2); MenB-4C and MenB-FHbp are not interchangeable (use same product for all doses in series)

Figure 24-6C Recommended adult immunization schedule.

(Continued)

Notes — Recommended Adult Immunization Schedule
United States, 2019

Pneumococcal vaccination

Routine vaccination

- **Age 65 years or older** (immunocompetent): 1 dose PCV13 if previously did not receive PCV13, followed by 1 dose PPSV23 at least 1 year after PCV13 and at least 5 years after last dose PPSV23
  - Previously received PPSV23 but not PCV13 at age 65 years or older: 1 dose PCV13 at least 1 year after PPSV23
  - When both PCV13 and PPSV23 are indicated, administer PCV13 first (PCV13 and PPSV23 should not be administered during same visit)

Special situations

- **Age 19 through 64 years with chronic medical conditions** (chronic heart [excluding hypertension], lung, or liver disease; diabetes), alcoholism, or cigarette smoking: 1 dose PPSV23
- **Age 19 years or older with immunocompromising conditions** (congenital or acquired immunodeficiency [including B- and T-lymphocyte deficiency, complement deficiencies, phagocytic disorders, HIV infection], chronic renal failure, nephrotic syndrome, leukemia, lymphoma, Hodgkin disease, generalized malignancy, iatrogenic immunosuppression [e.g., drug or radiation therapy], solid organ transplant, multiple myeloma) or anatomical or functional asplenia (including sickle cell disease and other hemoglobinopathies): 1 dose PCV13 followed by 1 dose PPSV23 at least 8 weeks later, then another dose PPSV23 at least 5 years after previous PPSV23; at age 65 years or older, administer 1 dose PPSV23 at least 5 years after most recent PPSV23 (note: only 1 dose PPSV23 recommended at age 65 years or older)
- **Age 19 years or older with cerebrospinal fluid leak or cochlear implant**: 1 dose PCV13 followed by 1 dose PPSV23 at least 8 weeks later; at age 65 years or older, administer another dose PPSV23 at least 5 years after PPSV23 (note: only 1 dose PPSV23 recommended at age 65 years or older)

Tetanus, diphtheria, and pertussis vaccination

Routine vaccination

- **Previously did not receive Tdap at or after age 11 years**: 1 dose Tdap, then Td booster every 10 years

Special situations

- **Previously did not receive primary vaccination series for tetanus, diphtheria, and pertussis**: 1 dose Tdap followed by 1 dose Td at least 4 weeks after Tdap, and another dose Td 6–12 months after last Td (Tdap can be substituted for any Td dose, but preferred as first dose); Td booster every 10 years thereafter
- **Pregnancy**: 1 dose Tdap during each pregnancy, preferably in early part of gestational weeks 27–36
- For information on use of Tdap or Td as tetanus prophylaxis in wound management, see www.cdc.gov/mmwr/volumes/67/rr/rr6702a1.htm

Varicella vaccination

Routine vaccination

- **No evidence of immunity to varicella**: 2-dose series VAR 4–8 weeks apart if previously did not receive varicella-containing vaccine (VAR or MMRV [measles-mumps-rubella-varicella vaccine] for children); if previously received 1 dose varicella-containing vaccine: 1 dose VAR at least 4 weeks after first dose
  - Evidence of immunity: U.S.-born before 1980 (except for pregnant women and health care personnel [see below]), documentation of 2 doses varicella-containing vaccine at least 4 weeks apart, diagnosis or verification of history of varicella or herpes zoster by a health care provider, laboratory evidence of immunity or disease

Special situations

- **Pregnancy with no evidence of immunity to varicella**: VAR contraindicated during pregnancy; after pregnancy (before discharge from health care facility), 1 dose VAR if previously received 1 dose varicella-containing vaccine, or dose 1 of 2-dose series VAR (dose 2: 4–8 weeks later) if previously did not receive any varicella-containing vaccine, regardless of whether U.S.-born before 1980

- **Health care personnel with no evidence of immunity to varicella**: 1 dose VAR if previously received 1 dose varicella-containing vaccine, or 2-dose series VAR 4–8 weeks apart if previously did not receive any varicella-containing vaccine, regardless of whether U.S.-born before 1980
- **HIV infection with CD4 count ≥200 cells/µL with no evidence of immunity**: Consider 2-dose series VAR 3 months apart based on individual clinical decision; VAR contraindicated in HIV infection with CD4 count <200 cells/µL
- **Severe immunocompromising conditions**: VAR contraindicated

Zoster vaccination

Routine vaccination

- **Age 50 years or older**: 2-dose series RZV 2–6 months apart (minimum interval: 4 weeks; repeat dose if administered too soon) regardless of previous herpes zoster or previously received ZVL (administer RZV at least 2 months after ZVL)
- **Age 60 years or older**: 2-dose series RZV 2–6 months apart (minimum interval: 4 weeks; repeat dose if administered too soon) or 1 dose ZVL if not previously vaccinated (if previously received ZVL, administer RZV at least 2 months after ZVL); RZV preferred over ZVL

Special situations

- **Pregnancy**: ZVL contraindicated; consider delaying RZV until after pregnancy if RZV is otherwise indicated
- **Severe immunocompromising conditions (including HIV infection with CD4 count <200 cells/µL)**: ZVL contraindicated; recommended use of RZV under review

Figure 24-6C Recommended adult immunization schedule.

(Continued)

connection to autism. Parents should expect that vaccinations given to their children are safe and effective. This is ensured by the Centers for Disease Control and Prevention (CDC) and other federal agencies through comprehensive pre-licensure trials and post-licensure monitoring.

CONTRAINDICATIONS AND PRECAUTIONS

Generally, contraindications dictate circumstances in which vaccines will not be given. Most contraindications and precautions are temporary, and the vaccine can be given at a later time. A **contraindication** is a condition in a recipient that greatly increases the chance of a serious adverse reaction. A **precaution** is a condition in a recipient that may increase the chance of an adverse event. Permanent contraindications to vaccination include the following:

- Severe allergy to a prior dose of vaccine or to a vaccine component
- Encephalopathy after pertussis vaccine

POINTS TO REMEMBER

Serious febrile illness is a contraindication to active immunization, especially with live virus vaccines. All vaccines can be administered to individuals with minor illnesses such as common diarrhea and mild upper respiratory disease, with or without fever.

POINTS TO REMEMBER

Vaccines must be kept in the refrigerator at temperatures between 2 and 8°C (35.6 and 46.4°F).

Current Vaccines in the United States

Many vaccines are available in the Unites States. Table 24-1 lists various vaccines, trade names, and routes of administration.

WHAT WOULD YOU DO?

The mother of a 9-month-old baby tells you that the baby has not received any vaccines. As a pharmacy technician, what would you do?

Table 24-1 Vaccines Currently Used in the United States

Vaccine	Trade Name	Route	Comments
Adenovirus	Adenovirus®	Oral	Live viral; approved for military, age 17 to 50 years
Anthrax	BioThrax®	IM	Inactivated bacterial; used against biological warfare emergencies
DTaP	Daptacel®, Infanrix®	IM	Inactivated bacterial; tetanus, diphtheria toxoids, plus acellular pertussis vaccine; minimum age 6 weeks
DT	generic only	IM	Inactivated bacterial toxoids; pediatric formulation (through age 6 years)

(Continued)

Table 24-1 Vaccines Currently Used in the United States *(Continued)*

Vaccine	Trade Name	Route	Comments
DTaP-IPV	Kinrix®, Quadracel®	IM	Inactivated bacterial and viral; licensed for fifth (DTaP) and fourth (IPV) booster at 4 to 6 years
DTaP-Hep B-IPV	Pediarix®	IM	Inactivated bacterial and viral; licensed for doses at 2, 4, and 6 months (through 6 years); not licensed for boosters
DTaP-IPV/Hib	Pentacel®	IM	Inactivated bacterial and viral; licensed for four doses at 2, 4, 6 months and at 15 to 18 months
Haemophilus influenzae type b (Hib)	PedvaxHIB®	IM	Inactivated bacterial
	ActHIB®	IM	Inactivated bacterial
	Hiberix®	IM	Inactivated bacterial; NOTE: the Hiberix trade name is a booster only, for an age range of 1 to 4 years
Hepatitis A (Hep A)	Havrix®	IM	Inactivated viral; pediatric and adult formulations; minimum age 12 months
Hepatitis A	Vaqta®	IM	Inactivated viral; pediatric and adult formulations; minimum age 12 months
Hepatitis B (Hep B)	Engerix-B	IM	Inactivated viral; three-dose series starts at birth; pediatric and adult formulations available
	Recombivax HB	IM	Inactivated viral; pediatric, adults, and dialysis formulations available; two pediatric doses = one adult dose
Hepatitis A-hepatitis B	Twinrix®	IM	Inactivated viral; pediatric dose of Hep A plus adult dose of Hep B; minimum age 18 years; three-dose routine series
Herpes zoster (shingles)	Zostavax®	Subcutaneous	Live attenuated viral; Licensed for 50 years or older; recommended for 60 years or older
	Shingrix®	IM	Non-live recombinant subunit; Licensed for 50 years or older
Human papillomavirus (HPV)	Gardasil®,	IM	Inactivated viral; Gardasil forms licensed for people 9 to 26 years of age
	Gardasil 9®	IM	
	Cervarix®	IM	Inactivated viral; Cervarix form licensed for females only, 9 to 26 years of age
Influenza (trivalent, types A and B)	Fluarix®	IM	Inactivated viral; minimum age 3 years
	Fluvirin®, Flucelvax®	IM	Inactivated viral; minimum age 4 years
	Fluzone®	IM	Inactivated viral, age range 6 months to 3 years based on amount in prefilled syringe
	Fluzone high-dose®, Fluad®	IM	Inactivated viral, licensed for 65 years or older

(Continued)

Table 24-1 Vaccines Currently Used in the United States *(Continued)*

Vaccine	Trade Name	Route	Comments
	Fluzone Intradermal®	Intradermal	Inactivated viral, age range 18 to 64 years
	Flublock®	IM	Recombinant, licensed for 18 years or older
	Flulaval®	IM	Inactivated viral, minimum age 6 months
	Afluria Quadrivalent®	IM	Inactivated viral, minimum age 18 years, non-quadrivalent form for 9 years or older
	FluMist Quadrivalent®	Intranasal	Live attenuated viral, ages 2 to 49 years
Japanese encephalitis	Ixiaro®	IM	Inactivated viral; licensed for 17 years or older; two-dose series
Measles-mumps-rubella	M-M-R II®	Subcutaneous	Live attenuated viral; minimum age 12 months; two-dose series
Measles-mumps-	ProQuad®	Subcutaneous	Live attenuated viral; ages 1 to 12 years; two-dose series
Meningococcal	Menactra®	IM	Inactivated bacterial; ages 9 months to 55 years
	Menveo®	IM	Inactivated bacterial; ages 2 to 55 years
	Bexsero Trumenba®	IM	Recombinant proteins; ages 10 to 25 years
Pneumococcal	Pneumovax 23®	Subcutaneous or IM	Inactivated bacterial; minimum age 2 years; usually given 1 year after Prevnar 13
	Prevnar 13®	IM	Inactivated bacterial; ages 6 weeks through 5 years and 50 years or older
Polio	Ipol®	Subcutaneous or IM	Inactivated viral; trivalent, types 1, 2, 3
Rabies	Imovax Rabies®, RabAvert®	IM	Inactivated viral
Rotavirus	Rota Teq®, Rotarix®	Oral	Live viral; Rota Teq: first dose between 6 weeks and 14 weeks 6 days; complete three-dose series by 8 months; Rotarix: same, but in a two-dose series
Tetanus (reduced), Diphtheria (Td)	Tenivac®	IM	Inactivated bacterial toxoids; adult formulation (7 years or older)
Tetanus (reduced), Diphtheria (reduced), Pertussis (Tdap)	Boostrix®, Adacel®	IM	Inactivated bacterial; tetanus and diphtheria toxoids plus pertussis vaccine; minimum age 10 years; Adacel: Acellular (ages 11 to 64 years)
Tetanus toxoid	Generic only	IM	Inactivate bacterial toxoid; for adults or children
Typhoid	Typhim Vi®	IM	Inactivated bacterial
	Vivotif Berna®	Oral	Live attenuated bacterial

(Continued)

Table 24-1 Vaccines Currently Used in the United States *(Continued)*

Vaccine	Trade Name	Route	Comments
Vaccinia (smallpox)	ACAM2000	Percutaneous	Live attenuated viral; minimum age 16 years
Varicella	Varivax®	Subcutaneous	Live attenuated viral; minimum age 12 months; two-dose series
Yellow fever	YF-Vax®	Subcutaneous	Live attenuated viral; minimum age 9 months

Vaccines for Special Groups Only

Some vaccines are targeted for selected groups of people such as travelers, medical professionals, drug addicts, male homosexuals, known contacts of disease carriers, certain at-risk individuals, and the elderly. Table 24-2 lists vaccines restricted to special groups.

In some cases, such as yellow fever or rabies, limitation of a vaccine to a select group reflects geographical restrictions, whereas in others it stems from problems in producing sufficient vaccine in time to meet the demand. For example, each influenza epidemic is caused by a different strain, requiring a new vaccine.

Table 24-2 Vaccines Restricted to Special Groups

Disease	Vaccine	Special Groups
Hepatitis B	Surface antigen	At risk (medical, nursing staff), drug addicts, male homosexuals, known contacts of carriers
Tuberculosis	BCG	United States: at-risk only
Influenza	Killed	At-risk; elderly
Rabies	Killed	At-risk postexposure (animal workers)
Hepatitis A	Killed (though an attenuated vaccine is available in China and India)	Travelers
Cholera	Killed or mutant	Travelers
Meningitis	Polysaccharide	Travelers
Typhoid (injectable) Typhoid (oral)	Killed or mutant attenuated	Travelers
Yellow fever	Attenuated	Travelers
Pneumococcal pneumonia	Polysaccharide	Elderly

Antitoxins

Antitoxins are forms of passive immunity. They provide immediate but short-term protection against serious symptoms because they contain antibodies, usually derived from horses, which neutralize dangerous toxins. The use of antitoxins to prevent diseases was discussed earlier in this chapter. An example is *tetanus*, caused by *Clostridium tetani*, which is commonly transferred into the body through contaminated wounds. Administration of the tetanus antitoxin can give short-term protection against this potentially life-threatening condition. Other common antitoxins include those for botulism and diphtheria. Trade names of antitoxins basically use the name of the condition they treat, such as *Diphtheria antitoxin, Botulismus antitoxin*, and *Tetanus antitoxin*.

Antivenins

Antivenins are suspensions of venom-neutralizing antibodies. They are prepared from the serum of immunized horses. They offer passive immunity and are administered to counteract poisons from snakes, spiders, or other venomous creatures. Antivenins are divided into two types: monovalent and divalent. The monovalent antivenin is only useful for specific species of creatures, while the divalent antivenin is effective against a variety of species. The most common use of antivenins in the United States is against black widow spiders, brown recluse spiders, rattlesnakes, copperheads, cottonmouths (water moccasins), and coral snakes. Other creatures for which antivenins are used when a bite or sting occurs include certain types of scorpions, frogs, and lizards. Antivenins are also referred to as *antivenoms*. Common antivenins include *Antivenin (Crotalidae) Polyvalent, Antivenin (Latrodectus Mactans), Crotalidae polyvalent immune FAB, Antivenin, Centruroides (Scorpion)*, and *CROFAB*.

Vaccine Storage

In order to preserve the effectiveness of vaccines, the CDC provides guidelines for their storage. While some vaccines must remain frozen until they are used, most are required to be stored at temperatures between 2 and 8°C (35.6 and 46.4°F). Examples of specific vaccine storage requirements include the following:

- Varicella vaccine: frozen until time of use

- MMR vaccine: may be stored in either a freezer or a refrigerator

- MMRV vaccine: must be frozen because it contains varicella

- All inactivated vaccines: must be stored in a refrigerator

- Certain live attenuated vaccines (influenza, rotavirus, typhoid, yellow fever): must be stored in a refrigerator, although the Flu-Mist influenza vaccine may be frozen in a special manufacturer-supplied freeze box; this is because the defrost cycle temperature of most frost-free freezers is too warm for Flu-Mist; therefore, the special freeze box contains specialized insulation to keep the vaccine at required temperatures.

WHAT WOULD YOU DO?

A hospital pharmacy technician received a call asking him or her to bring a varicella vaccine to the seventh floor. He or she immediately removed the vaccine and put it onto the pharmacy counter. Meanwhile, the pharmacist assigned him or her to compound an emergency medication *stat*. An hour later, he or she was called again about bringing the varicella vaccine, which was still lying on the pharmacy counter. If you were this pharmacy technician, what would you do?

Medications Used to Treat Lymphatic System Disorders

The treatment of lymphatic disorders depends on each condition's etiology and the signs and symptoms. For example, for inflammation or infections such as lymphadenitis or lymphedema, medications include antibiotics, analgesics, and anti-inflammatories. For lymphomas, chemotherapy usually involves combinations of medications administered concurrently (see Table 24-3).

MEDICATION ERROR ALERT

The chemotherapy medications most commonly involved in errors and patient harm or even death include amphotericin B, liposomal amphotericin, carboplatin, cisplatin, docetaxel, paclitaxel, doxorubicin hydrochloride, and liposomal doxorubicin.

Table 24-3 Medications Used for Lymphomas

Generic Name	Trade Name	Route of Administration	Average Adult Dosage
Chemotherapy (for Hodgkin's Lymphomas)			
(ABVD Combination Therapy)			(Based on patient's height, weight, referred to as *body surface area* or *BSA*)
doxorubicin	Adriamycin®		
bleomycin	Blenoxane®		
vinblastine	Velban®	IV	25 mg/m^2
dacarbazine	DTIC-Dome®	IV	10 units/m^2
		IV	6 mg/m^2
		IV	375 mg/m^2
Chemotherapy (for Non-Hodgkin's Lymphomas)			
(CHOP Combination Therapy)			
cyclophosphamide	Cytoxan®	PO/IV	PO: 1 to 5 mg/kg/day; IV: 40 to 50 mg/kg over two to five days in divided doses
hydroxydaunorubicin (doxorubicin)	Adriamycin®	IV	10 units/m^2
vincristine	Vincasar PFS®, Oncovin®	IV	1.4 to 2 mg/m^2
prednisone or prednisolone	Deltasone® or Prelone®	PO	60 to 100 mg/m^2
rituximab	Rituxan®	IV	375 mg/m^2

Summary

Viruses, bacteria, fungi, protozoa, and multicellular parasites can cause many different diseases. The immune system combats these disease-causing microbes. Its primary function is to eliminate infectious agents and minimize the damage they cause. The immune system includes the lymphatic system, and it utilizes cells, biochemicals, vessels, and organs to maintain immunity. The lymph nodes, thymus, and spleen have major lymphatic functions. Special proteins are formed in response to particular foreign substances. These proteins are called antibodies, and active production of antibodies results in acquired immunity. Antibodies are also known as immunoglobulins. Immunoglobulins are used in vaccinations against disease. Innate immunity is a rapid cellular response.

Diseases that are commonly vaccinated against include diphtheria, tetanus, pertussis, poliomyelitis, measles, mumps, rubella, *Haemophilus influenzae* infection, varicella, herpes zoster, and human papillomavirus. Vaccines used for special groups include **hepatitis**, influenza, H1N1 influenza A, H5N1 influenza A, pneumonia, Lyme disease, meningitis, rabies, yellow fever, tuberculosis, smallpox, **anthrax**, and rotavirus. There are three major forms of the influenza virus (A, B, and C). Disorders of the immune system include lymphomas (Hodgkin's disease and non-Hodgkin's lymphoma), along with cancer affecting the lymph nodes. Autoimmune disorders include type 1 diabetes mellitus, rheumatoid arthritis, autoimmune thyroiditis, and multiple sclerosis.

Antibodies that neutralize toxins are called antitoxins. Both antitoxins and antivenins are forms of passive immunity that protect against various toxins and poisons, such as those from snakes, spiders, and other creatures. The importance of correct vaccine storage cannot be overemphasized. While many vaccines may be stored in refrigerators, others require freezing before they are used. Inadequate storage of vaccines may lead to breakdown of their components, reducing effectiveness, and potentially resulting in serious harm.

REVIEW QUESTIONS

1. The largest immunoglobulin in molecular structure is:

   A.   IgD.
   B.   IgE.
   C.   IgM.
   D.   IgG.

2. Which of the following is a live attenuated bacterial vaccine?

   A.   Cholera
   B.   Anthrax
   C.   Pertussis
   D.   Typhoid (oral)

3. The first immunoglobulin produced by the body when challenged by antigens during the initial antigen exposure is:

   A.   IgG.
   B.   IgA.
   C.   IgM.
   D.   IgE.

4. The most common category of non-Hodgkin's lymphoma is:

   A.   indolent lymphoma.
   B.   follicular lymphoma.
   C.   lymphocytic lymphoma.
   D.   Hodgkin's lymphoma.

5. Which of the following cytokines is most critical for activation of the immune response?

    A. Interleukin-2
    B. Interleukin-9
    C. Interleukin-1
    D. Tumor necrosis factor

6. Which of the following is the body's first line of defense against pathogens?

    A. Antibody molecules
    B. Phagocytes
    C. Unbroken skin
    D. Neutrophils

7. Which of the following is not an autoimmune disorder?

    A. Type 1 diabetes mellitus
    B. Rheumatoid arthritis
    C. Hodgkin's disease
    D. Multiple sclerosis

8. Which of the following is not a live attenuated virus vaccine?

    A. Measles
    B. Varicella
    C. Yellow fever
    D. Hepatitis B

9. The process of weakening pathogens is known as:

    A. inoculation.
    B. attenuation.
    C. habituation.
    D. insemination.

10. Antibodies that neutralize toxins are called:

    A. antitoxins.
    B. antigens.
    C. exotoxins.
    D. antioxidants.

11. Which of the following is an example of a live attenuated vaccine?

    A. Influenza
    B. Rabies
    C. Pertussis
    D. Measles/mumps/rubella (MMR)

12. Which of the following is an example of type IV or "delayed" hypersensitivity?

    A. Graft rejection
    B. Rhinitis
    C. Serum sickness
    D. Asthma

13. Natural passive acquired immunity results from:

    A. ingestion of colostrum.
    B. a vaccine.
    C. a gamma globulin injection.
    D. having the mumps.

14. Which of the following organs is involved in the maturation of T lymphocytes?

    A. Thyroid
    B. Spleen
    C. Thymus
    D. Lymph nodes

15. Which of the following is a contraindication to an immunization?

    A. Measles vaccine in a 4-year-old girl
    B. Influenza vaccine in a pregnant woman
    C. Herpes zoster vaccine in an elderly patient
    D. Encephalopathy after pertussis vaccine

CRITICAL THINKING

A 72-year-old man went to a retail pharmacy to receive a flu vaccine. The pharmacist asked if he wanted a higher dose vaccine. The man said yes. After five days, he experienced body ache, coughing, and fatigue.

1. Why did the pharmacist offer this individual a higher dose vaccine?

2. Describe how the immune system will fight off a viral infection.

3. What other vaccines should elderly people receive?

WEB LINKS

American Lyme Disease Foundation: www.aldf.com

Cellular Information Related to Immunology: www.cellsalive.com

Immunization Schedules: www.cdc.gov/vaccines/schedules/

ImmYouNity: www.vaccines.com/dtap-tdap-vaccine-information.cfm

Nature Reviews: www.nature.com/nri

Immunization Action Coalition: www.immunize.org

MedicineNet.com: www.medicinenet.com

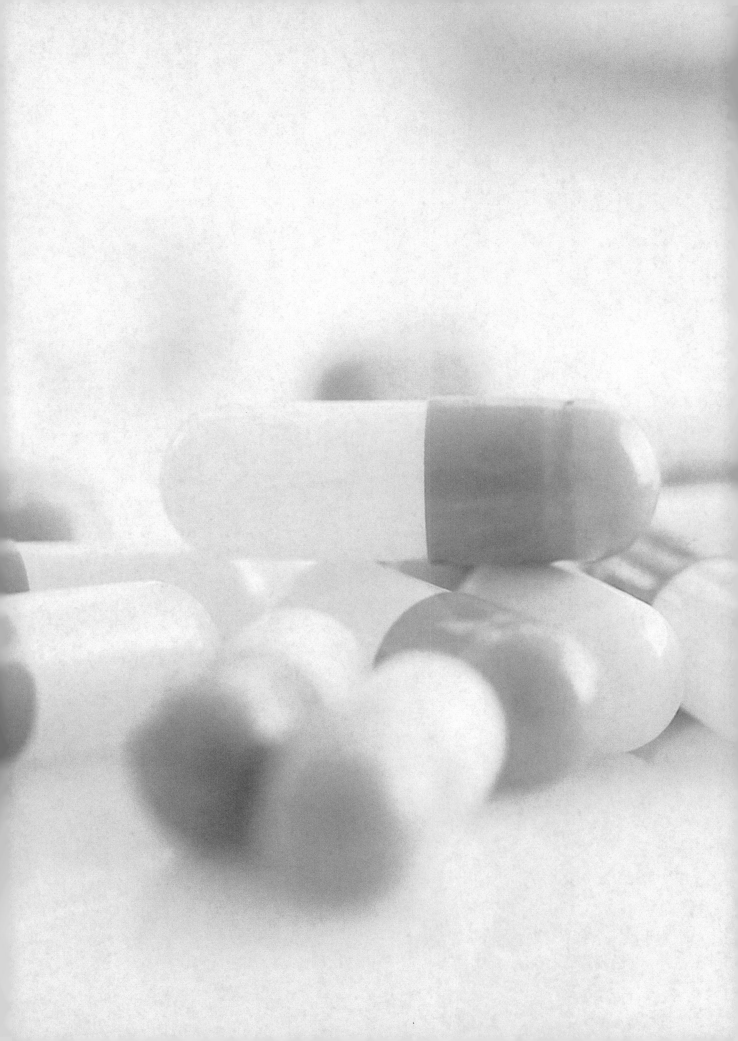

CHAPTER 25

Therapeutic Drugs for the Respiratory System

OUTLINE

Anatomy and Physiology of the Respiratory System

Disorders of the Respiratory System

OBJECTIVES

Upon completion of this chapter, the reader should be able to:

1. Identify the general functions of the respiratory system.
2. Describe the structure of the trachea and bronchi.
3. Explain the anatomy of the lungs.
4. Describe the risk factors for COPD.
5. Identify the pathophysiology of atelectasis.
6. Explain atypical pneumonia.
7. List four medications used to treat chronic asthma.
8. Describe allergic rhinitis.
9. Identify the treatment regimens for tuberculosis.
10. Describe various types of lung cancer.

KEY TERMS

alveolar sacs (alveoli)	bronchioles	exhalation	ventilation
antihistamines	bronchodilators	inhalation	
antitussives	dry powder inhaler (DPI)	larynx	
barrel chest	emphysema	metered dose inhaler (MDI)	

Overview

The most important function of the respiratory system is the inspiration of oxygen and the expiration of carbon dioxide. Therefore, the respiratory tract must exchange gases and supply oxygen to the body. Most of the oxygen binds with hemoglobin so that the blood can transport it. Breathing helps to rid the body of carbon dioxide and other wastes, maintaining the needed environment for cellular metabolism. The respiratory system functions automatically, at a rate of approximately 16 inspiration-expiration cycles per minute while at rest. This totals about 23,000 cycles per day. The effectiveness of the respiratory system affects the body's ability to function correctly and maintain homeostasis. It supplies oxygen for cellular respiration and the total breakdown of glucose by the body cells, which generates energy.

The respiratory system consists of the nasal passages, mouth, pharynx, **larynx**, trachea, bronchi, and lungs, as well as the accessory organs, such as the skeletal muscles of the chest wall and the diaphragm (see Figure 25-1).

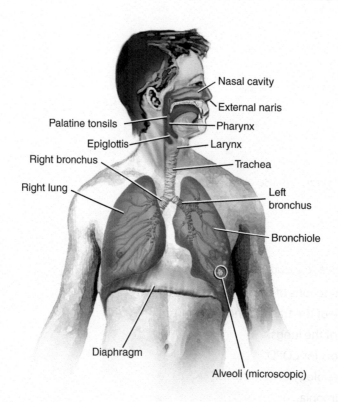

Figure 25-1 The respiratory system.

POINTS TO REMEMBER

During inspiration, most of the oxygen is absorbed into the blood circulation where it binds with hemoglobin to reach various tissues.

Anatomy and Physiology of the Respiratory System

The respiratory system is made up of two primary divisions: the portion where air is conducted, and the portion where gases are exchanged. The air-conducting portion consists of many passageways in which air is transported into and out of the lungs. The passageways begin as larger structures, progressively branching into smaller structures, which become more numerous. The lungs make up the gas-exchange division of the respiratory system, containing millions of microscopic alveoli. These tiny, thin-walled structures contain many capillaries that absorb oxygen from incoming air while releasing carbon dioxide. This is a basic explanation of the process of gas exchange.

The upper respiratory tract contains the nasal cavity, sinuses, mouth, pharynx, and larynx (see Figures 25-2 and 25-3). The lower respiratory tract is made up of the trachea and the lungs and is essential for the exchange of oxygen and carbon dioxide. The lower end of the trachea separates into the right and left bronchi. As the bronchi enter the lungs, they subdivide into bronchial tubes and small **bronchioles**. At the end of each bronchiole is an alveolar duct, which ends in the previously described sac-like clusters, called **alveolar sacs (alveoli)** (see Figure 25-4).

POINTS TO REMEMBER

Carbon dioxide is the most important chemical regulator of respiration.

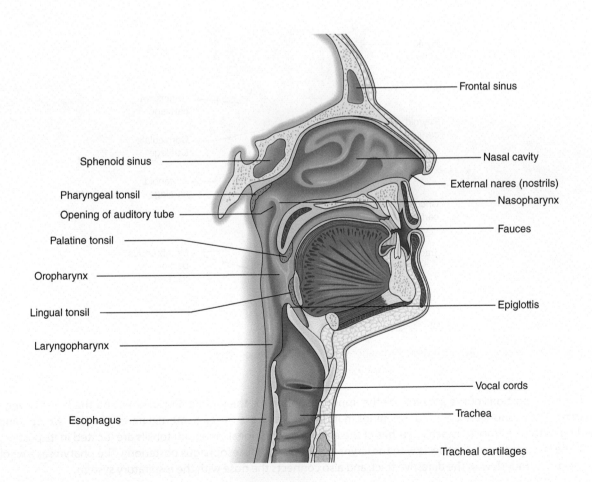

Figure 25-2 Sagittal view of the nasal cavity and pharynx.

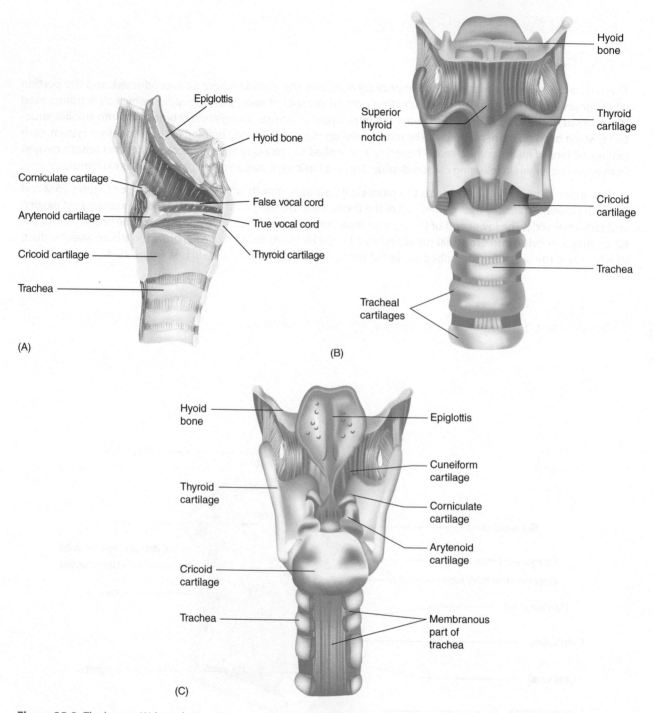

Figure 25-3 The larynx: (A) lateral view, (B) anterior view, and (C) posterior view.

The three portions of the pharynx are the upper nasopharynx, the middle oropharynx, and the lower laryngopharynx. The nasopharynx has four openings in its walls, which are the two internal nares and the two openings leading to the auditory (eustachian) tubes of the ears. The pharyngeal (adenoid) tonsils are located in its posterior wall. The laryngopharynx connects with the larynx anteriorly and the esophagus posteriorly. The pharynx as a whole connects the mouth with the digestive tract, and also connects the nose with the respiratory system.

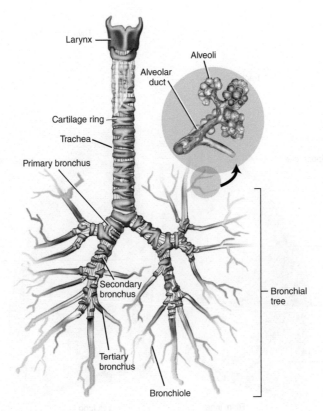

Figure 25-4 The bronchi, bronchioles, and alveoli.

MEDICAL TERMINOLOGY REVIEW

nasopharynx:

naso- = *nose*

-pharynx = *throat*

the upper part of the throat, behind the nose

LUNGS

The lungs are two large organs in the thoracic cavity that are sac-like in appearance. Overall, the lungs are cone-shaped, and they fill the pleural divisions of the thoracic cavity. They are enclosed and protected by two layers of pleural (serous) membrane. The outer layer joins the lung to the wall of the thoracic cavity. This layer is known as the parietal pleura. The inner visceral pleura cover the lungs. In between the two layers, there is a small pleural cavity that contains a lubricating fluid secreted by the membranes. This fluid helps to prevent friction so that the membranes can slide past each other during breathing. It also helps to hold the two pleural membranes together in each lung.

MEDICAL TERMINOLOGY REVIEW

pleural:

pleur/o = *pleura*

-al = *pertaining to*

pertaining to the pleura

The right lung has three lobes, while the left lung has only two since it must accommodate the heart within the chest (see Figure 25-5). The right lung is, therefore, wider and thicker than the left lung. However, it is slightly shorter than the left lung because the diaphragm muscle is located higher on the right side of the chest, because of the need to allow room for the liver.

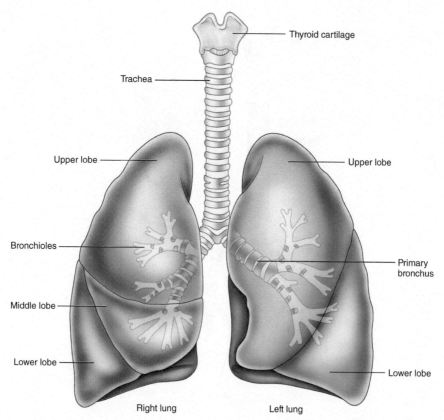

Figure 25-5 The branching bronchi and the lobes of the lungs.

The bronchioles are small ducts that lead to the alveoli (see Figure 25-6). Their walls are made up mostly of smooth muscle. This muscle allows the bronchioles to open and close, controlling airflow in the lungs. They open wider during exercise or because of stressful situations, so that airflow can increase. The terminal bronchioles are divided into microscopic respiratory bronchioles, which then divide into between 2 and 11 alveolar ducts. Each alveolus resembles a grape, and is an out-pouching that has an epithelial lining. There are more than 300 million alveoli in the lungs.

The alveoli are supported by a thin basement membrane that is highly elastic. Each alveolar sac consists of two or more alveoli sharing a single opening. Gas exchange occurs by diffusion across the alveoli and the walls of the capillaries surrounding them. Surfactant works by reducing the surface tension, keeping the alveoli open. Lack of enough surfactant may lead to respiratory distress syndrome, which primarily occurs in premature babies. Alveolar macrophages, also called dust cells, move through the alveoli to phagocytize particulates that are not filtered by the upper respiratory system.

THE PROCESSES OF RESPIRATION

Respiration supplies oxygen to and removes carbon dioxide from the body's trillions of cells. The three basic processes of respiration are ventilation, external respiration, and internal respiration. **Ventilation** (breathing) is the movement of air between the lungs and the external atmosphere. It is divided into **inhalation** (inspiration), which moves air inward, and **exhalation** (expiration), which moves air outward (see Figure 25-7). External respiration is the exchange of gases between the lungs and the blood. Internal respiration is the exchange of gases between the blood and body cells.

Inhalation occurs when the diaphragm and external intercostal muscles contract. The diaphragm is dome-shaped, and its contraction moves it downward as it flattens. The height of the thoracic cavity then increases. At the same time, the external intercostal muscles contract to lift the rib cage, pushing the sternum forward. Exhalation occurs as the diaphragm and external intercostal muscles relax and the rib cage descends. The space then decreases and the gases in the lungs are more compressed, increasing pressure.

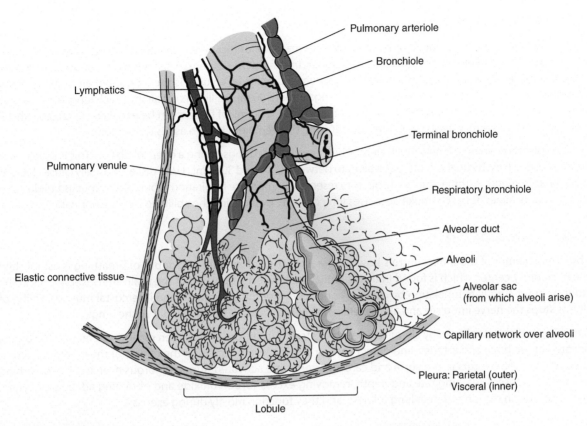

Figure 25-6 Anatomy of a lobule of a lung.

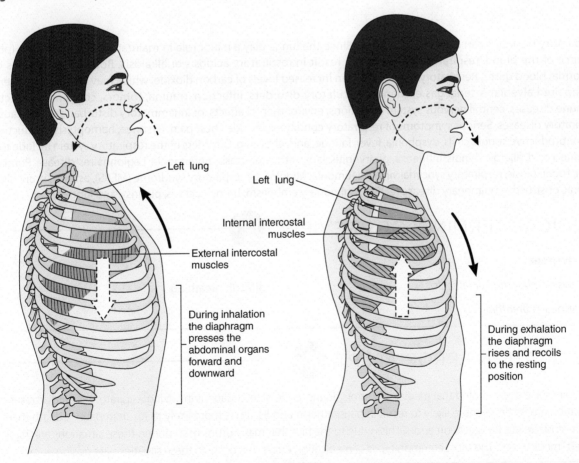

Figure 25-7 The two phases of ventilation: inhalation and exhalation.

MEASURING AIR FLOW

To determine lung health, controlled measurements are made of lung capacity. Machines are used to record how much air moves into and out of the lungs at various times. Important measurements include tidal volume, expiratory reserve volume, residual volume, and inspiratory reserve volume. Tidal volume is the amount of air moving in and out during passive breathing. At rest, every breath brings about 500 mL (milliliters) of air into each lung. After passive exhalation, about 2400 mL of air is still inside the lungs. About 1200 mL of this air can be expelled via forced exhalation. This is called expiratory reserve volume. The 1200 mL that remain is known as residual volume.

Inspiratory reserve volume is how much air may be drawn into the lungs during a deep inhalation. This is usually four to six times as much as the tidal volume, equivalent to between 2000 and 3000 mL. Lung diseases usually cause changes in these measurements. Asthma reduces inspiratory reserve volume since inspiration is blocked by mucus buildup and constricted bronchioles. Tobacco smoke decreases lung capacity by reducing the ability to breathe normally.

BREATHING CONTROL

The breathing center of the brain controls how we breathe. The normal rate and depth of breathing is established by the inspiratory center, which is found in the medulla, the lowermost portion of the brain stem. Nerve cells in the breathing center stimulate inhalation by causing contractions of the diaphragm and intercostal muscles. Filling of the lungs stops the nerve impulses and allows relaxation of the muscles, forcing air out of the lungs.

Breathing can also be altered by chemical receptors, stretch receptors, and oxygen receptors. Chemical receptors are located in the brain and arteries, and detect carbon dioxide levels, changing the effects of the breathing center as needed. Chemoreceptors in the aorta and carotid arteries are activated during vigorous exercise. The breathing center then increases breathing rate and depth, removing excess carbon dioxide and obtaining adequate oxygen. Stretch receptors in the lungs detect lung fullness, and they function mostly during exercise.

Disorders of the Respiratory System

Respiratory disorders can be acute or chronic. Since the lungs play a major role in maintaining the acid-base (pH) balance of the blood, respiratory disorders can result in respiratory acidosis or alkalosis. Both are conditions of abnormal blood gases. Respiratory failure results in increased levels of carbon dioxide, which may be a development of impaired alveolar-arterial gas exchange. Circulatory disorders, infection, trauma, tumors, congenital defects, immune diseases, central nervous system conditions, environmental effects, or inflammatory disturbances may cause respiratory diseases. Serious symptoms of respiratory conditions include chest pain, dyspnea, hemoptysis, productive or nonproductive cough, chills, dysphonia, fever, fatigue, and wheezing. Disorders of the respiratory system include the common cold, allergic rhinitis, influenza, pharyngitis, laryngitis, atelectasis, pneumonia, Legionnaires' disease, Pontiac fever, tuberculosis, respiratory syncytial virus pneumonia, Middle East respiratory syndrome (MERS), asthma, bronchitis, chronic obstructive pulmonary disease (COPD), pulmonary embolism, bronchiectasis, pleurisy, and lung cancer.

MEDICAL TERMINOLOGY REVIEW

dyspnea:

dys- = *abnormal or difficult*

-pnea = *breathing*

difficult breathing

MEDICATION ERROR ALERT

Studies have documented that medication errors during "code blue" situations involving respiratory or cardiac resuscitation are 39 times more likely to result in patient harm and 51 times more likely to result in patient death than non-code-related medication errors. This is due to the fact that many drugs used during these situations are "high alert" medications. The most common types of medication errors that occur in these situations are dosing errors.

COMMON COLD

An upper respiratory tract infection is generally referred to as the common cold. It involves an acute inflammatory process affecting the mucous membrane lining the upper respiratory tract. It is actually a group of illnesses caused by nearly 200 different viruses. In adults, rhinoviruses cause about 50% of all colds.

Symptoms may include nasal congestion and discharge, sneezing, sore throat, eye watering, hoarseness, and coughing. Additional symptoms may include fever, chills, or headache. Colds usually resolve within 4 to 10 days. Though there is no cure, treatment includes sufficient fluid consumption, rest, use of a vaporizer, and over-the-counter cold medicines, cough syrups, and analgesics. Also, zinc lozenges may slightly shorten the course of the common cold. Agents that relieve or prevent coughing are called **antitussives**. The initial stimulus for cough probably arises in the bronchial mucosa, where irritation results in bronchoconstriction. Antitussives are classified into two major groups: opioid and nonopioid. The cough suppression agents are classified in Table 25-1.

ALLERGIC RHINITIS

Allergic rhinitis is a reaction to airborne (inhaled) allergens. Depending on the allergen, the resulting rhinitis and conjunctivitis may occur seasonally, in which case it is commonly referred to as hay fever. It may start or worsen at a particular time of the year, triggered by the different blooming times of tree pollen, grasses, and weeds. It may also

Table 25-1 Antitussives and Related Medications

Generic Name	Trade Name	Route of Administration	Average Adult Dosage
Opioid Antitussives			
codeine	(generic only)	PO	15 mg q6h prn, may be increased up to 20 mg q4h (maximum 120 mg/day)
hydrocodone/ homatropine	Hycodan®, others	PO	1 tablet or 1 teaspoonful (5 mL) q4 to 6h prn (maximum 30 mL/day or 6 tablets/day)
Nonopioid Antitussives			
benzonatate	Tessalon®	PO	1 capsule (100 mg) tid prn (maximum 600 mg/day)
dextromethorphan	Delsym®, Robitussin DM®, others	PO	2 capsules (10 to 200 mg) q4h (maximum 12 capsules/day); or 10 to 20 mL of liquid q4h (maximum 120 mL/day)
Expectorant			
guaifenesin	Mucinex®	PO	1 or 2 tablets q12h with water (maximum 4 tablets/day)
Mucolytic			
acetylcysteine	Acetylcysteine Solution®	Inhalation	3 to 5 mL of 20% solution or 6 to 10 mL of 10% solution bid or qid

be year-round when the affected person is sensitive to indoor allergens such as dust mites, cockroaches, mold, or pet dander. Allergic rhinitis is the most common atopic allergic reaction, and it affects more than 20 million people in the United States.

Signs and symptoms include repeated sneezing that is most common just after awakening, runny nose, postnasal drip, itching, eye watering and reddening, dark circles under the eyes, coughing, wheezing, and loud breathing. Treatment of allergic rhinitis involves avoidance of all triggers of the condition, immunotherapy, over-the counter medications (**antihistamines**, decongestants, eye drops), prescription types of these medications, and cleaning of the nasal passages. Table 25-2 summarizes medications used for treating allergies.

INFLUENZA

Influenza, commonly called the flu, is a highly contagious viral respiratory infection. Three strains of a myxovirus cause influenza, but new strains evolve continually. As a result, annual modifications of the influenza vaccine are made, and the elderly, young children, and any person with debilitation, which increases risks of infection with influenza, should receive the vaccine. Examples of types of flu include Asian flu and bird flu. Airborne droplets transmit influenza. Symptoms of influenza include chills, fever, cough, sore throat, headache, fatigue, and muscle aches.

Treatment for influenza includes bed rest and adequate fluid intake, since in most cases the infection is self-limiting. Decongestants may be used on a limited basis, and additional treatments include antihistamines, saline sprays, cough medicines, nonsteroidal anti-inflammatory drugs (NSAIDs), salt-water gargles, and throat lozenges. However, severe cases may require antiviral medications. Antibiotics are not effective for treating influenza.

Table 25-2 Medications Used to Treat Allergies

Generic Name	Trade Name	Route of Administration	Average Adult Dosage
Corticosteroids			
beclomethasone	Beconase AQ®, Qnasl®	Intranasal	One to two sprays in each nostril bid
budesonide	Rhinocort Allergy®	Intranasal	One spray in each nostril once daily
flunisolide	Nasalide®	Intranasal	Two sprays in each nostril bid
fluticasone	Flonase Allergy Relief®	Intranasal	Two sprays in each nostril once daily or one spray in each nostril bid
mometasone	Nasonex®	Intranasal	Two sprays in each nostril once daily
triamcinolone	Nasacort Allergy 24HR®	Intranasal	Two sprays in each nostril once daily
Antihistamines			
desloratadine	Clarinex®	PO	5 mg once daily
fexofenadine	Allegra Allergy®, Allegra 24 Hour®	PO	Allergy: 60 mg bid; 24 Hour: 180 mg once daily
levocetirizine	Xyzal®	PO	2.5 to 5 mg once daily
olopatadine	Patanase®	Intranasal	Two sprays in each nostril bid
Leukotriene Receptor Antagonists			
montelukast	Singulair®	PO	10 mg once daily

Antihistamines appear to compete with histamine for cell receptor sites on effector cells. Thus, histamine-related allergic reactions and tissue injury are blocked or diminished in intensity. Most antihistamines have a sedating effect and should be used carefully, although some newer antihistamines with a much lower level of sedating effect are now available. These include cetirizine, loratadine, and fexofenadine. Of this group, loratadine and fexofenadine have the lowest sedating effect. Table 25-3 lists some examples of antihistamines.

WHAT WOULD YOU DO?

You are working in a hospital pharmacy when the pharmacist asks you to get a vial of influenza vaccine for a patient. Upon opening the refrigerator that contains the vaccine, you notice that the temperature inside doesn't seem much cooler than the room temperature of the pharmacy. What would you do?

Table 25-3 Examples of Antihistamines

Generic Name	Trade Name	Route of Administration	Average Adult Dosage
First-Generation Drugs			
brompheniramine	Dimetane®	PO	4 to 8 mg q6h prn
dexchlorpheniramine	Polaramine®	PO	2 mg (1 teaspoonful) q4 to 6h, or 4 to 6 mg of timed-release preparation at bedtime, or q8 to 10h
dimenhydrinate	Dramamine®	PO	50 to 100 mg q4 to 6h; (maximum 400 mg/day)
diphenhydramine	Benadryl®	PO	25 to 50 mg q4 to 6h prn (maximum 300 mg/day)
Second-Generation Drugs			
cetirizine	Zyrtec®	PO	5 to 10 mg daily (maximum 10 mg/day)
fexofenadine	Allegra®	PO	60 mg bid or 180 mg once daily with water
loratadine	Claritin®	PO	1 tablet (10 mg) daily (maximum)
Second-Generation Drugs with Decongestant			
fexofenadine/ pseudoephedrine	Allegra D®	PO	1 tablet (180 mg fexofenadine/240 mg pseudoephedrine) per day
loratadine/ pseudoephedrine	Claritin D®	PO	1 tablet (5 to 120 mg) bid or 1 tablet (10 to 240 mg) once daily

PHARYNGITIS

Pharyngitis is defined as inflammation or infection of the pharynx, which may be acute or chronic. It is usually caused by a viral or bacterial infection. Chronic pharyngitis can also be linked to syphilis or tuberculosis.

Signs and symptoms of pharyngitis may include throat soreness, dryness, burning, or the sensation of a lump or object. Signs vary due to the cause and may include chills, dysphonia, fever, dysphagia, and cervical lymphadenopathy. The pharyngeal mucosa is red and swollen, and tonsillar exudate is sometimes present. For viral causes, treatment includes lozenges, mouthwashes, ice collars, salt-water gargles, and aspirin. However, aspirin is not given to children due to the potential for Reye's syndrome. If the cause is an acute bacterial infection, systemic administration of antibiotics or sulfonamides is necessary. If streptococcal pharyngitis is documented, treatment will consist of a course of antibiotics lasting 7 to 10 days. For chronic tonsillitis, adenoiditis, and adenoid hypertrophy, surgical excision may be indicated. This may be followed by large amounts of fluids and bed rest.

LARYNGITIS

Laryngitis is defined as inflammation of the larynx and vocal cords. It can be caused by acute or chronic viral or bacterial infections. The most common causes of laryngitis include the common cold, pharyngitis, tonsillitis, and sinusitis. It may also be linked to bronchitis, influenza, pertussis, measles, pneumonia, diphtheria, mononucleosis, syphilis, and tuberculosis. Occasionally, the cause is simple irritation without any infection.

Signs and symptoms of laryngitis usually include hoarseness and aphonia (loss of voice). Other signs include fever, malaise, dysphagia, sore throat, and flu-like symptoms if the condition is severe. For viral laryngitis, treatment includes complete voice rest, bed rest in an adequately humidified room, adequate fluid intake, avoidance of smoking or drinking alcohol, and use of cough syrup or throat lozenges. The condition usually resolves in four to five days.

MEDICAL TERMINOLOGY REVIEW

laryngitis:

laryng/o = *larynx*

-itis = *inflammation*

inflammation of the larynx

ATELECTASIS

Atelectasis is defined as a collapsed or airless state of pulmonary tissues. It is caused by a bronchial tree obstruction. This may include foreign bodies, mucus plugs, or bronchogenic cancer. Atelectasis may be caused by fluid accumulation in the pleural cavity, which is called pleural effusion.

Signs and symptoms of atelectasis include partial or complete lung collapse. It leads to hypoxia and dyspnea. When a small amount of a lung is involved, only dyspnea may be present. Other signs may include cyanosis, substernal retraction, and diminished breath sounds. There may be a mediastinal shift toward the side of collapse that is revealed in chest radiography. The patient with atelectasis may have anxiety, diaphoresis, and tachycardia. Treatments of atelectasis include airway suctioning, spirometry, and antibiotics (if an infection is present). In infants, tracheal suctioning is indicated, usually followed by oxygen administration.

MEDICAL TERMINOLOGY REVIEW

atelectasis:

atel/o = *incomplete*

-ectasis = *dilation*

incomplete dilation (collapse) of the lung

PNEUMONIA

Pneumonia is defined as infective lung inflammation, usually caused by viral or bacterial infections. Common causative organisms include pneumococci, staphylococci, streptococci, *Haemophilus influenzae* type B, *Klebsiella pneumoniae*, and various other Gram-negative organisms. Adenoviruses, influenza viruses, and respiratory syncytial viruses may also cause pneumonia. Atypical pneumonia (previously called "walking pneumonia") is unique in that the patient is not significantly ill, but x-rays show serious abnormalities. Organisms such as legionella, mycoplasma, and chlamydia often cause this type of pneumonia. Additional causes of pneumonia include inhalation of poisonous gases or aspiration of foreign matter.

Signs and symptoms of pneumonia may be unilateral or bilateral and related to a portion of a lung or an entire lung. Symptoms include cough, fever, and shortness of breath, chills, sweating, chest pain, cyanosis, and blood in the sputum. In younger patients, there may be shallow, rapid respirations. Treatment of pneumonia is based on the cause. Commonly used medications include organism-specific antibiotics, penicillin, tetracyclines, erythromycin, and sulfonamides. Additional treatment measures include aspirin, oxygen administration, bed rest, adequate fluid intake, high-calorie diets, and postural drainage.

MEDICAL TERMINOLOGY REVIEW

pneumonia:

pneumon/o = *lung*

-ia = *condition*

condition of lung inflammation

ASTHMA

Asthma is a respiratory condition characterized by difficulty in exhaling and by wheezing. *Bronchial asthma*, normally called simply *asthma*, is caused by smooth muscle spasms in the bronchi that reduce airflow. This condition causes inflammation and accumulation of mucus in the air passages. Asthma is more common in children than in adults but may affect people of any age. It is not contagious. Though male children are affected more than female children, this is reversed in adults. African Americans and Puerto Ricans have the highest risks for asthma. In susceptible individuals, causes of asthma attacks include allergic reactions, exercise, changes in weather or altitude, and upper respiratory infection. A hereditary factor is strongly implicated. Asthma is a primary reason for emergency room visits, hospitalization, and lost days from school or work, affecting patients as well as caregivers.

The most important risk factors for asthma are history of atopic diseases, which include allergic rhinitis, dermatitis, and conjunctivitis, along with colds and other respiratory infections in childhood. *Respiratory syncytial virus* is the most common cause of bronchiolitis, which is inflammation of the small airways in children under 12 months of age. This virus is linked to wheezing in later childhood. The patient must avoid triggers such as known allergens and infection. Secondhand smoke should also be avoided. Exercise-induced asthma can be reduced by warming up for a period of 10 minutes before strenuous exercise and by using acute relief therapies such as short-acting beta-2-agonists, systemic corticosteroids, or anticholinergic agents. Signs and symptoms of asthma include chronic coughing, which may be productive or nonproductive, severe wheezing, and rapid, shallow respirations. This may lead to pallor, rapid pulse, severe sweating, and limited ability to speak because of the need for oxygen. The child is usually anxious, exhausted, and complains of a tight chest.

There is no cure for asthma. An exacerbation is also called an asthma *attack* or *episode*. If chronic, treatment includes regular medications to relax and widen the bronchi, as well as to release excessive mucus. Medications include albuterol, cromolyn sodium, aerosol corticosteroids, and theophylline. Allergy shots are desensitization injections that may be used as immunotherapy. For severe, acute attacks, inhalation therapy and epinephrine injections are indicated. For severe, persistent asthma, long-acting beta-2-agonists are prescribed along with inhaled corticosteroids. These beta-2-agonists should never be used on their own. For status asthmaticus, which may lead to fatal respiratory failure, hospitalization is required.

POINTS TO REMEMBER

Allergens are found in dust, pet dander, and cockroaches. In some cases, all carpeting may be removed from the home of an asthma patient. If this is not possible, vacuuming should occur weekly. Bedding and children's stuffed animals must be washed every week. Bedding that has feathers should be replaced, and dust-proof-pillow cases and mattress covers should be used.

Corticosteroids are the most potent and consistently effective anti-inflammatory agents that are currently available to use for asthma. There are three commonly used devices for inhalation administration, including metered dose inhalers, dry powder inhalers, and nebulizers. Drug administration with a **metered dose inhaler (MDI)** is often accomplished with one or two puffs from a handheld pressurized device (see Figure 25-8).

A **dry powder inhaler (DPI)** delivers medication in the form of micronized powder into the lungs. Medications such as cromolyn and albuterol are available for use this way. DPIs are breath-activated and are easier to use than MDIs. A nebulizer uses a small machine that converts a solution into a mist. The mist droplets are inhaled either through a facemask or through a mouthpiece. **Bronchodilators** are agents that widen the diameter of the bronchial tubes. They include beta-adrenergic agonists, theophylline, anticholinergics, and xanthine derivatives. *Peak flow meters* are used for patients aged five and older to assess air movement out of the lungs, primarily for moderate to severe persistent asthma or history of severe exacerbations. Examples of medications for treating asthma are summarized in Table 25-4.

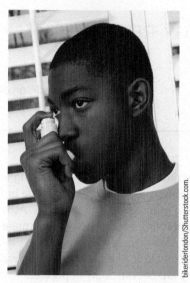

bikeriderlondon/Shutterstock.com.

Figure 25-8 . The metered dose inhaler aerosolizes medication for inhalation directly into the airways.

Table 25-4 Medications Used to Treat Asthma

Generic Name	Trade Name	Route of Administration	Average Adult Dosage
Beta-Agonists (short-acting)			
albuterol beta-2 selective	ProAir HFA®, Ventolin HFA, Proventil HFA, VoSpire ER	Inhalation	Two inhalations q4 to 6h
levalbuterol beta-2 selective	Xopenex®, Xopenex HFA®	Inhalation	0.63 mg tid via nebulizer
Beta-Agonists (long-acting)			
arformoterol beta-2 selective	Brovana®	Inhalation	15 mcg bid via nebulizer
formoterol beta-2 selective	Perforomist®	Inhalation	20 mcg bid via nebulizer
salmeterol beta-2 selective	Serevent Diskus®	Inhalation	One inhalation bid
Anticholinergics			
ipratropium	Atrovent HFA®	Inhalation	Two inhalations qid
tiotropium	Spiriva®	Inhalation	Two inhalations once daily using Handihaler device
Bronchodilators			
albuterol	Proventil®	MDI, Inhalation Capsules (IC), Nebulizer	MDI: Two puffs q4 to 6h prn; IC: 200 mg q4 to 6h, may be increased to 400 mcg q4 to 6h; Nebulizer: 2.5 mg q6 to 8h prn (2.5 to 5 mg once, then 2.5 mg q20min)
metaproterenol	Alupent®	MDI	Two to three inhalations q3 to 4h (maximum 12 inhalations/day)
terbutaline	Terbutaline Sulfate®	PO	5 mg tid at 6-hour intervals; may be decreased to 2.5 mg/dose prn (maximum 15 mg/day)

(Continued)

Table 25-4 Medications Used to Treat Asthma (*Continued*)

Generic Name	Trade Name	Route of Administration	Average Adult Dosage
Methylxanthines			
dyphilline	Lufyllin®	PO	Up to 15 mg/kg q6h
theophylline	Elixophyllin®, Theochron®, Theo-24®	PO	16 mg/kg/day (maximum 400 mg/day)
Leukotriene Receptor Antagonists			
montelukast	Singulair®	PO	10 mg once daily
zafirlukast	Accolate®	PO	20 mg bid
zileuton	Zyflo CF®	PO	600 mg qid
Phosphodiesterase-4 Inhibitor			
roflumilast	Daliresp®	PO	500 mcg once daily
Anti-IgE Antibody			
omalizumab	Xolair®	Subcutaneous	75 to 375 mg q2 to 4 weeks
Mast Cell Stabilizer			
cromolyn sodium	Gastrocrom®, NasalCrom®	Intranasal	Once spray into each nostril tid to qid (maximum 6 times per day)
Mucolytic			
acetylcysteine	Acetadote®, Cetylev®	IV, PO	Acetadote: 300 mg/kg in three doses over 21 hours; Cetylev: 140 mg/kg
Combination Products			
albuterol/ipratropium	Combivent Respimat®, Duoneb®	Inhalation	One inhalation qid (maximum 6 times per day)
budesonide/ formoterol	Symbicort®	Inhalation	Two inhalations bid
formoterol/ mometasone	Dulera®	Inhalation	Two inhalations bid
fluticasone/ salmeterol	Advair Diskus®, Advair HFA®	Inhalation	Two inhalations bid
Corticosteroids			
beclomethasone	Vanceril®, Beclovent®	MDI (inhalation)	Two inhalations (40 mcg each) bid or two inhalations (80 mcg each) bid (maximum 640 mcg/day)
budesonide	Pulmicort Turbuhaler®	DPI	One to four inhalations (200 mcg each) (maximum 400 mcg bid if using bronchodilators alone, maximum 800 mcg bid if also using inhaled or oral corticosteroids)
ciclesonide	Alvesco®	Inhalation	80 to 320 mcg bid based on use of bronchodilators or other corticosteroids
dexamethasone	Decadron®	MDI, DPI	0.75 to 9 mg/day
fluticasone	Flovent®	MDI	88 to 440 mcg bid (maximum 440 mcg bid if using bronchodilators alone or also taking inhaled corticosteroids; maximum 880 mcg bid if also taking oral corticosteroids)
prednisolone	Prelone®	PO	200 mg/day for one week, then 80 mg every other day for one month
prednisone	Deltasone®, Meticorten®	PO	Initial: 5 to 60 mg/day

WHAT WOULD YOU DO?

A friend who has been taking montelukast sodium (Singulair®) for his asthma has begun making strange statements about death. He has stated that he believed no one would miss him at his job if he "jumped in front of a train." You also know that his parents are dead and that he is estranged from his one sibling, a sister. Based on your knowledge, as a pharmacy technician, about the adverse effects of his medication, what would you do?

CHRONIC BRONCHITIS

Chronic bronchitis is inflammation of the bronchi caused by irritants or infection. A form of COPD, bronchitis may be classified as acute or chronic. In chronic bronchitis, hypersecretion of mucus and chronic productive cough lasts for three months of the year and occurs for at least two consecutive years. Common causes of chronic bronchitis include exposure to irritants, cigarette smoking, genetic predisposition, exposure to noxious gases, and respiratory tract infection.

Signs and symptoms of bronchitis include a deep and persistent cough that is productive. The sputum will be thick yellow, or darken even to appear gray. Additional symptoms include shortness of breath, wheezing, fever, and upper chest pain that is worsened when coughing. Inflammation may persist and worsen, causing obstructive and asthmatic symptoms. In the final stages, there may be nearly continuous coughing, shortness of breath, and wheezing. Treatment for chronic bronchitis is based on the stage at diagnosis. Acute infections must be quickly treated. For hypoxemia, low-flow oxygen therapy may be used. To loosen and expectorate thick mucus, postural drainage and percussion may be administered. For inflammation, aerosolized corticosteroids may be indicated. The patient should avoid smoking, and others who smoke should stay away from crowds of people and completely avoid anyone with a cold.

MEDICATION ERROR ALERT

Many inhalation products intended for use by nebulization are packaged in unit-dose containers that are very similar to those that contain other medications. For example, ipratropium (Atrovent HFA®), used for chronic bronchitis and other respiratory conditions, may have the drug name, concentration, lot number, and expiration date embossed into the plastic with transparent, raised letters that are difficult to read.

CHRONIC OBSTRUCTIVE PULMONARY DISEASE

COPD results from **emphysema**, chronic bronchitis, asthma, or a combination of these disorders. COPD is the most common lung disease, and its incidence is increasing. Cigarette smoking, recurrent or chronic respiratory tract infections, air pollution, allergies, and hereditary factors are common causes of COPD.

Signs and symptoms of COPD are those of chronic bronchitis as well as emphysema. These may include dyspnea, tachypnea, wheezing, coughing, the formation of a **barrel chest** due to overuse of accessory muscles to expel trapped air, shortness of breath, pursed lips, circumoral cyanosis, symptoms of right ventricular heart failure, and digital clubbing. Treatment of COPD is similar to that for chronic bronchitis and emphysema, and it may include avoidance of cigarette smoke and other irritants, avoidance of exposure to infections, annual influenza virus vaccinations, and supplemental oxygen. Medications include albuterol, terbutaline sulfate, metaproterenol sulfate, theophylline, expectorants, and antibiotics. Pulmonary rehabilitation, progressive exercise training, and surgery may be indicated. Refer back to Table 25-4 (medication for asthma), since these medications are also used for COPD.

POINTS TO REMEMBER

COPD is more prevalent in urban than in rural environments, and it is also related to occupational factors such as exposure to mineral or organic dusts.

MEDICATION ERROR ALERT

While most people would not believe that oxygen therapy could be anything except helpful for COPD, there are still dangers when using oxygen. Oxygen therapy should only be prescribed when a patient's oxygen saturation is 88% or lower at rest, based on the fact that oxygen saturation of 93% or higher is normal if you are at sea level. Prescribed *supplemental oxygen* is often overused, such as when a patent experiences "shortness of breath," which is actually *not usually caused by low oxygen levels.* An oximeter is used to easily measure oxygen saturation.

TUBERCULOSIS

Tuberculosis is a chronic bacterial infection that most commonly affects the lungs but can also affect the liver, spleen, bone marrow, lymph nodes, and meninges. It is caused by *Mycobacterium tuberculosis,* which is transmitted by ingestion or inhalation of infected droplets. Early signs and symptoms include chest pain, fever, loss of appetite and accompanying weight loss, and pleurisy. Lung tissue reacts to the bacterium by producing cells with phagocytic activities, forming tubercles, which without treatment enlarge and merge to form dead tissue areas that can fill the lung cavity. The patient experiences hemoptysis as a result.

The primary lesion of tuberculosis is located in the lungs. The patient's resistance to secondary tuberculosis depends on general health and environment. In the United States, certain groups within the general population are more prone to acquire active tuberculosis. These people include the following:

- Patients with AIDS
- Drug abusers
- Homeless shelter residents
- Nursing home residents

Antitubercular drugs are used to treat tuberculosis. Primary antitubercular drugs include isoniazid, ethambutol, rifampin, pyrazinamide, and streptomycin (Table 25-5).

Table 25-5 Medications Used to Treat Tuberculosis

Generic Name	Trade Name	Route of Administration	Average Adult Dosage
ethambutol	Myambutol®	PO	Once daily: 40 to 55 kg—800 mg; 56 to 75 kg—1200 mg; 76 to 90 kg—1600 mg; 3 times weekly direct observed therapy: 40 to 55 kg—1200 mg; 56 to 75 kg—2000 mg; 76 to 90 kg—2400 mg; 2 times weekly direct observed therapy: 40 to 55 kg—2000 mg; 56 to 75 kg—2800 mg; 76 to 90 kg—4000 mg
ethionamide	Trecator®	PO	15 to 20 mg/kg once daily or in divided doses
isoniazid (INH)	Isoniazid®	PO, IM	5 mg/kg PO or IM daily for up to six months; 3 times weekly direct observed therapy: 15 mg/kg/dose; 2 times weekly direct observed therapy: 15 mg/kg/dose; once weekly direct observed therapy: 15 mg/kg/dose
pyrazinamide (PZA)	Pyrazinamide®	PO	Once daily: 40 to 55 kg—1000 mg; 56 to 75 kg—1500 mg; 76 to 90 kg—2000 mg; 3 times weekly direct observed therapy: 40 to 55 kg—1500 mg; 56 to 75 kg—2500 mg; 76 to 90 kg—3000 mg; 2 times weekly direct observed therapy: 40 to 55 kg—2000 mg; 56 to 75 kg—3000 mg; 76 to 90 kg—4000 mg

(Continued)

Table 25-5 Medications Used to Treat Tuberculosis (*Continued*)

Generic Name	Trade Name	Route of Administration	Average Adult Dosage
rifabutin	Mycobutin®	PO	5 mg/kg once daily as a substitute for rifampin
rifampin	Rifadin®	PO, IV	10 mg/kg/day (maximum 600 mg/day); or 600 mg once daily
rifapentine	Priftin®	PO	600 mg twice per week for two months
streptomycin	Streptomycin®	IM	15 mg/kg/day (maximum 1 g)

WHAT WOULD YOU DO?

You are a hospital pharmacy technician who discovers that a patient diagnosed with tuberculosis has been seen smoking in the stairwell that is open to the outside air. Understanding the treatment requirements for tuberculosis, the seriousness of this condition, and the medications used for treatment, what would you do in this scenario?

LUNG CANCER

Lung cancer accounts for nearly 30% of all cancer deaths. It is the most common cause of cancer death for men and women throughout the world. It is usually caused by repeated carcinogenic irritation of the bronchial epithelium. This leads to increased rates of cell division. There are four major histologic types. The most common form is adenocarcinoma (40%), followed by squamous cell carcinoma (30%), small cell carcinoma (20%), and large cell carcinoma (10%). Adenocarcinoma, squamous cell carcinoma, and large cell carcinoma are collectively called non-small-cell lung cancer and have similar patterns of development and treatments. Small cell lung cancer is almost totally related to smoking, grows quickly, and metastasizes rapidly. Cigarette smoking is the overwhelming predisposing factor for lung cancers, responsible for 87% of all types. Smokers are 10 to 30 times more likely to develop lung cancer than those who do not smoke. Total lifetime smoking history increases risks.

The most common sign of lung cancer is coughing. Since there is often coexisting COPD, any changes must be documented. Additional signs and symptoms include dyspnea, hemoptysis, chest pain, and weight loss. The brain is the most common site of metastasis, but other sites include the liver, bones, and skin. Signs of metastasis include headache, weakness, mental status changes, and seizures. Lung cancer may be discovered in a patient without symptoms because of an abnormal chest x-ray. Treatments for lung cancer are based on the type and stage of tumors. In early stages, surgical resection with or without radiation or chemotherapy is preferred for non-small-cell tumors. Partial or total removal of a lung may be needed. For small cell lung cancer, medications include cisplatin plus etoposide or irinotecan, along with radiation therapy. Relapse for this form is common, and prognosis is much poorer than for the others.

Summary

The respiratory system is primarily made up of two divisions: the portion where air is conducted (various respiratory passageways) and the portion where gases are exchanged (the lungs). The upper respiratory tract contains the nasal cavity, sinuses, mouth, pharynx, and larynx. The lower respiratory tract is made up of the trachea and the lungs. In the nose, coarse hairs filter out large dust particles, while smaller particles are trapped by mucus secreted from the mucous membranes. Once air enters the nose and mouth, it is drawn backward into the pharynx.

The right and left primary bronchi divide off of the trachea and enter the lungs, where they branch extensively. The right lung has three lobes, while the left lung has only two, since it must accommodate the heart within the chest. The bronchioles are small ducts that lead to the alveoli, where gas exchange occurs via diffusion. Respiration supplies oxygen to and removes carbon dioxide from the cells of the body. Inhalation occurs when the diaphragm and external intercostal muscles contract. Exhalation occurs as the diaphragm and external intercostal muscles relax and the rib cage descends. The breathing center of the brain controls how we breathe, and it is found in the brain stem (medulla). Respiratory disorders include common cold, allergic rhinitis, influenza, pharyngitis, laryngitis, atelectasis, pneumonia, asthma, bronchitis, chronic obstructive pulmonary disease, bronchiectasis, tuberculosis, and lung cancer.

REVIEW QUESTIONS

1. Which of the following defines "inspiratory reserve volume"?

    A. Amount of air drawn into the lungs during a deep inhalation
    B. Amount of air moving in and out during passive breathing
    C. Amount of air that can be expelled during forced exhalation
    D. Amount of air that remains after complete exhalation

2. The upper respiratory tract contains all of the following, *except the:*

    A. sinuses.
    B. pharynx.
    C. trachea.
    D. nasal cavity.

3. Guaifenesin is classified as an:

    A. opioid antitussive.
    B. nonopioid antitussive.
    C. mucolytic.
    D. expectorant.

4. Which of the following is not a risk factor for COPD?

    A. Allergies
    B. Air pollution
    C. Cigarette smoking
    D. Chest trauma

5. Which of the following occurs in atelectasis?

    A. Mediastinal shift toward the side of lung collapse
    B. Mediastinal shift away from the side of lung collapse
    C. Relaxation of the diaphragm
    D. Contraction of the diaphragm

6. Structures formed by branching of the trachea within the mediastinum are the:

    A. bronchioles.
    B. alveoli.
    C. primary bronchi.
    D. secondary bronchi.

7. The actual sites of gas exchange within the lungs are the:

    A. pleural spaces.
    B. alveoli.
    C. terminal sacs.
    D. alveolar ducts.

8. Which of the following is another name for "walking pneumonia"?

   A. Atypical pneumonia
   B. Lobar pneumonia
   C. Bilateral pneumonia
   D. Viral pneumonia

9. Which of the following is not a bronchodilator used for chronic asthma?

   A. Terbutaline sulfate (terbutaline)
   B. Alupent (metaproterenol)
   C. Singulair (montelukast)
   D. Proventil (albuterol)

10. Which of the following is the trade name of cetirizine?

    A. Claritin
    B. Zyrtec
    C. Dramamine
    D. Allegra

11. Amantadine (Symmetrel) is used to treat which for the following conditions?

    A. Influenza
    B. Asthma
    C. Atelectasis
    D. COPD

12. Which of the following medications is a mast cell stabilizer?

    A. Daliresp (roflumilast)
    B. Xolair (omalizumab)
    C. Gastrocrom (cromolyn)
    D. Accolate (zafirlukast)

13. Which of the following is an example of an inhaled anticholinergic?

    A. Serevent Diskus
    B. Accolate
    C. Brovana
    D. Spiriva

14. Which of the following is not a primary drug used to treat tuberculosis?

    A. Ethambutol
    B. Rifampin
    C. Aceylcysteine
    D. Isoniazid

15. The most common type of lung cancer is:

    A. small cell carcinoma.
    B. large cell carcinoma.
    C. squamous cell carcinoma.
    D. adenocarcinoma.

CRITICAL THINKING

A 72-year-old man with a history of cigarette smoking (for 40 years) was administered and evaluated to rule out pneumonia as the cause of respiratory symptoms.

1. Explain the effects of cigarette smoking on the respiratory system.

2. If the patient has bacterial pneumonia, what would the treatments be?

WEB LINKS

American Lung Association: www.lung.org

American Academy of Allergy, Asthma, and Immunology: www.aaai.org

Asthma Information and Resources: www.asthma.com

COPD Information: www.copd.com

Emphysema: www.webmd.com/lung/copd/what-is-emphysema#1

Help for Tobacco Addiction: www.smokehelp.org

CHAPTER 26

Therapeutic Drugs for the Urinary System

OUTLINE

Anatomy and Physiology of the Urinary System
   Kidneys
   Functions of the Kidneys
   Hormones
Disorders of the Urinary System
   Renal Calculi
   Glomerulonephritis
   Renal Failure
   Diabetic Nephropathy
   Neurogenic Bladder
   Urinary Tract Infections

OBJECTIVES

Upon completion of this chapter, the reader should be able to:

1. Describe the structures of the urinary system.
2. Explain the functions of the urinary system.
3. Describe glomerular filtration, tubular secretion, and tubular reabsorption.
4. Explain hormones that affect the nephron.
5. Describe the complications of type 1 diabetes mellitus in the urinary system.
6. Explain acute glomerulonephritis.
7. Describe the treatment of renal failure.
8. Explain the causes of neurogenic bladder.
9. Name two examples of trade names of thiazide and loop diuretics.
10. Describe the most common cause of urinary tract infections.

KEY TERMS

angiotensinogen	**glomerulus**	**renal corpuscle**	**renin**
detrusor muscle	**hematuria**	**renal tubule**	**uremia**
erythropoietin	**lithotripsy**		

Overview

The urinary system functions in the production, storage, and excretion of urine. Together, these processes maintain homeostasis and prevent the body from becoming toxic. The urinary system cleanses the blood of the waste products of metabolism. It regulates water, salts, and acids in body fluids. The kidneys produce urine as well as play a role in regulating systemic blood pressure. The accessory structures of the urinary system transport and store urine in the bladder until it is voluntarily excreted through the urethra.

Anatomy and Physiology of the Urinary System

The urinary system consists of two kidneys, two ureters, the urinary bladder, and the urethra. One of the most important functions of the urinary system is filtration, which removes waste products from the blood. Removal of these waste materials results in the production and excretion of urine from the body. Each kidney contains approximately 1 million microscopic nephrons, which are the actual units of kidney function. They conduct the processes of filtration, reabsorption, and secretion of urine. Urine is then transported to the renal pelvis, and on to the ureters. Other functions of the kidneys include secretion of **renin**, which raises blood pressure, and **erythropoietin**, a hormone that stimulates red blood cell production as well as helps in activating vitamin D.

Urinary system function is often evaluated by urinalysis and blood tests. When normal, the urinary system conducts filtration, absorption, and elimination of metabolic wastes while balancing fluids and electrolytes. Tests for urinary disorders include culture and sensitivity tests for the use of proper antibiotics, radiologic tests for structural abnormalities, *cystoscopy* for internal examination of the bladder and urethra, and biopsy of lesions.

KIDNEYS

The kidneys are the most important excretory organs, removing a large amount of dissolved wastes from the body. The kidneys are vital for regulating the normal chemical composition of the blood. The two kidneys are positioned on either side of the vertebral column. The right kidney is lower than the left because of the location of the liver.

A renal artery serves each kidney, entering at the indented portion. Filtered blood then leaves the kidneys via the renal veins, draining into the inferior vena cava and flowing back to the heart. The wastes that are extracted from the blood are eliminated in the urine, which is made up of water, nitrogenous wastes, hormones, ions, and various other substances. The renal cortex contains many filtering nephrons. The inner portion of each kidney is the renal medulla (see Figure 26-1).

Nephrons

A kidney contains about 1 million microscopic nephrons. Most nephrons are located in the cortex. Each nephron consists of a **renal corpuscle** and a **renal tubule** (see Figure 26-2).

A renal corpuscle is composed of a cluster of blood capillaries called a **glomerulus**. Glomerular capillaries filter fluid, which is the first step in urine formation. The renal tubule leads away from the glomerular capsule and coils into a portion called the proximal convoluted tubule. The next section of this tubule is the descending limb of Henle, which bends into a U-shaped structure known as the loop of Henle. From the loop of the Henle, the tubule ascends to the distal convoluted tubule. The renal tubule ends by merging with a large, straight collecting duct, also called a collecting tubule. Urine is transported to the urinary bladder via the ureters, and the bladder stores the urine. The bladder opens into each ureter as well as the urethra, meaning that it has three openings. The openings outline a smooth triangular region known as the *trigone*, which is a common site of bladder infections. There are three layers of smooth muscle in the bladder, which form the **detrusor muscle**. The anatomy of the urinary bladder in a male is shown in Figure 26-3.

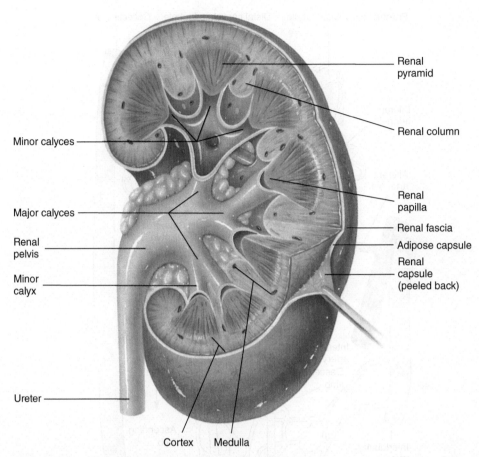

Figure 26-1 The internal anatomy of a kidney.

FUNCTIONS OF THE KIDNEYS

The primary functions of the kidneys include glomerular filtration, tubular reabsorption, and tubular secretion. Large amounts of blood are filtered by the nephrons. From this, 1 to 2 L of urine are produced every day, based on the quantity of fluids consumed. Substances filtered by the nephrons include water, sodium, glucose, waste products such as urea, and phenol. Blood filtration includes the processes of glomerular filtration, tubular reabsorption, and tubular secretion (see Figure 26-4).

Glomerular Filtration

Glomerular filtration is the first step of blood purification, and it is relatively simple. When blood flows through the glomerular capillaries, the capillary walls filter water and dissolved materials that it contains. This liquid forms the glomerular filtrate, which travels through the inner layer of the Bowman's capsule. Because of the barrier formed by this structure, red blood cells and larger proteins cannot escape. The filtrate then passes to the proximal convoluted tubule, loop of Henle, and distal convoluted tubule.

POINTS TO REMEMBER

The glomerular filtration rate (GFR) is the best estimate of kidney function. It estimates how much blood passes through the glomeruli every minute.

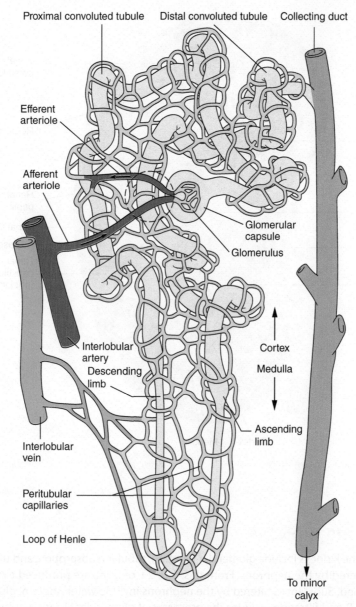

Figure 26-2 The anatomy of a nephron, the functional unit of a kidney.

Tubular Reabsorption

Most fluid filtered by the glomeruli is reabsorbed from the renal tubule back to the bloodstream. Tubular reabsorption describes this movement of water, molecules, and ions from the renal tubule to the bloodstream. It mostly occurs in the proximal convoluted tubule. Water, important nutrients, and ions leave the renal tubule to enter the capillary networks surrounding the nephrons. These capillaries branch from the efferent arterioles and soon empty into the renal veins to return nutrients to the body. Tubular reabsorption conserves water, ions, and nutrients that may have been filtered out in the glomerulus. Waste products such as urea and uric acid stay in the glomerular filtrate to be excreted in the urine. Tubular reabsorption assists in the control of blood pH. Because of tubular reabsorption, of the 45 gallons (180 L) of filtrate produced daily in the glomeruli, only about 1% actually leaves the kidneys as urine.

Tubular Secretion

Tubular secretion is the next step in blood purification, in which wastes are removed from the blood. These are primarily the wastes that were not filtered in the glomeruli. Unfiltered blood leaves the glomeruli via the efferent arterioles, flowing into the peritubular capillaries around the nephrons. Some wastes move through the capillary

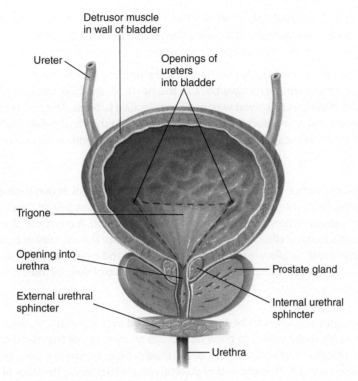

Figure 26-3 The anatomy of the urinary bladder in a male.

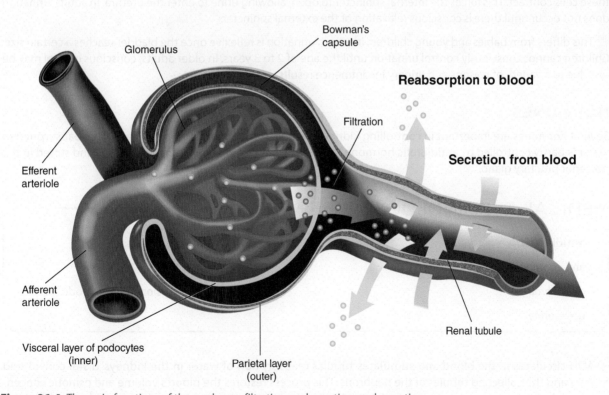

Figure 26-4 The main functions of the nephrons: filtration, reabsorption, and secretion.

walls into the nephron; this is the actual definition of tubular secretion and occurs in the distal convoluted tubule. This process also helps regulate the hydrogen concentrations of the blood. If the blood is excessively acidic, hydrogen ions move from the blood into the urine to reduce the acidity.

Through this process and others previously outlined, blood emptying into the renal vein is highly cleansed. This blood then moves through the inferior vena cava back to the heart. Meanwhile, the urine leaving the nephrons is made up mostly of water and various dissolved wastes. The collecting tubules descend through the renal medulla, converge, and form the larger collecting ducts. These ducts empty into the renal pelvis. During this part of the process, much of any remaining water escapes by osmosis to concentrate the urine further and conserve body water.

Micturition

In micturition, also known as urination or voiding, the bladder expels urine. This action is caused by both involuntary and voluntary nerve impulses. Since the average capacity of the bladder is about 500 mL, once it reaches 200 to 400 mL of urine, its stretch receptors transmit nerve impulses to the lower spinal cord. A conscious desire to urinate is initiated, along with an unconscious micturition reflex. During urination, the detrusor muscle contracts along with the muscles of the pelvic floor and abdominal wall. To allow urine to leave the bladder and move through the urethra to the outside of the body, the external urinary sphincter must relax. This muscle is made up of skeletal muscle surrounding the urethra.

Urine Control

The kidneys, moving through the ureters to be temporarily stored in the urinary bladder, continuously produce urine. Two sphincters act as muscular valves to prevent leakage of urine out of the bladder. The first is the internal sphincter, made up of the smooth muscle in the neck of the urinary bladder where it joins the urethra. The second is the external sphincter, made up of a flattened band of skeletal muscle that forms the floor of the pelvic cavity. When both sphincters relax, the urine is pushed into the urethra to exit the body.

When urine accumulates in the bladder and reaches between 200 and 300 mL, urination is stimulated. Stretch receptors in the bladder detect distention and send impulses over the sensory nerves to the spinal cord, stimulating additional nerve cells. The impulses travel along nerves terminating on the muscle cells of the bladder wall, and these cells contract. This forces the internal sphincter to open, allowing urine to enter the urethra. In adults, urination does not occur until there is conscious relaxation of the external sphincter.

This differs from babies and young children, in whom urination is reflexive once the bladder reaches a certain size. Children cannot consciously control urination until the age of 2 to 3 years. In older adults, conscious control may be lost due to a variety of reasons and urinary incontinence results.

HORMONES

Several hormones are important in controlling kidney function and maintaining homeostasis. The reabsorption of water is partly controlled by antidiuretic hormone (ADH), which is released by the hypothalamus and stored in the posterior pituitary gland.

MEDICAL TERMINOLOGY REVIEW

antidiuretic:

anti- = *against*

di- = *through*

ur- = *urine*

-etic = *pertaining to*

pertaining to suppression of urine production

ADH circulates in the blood and stimulates tubular reabsorption of water in the kidneys' distal convoluted tubules and the collecting tubules of the nephrons. This process restores the blood's volume and osmotic concentration, unless a person is excessively dehydrated. Conversely, excessive intake of water increases blood volume and decreases osmotic concentration, causing a reduction in ADH secretion. Falling ADH levels in the blood decrease tubular reabsorption, and more water is lost through the urine. Therefore, blood volume and osmotic concentration are restored, and urine output is increased.

The second important hormone that helps to regulate water balance is aldosterone. This steroid hormone is produced by the adrenal glands. Two factors control aldosterone levels in the plasma: blood pressure, and the volume of fluid inside the nephrons. A decrease in blood pressure and filtrate volume in the nephrons causes certain kidney cells to produce renin, an enzyme. Once in the bloodstream, renin comes into contact with **angiotensinogen**, a large plasma protein produced by the liver. Renin removes a segment of angiotensinogen to produce angiotensin I, a small peptide molecule. This inactive molecule is required to be converted to an active form, which is known as angiotensin II. The conversion is achieved by enzymes found when the blood flows through the lungs.

Aldosterone secretion is stimulated by angiotensin II. The aldosterone circulates in the bloodstream, and upon reaching the kidneys, stimulates nephron cells to increase sodium reabsorption. Since water follows sodium, it moves out of the nephrons into the peritubular capillaries, increasing blood volume and blood pressure, to shut down this feedback loop. The kidneys, by themselves, secrete erythropoietin, which stimulates red blood cell formation in the red bone marrow.

POINTS TO REMEMBER

Aldosterone is the most potent hormone regulating the body's electrolyte balance. It also partially regulates water absorption, since water follows sodium transport.

WHAT WOULD YOU DO?

A patient who has only one functioning kidney is prescribed a sulfonamide by a new physician. About to process the prescription, you carefully check the patient record and confirm that most sulfonamides can damage the filtering units of the kidneys. Since the patient only has one functioning kidney, what would you do?

Disorders of the Urinary System

The urinary system produces, stores, and eliminates urine from the body. It is composed of the kidneys, ureters, bladder, and urethra. Renal disorders include calculi, glomerulonephritis, renal failure, diabetic nephropathy, neurogenic bladder, and urinary tract infections.

RENAL CALCULI

Renal calculi, commonly known as kidney stones, are usually made up of calcium salts and other substances. Kidney stones may be of various sizes and numbers and may be found in different locations (see Figure 26-5). They are more common in males than in females, usually occurring between the ages of 30 and 50 years. Though usually of unknown cause, precipitating factors include chronic urinary tract infections, dehydration, immobility, or prolonged bed rest. Extended immobility causes the bones to release calcium, which may form kidney stones. Less common causes include hyperparathyroidism, gout, severe bone disease, and other metabolic disorders.

Signs and symptoms of kidney stones include **hematuria** and renal or urinary colic, which is severe, spasmodic pain in the flanks due to contractions in a ureter that is obstructed. It is often more severe than any other type of pain. Treatment of an acute attack of renal calculi includes analgesics and increased fluid intake to help pass the stone. Sometimes, the urine is strained in a filter to catch the stone so that it can be identified. Stones are usually as

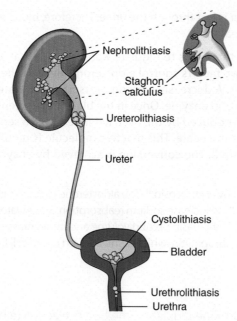

Figure 26-5 Types and location of renal calculi.

small as a grain of salt or as large as a small piece of rice, yet still are able to cause severe pain. Total obstruction of the urinary tract requires emergency surgery so that kidney damage can be prevented. One technique is the stone basket procedure; it involves passing a retrieval instrument through the urethra, bladder, and ureter to remove the stone. Another technique, called **lithotripsy**, involves exposure to external shock waves while the patient is placed in a tub of water. The shock waves break the stones into smaller pieces so that they will either pass or can be retrieved.

POINTS TO REMEMBER

The tendency to form kidney stones is inherited, particularly for stones that contain calcium, which account for more than half of all cases.

POINTS TO REMEMBER

Lithotripsy fragments and disintegrates kidney stones by using a high-voltage spark or an electromagnetic impulse outside of the body. This focuses the shock waves on the kidney stones.

WHAT WOULD YOU DO?

Calcium stones are the most common type of kidney stone. You notice that your father has been prescribed allopurinol because he has a calcium kidney stone. Knowing that this medication is designed to prevent kidney stones made of uric acid, not calcium, what would you do?

GLOMERULONEPHRITIS

Glomerulonephritis is a bilateral inflammation of the glomeruli (capillary tufts in the kidney nephrons). Typically this occurs after a streptococcal infection, and acute glomerulonephritis is sometimes called acute poststreptococcal glomerulonephritis. Glomerulonephritis can also be idiopathic, or it may be caused by an immune reaction that produces circulating antigen-antibody complexes that become trapped in the glomerular capillaries. The antigen may be linked to the presence of a tumor. The glomerular injury decreases blood filtration rates, causing water and salts to be retained.

Acute glomerulonephritis is most common in boys between ages 3 and 7 years. Most cases resolve within two weeks, and the patient experiences a spontaneous recovery. Chronic glomerulonephritis is a slowly progressive, noninfectious disease that may result in irreversible renal damage and renal failure. This form of glomerulonephritis is often linked to immune reactions, though primary renal disorders and multisystem diseases such as systemic lupus erythematosus may be implicated.

Signs and symptoms of acute glomerulonephritis include proteinuria, hypertension, edema, and decreased urine volume. Hematuria may be slight or severe, but often the urine is dark or coffee colored. No specific therapy is available if the condition is post-streptococcal, except for administration of antibiotics. Diuretics may control edema and hypertension. Sodium intake is restricted, and sometimes corticosteroids are administered if there is a suspected immune reaction.

Signs and symptoms of chronic glomerulonephritis include hypertension, hematuria, oliguria, proteinuria, edema, and azotemia (high levels of nitrogen-containing compounds in the blood). Treatment is aimed at controlling edema and hypertension while preventing uremia and congestive heart failure. Medications include antihypertensives, diuretics, and if needed, antibiotics. Dietary restriction of protein, salt, and fluid intake may be required. To reduce excess protein in the urine, angiotensin-converting enzyme (ACE) inhibitors may be administered. In some cases, the patient requires dialysis or kidney transplantation. Table 26-1 summarizes examples of diuretics.

Table 26-1 Examples of Diuretics

Generic Name	Trade Name	Route of Administration	Average Adult Dosage
Thiazide Diuretics			
chlorothiazide	Diuril®	PO, IV	500 to 1000 mg once or twice daily
chlorthalidone	Thalitone®	PO	Initial dose: 50 to 100 mg/day; Maint: 25 to 100 mg/day or 50 to 200 mg every other day
metolazone	Zaroxolyn	PO	2.5 to 10 mg/day (maximum 20 mg daily)
Loop Diuretics			
bumetanide	Bumex®	PO	0.5 to 2 mg/day
ethacrynic acid	Edecrin®	PO	50 to 100 mg on continuous or intermittent dosage schedule; dosage adjustments are usually in 25 to 50 mg increments to avoid fluid and electrolyte imbalances
furosemide	Lasix®	PO	20 to 80 mg as a single dose; may be repeated in 6 to 8 hours, or dose may be increased by 20 to 40 mg; after this, determined dose should be given once or twice daily no shorter than 6 hours apart (maximum 600 mg/day)
torsemide	Demadex®	PO	10 to 20 mg once daily (maximum 200 mg/day)
Potassium-Sparing Diuretics			
amiloride	Midamor®	PO	5 to 10 mg 1 to 2 times/day (maximum 20 mg daily)
spironolactone	Aldactone®	PO	After dosage testing, initial daily dose: 100 mg in one to two doses, with average range 25 to 200 mg/day
triamterene	Dyrenium®	PO	100 mg bid after meals (maximum 300 mg/day)
Carbonic Anhydrase Inhibitors			
dichlorphenamide	Keveyis®	PO	50 mg bid (maximum 200 mg/day)
methazolamide	Methazolamide®	PO	50 to 100 mg bid or tid

RENAL FAILURE

Acute renal failure is a sudden interruption of renal function. It can be caused by obstruction, poor circulation, or underlying kidney disease. The condition is usually reversible with treatment. If not treated, it may progress to end-stage renal disease, characterized by **uremia**, and death. Acute renal failure may occur over a period of hours to days.

Signs and symptoms of acute renal failure begin with gastrointestinal disturbances, headache, oliguria, drowsiness, and other alterations of consciousness. Additional symptoms may develop based on underlying causes, blood-urea-nitrogen (BUN) levels, and the amount of impairment that exists. Treatment focuses on the underlying cause, with the overall goal being to reverse the decreased renal perfusion. Monitoring of all body systems is critical, and the patient should be evaluated to determine if dialysis is appropriate. Fluid intake and output are controlled, and nutritional support focuses on protein balance in order to prevent metabolic acidosis. This means that a high-carbohydrate/low-protein diet should be administered. Sodium and potassium intake are also controlled. Medications include antihypertensives, anti-infective agents, and diuretics.

Chronic renal failure is usually the end result of gradual tissue destruction and loss of renal function. It can also result from a rapidly progressing disease of sudden onset that destroys the nephrons, causing irreversible kidney damage. Either type of renal failure will lead to accumulation of water and toxic wastes, causing death within two to three days, with death actually occurring from concentration of potassium ions. Excessive potassium causes the heart to go into fibrillation.

Signs and symptoms of chronic renal failure include weakness, tiredness, and lethargy. Hypertension and edema then develop, followed by arrhythmias, dyspnea, muscle weakness, metabolic acidosis, hair and skin changes, and ulceration of the gastrointestinal mucosa. Treatment focuses on the underlying causes, and often includes dialysis. Some patients may be candidates for kidney transplantation. Diet and nutritional changes are indicated, and fluid intake and output are regulated. Medications include antihypertensives, diuretics, anti-infective agents, and antiemetics. If severe anemia develops, erythropoietin is given to help form new red blood cells. If bone degeneration is present, vitamin D supplementation may be used. Care is basically supportive, to provide patient comfort.

POINTS TO REMEMBER

Renal failure, in its end stages, results in reduction of kidney function to less than 10% of normal. As wastes and toxins accumulate in the blood, the patient becomes confused or delirious, drowsy, lethargic, numb, and eventually unresponsive.

MEDICATION ERROR ALERT

Acute renal failure may be caused by high doses of nonsteroidal anti-inflammatory drugs. An example is a 20-day-old infant who received a 10-mg/kg dose of indomethacin after surgery for Fallot's tetralogy. This dose is 50 to 100 times higher than the therapeutic dose for an infant. The child presented with acute renal failure requiring continuous hemodialysis to restore normal renal function.

DIABETIC NEPHROPATHY

Diabetic nephropathy involves renal changes referred to as glomerulosclerosis, which is an eventual development in all patients with type 1 diabetes as well as many patients with type 2 disease. Lesions of the glomeruli cause the GFR to decrease over time, influenced by insufficient control of blood glucose levels and blood pressure.

Signs and symptoms of diabetic nephropathy include hypertension, urinary retention, nausea, and proteinuria. Complications include urinary tract infections. The disorder is irreversible, and treatment plans are individualized based on each patient's susceptibility to renal failure. Infections must be treated promptly. Medications for diabetic nephropathy include ACE inhibitors and diuretics. Fluid intake and output must be balanced, and the diet should contain low amounts of proteins and fats. The patient should be evaluated for dialysis or kidney transplantation.

MEDICATION ERROR ALERT

Medication errors occur frequently in treatment of patients with diabetic nephropathy and other forms of renal insufficiency. Serious adverse events may occur. Various risk factors may affect the susceptibility of patients with renal dysfunction to drug toxicity. The use of computerized systems has decreased the frequency of adverse events resulting from medication errors in patients with these renal conditions.

NEUROGENIC BLADDER

Neurogenic bladder is a dysfunction of urinary bladder control that results in difficulty emptying the bladder or urinary incontinence. It may develop because of damage to the brain, spinal cord, or nerves that supply the lower urinary tract. Damage may be the result of cerebrovascular accident, spinal cord trauma, neuropathies, tumors, herniated lumbar disks, poliomyelitis, myelomeningocele, or spinal cord lesions.

Signs and symptoms of neurogenic bladder vary, based on the underlying causes. Patients may report hesitancy, decreased volume of the urine stream, urinary retention, sensation of fullness, slight incontinence, lack of sensation, uncontrolled bladder contractions, and spontaneous voiding. Neurogenic bladder can result in renal failure. Patients with autonomous neurogenic bladder are unable to void without the application of pressure to the suprapubic area. Treatment focuses on preventing urinary tract infections and restoring as much normal function as possible. Various types of catheterization are used. In specific cases, medications include parasympathomimetic (anti-muscarinic) agents (see Table 26-2). Surgery and external collection devices may also be used.

Table 26-2 Examples of Anticholinergics (Anti-muscarinics) Used for Incontinence

Generic Name	Trade Name	Route of Administration	Average Adult Dosage
darifenacin	Enablex®	PO	7.5 to 15 mg once daily, with water
fesoterodine	Toviaz®	PO	4 to 8 mg once daily
oxybutynin	Ditropan®	PO	2.5 to 5 mg bid to tid (maximum 5 mg qid)
	Ditropan XL®	PO	5 to 10 mg/day, adjusted in 5 mg increments (maximum 30 mg/day)
	Oxytrol®	Transdermal patch	Apply q3 to 4d, changing sites
	Gelnique®	Topical gel	Apply one packet (84 mg) once daily, changing sites
solifenacin	Vesicare®	PO	5 to 10 mg once daily
tolterodine	Detrol®	PO	1 to 2 mg bid
	Detrol LA®		2 to 4 mg once/day, with water
trospium	Sanctura®	PO	20 mg bid on an empty stomach
	Sanctura XR®		60 mg every morning, with water, on an empty stomach

POINTS TO REMEMBER

Neurogenic bladder, in the United States, is most commonly linked to multiple sclerosis (40% to 90%), Parkinson's disease (37% to 72%), and stroke (15%).

MEDICATION ERROR ALERT

A patient brought a prescription for the diuretic *metolazone*, 2.5 mg/day, to his or her community pharmacy. The pharmacy technician misread the name as *methotrexate*, which is an antimetabolite. Fortunately, the Drug Utilization Review (DUR) step in the computer program displayed an alert message to verify the drug name again and displayed dosing information about methotrexate, which was very different to the prescribed dosage. If this error had gone undetected, the patient could have suffered ulcerations of the digestive tract, bone marrow suppression, hepatotoxicity, and even death.

WHAT WOULD YOU DO?

A patient was prescribed phenazopyridine, a urinary analgesic. You, the pharmacy technician, notice in the patient record that he or she is also taking leflunomide for his or her rheumatoid arthritis. There is a major drug interaction between these two agents. What would you do?

URINARY TRACT INFECTIONS

A urinary tract infection (UTI) may be of bacterial or fungal origin. It can occur anywhere in the urinary tract. The most common cause of a UTI is *Escherichia coli* (*E. coli*) that enters the urinary tract from the colon. *Urethritis* is an infection of the urethra. *Cystitis* is infection and inflammation of the bladder. *Pyelonephritis* is infection and inflammation of the kidney. Sexually transmitted diseases (STDs) are common causes of UTIs (Chapter 28). Risks for UTIs include a compromised immune system and diabetes mellitus, because of elevated urine glucose. Symptoms are varied. They include a painful burning sensation during urination, fever, and lack of urine output, cloudy or bloody urine, nausea, vomiting, and sometimes, confusion. Medications used to treat UTIs are summarized in Table 26-3.

Table 26-3 Examples of Antibiotics and Urinary Analgesics Used for Urinary Tract Infections

Generic Name	Trade Name	Route of Administration	Average Adult Dosage
Antibiotics			
Sulfonamides with Trimethoprim			
sulfamethoxazole/ trimethoprim	Septra DS®, Bactrim DS®	PO	160 to 800 mg (one double-strength tablet) q12h for 10 to 14 days
Penicillins			
amoxicillin	Amoxil®	PO	500 to 875 mg q12h or 250 to 500 mg q8h
Penicillin and Beta-Lactamase Inhibitor Combination			
amoxicillin/clavulanate	Augmentin®	PO	500 to 875 mg q12h or 250 to 500 mg q8h
Penicillin and Aminoglycoside Combination			
ampicillin/gentamicin	Omnipen + Garamycin®	IV	1 to 2 g ampicillin q6h with 1.5 mg/kg gentamicin q8h

(Continued)

Table 26-3 Examples of Antibiotics and Urinary Analgesics Used for Urinary Tract Infections *(Continued)*

Generic Name	Trade Name	Route of Administration	Average Adult Dosage
First-Generation Cephalosporins			
cephalexin	Keflex®	PO	1 to 4 g/day in divided doses (usually, 250 mg q6h)
cefadroxil	Duricef®	PO	1 to 2 g/day in one or two doses
Second-Generation Cephalosporins			
cefaclor	Ceclor®	PO	250 to 500 mg q8h for 3 to 10 days
cefuroxime	Ceftin®	PO	250 mg bid for 7 to 10 days
loracarbef	Lorabid®	PO	200 mg q24h for 7 days, or 400 mg q12h for 14 days
Third-Generation Cephalosporins			
cefpodoxime	Vantin®	PO	100 mg q12h for 7 days
ceftriaxone	Rocephin®	IV or IM	1 to 2 g once or in divided doses bid (maximum 4 g/day)
Fluoroquinolones			
ciprofloxacin	Cipro®	PO	250 mg bid for three days
levofloxacin	Levaquin®	PO	250 mg once daily for three days
norfloxacin	Noroxin®	PO	400 mg q12h for 3 to 21 days prn
ofloxacin	Floxin®	PO	200 mg q12h for 10 days
Nitrofurantoins			
nitrofurantoin	Macrodantin®	PO	50 to 100 mg q6h
nitrofurantoin	Macrobid®	PO	100 mg q12h for seven days
Tetracyclines			
tetracycline	Sumycin®	PO	250 to 500 mg q6h (maximum 2 g/day)
doxycycline	Vibramycin®	PO	100 mg q12h for first day, then 100 mg/day
minocycline	Minocin®	PO	Initial dose: 200 mg, followed by 100 mg q12h
demeclocycline	Declomycin®	PO	150 mg qid or 300 mg bid
Miscellaneous Antibiotics			
fosfomycin	Monurol®	PO	3 g (dissolve one sachet) × one dose
trimethoprim	Trimpex®	PO	100 mg q12h or 200 mg/day, for 10 days
Urinary Analgesics			
flavoxate	Urispas®	PO	1 to 2 (100 mg each) tablets tid to qid
methenamine	Urised®	PO	1 tablet or capsule
phenazopyridine	Pyridium®	PO	qid (tablets of various mg available) 190 to 200 mg tid after meals; do not administer for more than two days if used with a urinary antibacterial drug

Summary

The urinary system consists of two kidneys, two ureters, the urinary bladder, and the urethra. The kidneys are the most important excretory organs, removing a large amount of dissolved wastes from the body, and are vital for regulating the normal chemical composition of the blood. The renal cortex of each kidney contains millions of filtering nephrons, which are made up of renal corpuscles and tubules. Urine produced by the nephrons flows out of the kidneys through the ureters, which transport it to the urinary bladder. The bladder is made up of smooth muscles that stretch as it fills with urine. Its walls then contract to force urine out through the urethra, a thin tube that differs in length between males and females.

The nephrons filter large amounts of blood to produce between 1 and 2 L of urine every day. There are three steps in blood purification: glomerular filtration, tubular reabsorption, and tubular secretion. Hormones that are important in controlling kidney function and maintaining homeostasis include antidiuretic hormone (ADH) and aldosterone.

Disorders of the urinary system are many, but this chapter discusses only renal calculi, glomerulonephritis, renal failure, diabetic nephropathy, neurogenic bladder, and urinary tract infections. Medications used to treat urinary system disorders include diuretics, antibiotics, analgesics, and anticholinergics.

REVIEW QUESTIONS

1. The outermost layer of kidney tissue is the:

    A. renal pelvis.
    B. renal medulla.
    C. renal cortex.
    D. major calyx.

2. Which of the following is not a treatment for renal failure?

    A. Diuretics
    B. Antihypertensives
    C. Corticosteroids
    D. Dialysis

3. The portion of the nephron that attaches to the collecting duct is the:

    A. minor calyx.
    B. distal convoluted tubule.
    C. loop of Henle.
    D. proximal convoluted tubule.

4. When the level of antidiuretic hormone increases:

    A. more salt is secreted by the nephrons.
    B. more urine is produced.
    C. less urine is produced.
    D. less water is reabsorbed by the kidneys.

5. The filtration of blood is primarily the function of the:

    A. renal corpuscle.
    B. loop of Henle.
    C. distal convoluted tubule.
    D. collecting duct.

6. How many liters of filtrate are produced by the kidneys every day?

    A. 50 L
    B. 80 L
    C. 150 L
    D. 180 L

7. Which of the following hormones is secreted by the kidneys?

   A. Estrogen
   B. Erythropoietin
   C. Aldosterone
   D. Antidiuretic hormone

8. Which of the following is the trade name of flavoxate?

   A. Urispas
   B. Urised
   C. Pyridium
   D. Trimpex

9. Which of the following is the first step of blood purification?

   A. Tubular reabsorption
   B. Micturition
   C. Glomerular filtration
   D. Tubular secretion

10. Which of the following disorders of the kidney is an eventual development of type 1 diabetes?

    A. Glomerulonephritis
    B. Glomerulosclerosis
    C. Renal calculi
    D. Neurogenic bladder

11. All of the following disorders may cause neurogenic bladder, *except*:

    A. stroke.
    B. spinal cord trauma.
    C. poliomyelitis.
    D. cystitis.

12. Thalitone® is the trade name of:

    A. chlorthalidone.
    B. ethacrynic acid.
    C. furosemide.
    D. spironolactone.

13. The most common cause of acute glomerulonephritis is:

    A. *Bordetella pertussis.*
    B. *Haemophilus influenzae.*
    C. streptococci.
    D. *Klebsiella.*

14. Which disorder of the kidney requires antihypertensive drugs?

    A. Glomerulonephritis
    B. Neurogenic bladder
    C. Renal calculi
    D. Polycystic kidney

15. Which of the following is the most common cause of urinary tract infections?

    A. Staphylococci
    B. Streptococci
    C. Pneumococci
    D. *E. coli*

CRITICAL THINKING

A 62-year-old woman who has been diagnosed with diabetes has been suffering from renal failure.

1. Which part of the urinary system is affected by diabetes?

2. What is the treatment of renal failure?

WEB LINKS

American Association of Kidney Patients: aakp.org

American Kidney Fund: www.kidneyfund.org

American Society of Nephrology: www.asn-online.org

Kidney Cancer Association: www.kidneycancer.org

National Kidney Foundation: www.kidney.org

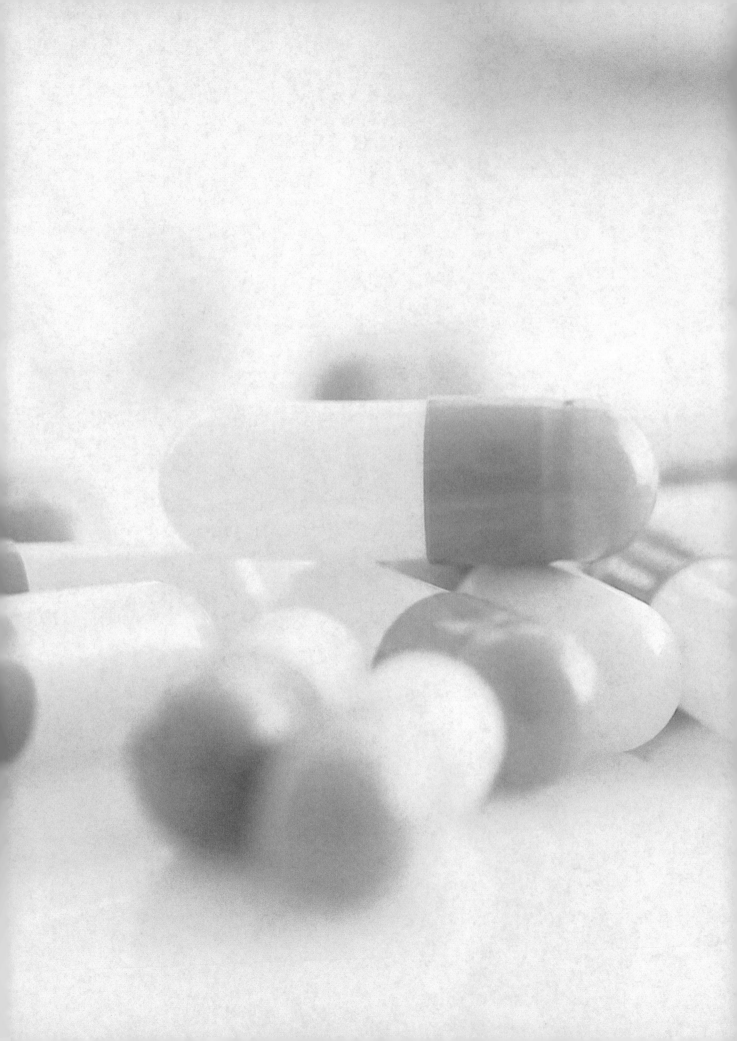

CHAPTER 27

Therapeutic Drugs for the Digestive System

OUTLINE

OBJECTIVES

Upon completion of this chapter, the reader should be able to:

1. Describe the general functions of the digestive system.
2. List the accessory organs of the digestive system.
3. Describe the three portions of the small intestine.
4. Explain the links between *Helicobacter pylori* and peptic ulcer.
5. Define gastroesophageal reflux disease (GERD) and its treatments.
6. Explain the common symptoms of Crohn's disease and its treatments.
7. Describe constipation and its treatments.
8. Compare colorectal cancer and liver cancer.

9. Name three trade names of proton pump inhibitors.

10. Name four examples of histamine (H₂) receptor antagonists.

KEY TERMS

cation	hemochromatosis	jejunum	pyloric sphincter
duodenum	hepatopancreatic ampulla	mesocolon	rugae
enamel	ileocecal sphincter	pepsin	toxemia
falciform ligament	ileum	pepsinogen	uvula
gallbladder	intrinsic factor	peristalsis	viremia
haustra	jaundice	peritonitis	

Overview

The digestive system comprises the alimentary canal, which is also referred to as the digestive tract, and the accessory organs of digestion. It regulates the ingestion, digestion, and absorption of nutrients. The accessory digestive organs are located outside the gastrointestinal (GI) tract, and they produce and secrete endocrine and exocrine enzymes. The purpose of the digestive system is to break down (digest) food into particles that are small and simple enough to be absorbed. Disorders of the digestive system affect ingestion and digestion of food, absorption of nutrients, and elimination of wastes. As a result, a variety of abnormalities may develop, including inflammation, tissue erosion, benign and malignant tumors, infection, interference with blood or nerve supplies, obstructions, malnutrition, and malabsorption.

Anatomy and Physiology of the Digestive System

The digestive system ingests food, digests it, absorbs the end products of digestion, and eliminates waste. The digestive system consists of the digestive tract (several organs) and accessory glands of digestion. It contains the digestive tube of the body through which food passes from the mouth to the esophagus, stomach, and intestines. The accessory glands include the salivary glands, liver, gallbladder, and pancreas (see Figure 27-1).

ORAL CAVITY

The oral cavity is also called the mouth or the buccal cavity. It is formed on the sides by the cheeks, on its roof by the hard and soft palates, and on its floor by the tongue (see Figure 27-2). From the posterior border hangs the cone-shaped **uvula**, which aids in swallowing, preventing food from backing up into the nasopharynx.

SALIVARY GLANDS

Three pairs of large salivary glands are responsible for most saliva secretion: the parotid, submandibular, and sublingual glands. They are located outside the oral cavity, and the saliva they produce travels through ducts that empty into the mouth (see Figure 27-3). A small amount of saliva is also released into the oral cavity from buccal glands lining the mouth. Saliva functions to dissolve foods. It contains amylase, which begins breaking down complex carbohydrates into simple sugars.

ESOPHAGUS

The esophagus is a muscular and collapsible tube. It secretes mucus and moves food to the stomach, but not to absorb any food or produce digestive enzymes. Muscle contractions collectively referred to as **peristalsis** push food through the esophagus in continuous, wave-like motions (see Figure 27-4).

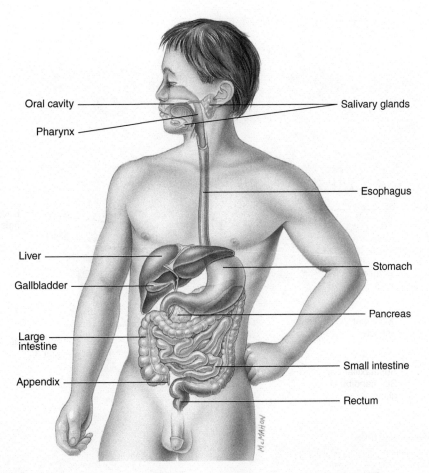

Oral cavity

Pharynx

Salivary glands

Esophagus

Liver

Gallbladder

Large intestine

Appendix

Stomach

Pancreas

Small intestine

Rectum

Figure 27-1 The digestive system.

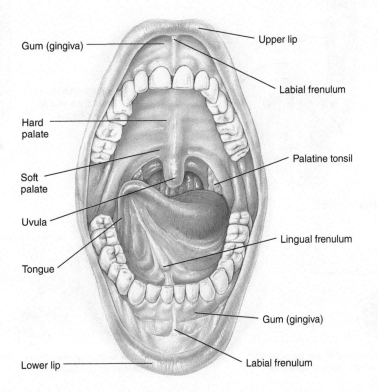

Gum (gingiva)

Upper lip

Labial frenulum

Hard palate

Soft palate

Uvula

Tongue

Palatine tonsil

Lingual frenulum

Gum (gingiva)

Lower lip

Labial frenulum

Figure 27-2 The tongue and oral cavity.

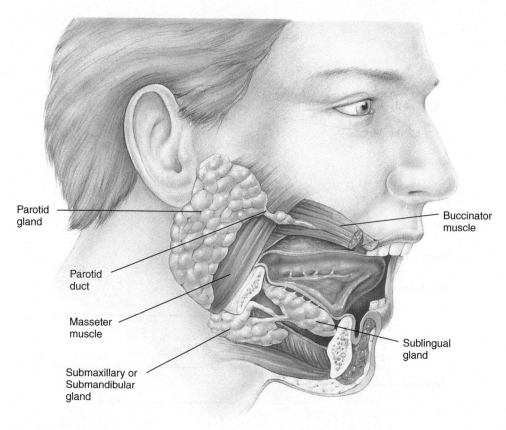

Figure 27-3 The salivary glands.

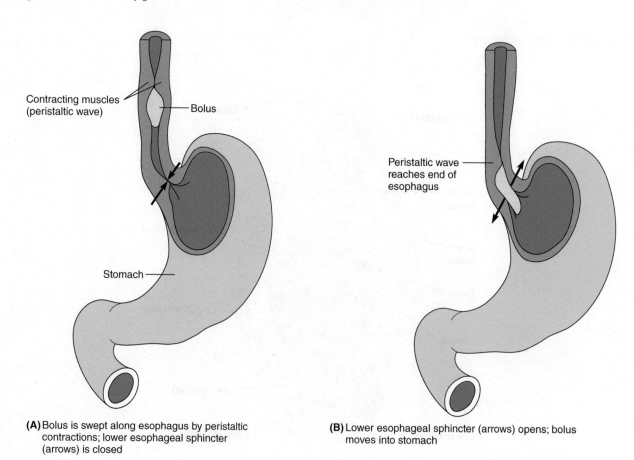

(A) Bolus is swept along esophagus by peristaltic contractions; lower esophageal sphincter (arrows) is closed

(B) Lower esophageal sphincter (arrows) opens; bolus moves into stomach

Figure 27-4 Food bolus passing from the esophagus into the stomach.

STOMACH

The stomach is able to stretch to accommodate a large amount of food. There are four parts of the stomach:

- *Cardia*—which surrounds the gastroesophageal sphincter

- *Fundus*—above and to the left of the cardia; it is a rounded area

- *Body*—below the fundus; it is the large central part of the stomach

- *Pylorus* (antrum)—the narrow inferior area connected, via the **pyloric sphincter**, with the **duodenum** of the small intestine

An empty stomach has large folds in its mucosa, which are called **rugae**. Filling of the stomach with food smoothes the rugae out until they actually disappear. There are many gastric glands in the stomach mucosa. They have three types of secreting cells (see Figure 27-5):

- *Chief cells*—which secrete the main gastric enzyme, **pepsinogen**

- *Parietal cells*—which secrete hydrochloric acid, activating pepsinogen to form **pepsin**, which begins the breakdown of proteins; the parietal cells also produce a glycoprotein known as **intrinsic factor**, which is required for the body's absorption of Vitamin B_{12}

- *Mucous cells*—which secrete mucus, protecting the stomach from digesting itself

Together, the secretions of these cells form gastric juice. There are three layers of the muscularis coat of the stomach: an outer longitudinal, a middle circular, and an inner oblique layer. They allow various types of stomach contractions to break up food into smaller pieces and mix it with gastric juice.

The stomach begins digesting proteins by utilizing secreted pepsin and hydrochloric acid. Because the hydrochloric acid of the stomach can cause erosion and ulcers, mucus is present to protect the stomach lining. Stomach contents then empty into the duodenum within 2 to 6 hours after being consumed. Carbohydrate-rich foods pass through the stomach first. Protein foods pass through next, since digestion of these foods starts in the stomach. Highly fatty foods pass through last. The stomach also absorbs some of the water and salts present in foods, as well as drugs such as aspirin and alcohol.

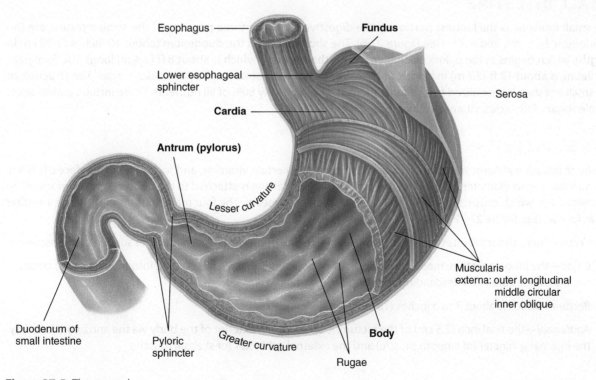

Figure 27-5 The stomach.

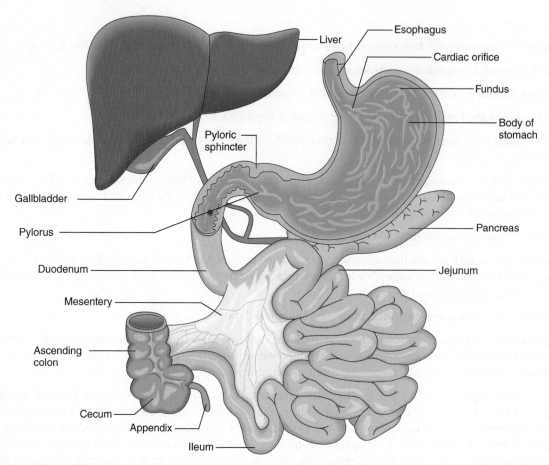

Figure 27-6 The small intestine.

SMALL INTESTINE

The small intestine is the longest portion of the digestive tract. The three portions of the small intestine are the duodenum, **jejunum**, and **ileum** (see Figure 27-6). The shortest part is the duodenum (about 10 inches or 25 cm in length), which begins at the pyloric sphincter. It joins the jejunum (which is about 8 ft [2.4 m] long). The final part, the ileum, is about 12 ft (3.7 m) in length, and it joins the large intestine via the **ileocecal sphincter**. The structure of the small intestine is specialized for the function of absorbing nearly 80% of all nutrients. These include amino acids, simple sugars, fatty acids, vitamins, minerals, and water.

LARGE INTESTINE

The large intestine absorbs water, absorbs and also produces certain vitamins, and forms and expels feces. It is 5 ft (1.5 m) long, and its diameter is 2.5 inches (6.4 cm). The large intestine is attached to the abdomen's posterior wall by the **mesocolon**, which consists of extensions of the visceral peritoneum. The four main sections of the large intestine are as follows (see Figure 27-7):

- *Cecum*—joins the small intestine via the ileocecal valve. The *appendix* is attached to the surface of the cecum

- *Colon*—the longest section, made up of consecutive pouches (**haustra**); it is divided into the ascending colon, the transverse colon, the descending colon, and the sigmoid colon

- *Rectum*—which is about 7 to 8 inches (18 to 20 cm) in length

- *Anal canal*—the final inch (2.5 cm) of the rectum; it opens to the exterior of the body via the anus, controlled by the internal sphincter (of smooth muscle) and the external sphincter (of skeletal muscle)

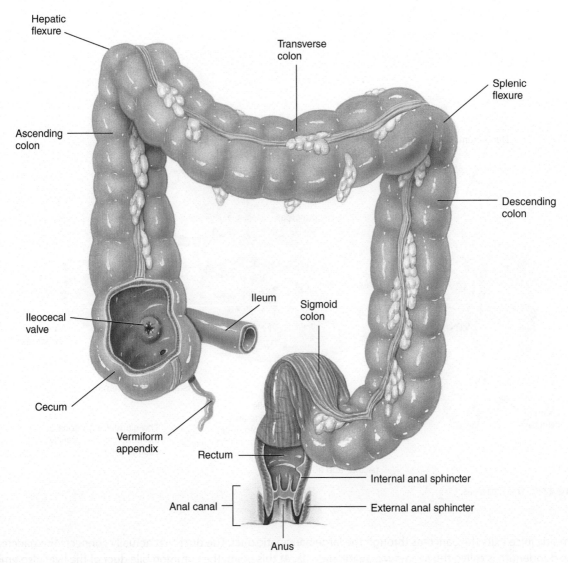

Figure 27-7 The large intestine.

Aside from extensive water absorption, the bacteria of the large intestine produce three important vitamins: K, biotin, and B$_5$. These are also absorbed by the large intestine, for various functions. Large intestinal glands also produce mucus.

POINTS TO REMEMBER

The large intestine houses more than 700 species of bacteria that perform many different functions.

ACCESSORY ORGANS

The accessory organs of the digestive system include the pancreas, liver, and gallbladder.

Pancreas

The pancreas lies beneath the stomach and is soft and oblong in shape. It is about 1 inch (2.5 cm) thick and 6 inches (15 cm) long. The pancreas is divided into a head, body, and tail (see Figure 27-8). The pancreas is made up of the islets of Langerhans. These islets secrete insulin and glucagon from beta and alpha cells. The *pancreatic acini* have exocrine functions. They release pancreatic juice, which consists of lipases, carbohydrases, proteases, and nucleases.

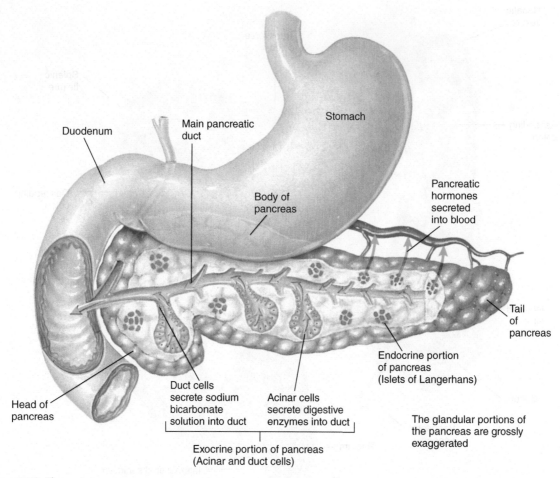

Duodenum

Main pancreatic duct

Stomach

Body of pancreas

Pancreatic hormones secreted into blood

Tail of pancreas

Endocrine portion of pancreas (Islets of Langerhans)

Duct cells secrete sodium bicarbonate solution into duct

Acinar cells secrete digestive enzymes into duct

The glandular portions of the pancreas are grossly exaggerated

Head of pancreas

Exocrine portion of pancreas (Acinar and duct cells)

Figure 27-8 The pancreas.

Pancreatic juice exits the pancreas through the large pancreatic duct. The duct that actually connects the pancreas to the duodenum is called the **hepatopancreatic ampulla**. At this point, the common bile duct of the liver also empties into the duodenum.

Liver

The liver is the largest gland in the body, and its basic functional unit is the *lobule*. The liver is an organ that performs over 500 functions. Among these functions, the liver produces bile to assist in digestion, metabolizes drugs, removes damaged blood cells from the circulation, stores and secretes glucose, and stores vitamins (A, D, E, and K), minerals (copper and iron), and fats and amino acids. It also synthesizes plasma proteins and clears the blood of toxic metabolic by-products. The liver is divided into two main lobes, which are separated by the **falciform ligament** (see Figure 27-9).

POINTS TO REMEMBER

The average adult liver is the heaviest organ in the body, weighing about 3 to 4 lb (1.4 to 1.8 kg).

Gallbladder

The **gallbladder** is located next to the liver. It is pear-shaped and is only about 3 to 4 inches (7.5 to 10 cm) in length. It acts as the storage place for bile, which it receives from the liver via the hepatic duct. The bile flows through the common bile duct to enter the duodenum. Obstruction of the cystic duct may lead to **jaundice**.

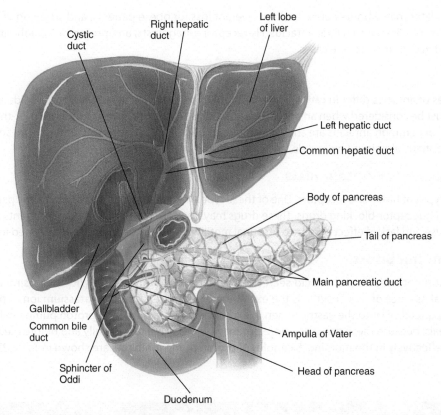

Figure 27-9 The liver.

Disorders of the Digestive System

The most common diseases and disorders of the gastrointestinal system include gastroesophageal reflux disease (GERD), peptic ulcers, Crohn's disease, diarrhea, constipation ulcerative colitis, and colorectal cancer. Disorders affecting the accessory organs of the digestive system include pancreatitis, pancreatic cancer, cholecystitis, viral hepatitis, and liver cancer.

MEDICATION ERROR ALERT

Digestive system conditions that are sometimes misdiagnosed include *hemochromatosis, Wilson's disease, celiac disease, Crohn's disease,* and *ulcerative colitis.* When a misdiagnosis occurs, it is possible for the wrong medications to be prescribed, resulting in a medication error, and treatments that may then be useless or even harmful.

GASTROESOPHAGEAL REFLUX DISEASE

GERD refers to backflow of stomach contents into the esophagus and past the lower esophageal sphincter, without associated vomiting. The condition commonly occurs in pregnant or obese patients, and it often occurs at night, since lying down after a meal often contributes to reflux. It can be confirmed using various studies, including barium swallow, endoscopy with esophageal biopsy, monitoring of esophageal pH, and various scanning tests.

Signs and symptoms of GERD include a burning sensation (known as heartburn) that may radiate to the chest or arms. Other symptoms include belching that expresses vomitus into the mouth, dysphagia, erosive esophagitis, erosion of tooth **enamel**, and dental caries. Complications may include esophageal stricture, mucosal ulceration, and pulmonary aspiration. Treatment includes elevation of the head of the bed by approximately 6 inches (15 cm), eating a light dinner no later than 3 hours before bedtime, weight loss for obese patients, and stopping of alcohol use and cigarette smoking. Medications include antacids, H_2-receptor antagonists, and proton pump inhibitors, with antireflux surgery used in extremely severe cases.

Antacids

The various types of antacids differ in **cation** content, neutralizing capacity, duration of action, side effects, and cost. These factors must be considered when an antacid is chosen for therapeutic use. Antacids are over-the-counter (OTC) drugs. Examples of common antacids are shown in Table 27-1. The most widely used antacids are sodium bicarbonate, calcium carbonate, aluminum hydroxide, and magnesium hydroxide.

Histamine Receptor Antagonists

There are three types of histamine receptors. One of these types mediates acid secretion by gastric parietal cells and is inhibited by the H_2-receptor-blocking drugs. These drugs may be preferred to other antiulcer agents because of their convenience of use and lack of effect on gastrointestinal motility. H_2-receptor antagonists are listed in Table 27-2.

Proton Pump Inhibitors

The final common pathway in gastric acid secretion is the proton pump—an H_1/K_1-adenosine triphosphatase. The physiological essence of this enzyme is the exchange of hydrogen ions for potassium ions. Thus, hydrogen is secreted by the parietal cell into the gastric lumen in exchange for potassium. The proton pump inhibitors should be taken before meals, because these drugs are more potent when they are taken orally and before meals. They are also absorbed more effectively in the morning. Examples of proton pump inhibitors are shown in Table 27-3.

Table 27-1 Examples of Common Antacids

Generic Name	Trade Name	Route of Administration	Average Adult Dosage
aluminum hydroxide	Amphojel®	PO	500 to 1500 mg 4 to 6 times/day prn, between meals and at bedtime
calcium carbonate	Tums®	PO	0.5 to 2 g prn
magaldrate	Riopan®	PO	480 to 1080 mg (5 to 10 mL)
magnesium hydroxide and aluminum hydroxide	Maalox®	PO	5 to 15 mL liquid prn (maximum 80 mL within 24 hours)
aspirin/citric acid/sodium bicarbonate	Alka Seltzer®	PO	300 mg to 2 g/day

Table 27-2 Examples of Histamine (H_2) Receptor Antagonists

Generic Name	Trade Name	Route of Administration	Average Adult Dosage
cimetidine	Tagamet®	PO, IM, IV	PO: 300 mg 4 times daily; IM/IV: 300 mg q6 to 8h
famotidine	Pepcid®	PO, IV	PO: 40 mg at bedtime or 20 mg bid; IV: 20 mg q12h
nizatidine	Axid®	PO	150 mg bid or 300 mg at bedtime
ranitidine	Zantac®	PO, IM, IV	PO: 150 mg bid or 300 mg at bedtime; IM/IV: 50 mg q6 to 8h

WHAT WOULD YOU DO?

Prior to getting to your pharmacy one morning, you read a newspaper article about an FDA warning about a link with certain proton pump inhibitors (PPIs) and adverse events such as arrhythmias and seizures. If a patient who had previously had arrhythmias came to your pharmacy with a prescription for lansoprazole, a PPI, what would you do?

Table 27-3 Examples of Proton Pump Inhibitors

Generic Name	Trade Name	Route of Administration	Average Adult Dosage
dexlansoprazole	Dexilant®	PO	30 mg once daily, for up to four weeks
esomeprazole	Nexium®	PO	20 mg once daily, for up to four weeks
lansoprazole	Prevacid®	PO	15 mg/day for four weeks
omeprazole	Prilosec®	PO	20 mg bid for four to eight weeks
omeprazole/sodium bicarbonate	Zegerid®	PO	20 mg once daily, for up to four weeks
pantoprazole	Protonix®	PO	40 mg once daily, for up to eight weeks
rabeprazole	AcipHex®	PO	20 mg/day for four weeks

PEPTIC ULCERS

Peptic ulcers are lesions in the mucosal membrane, which can develop in the lower esophagus, stomach, or duodenum. Ulcers may be acute or chronic. About 80% of all peptic ulcers are duodenal ulcers, which affect the proximal part of the small intestine; they occur most commonly in men aged 20 to 50 years. Gastric ulcers are most common in middle-aged and elderly men, especially those who are chronic users of nonsteroidal anti-inflammatory drugs (NSAIDs), alcohol, or tobacco. Peptic ulcers may be caused by *Helicobacter pylori* infection because it induces inflammation.

Signs and symptoms of peptic ulcers of the stomach include heartburn, epigastric pain, and uncomfortable fullness after eating. Signs and symptoms of peptic ulcers of the duodenum include midepigastric pain, heartburn, and, sometimes, severe upper abdominal pain with nausea and vomiting. Most severe attacks occur approximately 2 hours after a meal. Complications of peptic ulcers include hemorrhage, shock, gastric perforation, and gastric outlet obstruction.

Treatment of peptic ulcers includes rest, medications, dietary changes involving eating smaller and less spicy meals, and lifestyle changes involving stopping smoking and drinking alcohol. Any irritating substance should be eliminated, and stress reduction along with increased physical activity is suggested. Medications may include sedatives, tranquilizers, histamine receptor-blocking agents, antacids, mucosal coating agents, and proton pump inhibitors. If *H. pylori* is present, antibiotics are used, often in combination with a proton pump inhibitor. For severe cases involving bleeding or perforation, surgery may be indicated, as well as intravenous fluid administration and blood replacement.

MEDICATION ERROR ALERT

Peptic ulcer disease and gastric cancer may have similar symptoms, so a correct diagnosis is essential to the correct medication therapy regimen. In a small number of cases, the two conditions may coexist. If gastric cancer is misdiagnosed as peptic ulcer disease, medications used to treat the nonexistent ulcer, such as the proton pump inhibitor omeprazole, may actually encourage cancer growth. Studies have shown omeprazole to have carcinogenic effects.

CROHN'S DISEASE

Crohn's disease is a condition of the intestinal tract characterized by patches of inflammation and even ulcers. Crohn's disease is also known as regional enteritis, granulomatous colitis, ileitis, and ileocolitis. This disease is most prevalent in adults aged 20 to 40 years. The exact cause is unknown, but it may be linked to infectious agents, immunological factors, diet, psychosomatic illness, allergies, autoimmune factors, and genetic causes.

Signs and symptoms include fever, diarrhea, and abdominal cramps more often in the right lower quadrant, weight loss, malaise, nausea, anorexia, abnormal appetite, and abdominal fullness. Perianal fissures and fistulas may develop, and complications include deep ulcerations, adhesions, symptoms of bowel obstruction, and abscesses.

Crohn's disease is not curable, but treatment is aimed at treating flare-ups and maintaining remission. Dietary supplements of vitamins, minerals, calories, and protein are indicated. Intravenous nutrition may be needed for severe diarrhea. Additional medications include anticholinergics, narcotic agents, antibacterials (especially sulfasalazine), corticosteroids, and immunosuppressants. Surgery may be required to remove the affected portion of the intestine. If extensive, a colostomy or ileostomy may also be needed.

ULCERATIVE COLITIS

Ulcerative colitis is an inflammatory disease that affects the mucosa of the colon. It is of uncertain cause, and is usually chronic, often prevalent within families. It produces edema and ulcerations (see Figure 27-10). Severity ranges from a mild, localized disorder to a severe disease that may cause a perforated colon, progressing to potentially fatal **peritonitis** and **toxemia**. Ulcerative colitis occurs primarily in young adults, with prevalence in women only slightly higher than in males. It is believed to have an autoimmune component. The condition is more common in whites and those of Jewish descent.

Onset of symptoms peaks between ages 15 and 20 years, and then again, between ages 55 and 60 years. Signs and symptoms include intermittent bloody diarrhea, abdominal cramping, urgency, stools containing mucus, and over time, loosening of the stool with more frequency. Cramping and rectal pressure, weight loss, fever, and malaise become prevalent. Sometimes, diarrhea alternates with constipation. Mucosal bowel ulceration causes blood and pus to be present along with mucus in the stool. If fulminant, severe complications include hemorrhage, perforation, and severe diarrhea.

Treatment of ulcerative colitis includes a balanced diet of foods that are nonirritating to the patient (usually, this means high in protein, vitamins, and calories but low in fats and bulk). Medications include anticholinergics,

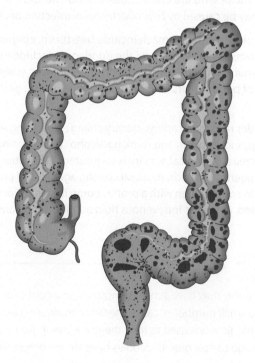

Figure 27-10 Ulcerative colitis.

5-aminosalicylates, which include Apriso® (mesalamine) and Colazal® (balsalazide), corticosteroids, and, in some cases, antidiarrheal agents. Imodium A-D® (loperamide) is indicated for relatively mild diarrhea, with higher doses needed for more severe diarrhea. For severe hemorrhage or perforation, surgical removal of the diseased colon is indicated. A proctocolectomy also may be required, in which the colon and rectum are removed; this is followed by ileostomy or ileoanal anastomosis. Since chronic ulcerative colitis is linked to colon cancer, the patient must be reexamined annually.

POINTS TO REMEMBER

Ulcerative colitis flare-ups are often categorized by bloody diarrhea, with or without the presence of whitish-colored mucus.

MEDICATION ERROR ALERT

The acne medication isotretinoin (Accutane®) should be avoided in patients with Crohn's disease or ulcerative colitis, as it has been shown to cause or exacerbate both of these conditions.

DIARRHEA

Diarrhea is the manifestation of many illnesses, and it is an abnormal increase in fluidity, frequency, or volume of bowel movements. General discomfort, abdominal cramping, and gas often accompany diarrhea. Its etiology includes infections (bacterial, viral, fungal, and parasitic), irritable bowel syndrome, inflammatory bowel disease (Crohn's disease and ulcerative colitis), toxins (food poisoning), drugs, and other causes. Treatment should be focused on the underlying cause.

The use of antidiarrheal agents is occasionally necessary for convenience or for conditions for which there is no primary treatment. The most commonly used antidiarrheals are anticholinergics, opioid narcotics, meperidine congeners (diphenoxylate), and loperamide. Opioid antidiarrheals are the most effective drugs for controlling diarrhea. Selected agents used to treat diarrhea are shown in Table 27-4.

CONSTIPATION

Constipation is difficult or infrequent passage of stool. Normal stool frequency ranges from two to three times daily to two to three times per week. Because constipation is a symptom rather than a disease, a medical evaluation should be undertaken in patients who develop constipation.

Table 27-4 Examples of Antidiarrheal Agents

Generic Name	Trade Name	Route of Administration	Average Adult Dosage
attapulgite	Donnagel®	PO	60 to 120 mL after each loose stool
bismuth subsalicylate	Pepto-Bismol®	PO	15 mL every 30 to 60 minutes or 2 tablets or 2 capsules every 30 to 60 minutes
diphenoxylate with atropine	Lomotil®	PO	5 to 20 mg/day
furazolidone	Furoxone®	PO	Tablets: 25 to 100 mg/day; liquid: 25 to 200 mg/day
loperamide	Imodium®	PO	4 mg as a single dose, then 2 mg after each episode of diarrhea

Various laxatives are used for treatment of constipation that either accelerate fecal passage or decrease fecal consistency. They work by promoting one or more of the mechanisms that cause diarrhea. Because of the wide availability and marketing of OTC laxatives, there is a potential that patients who use these agents to self-medicate symptoms will not seek an appropriate diagnosis. Some examples of laxatives and stool softeners are shown in Table 27-5.

COLORECTAL CANCER

Colorectal cancer is an extremely common malignancy that usually occurs due to a transformation of adenomatous polyps. Most (80%) of the cases are sporadic, with 20% related to genetics. Risk factors include chronic ulcerative colitis and Crohn's disease. Signs and symptoms include occult bleeding, fatigue, weakness, obstruction, and colicky abdominal pain. Prognosis depends on the stage of the cancer. For treatment of colorectal cancer, bowel resection surgery is attempted in 70% of patients presenting without metastatic disease. Additionally, chemotherapy and radiation therapy is used.

Table 27-5 Examples of Laxatives and Stool Softeners

Generic Name	Trade Name	Route of Administration	Average Adult Dosage
Bulk-Forming Laxatives			
methylcellulose	Citrucel®	PO	500 to 6000 mg/day
polycarbophil	Mitrolan®	PO	2 tablets up to 4 times daily
psyllium seed	Metamucil®, Perdiem®	PO	1 tsp in 8 oz water up to 4 times daily
Saline and Osmotic Laxatives			
magnesium citrate	Citrate of Magnesia®	PO	1000 to 6000 mg/day
lactulose	Cephulac®	PO, Rectal	30 to 150 mL/day
polyethylene glycol	MiraLax®	PO	17 g of powder in 4 to 8 oz of fluid/day
Stimulant Laxatives			
bisacodyl	Dulcolax®	PO, Rectal	PO: 10 to 15 mg; Rectal: one suppository
castor oil	Emulsoil®	PO	45 to 60 mL/day
senna	Senokot®	PO	10 to 15 mL or 2 tablets at bedtime
Oral Lubricant Laxatives			
mineral oil	Kondremul®, Agoral®, Petrolagar®	PO	2 to 15 tsp/day
Stool Softeners			
docusate calcium	Surfak®	PO, Rectal	240 mg/day
docusate potassium	Dialose®	PO, Rectal	PO: 1 to 3 capsules daily; Rectal: one suppository
docusate sodium	Colace®	PO, Rectal	1 to 4 tablets or capsules/day
Opioid Antagonist			
naloxegol	Movantik®	PO	25 mg once daily; if not tolerated, reduce to 12.5 mg

PANCREATITIS

Pancreatitis is defined as acute or chronic inflammation of the pancreas. The condition may affect other organs as well. Activated pancreatic enzymes leaking from the acinar cells into the surrounding tissues may cause acute pancreatitis. The condition may be related to alcoholism, biliary tract disease, infection, trauma, highly elevated blood calcium levels, structural abnormalities, hemorrhage, drugs, or hyperlipidemia. When the patient is not alcoholic, gallstones are often causative, with less common causes including endocrine or metabolic disorders. The condition may also be of unknown origin. Smoking often worsens the condition in alcoholic individuals and when the cause is not known.

Signs and symptoms of pancreatitis are linked to the organ becoming edematous, inflamed, hemorrhagic, and necrotic. Acute pancreatitis causes sudden and severe abdominal pain radiating to the back, nausea, vomiting, worsening of pain when walking or lying supine, and lessening of pain when sitting or leaning forward. The patient has diaphoresis, tachycardia, and breathes with rapid and shallow efforts. Body temperature rises as blood pressure falls. The abdomen feels tender mostly in the upper portion, bowel sounds are reduced, and mild jaundice often develops. Chronic pancreatitis may cause constant back pain, recurring yet mild symptoms of acute pancreatitis, anorexia, nausea, vomiting, constipation, flatulence, and weight loss.

Treatment of pancreatitis consists of supportive care in most cases, as most cases are mild and lack local or systemic complications. However, acute pancreatitis may require emergency administration of intravenous fluids and electrolytes. The patient should not receive anything by mouth, and a nasogastric suction tube using intermittent suction may be placed for approximately one week. Adequate meperidine hydrochloride or other pain medications are administered. For bacterial infections, antibiotics are given. Anticholinergics help to slow bowel motility and reduce secretions from the pancreas. Electrolytes, hematocrit, serum amylase and lipase, glucose, and serum calcium must be monitored. If an abscess develops, prompt percutaneous or surgical drainage is required. For chronic pancreatitis, the patient requires monitoring for malabsorption, steatorrhea, and impaired glucose tolerance, which indicates diabetes mellitus. For an obstructed pancreatic duct, surgery may be required.

POINTS TO REMEMBER

Chronic pancreatitis often develops in people between the ages of 30 and 40 years and is usually caused by years of heavy alcohol abuse, which eventually destroys the pancreas.

WHAT WOULD YOU DO?

A woman is prescribed Yaz®, an oral contraceptive. Upon checking her patient record, you notice that she has a high cholesterol level. The drug carries an FDA warning concerning increased occurrence of pancreatitis when used by women with high cholesterol. If you were the pharmacy technician in this scenario, what would you do?

CHOLECYSTITIS

Cholecystitis is defined as acute or chronic inflammation of the gallbladder. It is often linked to an obstruction of the cystic duct by a gallstone. Sometimes, however, it is caused by trauma, infection, or other damage to the gallbladder. The condition may become chronic.

Signs and symptoms include colicky pain in the upper right abdominal quadrant that intensifies as it radiates to the right lower shoulder area. There is often nausea, vomiting, protecting of the muscles in the affected area, and shallow respirations. Additional signs include fever, clay-colored stools, jaundice, darkened urine, and pruritus. An acutely inflamed gallbladder may rupture, resulting in peritonitis. Sometimes the condition subsides on its own, with pain resolving in several days.

MEDICAL TERMINOLOGY REVIEW

cholecystalgia:

cholecyst/o = *gallbladder*

-algia = *pain*

gallbladder pain

Treatment for cholecystitis begins with elimination of fatty foods. If acutely ill and persistently vomiting, the patient is fed by a nasogastric tube. Intravenous supplementation of fluids and electrolytes is administered. Once stabilized, the patient is scheduled for cholecystectomy. Medications may include antibiotics, antiemetics, and analgesics.

VIRAL HEPATITIS

Viral hepatitis is a viral infection that produces inflammation of the liver, resulting in hepatic cell destruction and necrosis. It is the 10th leading cause of death among adults in the United States. Viral hepatitis is classified into six types: A, B, C, D, E, and G. Each type is commonly abbreviated in a way that indicates the causative virus, such as "HAV" for hepatitis A, "HBV" for hepatitis B, and so on.

- *Hepatitis A*—Transmitted by fecal-oral contamination, this form is not usually considered an important risk to health care workers. It is also known as acute infective hepatitis. The HAV vaccine is either administered alone (under the trade names Havrix® and Vaqta®) or in combination with the HBV vaccine (under the trade name Twinrix®). With the advent of vaccination, there has been a dramatic decline in the incidence of HAV infections, and a large reduction in infections among populations at highest risk in the United States, which include Native Americans and Alaskan Natives. The HAV vaccine is now recommended for all American children between 12 and 23 months of age.

- *Hepatitis B*—This form is the primary blood-borne hazard for health care workers and may be transmitted through contaminated plasma and serum, contaminated needles, cuts caused by contaminated sharps, sexual contact, and contaminated material being splashed into the eyes, nose, mouth, or broken skin. Since this form is also sexually transmitted, it will be discussed in detail in Chapter 28.

- *Hepatitis C*—Also known as *non-A, non-B hepatitis*, this chronic form is mostly transmitted by blood infusion or intravenous drug use, shared needles, and sexual contact. Therefore, it will also be discussed in Chapter 28.

- *Hepatitis D*—Also known as delta hepatitis, this form occurs only in patients who are infected with HBV. Therefore, the HBV vaccine can prevent this form as well. HDV is transmitted through sharing of needles and sexual contact. It is not common in the United States and is diagnosed by detecting HDV serum antibodies.

- *Hepatitis E*—This form is acute and common in Africa, South America, and Southeast Asia. It is similar to HAV and often occurs in the rainy season or after natural disasters as a result of fecally contaminated food or water. No serological test is available to detect HEV. This form is most dangerous in pregnant women, in whom it is associated with an increased mortality rate.

- *Hepatitis G*—This form is caused by the single-stranded RNA *flavivirus* and is usually spread by contact with blood, and possibly semen. Its incubation period may last for weeks, and it usually causes only mild symptoms. There is no vaccine, and **viremia** may persist for months or years.

Signs and symptoms of hepatitis differ slightly among its various forms but generally include abrupt onset of headache, anorexia, fever, malaise, dark urine, nausea, and clay-colored stools. Resulting jaundice causes the skin and sclera of the eyes to become yellowed. Abdominal discomfort, myalgia, and liver enlargement often occur, though hepatitis may be symptomatic, especially in children.

MEDICAL TERMINOLOGY REVIEW

hepatitis:

hepat = *liver*

-itis = *inflammation*

inflammation of the liver

Treatment for hepatitis includes rest, intramuscular immune globulins, isolation to prevent cross infection, antiemetics, analgesics, restricted physical activity, a diet low in fats and high in carbohydrates, and complete avoidance of alcohol.

POINTS TO REMEMBER

Viral hepatitis is the leading cause of liver cancer, and the most common reason for liver transplantation. More than 4 million Americans have chronic hepatitis, with most unaware that they are infected.

LIVER CANCER

Chronic liver disease often results in *hepatocellular carcinoma*, a primary type of liver cancer. It is most commonly linked to hepatitis B viral infection but may also be linked to cirrhosis, hereditary **hemochromatosis**, and exposure to *aflatoxins*, which are produced by molds that may contaminate corn, peanuts, soybeans, and other foods. Primary liver cancer is rare in developed countries. Secondary liver cancer is more common, usually metastasizing from the colon, lung, breast, or prostate gland.

MEDICAL TERMINOLOGY REVIEW

hepatectomy:

hepat- = *liver*

surgical removal of (a part of) the liver

-ectomy = *surgical removal*

Signs and symptoms of liver cancer may mimic those of various chronic liver diseases. Symptoms may include upper abdominal pain, early feelings of fullness when eating, weight loss, and an abdominal mass that can be palpated. Additional signs include ascites, hepatomegaly, jaundice, and splenomegaly. There may be unexplained changes in tissues not located near the tumor or its metastases.

Treatment includes partial surgical hepatectomy of the liver, though many patients are not able to have this surgery owing to the extent of the tumor or because of underlying liver disease. If the tumor is less than 5 cm in diameter, has no microvascular involvement, and no extrahepatic spread, liver transplantation may be considered. For nonmetastatic liver cancer, other options include percutaneous ethanol injection and radiofrequency ablation.

Summary

The digestive system ingests food, digests it, absorbs the end products of digestion, and eliminates waste. Mechanical digestion is the breakdown of large food particles into smaller pieces by physical means. Chemical digestion is the chemical alteration of food. The alimentary tract includes the mouth, esophagus, stomach, and intestines. Accessory organs include the salivary glands, liver, gallbladder, and pancreas. The teeth break up food by chewing. The esophagus passes food to the superior part of the stomach using muscle contractions collectively known as peristalsis, which also exists in lower parts of the gastrointestinal tract.

The pancreas releases digestive enzymes, and it also secretes glucagon and insulin, which are hormones controlling and regulating blood glucose levels. The liver aids in digestion as well as many other life-sustaining functions. It produces plasma proteins and heparin, phagocytizes bacteria and worn-out red blood cells, stores glycogen as well as vitamins and minerals, inactivates toxins and poisons, and produces bile salts. The large intestine absorbs water, absorbs and produces vitamins, and forms and expels feces.

Common disorders of the digestive system include gastroesophageal reflux disease, peptic ulcers, Crohn's disease, ulcerative colitis, diarrhea, constipation, colorectal cancer, and various forms of viral hepatitis. Gastric ulcers are most common in middle-aged and elderly men, especially in chronic users of nonsteroidal anti-inflammatory drugs, alcohol, or tobacco. Other conditions affecting the digestive system include pancreatitis and cholecystitis. Common medications used to treat digestive system disorders include antacids, histamine receptor antagonists, proton pump inhibitors, antidiarrheal agents, laxatives, and stool softeners.

REVIEW QUESTIONS

1. The accessory glands of the digestive system include all of the following, *except the:*

   A. liver.
   B. pancreas.
   C. spleen.
   D. salivary glands.

2. Which of the following nutrients begins digestion in the mouth *chemically*?

   A. Simple sugars
   B. Amino acids
   C. Triglycerides
   D. Fatty acids

3. Which of the following is not one of the salivary glands?

   A. Sublingual
   B. Parotid
   C. Sebaceous
   D. Submandibular

4. Which of the following cells in the stomach secretes pepsinogen?

   A. Parietal
   B. Chief
   C. Alpha cells
   D. Beta cells

5. Which of the following is a risk factor for liver cancer?

   A. Gallstones
   B. Diabetes mellitus
   C. Corticosteroids
   D. Hepatitis B

6. The longest portion of the digestive tract is the:

   A. colon.
   B. duodenum.
   C. ileum.
   D. jejunum.

7. Which of the following is a risk factor for colorectal cancer?

   A. Peptic ulcer
   B. Ulcerative colitis
   C. Pancreatitis
   D. Hepatitis B

8. The most common site of peptic ulcers is which part of the digestive tract?

   A. Esophagus
   B. Stomach
   C. Duodenum
   D. Colon

9. Peptic ulcer disease may be caused when *H. pylori* induces which of the following?

   A. Inflammation
   B. Viral infections
   C. Pepsin
   D. Hydrochloric acid

10. Which of the following parts of the small intestine is involved in Crohn's disease?

     A. Duodenum
     B. Jejunum
     C. Ileum
     D. Cecum

11. Severe complications of ulcerative colitis include all of the following, *except:*

     A. diarrhea.
     B. heartburn.
     C. hemorrhage.
     D. perforation.

12. Which of the following is the trade name of oral antacid calcium carbonate?

     A. Maalox®
     B. Tums®
     C. Amphojel®
     D. Alka Seltzer®

13. Which of the following drugs is an example of proton pump inhibitors?

     A. Zantac®
     B. Prilosec®
     C. Furoxone®
     D. Colace®

14. Which of the following drugs is a stimulant laxative?

     A. Dialose®
     B. Mitrolan®
     C. Dulcolax®
     D. Lomotil®

15. All of the following are examples of H_2-receptor antagonists, *except:*

     A. Prevacid®.
     B. Pepcid®.
     C. Tagamet®.
     D. Axid®.

CRITICAL THINKING

A 27-year-old nurse was diagnosed with viral hepatitis, despite receiving two series of immunizations 15 years earlier. She had been married for 5 years prior to diagnosis, with no children.

1. Compare hepatitis B and hepatitis C, and their routes of transmission.

2. Explain the complete series of vaccines for hepatitis B.

WEB LINKS

Crohn's & Colitis Foundation of America: www.crohnscolitisfoundation.org

Digestive Health Probiotic: www.drugs.com/cdi/digestive-health-probiotic.html

Digestive System Disorders: www.digestivesystemdisorders.org

National Digestive Diseases Information Clearinghouse: www.niddk.nih.gov/health-information/digestive-diseases

Nutrition.gov: www.nutrition.gov/subject/nutrition-and-health-issues/digestive-disorders

CHAPTER 28

Therapeutic Drugs for the Reproductive System

OUTLINE

OBJECTIVES

Upon completion of this chapter, the reader should be able to:

1. Describe the structures of the female reproductive system.
2. Describe the hormones of the ovaries and testes.
3. Explain the treatments for infertility.
4. Explain monophasic and biphasic contraceptives.
5. Describe the menstrual cycle.
6. Identify various types of androgens.
7. Describe the causes and treatments of benign prostatic hyperplasia.
8. Describe the three types of estrogen/progestin formulations.
9. Explain erectile dysfunction and its treatments.
10. Describe chlamydia and its complications without treatment.

KEY TERMS

amenorrhea	endometrium	menses	semen
chancre	fallopian (uterine) tubes	myometrium	seminiferous tubules
corpus albicans	genitourinary	oligomenorrhea	spermatogonia
corpus luteum	gummas	ovulation	tunica albuginea
cryptorchidism	infundibulum	perimetrium	vas deferens
endometriosis	menorrhagia	prostate gland	

Overview

Human reproduction begins with the joining of one male and one female sex cell. The female reproductive system includes the ovaries, eggs, female sex hormones, uterus, vagina, and other accessory glands and structures. The male reproductive system includes the testes, sperm, male sex hormones, scrotum, penis, and other accessory glands and structures.

Anatomy and Physiology of the Reproductive System

The anatomy and physiology of the female and male reproductive systems differ significantly. Therefore, we will discuss them separately.

FEMALE REPRODUCTIVE SYSTEM

The main female sex organs are the ovaries (gonads). They produce ova (eggs) as part of their exocrine function. They also have an endocrine function, producing the female sex hormones estrogen and progesterone. A mature *follicle* containing a mature egg is called a graafian follicle, and is basically an endocrine gland, secreting estrogen in preparation of ejecting the egg. This process of ejection is known as **ovulation**. Once the egg ruptures outward, the follicle forms the corpus luteum (yellow body) and produces progesterone. It eventually deteriorates to form the corpus albicans (white body).

The remainder of the female reproductive system consists of ducts and organs, which nurture and transport the eggs. These include the uterine (fallopian) tubes, uterus, and vagina (see Figure 28-1). Estrogen controls the appearance of female sexual characteristics and also regulates the menstrual cycle. Progesterone plays many roles but is primarily responsible for maintaining the proper uterine environment needed to support pregnancy.

The ova are transported from the ovaries to the uterus through the **fallopian (uterine) tubes**, one of which connects to each ovary. Each tube has a funnel-shaped open end known as the **infundibulum**. Fertilization most commonly occurs in the upper third part of the fallopian tube. After ovulation, fertilization may occur at any time within 24 hours. A fertilized ovum moves down the fallopian tube to enter the uterus within seven days.

MEDICAL TERMINOLOGY REVIEW

ovulation:

ov/o = *ovum; egg*   process of releasing amature ovum

-lation 5 = *process*

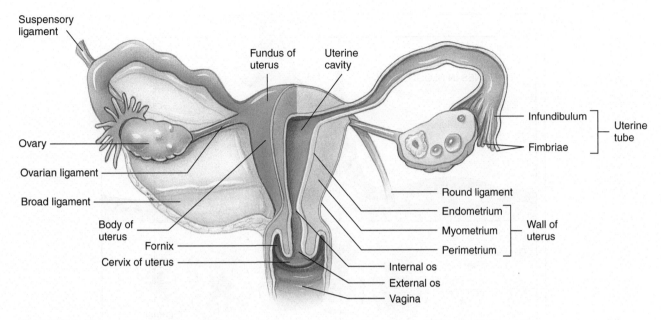

Figure 28-1 The position of the ovaries, uterine tubes, uterus, and vagina of the female reproductive system.

The uterus is divided into a fundus, body, cervix, and isthmus. The fundus is dome-shaped, and it lies above the fallopian tubes. The main portion of the uterus is known as the body. The cervix is the thin, inferior area opening into the vagina. The isthmus is small and constricted, lying between the body and the cervix. The inner portion of the body of the uterus is described as the uterine cavity, while the inner cervix is called the cervical canal.

There are three layers of uterine tissue: the endometrium, myometrium, and perimetrium. The inner **endometrium** is a mucosal layer in which a fertilized ovum buries itself during implantation. The middle **myometrium** is made up of smooth muscle that functions to move the baby out of the womb during delivery. The outer **perimetrium** is composed of serous membrane.

Menstruation is also known as the menstrual cycle or **menses**. The lining of the uterus is shed in a continuous cycle because of alterations in hormone levels. Though a menstrual cycle of 28 days is most common, it may range between 24 and 35 days. There are three phases: the menstrual phase, proliferative phase, and secretory phase (see Figure 28-2).

The menstrual phase is the actual time of menstruation and lasts from day one to day five. The thick endometrial uterine lining is shed, accompanied by blood, tissue fluid, epithelial cells, and mucus. Bleeding may last from three to five days, with these substances exiting through the vagina as the menstrual flow. The ovarian cycle is also occurring at this time, with the primary follicles beginning their development. In the earliest parts of this phase, between 20 and 25 primary follicles start producing low levels of estrogen. The transparent zona pellucida, a membrane, develops around each ovum. At about day four or five, approximately 20 primary follicles develop into secondary follicles and secrete a follicular fluid forcing the ovum to the edge of the secondary follicle. Only one follicle will actually mature through the process of meiosis; the others experience cellular death or atresia.

The proliferative phase varies in length, usually lasting from day 6 to day 14 of the 28-day cycle. Estrogen levels from the follicles increase, causing the endometrial lining to become thicker. The rupturing of the Graafian follicle releases the ovum into the pelvic cavity on day 14.

The secretory phase is nearly always the same length, lasting from day 15 to day 28. It is the time between ovulation and the beginning of the next menstrual cycle. Blood estrogen levels drop slightly, and development of the **corpus luteum** occurs in response to secretion of luteinizing hormone (LH). The corpus luteum then secretes more progesterone, and some estrogen. The progesterone aids the endometrium in receiving a fertilized ovum by increasing its size and causing it to secrete nutrients, which flow into the uterine cavity. Without fertilization and implantation, the corpus luteum degenerates into the **corpus albicans** and another menstrual cycle begins.

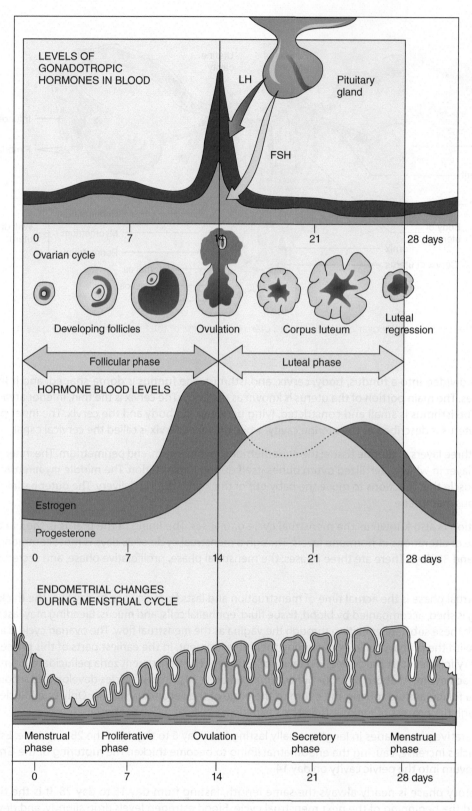

Figure 28-2 The menstrual cycle.

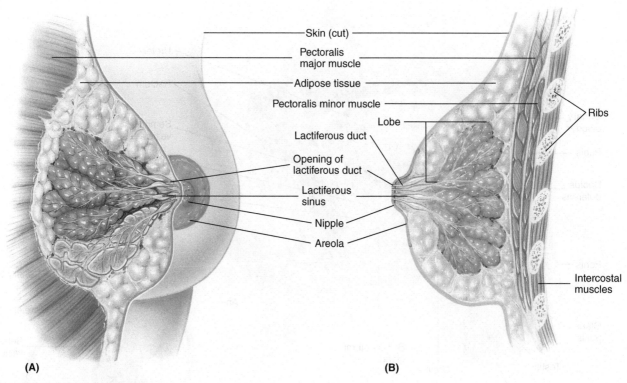

Figure 28-3 The mammary glands.

However, when fertilization and implantation do occur, the corpus luteum continues to exist for approximately four months, continuing to secrete progesterone and some estrogen. It is maintained by human chorionic gonadotropin, which is released from the developing placenta. A developed placenta also secretes estrogen to support the pregnancy, and progesterone to both support pregnancy and cause breast development so that the mammary glands can produce milk.

Though mammary glands are present in both sexes, they are normally functional only in females, producing milk to nourish a newborn baby. They increase in size because of estrogen secretion during puberty, and are actually modified sweat glands (see Figure 28-3). The mammary glands function, under the influence of hormones from the pituitary gland (prolactin and oxytocin), to secrete and eject milk during the process of lactation.

MALE REPRODUCTIVE SYSTEM

The main male sex organs are the testes, also called the male gonads. They produce sperm as well as male sex hormones. The scrotum supports the testes, for developing sperm cells (see Figure 28-4). A series of ducts transport sperm into the female reproductive tract during intercourse. Accessory glands secrete substances that combine to form **semen**. In addition to being the organ of urination, the penis serves to transport sperm and also to penetrate the vagina for reproduction.

The testes are located within the scrotum because sperm need a temperature that is lower than normal body temperature. The scrotal environment is approximately 3 degrees (Fahrenheit) less than body temperature. They are the male gonads, producing the male sex hormone (testosterone) and sperm (see Figure 28-5). The **tunica albuginea** is white connective tissue covering each testes, which extends inward, dividing each testis in many smaller lobules. Each lobule contains one to three tightly coiled, convoluted **seminiferous tubules**, which produce sperm via spermatogenesis. This process begins with immature sperm cells called **spermatogonia**. The resulting cells now contain 23 instead of 46 chromosomes and are called spermatids. These are the cells that will eventually mature into sperm cells.

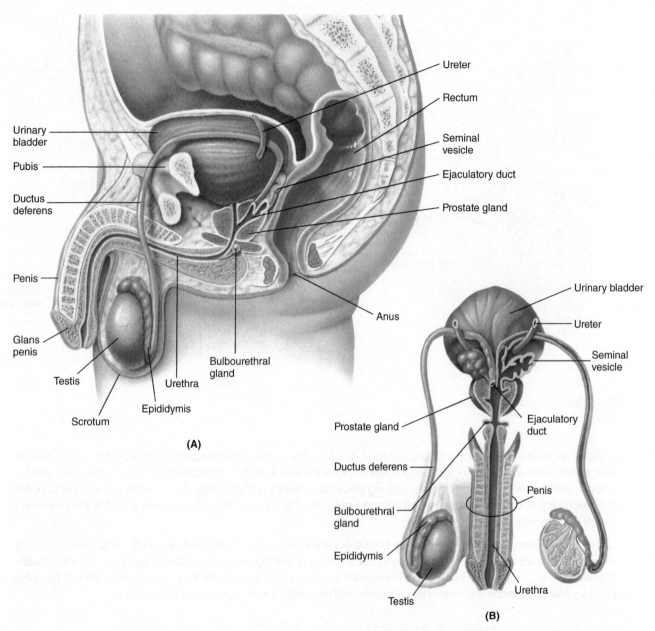

Figure 28-4 The organs and ducts of the male reproductive system.

MEDICAL TERMINOLOGY REVIEW

spermatogonia:

spermato- = *semen*

-gonia = *seeds*

any male gonadal cells that are progenitors of spermatocytes

Clusters of interstitial cells of Leydig lie in the testicular lobules, between the seminiferous tubules and soft connective tissues. These interstitial cells produce testosterone. Since the testes produce both sperm and testosterone, they are like the ovaries in the female reproductive system, and have both exocrine and endocrine functions. The **prostate gland** encircles the prostatic urethra just under the bladder, secreting an alkaline fluid that comprises 13% to 33% of semen.

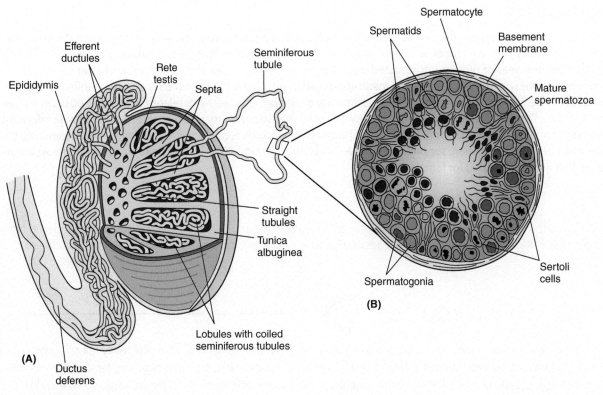

Figure 28-5 The anatomy of a testis.

POINTS TO REMEMBER

The epithelial cells of the seminiferous tubules can give rise to testicular cancer, a common cancer in young men. In most cases, the first sign is a painless enlargement of one of the testicles.

POINTS TO REMEMBER

All male patients, after age 55, should be checked for blood testosterone levels. If levels are low, the urologist may consider testosterone therapy. If high, the individual should not use testosterone to increase libido. In January 2014, the FDA issued an alert that high testosterone levels are linked to higher risk of stroke, heart attack, and death. Normal testosterone levels are between 300 and 1200 ng/dL (nanograms per deciliter).

POINTS TO REMEMBER

A vasectomy is a surgical procedure in which the **vas deferens** is cut or cauterized through a small incision in the scrotum. A post-vasectomy male will produce fluids and is able to ejaculate, meaning that libido is normal, and erections still occur. There is now simply no sperm in the semen. All secondary male sexual characteristics are also maintained.

Disorders of the Reproductive System

Disorders of the reproductive system include infertility, pelvic inflammatory disease (PID), dysfunctional uterine bleeding, menopause, hypogonadism, benign prostatic hyperplasia (BPH), prostate cancer, erectile dysfunction, and sexually transmitted infections (STIs).

INFERTILITY

The term *infertility* is usually defined as inability of a couple to conceive after one year of unprotected intercourse. Female infertility accounts for 60% to 70% of infertility among couples. Infertility treatment evaluations usually begin after one year of regular unprotected intercourse, in women under the age of 35, and after six months in women over the age of 35. In many cases, medications can correct anovulation, which is a cause of infertility. Various drugs promote ovarian follicle maturation and stimulate ovulation. **Endometriosis** related to PID may obstruct the fallopian tubes. Females with irregular menstrual cycles or no menstruation may also be infertile. For female infertility, medications are available that work in a variety of ways. These include reducing high prolactin levels, promoting follicle maturation and ovulation, suppressing follicle-stimulating hormone (FSH), and preventing premature ovulation. Table 28-1 lists agents used for female infertility.

POINTS TO REMEMBER

Infertility is the failure to conceive after one year of well-timed intercourse. A workup should be considered after six months if the woman is between the ages of 35 and 40 years, but immediately if she is at least 40 years old.

WHAT WOULD YOU DO?

You overhear a young woman who is purchasing various herbal supplements at your pharmacy tell an accompanying friend that her infertility can be "cured" by taking them. You are aware that no herbal supplements have been proven to successfully treat infertility. If you were the pharmacy technician in this situation, what would you do?

Table 28-1 Medications Used for Female Infertility

Generic Name	Trade Name	Route of Administration	Average Adult Dosage
Ergoline Derivative and Dopamine Agonist			
bromocriptine	Parlodel®	PO	1.25 to 2.5 mg/day
Selective Estrogen Receptor Modulator			
clomiphene	Clomid®	PO	50 mg/day for five days
Progestin			
progesterone	Crinone®	Intravaginal	Gel: 90 mg once daily or bid; insert: 100 mg bid to tid
Ethisterone Derivative and Synthetic Steroid			
danazol	Danocrine®	PO	800 mg/day in two divided doses
Follicle-Stimulating Hormone (FSH) and Luteinizing Hormone (LH) Enhancing Drugs			
chorionic gonadotropin	Novarel®	IM	5000 to 10,000 USP units one day following last dose of menotropins
choriogonadotropin alfa (r-HCG)	Pregnyl®	Subcutaneous	250 mcg once after last dose of an FSH agent
follitropin alfa	Gonal-F®	Subcutaneous	75 to 300 international units/day
follitropin beta	Follistim®	Subcutaneous	150 international units/day
menotropins	Repronex®	IM, subcutaneous	150 international units/day for five days
urofollitropin	Bravelle®	Subcutaneous	150 international units/day

(Continued)

Table 28-1 Medications Used for Female Infertility *(Continued)*

Gonadotropin-Ovulation Stimulator			
menotropins	Menopur®	Subcutaneous	150 units daily for first five days, adjusted based on ultrasound
Gonadotropin-Releasing Hormone (GnRH) Antagonists			
cetrorelix acetate	Cetrotide®	SC	0.25 mg once daily or 3 mg once during the early to mid-follicular phase
GnRH Analogs and Agonists			
goserelin acetate	Zoladex®	SC	3.6 mg/day every 28 days
leuprolide	Lupron®	IM	3.75 mg once a month for up to six months
nafarelin	Synarel®	Intranasal spray	1600 mcg/day, via two sprays of 200 mcg into each nostril in the morning and two sprays into each nostril in the evening

Male infertility accounts for 30% to 40% of infertility. For male infertility, before any medication is used, a psychological etiology must be ruled out. The most common physical causes include oligospermia, azoospermia (due to obstructions), and erectile dysfunction, which make intercourse difficult or impossible. Human chorionic gonadotropin, menotropins, antiestrogens, testolactone, and nutritional supplements are all used for male infertility. For erectile dysfunction (impotence), medications include enzyme phosphodiesterase-5 inhibitors, and in rare cases the drugs alprostadil and papaverine/phentolamine.

Androgens such as testosterone are used to treat hypogonadism, **cryptorchidism**, and breast cancer. Lack of sufficient testosterone secretion in the testes may cause hypogonadism, which is either congenital or acquired later in life. Androgens have other essential physiological effects, including synthesis of erythropoietin and anabolism of skeletal muscle. Selected androgens and gonadotropins are listed in Table 28-2.

Use of testosterone and other androgens is contraindicated in patients with known hypersensitivity to any contained ingredients; in women during pregnancy and lactation; in men with cancer of the breast or suspected cancer of the prostate; in patients with pituitary insufficiency, a history of myocardial infarction, hypercalcemia, prostatic hyperplasia, hepatic dysfunction, or nephrosis; and in infants and young children. Androgens should be used with caution in elderly patients; in diabetic patients; in those who have hypertension, coronary artery disease, renal disease, hypercholesterolemia, or gynecomastia; and in prepubertal males.

Adverse reactions in males include gynecomastia, excessive frequency and duration of penile erection, oligospermia, hirsutism, male-pattern baldness, acne, increased or decreased libido, headache, anxiety, and depression. In females, adverse reactions include amenorrhea, menstrual irregularities, inhibition of gonadotropin secretion, and virilization (deepening of the voice, clitoral enlargement, increased growth of facial and body hair, and male-type baldness).

WHAT WOULD YOU DO?

Your middle-aged brother wants to try AndroGel® because he has low testosterone. You know that he had a mild heart attack two years ago. He insists that he is going to "reverse his aging process" and asks you for your professional opinion. What would you do?

PELVIC INFLAMMATORY DISEASE

PID is an infection of the uterine lining that may spread into the fallopian tubes. Though usually caused by gonorrhea and chlamydia, the initial infection often becomes multi-bacterial, involving aerobic as well as anaerobic organisms. If abscesses form, it may become life threatening. PID is most common in younger, sexually active women with more than one sexual partner.

Table 28-2 Androgens and Gonadotropins Used for Male Reproductive Disorders

Generic Name	Trade Name	Route of Administration	Average Adult Dosage
Androgens			
danazol	Danocrine®	PO	200 to 400 mg bid for three to six months
fluoxymesterone	Androxy®	PO	5 to 20 mg/day
methyltestosterone (capsules)	Android®, Testred®, Virilon®	PO	10 to 50 mg/day
methyltestosterone (tablets)	Methitest®	Buccal	5 to 25 mg/day
oxandrolone	Oxandrin®	PO	2.5 to 20 mg/day divided 2 to 4 times/day for two to four weeks
oxymetholone	Androl-50®	PO	1 to 5 mg/kg/day
testosterone (buccal)	Striant®	Buccal	30 mg q12h
testosterone (transdermal)	Testoderm TTS®, Androderm®, others	Transdermal	Testoderm TTS patch: apply one patch/day; (Androderm patch): apply one 2.5 to 7.5 mg patch/day
testosterone (pellets)	Testopel®	Implantable pellets	150 to 450 mg in subdermal fat q3 to 6 months
testosterone (gel)	AndroGel®, Testim®	Gel	Apply 5 g/day (maximum 10 g/day)
testosterone cypionate	Depotest®, Andro-Cyp®, Depo-Testosterone®	IM	50 to 400 mg q2 to 4 weeks
testosterone enanthate	Andro LA®, Delatest®, Delatestryl®	IM	50 to 400 mg q2 to 4 weeks
Gonadotropin			
human chorionic gonadotropin	Pregnyl®	IM	500 to 1000 units 3 times/week for three weeks, then same dose twice/week for three weeks

Signs and symptoms include foul-smelling vaginal discharge and abdominal pain, chills, fever, malaise, and backache. Pain may be severe enough to affect normal walking. Abscesses may cause a soft, tender pelvic mass that can be palpated. There is usually elevation of the white blood cell count. Early diagnosis is essential. Adhesions forming in or around the fallopian tubes may cause infertility or increase risks for ectopic pregnancy. Treatment for PID must be prompt in order to avoid widespread damage to the reproductive system, including adhesions caused by inflammation. Treatment requires dual therapy active against *Neisseria gonorrhoeae* and *Chlamydia trachomatis*. If there is a tubo-ovarian abscess, antimicrobial therapy must also target anaerobic microorganisms. Intramuscular, oral, or intravenous medications include ceftriaxone, levofloxin, doxycycline, metronidazole, cefoxitin, probecencid, ceftizoxime, cefotaxime, cefotetan, clindamycin, gentamicin, and ampicillin/sulbactam.

POINTS TO REMEMBER

Pelvic inflammatory disease has been linked to the development of pelvic abscesses caused by infection with the bacterium *Actinomyces* in women who use intrauterine devices.

DYSFUNCTIONAL UTERINE BLEEDING

Dysfunctional uterine bleeding involves hemorrhaging in abnormal amounts or on a noncyclical basis. The condition may be excessive, prolonged, or unpatterned, and not related to structural or systemic diseases. It may be either ovulatory with heavy, cyclical bleeding or anovulatory with irregular bleeding. This disorder can be caused by early abortion, pelvic neoplasms, infection, pregnancy, and thyroid disorders. The disorder may involve **amenorrhea**, breakthrough bleeding between menstrual periods, endometrial carcinoma, **menorrhagia, oligomenorrhea**, post-menopausal bleeding, or premenstrual syndrome (PMS). Dysfunctional uterine bleeding is often caused by an imbalance between estrogen and progesterone levels. Sometimes, oral contraceptives are prescribed to help balance these levels. For abnormalities of the uterus, progestins are the preferred treatment. Estrogens and progestins used for various therapies are listed in Table 28-3.

Table 28-3 Examples of Estrogens and Progestins Used for Various Therapies			
Generic Name	**Trade Name**	**Route of Administration**	**Average Adult Dosage**
Estrogens			
conjugated estrogen	Premarin®	PO	0.3 to 1.25 mg/day for 21 days every month
	Premarin Vaginal®	Vaginal cream	0.5 g/day, or twice weekly, for 21 days every month
esterified estrogen	Menest®	PO	1.25 mg daily (three weeks on, one week off, cycle)
estradiol	Climara®, Estraderm®, Estrace®, Vivelle®	PO, Transdermal patch, Topical gel, Intravaginal cream	PO: 0.5 to 2 mg/day; Transdermal patch: once weekly (Climara) or twice weekly (0.025 to 0.1 mg/day); topical gel: 1.25 g/day; intravaginal cream: insert 2 to 4 g/day for two weeks, then reduce to half the initial dose for two weeks, then use 1 g 1 to 3 times/week
estradiol cypionate	(Depo-Estradiol®)	IM	1 to 5 mg q3 to 4 weeks
estradiol valerate	Delestrogen®, Duragen-10®, Valergen®	IM	10 to 20 mg q4week
estropipate	Ogen®	PO	0.75 to 6 mg/day for 21 days every month
Progestins			
medroxyprogesterone	Depo-Provera®, Depo-subQ-Provera®, Provera®, Cycrin®	PO, IM, SC	PO: 5 to 10 mg/day on days 1 to 12 of menstrual cycle; IM (Depo-Provera): 150 mg/day for three months, give first dose during first five days of menstrual period or within first five days postpartum if not breastfeeding; SC (depo-subQ-Provera): 104 mg/day for three months, give first dose during first five days of menstrual period or at sixth week postpartum if not breastfeeding
norethindrone	Micronor®, Nor-Q.D.®	PO	0.35 mg/day beginning on day one of menstrual cycle

(Continued)

Table 28-3 Examples of Estrogens and Progestins Used for Various Therapies *(Continued)*

Generic Name	Trade Name	Route of Administration	Average Adult Dosage
progesterone	Crinone®, Endometrin®, Prochieve®, Prometrium®	IM (for amenorrhea or functional uterine bleeding); intravaginal or oral tablets (as assisted reproductive technology)	IM: 5 to 10 mg/day; intravaginal: 90 mg gel once daily; oral tablets: 100 mg, 2 to 3 times/day
Estrogen–Progestin Combinations			
conjugated estrogens (equine)/ medroxyprogesterone	Premphase®, Prempro®	PO, intravaginal cream	PO (Premphase): estrogen 0.625 mg/day on days 1 to 28; add 5 mg medroxyprogesterone daily on days 15 to 28; PO (Prempro): estrogen 0.3 mg and medroxyprogesterone 1.5 mg/day; intravaginal cream: insert 0.5 to 2 g/day for two to three months
estradiol/ levonorgestrel	Climara Pro®	Transdermal patch	0.045 mg estradiol/0.015 mg levonorgestrel; replace/apply one patch/ week
estradiol/ norgestimate	Prefest®	PO	1 tablet (1 mg estradiol) for three days, followed by 1 tablet (1 mg estradiol combined with 0.09 mg norgestimate) for three days; regimen repeated continuously with no interruption
ethinyl estradiol/ norethindrone acetate	Activella®	PO, transdermal patch	PO: 1 tablet/day (containing 0.5 to 1 mg of estradiol and 0.5 to 1 mg of norethindrone); transdermal patch: one patch twice weekly

MENOPAUSE

Menopause is also referred to as climacteric, and it is defined as cessation of menstrual periods for one year, with signs of ovarian failure. It usually occurs between the ages of 50 and 51 years and is only considered premature when it occurs before the age of 40. Fluctuations in a woman's menstrual cycle hormones begin in her 30s, causing ovarian production of viable eggs to decline. Ovulation eventually ceases along with menstruation. Menopause may also be induced by chemotherapy, radiation treatments, or total hysterectomy.

Signs and symptoms of menopause often begin by age 45, including fluctuations in menstrual cycle and flow. Menstrual flow becomes lighter and periods, less frequent. Accompanying symptoms that are linked to hormonal changes may range from mild to unbearable and include hot flashes, night sweats, skin changes, vaginal dryness, depression, memory deficits, anxiety, sleep disorders, and decreased libido. Treatment of menopausal complaints is designed to manage these symptoms until they eventually subside. This usually involves use of estrogen-containing products, though these have been linked to an increased incidence of various cancers. Vaginal lubricants may aid menopausal women. For treatment of menopause-related osteoporosis, which was discussed in Chapter 21, bisphosphonates and medications such as ibandronate (Boniva®) and risedronate (Actonel®) are used. Calcium and vitamin D supplements, and weight-bearing exercises, are also recommended.

Hormone replacement therapy, consisting of estrogen alone or combined with a progestin, has been prescribed for many years for women during menopause. However, this type of treatment has many good and bad effects. The

Women's Health Initiative evaluated the effects of estrogen replacement on its own, as well as estrogen-progestin replacement. This evaluation found that women taking estrogen alone experienced a higher risk of stroke and thromboembolic disease but did not experience a higher risk for breast cancer or myocardial infarction. In contrast, women taking estrogen-progestin experienced a decreased risk of hip fractures and colorectal cancer, but they also experienced a much higher risk of myocardial infarction, stroke, breast cancer, dementia, and venous thromboembolism. These findings emphasized that the potential benefits of long-term hormone replacement therapy may not outweigh the risks for some women. However, hormone replacement does help to relieve immediate and distressing menopausal symptoms for many women.

Currently, short-term use of these therapies is recommended in menopausal women who do not have a history of cardiovascular disease or cancer. Estrogens are also used in the treatment of female hypogonadism, primary ovarian failure, and as replacement therapy after surgical removal of the ovaries (usually combined with a progestin).

WHAT WOULD YOU DO?

Prempro® is a combination drug that contains both estrogen and progestin. Millions of women have taken it to relieve the distressing symptoms of menopause. An elderly woman comes to your pharmacy counter with a prescription for a cancer medication. She is angry and tells you, the pharmacy technician, that she took Prempro® for years during her menopause, and now she has "cancer because of it." She is concerned because her 50-year-old daughter has recently been prescribed Prempro®. The woman asks you for your opinion. What would you do?

HYPOGONADISM

Hypogonadism is a lack of estrogen production from the ovaries or testes. In women, symptoms include lack of menstruation and breast development, a short stature, hot flashes, loss of menstruation and body hair, and decreased libido. In adult females, hypogonadism can cause infertility as well as an early form of menopause, the natural transition that occurs between ages 50 and 60. Menopause increases risks for osteoporosis and heart disease once the process is complete. A type of female hypogonadism, known as Turner syndrome, is due to a genetic defect. In infant girls, the hands and feet are swollen and the neck appears thick and webbed. In older females, there may be eyelid drooping, absent or incomplete pubertal development, with small breasts and scant pubic hair. There may be an absence of menstruation, short height, and vaginal dryness. Body image may be improved using hormonal therapies, though treatment cannot make the patient fertile. Hormone replacement therapy may reduce symptoms, and include estrogen, progestin, and even low-dose testosterone.

In males, hypogonadism causes a lack of sufficient amounts of testosterone to be produced. This can occur during fetal development, in puberty, or adulthood. Male hypogonadism may be caused by fetal underdevelopment of the genitals, impaired growth in puberty, bacterial or viral infections, and injury to the glands producing testosterone, by tumors or trauma. The affected individual has impaired muscle and body hair development, gynecomastia, erectile dysfunction, and sexual difficulties. If caused by an anterior pituitary tumor, it is known as *central hypogonadism*. The signs and symptoms are headaches, double or impaired vision, and milky breast discharge. Lack of testosterone can cause fatigue and problems with concentration. Androgens can be used, administered orally or via transdermal or intramuscular routes. Today, natural testosterone is chemically synthesized in laboratories.

BENIGN PROSTATIC HYPERPLASIA

BPH is nonmalignant, noninflammatory hypertrophy of the prostate gland. Enlargement of the prostate gland is a common condition in men after age 50, and frequency of this condition increases with age. BPH usually progresses to the point of causing compression of the urethra, or neck of the bladder, with urinary obstruction. Its cause is not fully understood but appears to be linked to aging as well as changes in hormones and metabolism.

Signs and symptoms include weak urine stream, difficulty in starting to urinate, or inability to fully empty the bladder. Additional symptoms include nocturia, urinary frequency, and fecal incontinence. Severe cases may include inflammation and symptoms that mimic renal disease.

Table 28-4 Medications Used to Treat Benign Prostatic Hyperplasia

Generic Name	Trade Name	Route of Administration	Average Adult Dosage
5-Alpha-Reductase Inhibitors			
dutasteride	Avodart®	PO	0.5 mg once daily
finasteride	Proscar®	PO	5 mg once daily
Alpha-1 Blockers			
alfuzosin	Uroxatral®	PO	10 mg once daily
doxazosin	Cardura®, Cardura XL®	PO	Cardura: 1 mg once daily, titrate up to 4 to 8 mg once daily; XL: 4 mg once daily with breakfast, titrate up to 8 mg once daily
tamsulosin	Flomax®	PO	0.4 mg once daily 30 minutes after same meal each day
terazosin	Hytrin®	PO	1 mg at bedtime, titrate up prn; to 10 mg (maximum 20 mg/day)
5-Alpha-Reductase Inhibitors/Alpha-1 Blockers			
dutasteride/tamsulosin	Jalyn®	PO	0.5 mg dutasteride/0.4 mg tamsulosin once daily, 30 minutes after same meal each day
Phosphodiesterase Type 5 Inhibitors			
tadalafil	Cialis®	PO	2.5 to 5 mg once daily before intercourse

Treatment of BPH usually begins when symptoms interrupt normal daily living. Patients should control fluid intake before going to bed and avoid medications such as decongestants that may cause urine retention. Medications include alpha-adrenergic blockers (tamsulosin hydrochloride, doxazosin mesylate, and terazosin hydrochloride) to relax tight prostate muscles and finasteride, which may actually shrink the prostate gland. Transurethral resection of the prostate is an effective surgical procedure in which the obstructive area of the prostate is removed. Agents used to treat BPH are summarized in Table 28-4.

PROSTATE CANCER

Prostate cancer is an extremely common, yet slow-growing cancer. It is fatal in only 3% of cases, yet is ranked as the second-leading cause of cancer death in men. Risk factors include age above 45, African American race, inherited gene mutations, and diets that are high in animal fat and low in vegetables or selenium.

Prostate cancer is often asymptomatic when it is diagnosed through annual digital rectal exam or by a high serum concentration of prostate-specific antigen (PSA). Digital rectal exam may detect nodules or areas of induration that are asymmetric. Recently, a new blood test has been developed that improves diagnostic accuracy, and it may reduce false positives and unnecessary biopsies. It is called the *Prostate Health Index (PHI)* test, and it uses three different prostate-specific markers. The PHI is more accurate than the PSA test.

If symptoms exist, they usually include weak or interrupted urine flow, difficulty starting or stopping urine flow, urinary frequency, urinary retention, dysuria, and hematuria. Sudden onset of erectile dysfunction may also indicate prostate cancer.

POINTS TO REMEMBER

PSA level is increased in patients with acute prostatitis. If a patient is suspected of having prostate cancer, the PSA test should not be performed until one month after treatment for prostatitis.

Treatment of prostate cancer is based on the Gleason score, which gauges histology, PSA level, the patient's age and overall health, and treatment risks and benefits. For early stages, options include radical prostatectomy, radiation therapy, hormone therapy, or observation to detect changes. Radical prostatectomy and radiation may cause erectile dysfunction and urinary abnormalities. To reduce androgen levels, orchiectomy or use of luteinizing hormone-releasing hormone (LHRH) may be indicated. If the disease is advanced, hormone therapy is preferred, which usually requires addition of a second type of hormone eventually, or chemotherapy. Patients must be reassessed every 6 to 12 months using follow-up PSA tests and digital rectal examinations. Hormonal prostate cancer treatments include LHRH, which includes leuprolide (Lupron Depot) and goserelin (Zoladex). These agents work by blocking hormone production in the testes. Another option involves the antiandrogens called flutamide (Eulexin) and nilutamide (Nilandron). These agents work by blocking the effects of testosterone.

ERECTILE DYSFUNCTION

Erectile dysfunction (ED) is the inability to achieve or maintain an erection. This is commonly called *impotence*. The condition is due to an insufficient amount of blood flowing to the penis, and not a lack of libido. It may occur only rarely, or be chronic. With continued aging, likelihood of experiencing ED is increased. There are also higher risks for developing prostate conditions and various diseases that affect erectile function. These include atherosclerosis, diabetes, cardiovascular disease, and hypertension. Agents used to treat erectile dysfunction are summarized in Table 28-5.

Table 28-5 Medications Used for Erectile Dysfunction

Generic Name	Trade Name	Route of Administration	Average Adult Dosage
sildenafil	Viagra®	PO	50 mg approximately 30 to 60 minutes prior to intercourse (maximum 100 mg once daily)
tadalafil	Cialis®	PO	10 mg approximately 30 minutes prior to intercourse (maximum 20 mg once daily); once-daily dosing: 2.5 to 5 mg/day
vardenafil	Levitra®	PO	10 mg approximately 1 hour prior to intercourse (maximum 20 mg once daily)

SEXUALLY TRANSMITTED INFECTIONS

STIs are very common in the United States, especially among teens and young adults aged 15 to 24 years. In this group, chlamydia is four times more common than in any other age group. Chlamydia and gonorrhea are almost equally as common in the 15-to-24 age group. Syphilis is more common in young adults between the ages of 20 and 29 years. Genital herpes, which is type 2, affects approximately 1 million people in the United States every year. Trichomoniasis is the most common curable STI in the United States, affecting about 3.7 million people (Centers for Disease Control and Prevention, 2012).

Viral Hepatitis

Acute viral hepatitis involves diffuse liver inflammation due to certain hepatotropic viruses, with diverse modes of transmission and epidemiologies. Chronic hepatitis lasts for six months or more. Common causes include the hepatitis B and C viruses, both of which may be sexually transmitted.

Hepatitis B

Hepatitis B is the primary blood-borne hazard for health care workers, and it may be transmitted through contaminated plasma and serum, contaminated needles, cuts caused by contaminated sharps, sexual contact, and contaminated material being splashed into the eyes, nose, mouth, or broken skin. HBV is also transmitted from infected mothers to their infants. The virus can survive for at least one week on an environmental surface, even if dried. HBV is also known as serum hepatitis. This severe infection may result in prolonged illness and can become chronic, causing liver tissue destruction, cirrhosis, and death. In the acute form, nearly one-third of the patients have no symptoms. Any initial symptoms last for between 2 and 14 days, and there is no specific treatment or medication that kills the virus. Approximately 90% of patients recover fully after acute HBV, but the remainders develop chronic HBV, increasing the risk of liver damage, cirrhosis, liver cancer, or liver failure.

The HBV vaccine is highly effective in providing immunity against HBV for at least seven years. A combination HBV and Hib conjugate vaccine is available. For hepatitis B, interferon alfa is used if the disease is persistent. Acute hepatitis B is usually self-resolved, but early antiviral treatment is used when the infection becomes fulminant, or when the immune system is compromised. Chronic hepatitis B patients with elevated serum alanine aminotraferse and HBV-DNA levels require treatment for six months to one year. Antivirals include lamivudine, adefovir, tenofovir, telbivudine, entecavir, interferon alpha-2a, and pegylated interferon alpha-2a.

Hepatitis C

Hepatitis C is also known as *non-A, non-B hepatitis*. This chronic form is mostly transmitted by blood infusion or intravenous drug use, shared needles, and sexual contact. Up until recently it was not curable. Diagnosis requires detection of HCV antibodies. For hepatitis C, glucocorticoids may help in reducing inflammation. However, major drug research is improving treatments for chronic hepatitis C. Today, certain combinations of antivirals can be curative. The mechanism of action of the *interferon alfa* is unspecific. Activated immune cells attack other virus-infected cells as well as normal, uninfected cells. Newer medications have more specific mechanisms, including ombitasvir, ritonavir, and sofosbuvir. They work by targeting key enzymes for viral replication, with less side effects and better outcomes. Recent medications are still very expensive, however. Table 28-6 summaries medications used to treat hepatitis B and hepatitis C.

WHAT WOULD YOU DO?

Statins, which are prescribed to lower cholesterol and reduce risks of cardiovascular disease, can interact with medications used to treat the hepatitis C virus, leading to serious adverse effects. If a patient came to your pharmacy with a prescription for an HCV medication and you noticed that the computer said he was taking statins, what would you do?

Table 28-6 Medications Used to Treat Hepatitis B and C

Generic Name	Trade Name	Route of Administration	Average Adult Dosage
Hepatitis B (only)			
Nucleoside Reverse Transcriptase Inhibitors (NRTIs)			
entecavir	Baraclude®	PO	0.5 to 1 mg once daily
lamivudine	Epivir-HBV®	PO	100 mg once daily
telbivudine	Tyzeka®	PO	600 mg once daily
Nucleotide Reverse Transcriptase Inhibitors (NTRTIs)			
adefovir	Hepsera®	PO	10 mg once daily
tenofovir	Viread®	PO	300 mg once daily
Both Hepatitis B and C			
Interferons			
interferon alfa-2b	Intron A®	IM, subcutaneous	5 million units/day or 10 million units 3 times/week for 16 weeks
interferon alfa-2a pegylated	Pegasys®	Subcutaneous	180 mcg once weekly, for 48 weeks

(Continued)

Table 28-6 Medications Used to Treat Hepatitis B and C *(Continued)*

Generic Name	Trade Name	Route of Administration	Average Adult Dosage
Hepatitis C (only)			
Antiviral			
ribavirin	Rebetol®	PO	800 to 1400 mg/day for 24 or 48 weeks, combined with pegylated interferons
Interferon			
interferon alfa-2b pegylated	PegIntron®	Subcutaneous	1 mcg/kg once weekly
Protease Inhibitors			
boceprevir	Victrelis®	PO	800 mg tid, added to PEG-INF plus ribavirin after four weeks of dual therapy
telaprevir	Incivek®	PO	1125 mg bid, added to PEG-INF plus ribavirin after 11 weeks of dual therapy
Combination Products			
ombitasvir, paritaprevir, ritonavir, dasabuvir	Viekira Pak®, Viekira XR®	PO	Ombitasvir/paritaprevir/ritonavir: 2 tablets q morning; dasabuvir: 1 tablet bid; extended release form: 3 tablets once daily
ledipasvir, sofosbuvir	Harvoni®	PO	1 tablet (90 mg ledipasvir/400 mg sofosbuvir) once daily

Chlamydia

Chlamydia, one of the most commonly reported infectious diseases in the United States, causes urethritis in men and ure-thritis and cervicitis (a common infection of the lower genital tract) in women. It is caused by *C. trachomatis*, an intracellular bacterium that is usually transmitted through sexual contact. Primary infection usually occurs around the genitals but may also be located in the oral or anal regions. Often, transmission occurs without either partner knowing they have chlamydia.

Chlamydia sometimes is referred to as the silent STI because it has no symptoms in more than 50% of the patients. In most women, there are no initial symptoms, but three out of four affected males have symptoms within three weeks of exposure. It is the leading cause of PID and a major cause of female sterility. In women, early symptoms include thick vaginal discharge with burning, abdominal pain, itching, and dyspareunia. In men, there is penile discharge with burning and itching, and burning during urination that is caused by urethritis. If a newborn acquires chlamydia from the mother during birth, the condition may lead to conjunctivitis, blindness, arthritis, or systemic infections.

Treatment involves antibiotics for both partners, starting with a single injection that is followed with a course of oral antibiotics (often, azithromycin or erythromycin). A seven-day regimen of doxycycline also may be used. If treatment is prompt, the infection may be cured and complications such as PID and abnormal pregnancies prevented. Follow-up test-ing should be conducted. To prevent reinfection, all sexual partners, within 60 days of symptom onset or diagnosis, must be evaluated and treated. For at least seven days after treatment onset, there must be abstinence from sexual intercourse. When a pregnant woman contracts chlamydia, treatment options are different; they include azithromycin and amoxicillin.

MEDICATION ERROR ALERT

There are common mistakes that occur in the treatment of chlamydia, such as the popular use of *ciprofloxacin*, even though there is increasing evidence that the causative bacteria are becoming resistant to this antibiotic. Also, treatments for chlamydia must be administered for an entire two-week period and follow-up appointments are essential to confirm that the disease has been cleared up.

Gonorrhea

Gonorrhea is a very common infection of the **genitourinary** tract. It is caused by *N. gonorrhoeae* and is usually transmitted sexually. Though the disease appears to be declining in prevalence, *N. gonorrhoeae* is increasingly resistant to the drugs that have traditionally been used for treatment. Because the infection may be transmitted during birth, prophylactic erythromycin salve is often administered to newborn infants to protect them from eye infections and possible future blindness.

Signs and symptoms of gonorrhea are similar to those of chlamydia, and they may include pus from the urethra or rectum, increased urinary frequency, dysuria, severe rectal pain and itching, anal bleeding, abnormal vaginal discharge, uterine bleeding, and pharyngitis. Gonorrhea may also infect the eyes or throat, or it may produce a widespread infection affecting all body systems. Based on the infection site, signs and symptoms arise in 2 to 8 days in males and in about 10 days in females. The most common sites of infection are the urethra, rectum, and oropharynx in both sexes, and in the endocervical canal in females.

Treatment for gonorrhea should be given to the affected individual and all sexual partners. Upon diagnosis, medications that should be administered include ceftriaxone, cefixime, ciprofloxacin, and doxycycline. Penicillin and tetracycline are not as widely used in the treatment of gonorrhea as in the past because many strains of the bacteria have become resistant to these agents. Follow-up cultures should be performed to assure a complete cure. Without treatment, complications include PID, septicemia, infertility, and septic arthritis.

MEDICAL TERMINOLOGY REVIEW

dysuria:

dys = *difficult*   -ia = *condition*

ur/o = *pertaining to urine*   difficult urination

Trichomoniasis

Trichomoniasis is a protozoal infection of the lower genitourinary tract. The condition usually affects the vagina in women and the urethra in men. It is caused by *Trichomonas vaginalis*, usually transmitted through sexual contact.

Initial symptoms for both male and female patients include urethritis with dysuria and itching. Between 20% and 50% of infected women are asymptomatic. Women may notice a profuse, greenish-yellow discharge from the vagina that has an unpleasant odor. Clinical examination often reveals a "strawberry cervix," caused by cervical micro hemorrhages. Men may have a whitish penile discharge but are usually asymptomatic. Nearly 15% of sexually active adults have trichomoniasis. Though trichomoniasis may subside on its own, lack of treatment means that the infection remains present and may become chronic.

MEDICAL TERMINOLOGY REVIEW

trichomoniasis:

trich/o = *hair-like*   -iasis = *condition*

mon/o = *single*   condition caused by a single-celled organism
                                                                with hair-like appendages

Treatment is based on positive laboratory culture. If positive, anti-infective medications called nitroimidazole are administered. Metronidazole or tinidazole may usually be given in a single large dose. Some patients require metronidazole twice a day for up to seven days. Patients must avoid drinking alcohol while taking metronidazole or tinidazole.

Genital Herpes

Genital herpes is an infection of the skin of the genital area. Ulcerations develop after skin-to-skin contact. These cause painful genital sores that are similar to cold sores. Genital herpes is caused by herpes simplex virus type 2 (HSV-2) and is a recurrent, incurable viral disease (see Figure 28-6). One out of every five adults carries the highly

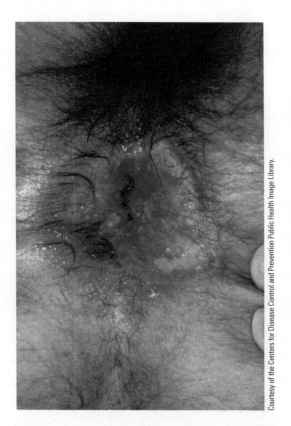

Courtesy of the Centers for Disease Control and Prevention Public Health Image Library.

Figure 28-6 Genital herpes.

contagious HSV-2. It is usually transmitted through sexual contact. Cross-infection with herpes simplex virus type 1 (HSV-1) may result from oral-genital or anal sex. In younger patients, genital herpes is often caused by HSV-1. Open lesions increase risks of contracting acquired immunodeficiency syndrome (AIDS) during intercourse between persons with HSV-2 and those positive for human immunodeficiency virus (HIV).

Signs and symptoms include one or more lesions resembling blisters on the genitals or around the anus. These may be painful, occurring 2 to 30 days following sexual contact with an infected individual. Symptoms may also include those resembling systemic influenza, fever, swollen glands, headache, and painful urination. Recurrent outbreaks may occur for months to years since the virus remains dormant in the nervous system between these recurrences.

Though genital herpes is incurable, prescription antiviral medications can reduce the duration and frequency of outbreaks. These medications include acyclovir, famciclovir, and valacyclovir. Affected women must be monitored for the development of cervical cancer, so a Papanicolaou (Pap) smear must be performed every six months. Since genital herpes can be transmitted to newborns from affected mothers during vaginal delivery, cesarean section may be indicated if the mother is infected with HSV-2. When suppressive therapy is used, this decreases reoccurrence by 70% to 80% in patients who have six or more outbreaks per year.

Syphilis

Syphilis is a chronic, systemic STI that develops in four stages. Infection with the *Treponema pallidum* spirochete usually occurs through sexual contact (or other direct contact) with infected lesions or infected body fluids. Congenital transmission of syphilis can also occur during pregnancy.

Primary Syphilis   Initial signs and symptoms of *primary syphilis* include the presence of a painless but highly contagious local lesion called a **chancre** on the male or female genitalia (see Figure 28-7). This occurs within 21 days but may range between 10 and 90 days. Affected areas may also include the perianal area, mouth, and throat. Chancres heal on their own within three to six weeks.

Secondary Syphilis   After the primary lesion heals, the causative organism has infiltrated the entire body, causing additional lesions to appear in the lymph nodes, skin (in a symmetrical pattern on the trunk, palms, and soles), brain,

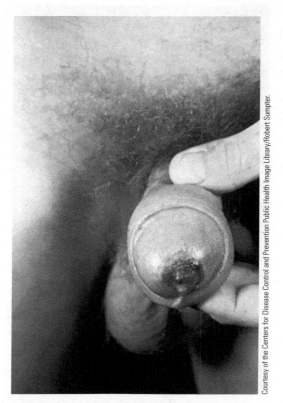

Courtesy of the Centers for Disease Control and Prevention Public Health Image Library/Robert Sumpter.

Figure 28-7 Primary syphilis: male.

cardiovascular system, spinal cord, and elsewhere. It is still contagious during this time, and symptoms include fever, joint aches, headaches, mouth sores, and rashes on the palms and soles. Secondary syphilis develops within two to eight weeks. A latent stage develops if there is no treatment or inadequate treatment within 4 to 10 weeks. After this, there are no signs and symptoms, but serology tests can confirm the disease. If a fetus is infected, death often occurs in utero, or the child is born with congenital syphilis, resulting in many abnormalities.

Tertiary Syphilis   The next stage is a latent period that may develop between 10 to 30 years after initial infection, often with no symptoms. It occurs in 25% to 30% of the patients. There is no central nervous system involvement. Tertiary syphilis may involve the skin, joints, or cardiovascular system.

Neurosyphilis   The final stage involves CNS lesions, called **gummas**, which cause potentially disabling, life-threatening tissue damage. If a fetus is infected, death often occurs in utero, or the child is born with congenital syphilis, resulting in many abnormalities. Gummas can affect up to 50% of the patients.

Syphilis is easily cured in the early stages using benzathine penicillin G antibiotic therapy. Other antibiotics such as doxycycline or tetracycline may also be used. Patients should be monitored with follow-up blood tests for up to one year. Without early treatment during the primary stage, syphilis becomes a systemic, chronic disease that can involve any organ or tissue. If neurosyphilis is present, the treatment is with aqueous crystalline penicillin G. Medications used to treat various STIs are summarized in Table 28-7.

Human Papillomavirus

Genital human papillomavirus (HPV) is the most common sexually transmitted disease in the United States. While only 30 types infect the genitals, there are over 100 types that have been discovered. This virus is extremely common in sexually active adults, and is usually self-limiting, transmitted often between sexual partners. It may cause genital warts and cervical cell changes that can lead to cervical cancer. Many forms of HPV do not produce signs and symptoms, and the virus is usually detected in a routine checkup. Many infected patients are unaware that they have the virus. Unless there are clinical signs of genital warts of cervical cancer, HPV is not treated, since it is self-limiting and no therapy effectively eradicates the virus.

POINTS TO REMEMBER

The Gardasil® vaccine is available for the prevention of HPV types 6, 11, 16, and 18. The HPV types 16 and 18 are associated with cervical cancer. Gardasil was initially approved for females between ages 9 and 26. It was then recommended for routine vaccination of females at ages 11 and 12. A newer form, Gardasil 9, is approved for females 27 through 45.

Table 28-7 Medications Used to Treat Sexually Transmitted Infections

Generic Name	Trade Name	Route of Administration	Average Adult Dosage
Vaginal Candidiasis			
clotrimazole	Gyne-Lotrimin®	Intravaginal	2%: one applicator full/day for three days; 1%: one applicator full/day for seven days
fluconazole	Diflucan®	PO	150 mg as a single dose
miconazole	Monistat®	Vaginal suppository	1200 mg inserted for one day
terconazole	Terazol®	Intravaginal	0.8% cream: one applicator full (5 g)/day at bedtime, for three days; 0.4% cream: one applicator full (5 g)/day for seven days
tioconazole	Vagistat-1®	Intravaginal	One applicator full (5 g) before bedtime as a single dose
Chlamydia			
azithromycin	Zithromax®	PO	1 mg once
doxycycline	Vibramycin®	PO	100 mg bid for seven days
erythromycin	E-Mycin®	PO	500 mg qid for seven days
levofloxacin	Levaquin®	PO	500 mg/day for seven days
ofloxacin	Floxin®	PO	300 mg bid for seven days
Bacterial Vaginitis			
clindamycin	Clindesse®	Intravaginal	One applicator full (5 g) at bedtime for seven days
metronidazole	Flagyl®, Metrogel Vaginal 0.75%®	PO, intravaginal	PO: 500 mg bid, for seven days; intravaginal: one applicator full (5 g)/day for five days
Genital Herpes			
acyclovir	Zovirax®	PO	400 mg tid for 7 to 10 days
famciclovir	Famvir®	PO	250 mg tid for 7 to 10 days
valacyclovir	Valtrex®	PO	1 g bid for 10 days
Gonorrhea			
cefixime	Suprax®	PO	400 mg once
cefixime/azithromycin	Zithromax®	PO	1 g once
ceftriaxone	Rocephin®	IM	250 mg once

(Continued)

Table 28-7 Medications Used to Treat Sexually Transmitted Infections *(Continued)*

Generic Name	Trade Name	Route of Administration	Average Adult Dosage
Syphilis			
benzathine/penicillin G	Bicillin L-A®	IM	2.4 million units once
Trichomoniasis Vaginalis			
metronidazole	Flagyl®, Metrogel Vaginal®	PO	2 g once
tinidazole	Tindamax®	PO	2 g once

Genital Warts

Genital warts are most often caused by human papillomavirus types 6 and 11. The majority of genital warts are flat and popular, upon the genital mucosa. They are sometimes, painful, itchy, or easily damaged. Visual inspection of the external genitalia is usually sufficient for diagnoses. HPV types 6 and 11 can be related to conjunctival, nasal, oral, and laryngeal warts. Biopsy is recommended when the diagnosis is uncertain, the lesions do not respond to standard treatments, they worsen during therapy, the patient's immune system is compromised, or the warts are pigmented, hardened, fixed, bleeding, or ulcerated. Treatments are aimed at removal of the warts, but this does not eliminate the HPV infection. Untreated warts can self-resolve, remain unchanged, or increase in both size and number. The Gardasil® vaccine protects against the development of genital warts.

Treatment options include podophyllin resin, podofilox, imiquimod, cryotherapy, and trichloroacetic or bichloroacetic acid. Podophyllin resin is a tincture of benzoin that must be applied by a health care professional. It disrupts viral activity and induces local tissue necrosis. Podofilox is a patient-applied solution or gel that cannot be used for perianal warts. Imiquimod (Aldara®) is also patient-applied, and it acts as an immune response modifier. Cryotherapy involves wart removal via freezing techniques with nitrogen. Trichloroacetic or bichloroacetic acids cause chemical coagulation of proteins in the warts.

Special Topic—Contraceptives

A woman's menstrual cycle is controlled by both estrogen and progesterone. Manipulating estrogen and progesterone levels can prevent pregnancy (a popular method of contraception). Oral contraceptives are the most commonly used drugs to prevent pregnancy.

Oral contraceptives include the following:

1. Estrogen and progestin combinations
2. Progestin-only preparations

Table 28-8 shows some examples of the most commonly used contraceptive agents.

Though oral contraceptives are available in many different formulations, they are all commonly referred to as "the pill." The most commonly used type of estrogen in oral contraceptives is ethinyl estradiol. The most commonly used progestin is norethindrone.

With correct use, oral contraceptives are nearly 100% effective. Most formulations that contain estrogen have only 20 mcg of the hormone. Usually, the patient begins taking the pill on day five of her menstrual cycle, taking one per day for 21 days. For the remaining seven days of the cycle, she takes a placebo pill. Use of these placebos ensures that the patient remembers to take a pill every day, and some placebos contain iron, to supplement loss of this mineral during menstruation.

The three types of estrogen/progestin formulations are monophasic, biphasic, and triphasic. The monophasic type is most commonly used, and it delivers a steady dose of hormones throughout the 21-day cycle. The biphasic type has increased amounts of progestin toward the end of the cycle, which nourishes the uterine lining more effectively. The triphasic type has varying amounts of estrogen and progestin. All three types have the same effectiveness. Progestin-only oral contraceptives are sometimes referred to as "minipills" and work differently, by producing mucus at the uterine entrance that makes it difficult for sperm to enter. They also often inhibit implantation of a fertilized ovum. Minipills are slightly less effective than estrogen/progestin formulations and cause more adverse effects, but is a better option if the patient has a higher risk of adverse effects caused by estrogen.

Adverse effects of oral contraceptives are varied and may include breast milk reduction, cancer, glucose elevation, hypertension, increased appetite, weight gain, fatigue, depression, acne, hirsutism, exacerbation of lupus

Table 28-8 Examples of Contraceptive Agents

Generic Name	Trade Name	Route of Administration	Average Adult Dosage
Monophasic Agents			
estrogen/progestin	Alesse-28®, Necon 1/35®, Ortho-Novum 1/35®	PO	One active tablet daily for 21 days, then placebo tablet or no tablets for seven days, repeat cycle
estinyl estradiol/ desogestrel	Desogen®, Ortho-Cept®	PO	One active tablet daily for 21 days, then placebo tablet or no tablets for seven days, repeat cycle
estinyl estradiol/ levonorgestrel	Alesse®, Levlen®, Nordette®	PO	One active tablet daily for 21 days, then placebo tablet or no tablets for seven days, repeat cycle
ethinyl estradiol/ drospirenone	Yasmin®	PO	One active tablet daily for 21 days, then placebo tablet or no tablets for seven days, repeat cycle
ethinyl estradiol/ norelgestromin	Ortho Evra®	Transdermal patch	Wear patch for 21 days, remove for seven days
Biphasic Agents			
ethinyl estradiol/ norethindrone	Ortho-Novum 10/11®	PO	One first-phase tablet/day for 10 days, then 1 second-phase tablet/day for 11 days; skip seven days before restarting
Triphasic Agents			
ethinyl estradiol/ levonorgestrel	Tri-Levlen®, Triphasil®	PO	One first-phase tablet/day for seven days, followed by 1 second-phase tablet/day for seven days, then one third-phase tablet/day for seven days; skip seven days before restarting
ethinyl estradiol/ norethindrone	Ortho-Novum 7/7/7®, Tri- Norinyl®	PO	One first "active" tablet starting on first Sunday after menstruation begins, or on that Sunday if menstruation begins that day; take one active table daily for 21 days followed by one green "reminder" table daily for seven days
Estrophasic Agents			
ethinyl estradiol/ norethindrone	Estrostep®	PO	1 tablet/day for 21 days; skip seven days before restarting

(Continued)

Table 28-8 Examples of Contraceptive Agents *(Continued)*

Generic Name	Trade Name	Route of Administration	Average Adult Dosage
Progestin-Only Agents			
norethindrone	Micronor®, Nor-Q.D.®	PO	0.35 mg/day starting on day one of menstrual flow, then continuing indefinitely
1norgestrel	Ovrette®	PO	0.075 mg/day starting on day one of menstrual flow, then continuing indefinitely
Long-Acting Agents			
ethinyl estradiol/ levonorgestrel (extended-cycle)*	Seasonique®	PO	1 tablet/day for 21 days; then 1 placebo tablet/day for seven days
etonogestrel/ethinyl estradiol**	NuvaRing®	Vaginal ring	Insert ring on first day of menstrual bleeding, and leave in place for three weeks; then remove for seven days
intrauterine progesterone contraceptive system	Progestasert®	IM, IUD	Insert device on seventh day of menstrual cycle; may leave in place up to five years
levonorgestrel	Mirena®	IUD	Device is inserted by a physician; may leave in place up to five years
medroxyprogesterone acetate	Depo-Provera®	IM	100 mg q3 months

*WARNING: This medication should not be used by patients who smoke cigarettes; this increases the risk of serious cardiovascular events, especially in women over the age of 35 years.

**WARNING: This medication is linked to thromboembolic disorders and other vascular problems.

erythematosus, menstrual irregularities, migraine headaches, nausea, edema, breast tenderness, and thromboembolic disorders. Also, estrogens are in pregnancy category X, with definite teratogenic effects. Therefore, any women who become pregnant while taking oral contraceptives containing estrogen must discontinue them immediately.

MEDICATION ERROR ALERT

Medication errors sometimes occur due to something as simple as incorrect packaging by a manufacturer. In 2012, medication lots of norgestrel/ethinyl estradiol (Lo/Ovral-28®) had to be recalled because the manufacturer packaged some tablets out of order and used inexact numbers of active and inactive tablets. Because of these errors the product provided inadequate contraception, which increased the risk of unintended pregnancies.

LONG-TERM CONTRACEPTIVES

Long-term contraceptives are also available for administration by deep intramuscular injection (providing three months of protection), skin implants (providing three years of protection), transdermal patches, vaginal implants (providing three weeks of protection), uterine implants (providing five years of protection), and as extended-regimen oral contraceptives. These oral contraceptives actually extend the time between menses so that only four periods occur every year.

POINTS TO REMEMBER

The risk of ovarian cancer may be reduced by the use of oral contraceptives, nonsteroidal anti-inflammatory drugs, and acetaminophen.

EMERGENCY CONTRACEPTIVES

For "emergency" contraception, an agent called Plan B® is used, which contains levonorgestrel. Two doses are taken, 12 hours apart, which act by preventing ovulation as well as by altering the endometrium of the uterus and preventing implantation. However, if implantation of a fertilized ovum has already occurred, this medication will not terminate the pregnancy. The medication must be administered as soon as possible after unprotected intercourse. It is less effective once 72 hours have passed, and it is ineffective if seven days have passed. Normally, about 8% of women who have unprotected sex become pregnant, and Plan B® reduces that number to between 1% and 2%. Medications used for emergency contraception and pharmacological termination of pregnancy is listed in Table 28-9.

Table 28-9 Medications Used for Emergency Contraception and Abortion

Generic Name	Trade Name	Route of Administration	Average Adult Dosage
Emergency Contraceptive			
levonorgestrel	Plan B®	PO	One dose of 1.5 mg within 72 hours of unprotected intercourse, followed by another dose 1.5 mg 12 hours later. Alternately, both doses may be taken at once, within 72 hours of unprotected intercourse
Pharmacological Agents That Terminate Early Pregnancy			
carboprost tromethamine	Hemabate®	IM	250 mcg (1 mL) initial dose, repeated at 1½ to 3½ hours intervals, if indicated by uterine response; may be increased to 500 mcg (2 mL) if uterine contractility is not adequate after several doses (maximum 12 mg); this drug should not be administered continuously for more than one month
dinoprostone	Cervidil®, Prepidil®, Prostin E$_2$®	Intravaginal	Insert suppository high in vagina; repeat every 2 to 5 hours until abortion occurs or membranes rupture (maximum 240 mg)
methotrexate/misoprostol	(generic only)	IM (methotrexate) + Intravaginal (misoprostol)	Methotrexate (50 mg/m^2), followed five days later by intravaginal misoprostol (800 mcg)
mifepristone/misoprostol	Mifeprex®	PO	Day one: 600 mg of mifepristone; day three, if abortion has not occurred: 400 mcg of misoprostol

Summary

The main female sex organs are the ovaries, which produce ova (eggs) as part of their exocrine function. They also have an endocrine function, producing the female sex hormones estrogen and progesterone. Female accessory organs include the fallopian tubes, uterus, vagina, and external genitalia. Menstruation is also known as the menstrual cycle or menses. The vagina not only passes the menstrual flow but is also the receptacle for the penis during sexual intercourse. The mammary glands produce milk to nourish a newborn baby.

The main male sex organs are the testes, which produce sperm as well as male sex hormones. The penis serves, along with being the organ of urination, to transport sperm and also to penetrate the vagina for reproduction. Together, these glands secrete the liquid portion of the semen, which contains the sperm and is produced during ejaculation.

Disorders of the reproductive system include infertility, pelvic inflammatory disease, dysfunctional uterine bleeding, menopause, hypogonadism, benign prostatic hyperplasia, prostate cancer, erectile dysfunction, and sexually transmitted diseases. Medications for reproductive system disorders include those for infertility, various reproductive disorders, benign prostatic hyperplasia, erectile dysfunction, hepatitis B and C, and sexually transmitted infections. There are also many different types of contraceptives.

REVIEW QUESTIONS

1. The muscular layer of the uterus is the:

   A. perimetrium.
   B. sarcometrium.
   C. endometrium.
   D. myometrium.

2. The average length of the menstrual cycle is:

   A. 10 days.
   B. 14 days.
   C. 21 days.
   D. 28 days.

3. Menstruation is triggered by a drop in the levels of:

   A. luteinizing hormone.
   B. follicle-stimulating hormone.
   C. estrogen.
   D. progesterone and estrogen.

4. Testosterone is secreted by the:

   A. interstitial cells.
   B. sustentacular cells.
   C. hypothalamus.
   D. hypophysis.

5. Which of the following is an example of a progestin?

   A. Norethindrone
   B. Estropipate
   C. Dinoprostone
   D. Carboprost

6. Oxymetholone is an example of a(n):

   A. progestin.
   B. androgen.
   C. GnRH analog.
   D. prostaglandin.

7. The silent STI is referred to as:

   A. gonorrhea.
   B. genital herpes.
   C. syphilis.
   D. chlamydia.

8. The trade name for tamsulosin is:

   A. Flomax.
   B. Cialis.
   C. Levitra.
   D. Cardura.

9. Which of the following is the trade name of tadalafil?

   A. Levitra
   B. Cialis
   C. Allegra
   D. Viagra

10. The most commonly used estrogen/progestin formulations are:

    A. monophasic.
    B. biphasic.
    C. triphasic.
    D. polyphasic.

11. Which of the following contraceptive agents is administered intramuscularly?

    A. Mirena
    B. Nuva Ring
    C. Depo-Provera
    D. Ovrette

12. Which of the following medications is not used for female infertility?

    A. Parlodel
    B. Clomid
    C. Andro LA
    D. Follistim

13. Which of the following is *not* an example of a contraceptive agent?

    A. Desogen®
    B. Ortho-Cept®
    C. Levitra®
    D. Yasmin®

14. The trade name of sildenafil is:

    A. Cialis®.
    B. Viagra®.
    C. Depotest®.
    D. Androderm®.

15. Which of the following medications is used for emergency contraception and abortion?

    A. Hemabate®

    B. Depo-Provera®

    C. Mirena®

    D. Progestasert®

CRITICAL THINKING

A 25-year-old woman who has had chlamydia is diagnosed with PID.

    1. What are the signs and symptoms of PID?

    2. What are the treatments of choice?

WEB LINKS

Infertility and Reproductive Disorders: academic.oup.com/humupd/article/22/1/104/2457870

MamasHealth.com: blog.mamashealth.com

Men's Health Center: www.webmd.com/men/default.htm

Pregnancy Week by Week: www.pregnancy.com

Women's Health Center: www.webmd.com/women/default.htm

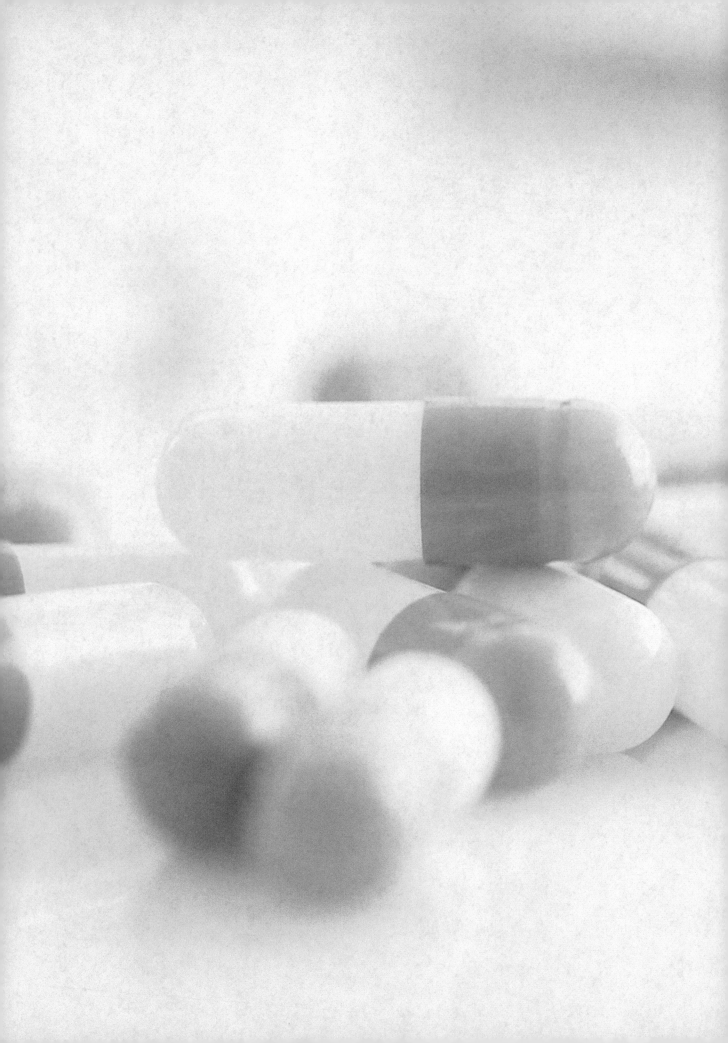

Therapeutic Drugs for the Eyes, Ears, and Nose

OBJECTIVES

Upon completion of this chapter, the reader should be able to:

1. Explain the structure and function of the eyes, ears, and nose.
2. Describe the three layers of the eyes.
3. Compare the structure of the middle and inner ears.
4. Identify the types of drugs that cause ototoxicity.
5. Define the term "conjunctivitis" and its treatments.

6. Differentiate between angle-closure and open-angle glaucoma.

7. Discuss the various treatments for glaucoma.

8. Identify various drugs used to treat otitis media and other ear disorders.

9. Describe the signs and symptoms of retinal detachment.

10. Explain drugs that are used for allergies and sinusitis.

KEY TERMS

aqueous humor	conjunctivitis	optic disc	sclera
auditory ossicles	cornea	organ of Corti	semicircular canals
auditory tube	eardrum	ototoxicity	suspensory ligaments
cerumen	external acoustic meatus	oval window	utricle
choroid	fovea centralis	pupil	uvea
ciliary body	labyrinth	retina	vitreous humor
cochlea	macula lutea	rods	
cones	macular degeneration	saccule	

Overview

The sense of vision is the dominant sense, with approximately 70% of all sensory receptors of the body found in the eyes. Almost 50% of the cerebral cortex is somewhat involved in visual processing. There are many eye disorders that can be critical, can cause blindness, including glaucoma, macular degeneration, and retinal detachment. The ears consist of three areas: external, middle, and inner. The middle ear is susceptible to various infections because of its specialized location. The inner ear is the center of the sense of hearing, and it can be harmed by many drugs due to their toxicity. The nose is the only external part of the respiratory system; it is surrounded by various cavities called sinuses. Common conditions involved with these structures include allergic rhinitis and bacterial sinusitis.

Anatomy and Physiology of the Eyes

Each eye is a hollow, spherical structure about 2.5 cm in diameter that is housed inside the bony orbits of the facial bones (see Figure 29-1). A single pair of optic nerves supplies the eyes. The wall of each eye has three distinct layers, which include sclera, choroid, and retina.

SCLERA

The outer layer of the eye is known as the **sclera**. The anterior portion of this outer layer bulges forward as the transparent **cornea**, which helps focus the entering light rays. The cornea is continuous with the sclera. However, the cornea does not contain blood vessels. The sclera is the white portion of the eye, consisting of tough and fibrous membranes. It is thinnest over the anterior surface and thickest at the back of the eye, where the optic nerve enters. A thin mucous membrane layer known as the conjunctiva lines the anterior eye and inner part of the eyelids. The conjunctiva covers the sclera, therefore, appearing white even though it is actually clear.

CHOROID

Each eye's vascular middle layer is called the **uvea**. It contains a layer just below the sclera that is known as the **choroid**, containing many capillaries providing blood and nutrients to the eye structures. The iris is the colored portion, which may be blue, brown, green, or hazel. The center of the iris contains a central opening called the **pupil**, which determines the amount of light that enters the eye. The pupil's diameter is controlled by contraction and relaxation of two sets of muscles inside the iris. The radial muscles dilate the pupil in dim light, and the circular muscles constrict it in bright light.

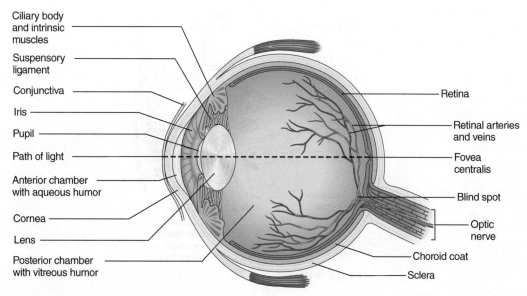

Figure 29-1 Structures of the eye.

Posterior to the iris, the lens is a clear, biconvex structure. It assists with focusing of images on the eye's sensitive nerve layer (the retina). On either side of the lens, the **ciliary body** secretes **aqueous humor**, a nutrient-rich watery fluid that bathes the anterior chamber of the eye. The ciliary body also has muscles that help to adjust the lens for viewing objects up close. Many **suspensory ligaments** radiate outward from the ciliary body, attaching to the lens to hold it in position. The ligaments react to the contraction and relaxation of the ciliary body muscles. Through their actions, the lens becomes thicker or thinner as required to help bend incoming light rays and focus images. Accommodation is the ability of the lens to focus on objects at different distances. In most adults, accommodation becomes less accurate with aging, and visual correction is needed.

Proper eye pressure is maintained by the aqueous humor, which is continually produced by the ciliary body and reabsorbed into the venous circulation. The posterior chamber of the eye, located behind the lens, contains the **vitreous humor**. This clear substance resembles jelly and helps to stabilize the eye and give physical support to the retina. The vitreous humor is not continually produced, and injury to the eye that causes the vitreous humor to escape may lead to blindness. The vitreous as well as aqueous humor aid in refracting light rays as they pass from the anterior eye to the retina.

RETINA

The inner layer of the eye is the **retina**, which contains sensitive nerve cells (photoreceptors) that alter the energy of light rays into nerve impulses (see Figure 29-2). The impulses then travel along the optic nerve at the back of the eye to the brain for interpretation. The retina's nerve cells are called **rods** and **cones**. The rods are located at the outer edges of the retina; they provide vision in dim light and are also involved in peripheral vision. The cones, which enable us to visualize colors, function in bright light and are also involved in central vision. Most cones are found in the **fovea centralis**, which is a small depression inside the **macula lutea**, a yellowish oval spot near the retina's center. Sharpest focus occurs when an image is focused directly on the fovea centralis. This is called central vision. The only part of the retina that is not sensitive to light is the **optic disc** (blind spot), since it contains no rods or cones. This is the area where the optic nerve leaves the eye, and its center point is where the artery supplying the retina enters.

Light rays enter the eyes, to be transmitted through the cornea, aqueous humor, pupil, lens, and vitreous humor. They reach the retina, are converted into impulses, and move from the optic nerve to the occipital lobe of the brain. This is the process of vision. At the optic chiasm, the nerve fibers cross, continuing to the thalamus. They synapse with neurons to send impulses to the right and left visual regions of the occipital lobe. Since these tracts cross, stimuli from the right visual fields are translated in the left occipital area, and vice versa (see Figure 29-3). In a final step, the signals received by the brain are combined and processed to produce the image that we "see."

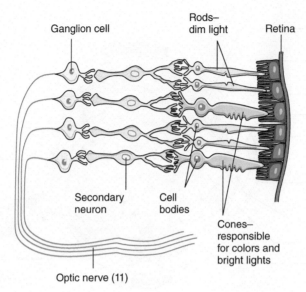

Figure 29-2 Layers of the retina.

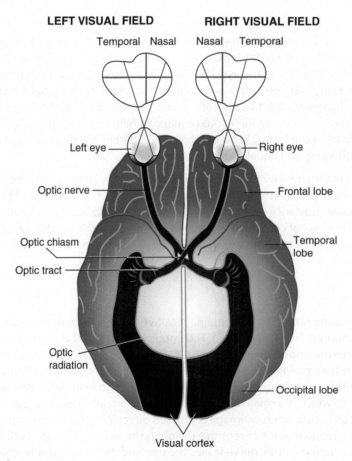

Figure 29-3 The vision pathway.

Disorders of the Eyes

The most common disorders of the eyes are conjunctivitis, glaucoma, macular degeneration, diabetic retinopathy, and retinal detachment.

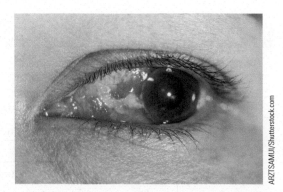

Figure 29-4 Conjunctivitis.

MEDICATION ERROR ALERT

Prescription and OTC eye drops may contain substances that cause allergic reactions, leading to surface irritation of the eyes. Continued use may result in increased inflammation, requiring medicated eye drops for treatment. Eye drops, in turn, may interact with other medications or health problems, resulting in systemic reactions.

CONJUNCTIVITIS

Conjunctivitis is a common condition in which the conjunctiva becomes inflamed (see Figure 29-4). It may result from bacterial or viral infection, or from irritation caused by allergies or chemicals. The most common causative bacteria include *Staphylococcus aureus*, *Streptococcus pneumonia*, *Haemophilus influenze*, and *Moraxella catarrhalis*. It is often transmitted when contaminated fingers, towels, or washcloths touch the eyes. Conjunctivitis may be unilateral or bilateral; it often starts in one eye and spreads to the other eye via the hands. It is important that infected individuals avoid sharing towels, clothes, or any personal items with other people, and they must seek treatment promptly. Signs and symptoms include redness, itching, and swelling of the conjunctiva. It is also known as "pink eye" and is extremely contagious.

MEDICAL TERMINOLOGY REVIEW

amblyopia:

ambly/o = *dull or dim*

-opia = *vision condition*

vision condition involving dulled sight with double images

MEDICAL TERMINOLOGY REVIEW

diplopia;

dipl/o = *double*

-opia = *vision condition*

condition of seeing double images

Treatment for conjunctivitis is varied, based on the cause. Any discharge should be removed from the eyes, which is accomplished with cool compresses. If the cause is a bacterial infection, topical antibiotics are prescribed. For allergic conjunctivitis, combination drugs containing an antihistamine and mast cell stabilizers are used. Table 29-1 summarizes ophthalmic antibiotics and Table 29-2 summaries topical medications used for allergic conjunctivitis.

Table 29-1 Ophthalmic Antibiotics

Generic Name	Trade Name	Average Adult Dosage
Aminoglycosides		
gentamicin	Genoptic®	Instill one to two drops 0.3% strength q4h
tobramycin	Tobrex®	Apply 0.5-inch ribbon of ointment, 0.3% strength, bid to tid
Fluoroquinolones		
besifloxacin	Besivance®	Instill one drop tid, 4 to 12 hours apart for seven days
ciprofloxacin	Ciloxan®	Instill one to two drops into conjunctival sac(s), 0.3% strength, q2h for two days; then one to two drops q4h for the next five days
gatifloxacin	Zymar®	Days one and two: instill one drop q2h up to 8 times daily; days three to seven, instill one drop up to qid
moxifloxacin	Vigamox®	Instill one drop 0.5% strength tid for seven days
norfloxacin	Chibroxin®	Apply one to two drops topically qid for up to seven days
ofloxacin	Ocuflox®	Days one and two: instill one to two drops 0.3% strength, q2 to 4h; days three to seven, instill one to two drops qid
polymyxin/trimethoprim	Polytrim®	Instill one drop in affected eye(s) q3h (maximum six doses/day) for 7 to 10 days
polymyxin B sulfate	Polymyxin B®	Dissolve 500,000 units in 20 to 50 mL sterile water for subconjunctival injection, for a 10,000 to 25,000 units per mL concentration
Macrolides		
azithromycin	AzaSite®	Days one and two: instill one drop bid, 8 to 12 hours apart; next five days, instill one drop once daily
erythromycin	Ilotycin®	Apply a 1-cm ribbon of ointment up to 6 times daily
Sulfonamide		
sulfacetamide	Bleph-10®	Instill one to two drops into conjunctival sac, 10% strength, q2 to 3h prn for 7 to 10 days
Miscellaneous Antibiotics		
bacitracin	generic only	Apply 1 to 3 times/day
polymyxin B/trimethoprim	Polytrim®	One drop in affected eye(s) q3h (maximum six doses/day) for 7 to 10 days
Antifungal		
natamycin	Natacyn®	One drop in conjunctival sac q1 to 2h; after three to four days reduce to 6 to 8 times daily (treatment lasts for two to three weeks)
Antivirals		
ganciclovir	Zirgan®	One drop of gel in affected eye(s) 5 times/day; then one drop tid for seven days
trifluiridne	Viroptic®	One drop in affected eye(s) q2h (maximum nine drops/day); then one drop q4h for seven days
Immunological Agent		
cyclosporine	Restasis®	One drop in each eye q12h

Table 29-2 Topical Medications Used to Treat Allergic Conjunctivitis

Generic Name	Trade Name	Average Adult Dosage
Decongestants		
naphazoline	Naphcon®, Clear Eyes Redness Relief®	Instill one or more drops prn into affected eye(s)
oxymetazoline	Visine-LR®	Instill one or more drops prn into affected eye(s)
phenylephrine	Refresh Redness Relief®	Instill one drop q3 to 5min to conjunctival fornix prn (maximum three drops per eye per day)
tetrahydrozoline	Visine®	Instill one drop per eye (maximum four drops per eye per day)
Decongestants and Antihistamines		
naphazoline/antazoline	Vasocon-A®	Instill one or more drops prn into affected eye(s)
naphazoline/pheniramine	Naphcon-A®, OPcon-A®, Visine-A®	Instill one or more drops prn into affected eye(s)
Histamine Antagonists		
alcaftadine	Lastacaft®	Instill one drop in each eye once daily
emedastine	Emadine®	Instill one drop in affected eye(s) up to qid
Histamine Antagonists and Mast Cell Stabilizers		
azelastine	Optivar®	Instill one drop bid
bepotastine	Bepreve®	Instill one drop into affected eye(s) bid
epinastine	Elestat®	Instill one drop in each eye bid
ketotifen	Zaditor®	Instill one drop bid, q8 to 12h, but no more than bid
olopatadine (0.1%)	Patanol®	Instill one drop bid, q6 to 8h
olopatadine (0.2%)	Pataday®	Instill one drop into affected eye(s) once/day
Mast Cell Stabilizers		
cromolyn	Crolom®	Instill one to two drops in each eye 4 to 6 times per day, at regular intervals
lodoxamide	Alomide®	Instill one to two drops in affected eye(s) qid; not to be used for longer than three months
nedocromil	Alocril®	Instill one to two drops in each eye bid, at regular intervals
pemirolast	Alamast®	Instill one to two drops in affected eye(s) qid

Allergic Conjunctivitis

Allergic conjunctivitis is inflammation of primarily the conjunctiva of the eye. When the eyes are exposed to allergens, they become red, itchy, and watery. This occurs most often in allergy season, when irritants or foreign objects cause mast cells to release histamine, resulting in inflammation. Seasonal allergies are allergic reactions to pollen from flowers, grasses, and trees. Additional causes include molds, pet dander, cigarette smoke, dust mites, and exhaust fumes. Oral medications are often used to resolve conjunctivitis and other allergy symptoms, along with topical medications. Ophthalmic antihistamines, decongestants, mast-cell stabilizers, and combination drugs are available. Non-pharmacologic therapies include avoiding allergen exposure and allying cold compresses three to four times daily.

GLAUCOMA

The term glaucoma describes a group of diseases affecting the optic nerve. Raised intraocular pressure is a significant risk factor for the development of glaucoma. If untreated, glaucoma leads to permanent optic nerve damage, which can progress to blindness. It is the second leading cause of blindness throughout the world. There is an estimated 60 million cases worldwide. This is expected to increase to 76 million in 2020, and 111 million in 2040. In the United States, approximately 3 million Americans are living with glaucoma, yet only about 50% know that they have the condition. Glaucoma is more common in patients older than 60 years of age, and among those over 80, one in 10 has the condition. Other risk factors for glaucoma include family history, nearsightedness, and the African American race. There are two primary types: chronic open-angle glaucoma and acute angle-closure glaucoma. To determine the extent and type of the disease, the pupils are dilated using a variety of medications (see Table 29-3).

Open-Angle Glaucoma

In chronic open-angle glaucoma, aqueous humor reabsorption is impaired by a blockage at the level of the trabecular meshwork of the eye. There is less aqueous humor than normal flowing out of the eye's anterior chamber. This results in a buildup of the humor and increased intraocular pressure. This condition may be secondary to trauma, occurring even years afterward. It may also be caused by overuse of topical steroids. About 2% of people in the United States who are older than age 40 have primary open-angle glaucoma, which is by far the most common form of the disease. Signs and symptoms of chronic open-angle glaucoma, which is the most common type and treatable type, usually appear after the condition has persisted for some time. Unfortunately, by the time symptoms appear, significant damage has usually occurred. Routine, regular ophthalmic examinations are the best way to detect glaucoma. In these examinations, the intraocular pressure is measured and the optic nerve is evaluated. Left untreated, this form of glaucoma eventually causes loss of peripheral vision. Central vision often remains clear for a long time, but will eventually be lost, as well.

Chronic open-angle glaucoma is usually treated with medications that decrease production of aqueous humor. These include carbonic anhydrase inhibitors, beta-blockers, and alpha-adrenergic agents. Treatment may also involve medications that increase uveoscleral outflow, such as prostaglandin analogs. Additional medications include cholinergic agonists, nonselective sympathomimetics, and osmotic diuretics. Laser treatments may succeed in opening the outflow system, and sometimes surgery is able to bypass this system. Most patients with this type of glaucoma can simply control the condition with eye drops.

Angle-Closure Glaucoma

Narrowing of the aqueous humor drainage system, which may also become completely closed, causes acute angle-closure glaucoma. This results in a fast and significant increase in intraocular pressure. Acute angle-closure

Table 29-3 Medications Used to Dilate the Pupils

Generic Name	Trade Name	Average Adult Dosage
Mydriatic (Sympathomimetic)		
phenylephrine	Mydfrin®	One drop of 2.5% or 10% solution prior to eye examination
Cycloplegics (Anticholinergics)		
atropine	Isopto Atropine®	One drop of 0.5% solution/day
cyclopentolate	Cyclogyl®	One drop of 0.5% to 2% solution 40 to 50 minutes prior to eye examination
homatropine	Isopto Homatropine®	One to two drops of 2% or 5% solution prior to eye examination
scopolamine hydrobromide	Isopto Hyoscine®	One to two drops of 0.25% solution 1 hour prior to eye examination
tropicamide	Mydriacyl®, Tropicacyl®	One to two drops of 0.5% to 1% solution prior to eye examination

glaucoma is a medical emergency that is often linked to blurred vision, headaches, severe eye pain, and eye redness. The patient is sensitive to light and may see "halos" around lights. A serious attack causes persistence and worsening of symptoms. Severe pain may develop, followed by nausea and vomiting. Elevated pressure causes haziness of the cornea. The pressure elevation in this form is usually much higher than in chronic open-angle glaucoma. Untreated acute angle-closure glaucoma eventually results in blindness. Fortunately, angle-closure glaucoma only accounts for about 10% of all glaucoma cases.

Early treatment of glaucoma is essential because the resulting visual loss usually cannot be reversed. While medications are used to treat this form, surgical procedures may be indicated. The primary treatment of acute angle-closure glaucoma is laser iridotomy, which makes a small opening in the iris that allows the filtering angle to open. Intraocular pressure is often lowered with medications prior to the procedure. Medications used for both forms of glaucoma are summarized in Table 29-4.

POINTS TO REMEMBER

The most common causes of blindness, worldwide, are loss of transparency of the cornea and glaucoma.

Table 29-4 Medications Used for Glaucoma

Generic Name	Trade Name	Average Adult Dosage
Carbonic Anhydrase Inhibitors		
acetazolamide	Diamox®	PO: 250 mg 1 to 4 times daily
brinzolamide	Azopt®	Instill one drop of 1% solution tid
dorzolamide	Trusopt®	Instill one drop of 2% solution in affected eye tid
methazolamide	Methazolamide®	PO: 50 to 100 mg bid to tid
Beta-Adrenergic Blockers		
betaxolol	Betoptic S®	Instill one drop of 0.5% solution bid
carteolol	Carteolol Hydrochloride®	Instill one drop of 1% solution in affected eye(s) bid
levobunolol	Betagan®	Instill one to two drops of 0.25% to 0.5% solution 1 to 2 times daily
metipranolol	OptiPranolol®	Instill one drop of 0.3% solution bid
timolol	Betimol®, Istalol®, Timoptic®	Instill one to two drops of 0.25% to 0.5% solution 1 to 2 times daily, or gel (salve): apply once daily
Combination Products		
brimonidine/timolol	Combigan®	Instill one drop in affected eye(s) bid, approximately 12 hours apart
timolol/dorzolamide	Cosopt®	Instill one drop in affected eye(s) bid
Alpha₂-Adrenergic Agonists		
apraclonidine	Iopidine®	Instill one drop of 0.5% solution bid
brimonidine	Alphagan®	Instill one drop of 0.2% solution bid
Prostaglandin Analogs		
bimatoprost	Lumigan®	Instill one drop of 0.03% solution daily in the evening

(Continued)

Table 29-4 Medications Used for Glaucoma (Continued)

Generic Name	Trade Name	Average Adult Dosage
latanoprost	Xalatan®	Instill one drop of 0.005% solution daily in the evening
tafluprost	Zioptan®	Instill one drop in conjunctival sac of affected eye(s) once daily in the evening
travoprost	Travatan Z®	Instill one drop of 0.004% solution daily in the evening
Cholinergic Agonists (Miotics)		
carbachol	Miostat®, Carboptic®	Instill one to two drops of 0.75% to 3% solution in lower conjunctival sac q4h, totaling tid
echothiophate iodide	Phospholine Iodide®	Instill one drop of 0.03% to 0.25% solution 1 to 2 times daily
pilocarpine	Isopto Carpine®, Pilopine®, Pilocar®	Acute glaucoma: instill one drop of 1% to 2% solution q5 to 10min for three to six doses; chronic glaucoma: instill one drop of 0.5% to 4% solution q4 to 12h
Nonselective Sympathomimetics		
dipivefrin HCl	Propine®	Instill one drop of 0.1% solution bid
Osmotic Diuretics		
isosorbide	Ismotic®	PO: 1 to 3 g/kg, 1 to 2 times daily
mannitol	Osmitrol®	IV: 1.5 to 2 mg/kg as a 15% to 25% solution over 30 to 60 minutes
Miscellaneous Hyperosmotic Agents		
glycerin (50%)	Generic only	PO: 1 to 1.5 g/kg
Corticosteroids—High Potency		
fluorometholone (0.1%)	Flarex®	One to two drops instilled into conjunctival sac(s) qid
prednisolone (1%)	Pred Forte®	Shake well, then instill one to two drops into the conjunctival sac bid to qid
rimexolone (1%)	Vexol®	Apply one to two drops into the conjunctival sac of affected eye qh for the first week, then one drop q2h during the second week, then taper until no longer needed
Corticosteroids—Intermediate Potency		
dexamethasone (0.1%)	Maxidex®	Shake well, then instill one to two drops into the conjunctival sac(s) (maximum 4 to 6 times daily)
difluprednate (0.05%)	Durezol®	Instill one drop into the conjunctival sac of affected eye qid, for 14 days, then tapered off
fluorometholone (0.1%)	FML®	Shake well, then instill one drop into the conjunctival sac bid to qid (up to one application q4h)
fluorometholone (0.25%)	FML Forte®	Instill one drop into the conjunctival sac bid to qid; do not discontinue therapy prematurely

(Continued)

Table 29-4 Medications Used for Glaucoma (Continued)		
Generic Name	**Trade Name**	**Average Adult Dosage**
loteprednol (0.2%)	Lotemax®	Apply 0.5 inch ribbon into the conjunctival sac(s) qid continuing for two weeks
loteprednol (0.5%)	Alrex®	Shake well, the instill one drop into the affected eye(s) qid
prednisolone acetate (0.12%)	Pred Mild®	Shake well, then instill one to two drops into the conjunctival sac bid to qid
Corticosteroids—Low Potency		
dexamethasone (0.05%) or (0.1%)	Decadron®, Maxidex®	0.75 to 9 mg/day based on disease state
medrysone (1%)	HMS®	Shake well, then instill one drop in conjunctival sac up to qid

MACULAR DEGENERATION

Macular degeneration is a medical condition that affects primarily older adults, resulting in thinning and atrophy of the retina. It can result in loss of central vision, making it difficult for the person to see fine details, read, or recognize the faces of others. It is the leading cause of blindness in people older than 50 years in the United States. Age-related macular degeneration starts with yellow deposits in the macula, which may be related to elevated cholesterol deposits. Age, genetic factors, and prolonged light exposure have been linked to its development. Proper intake of beta-carotene, zinc, and vitamins A, C, and E can reduce the risk of developing this condition and slow its progression.

Treatment for macular degeneration is aimed at slowing the deterioration it causes, as there is no cure. It may be treated with laser photocoagulation, photodynamic therapy, injection of antiangiogenic factors, or all of these therapies combined.

POINTS TO REMEMBER

Risk factors for macular degeneration include obesity, cigarette smoking, Chlamydia pneumoniae infection, family history, excessive sunlight exposure, hyperopia, hypertension, short stature, and blue or light-colored irises.

DIABETIC RETINOPATHY

Diabetic retinopathy affects the retinal blood vessels and usually occurs between 8 and 10 years after onset of diabetes mellitus (see Figure 29-5). It is most prevalent in diabetic patients who do not control their blood glucose levels, though anyone with diabetes is at risk for developing the condition. This is because diabetes causes vascular changes that can lead to poor circulation throughout the body, including in the retinal blood vessels.

Signs and symptoms of diabetic retinopathy include hemorrhages, microaneurysm, dilation of retinal veins, and neovascularization. The condition usually develops in both eyes. Visual clarity is lost, and blindness often results.

Treatment usually involves laser photocoagulation. Vision may be maintained with treatment, though retinopathy often recurs. A vitrectomy may be needed in cases of vitreous hemorrhage or proliferative disease.

RETINAL DETACHMENT

Retinal detachment involves separation (elevation) of the retina from the choroid (see Figure 29-6). Risk factors for retinal detachment include extreme nearsightedness and a history of eye trauma. The condition usually begins when a tear in the retina allows fluid to leak underneath it, causing separation from the choroid. Once separated, this portion of the retina no longer has visual function. Continued elevation of the retina causes the visual loss to progress.

Signs and symptoms of retinal detachment may be partial or complete loss of vision. Early diagnosis and treatment of retinal detachment is imperative. Treatment includes photocoagulation or surgery, performed quickly

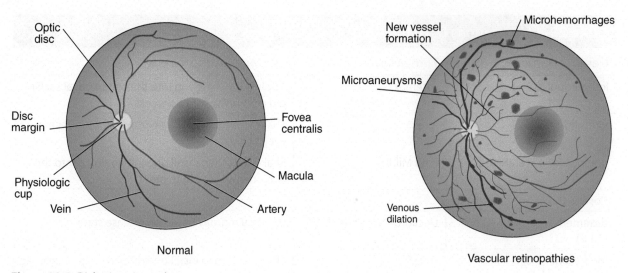

Figure 29-5 Diabetic retinopathy.

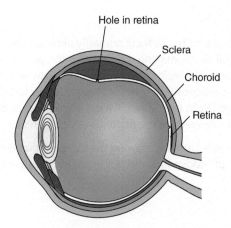

Figure 29-6 Retinal detachment.

to prevent additional detachment. If there are retinal tears but no significant detachment, photocoagulation or cryotherapy may be used. Photocoagulation easily seals retinal tears.

POINTS TO REMEMBER

Preeclampsia and eclampsia may be associated with exudative retinal detachment. There is no indicated intervention, and prognosis is usually good.

DRY EYES

The environment, other medical conditions, or side effects of medications may cause occasional or constant dry eyes. Lack of adequate tearing causes the eyes to lose lubrication and protection, and also for debris to build up. There is often irritation and temporary blurred vision. Prevalence of dry eye is in 5% to 35% of people, based on age. It is most common in older people, prevalence being more in females than in males. Sometimes, severe chronic dry dye can lead to additional eye damage when not treated. Non-pharmacologic treatments include increased dietary intake of omega-3 fatty acids or fish oil supplements; avoiding dryness, dust, and wind; using a home humidifier; applying warm eye compresses; avoiding cigarette smoke; and reducing time spent in front of computer screens or televisions. When these measures fail, *artificial tear medications* may be required.

Artificial Tears

Artificial tear substitutes lubricate the eyes and provide temporary relief from dry eye. These medications do not treat any underlying causes. For severe or chronic dry eyes, the patient may require treatment from an ophthalmologist. There are many over-the-counter (OTC) products available, in drop, gel, or ointment forms. They may be used as often as every 30 minutes with few side effects apart from mild stinging. The reason for this is a slight difference in pH between normal and artificial tears. Therefore, preservative-free artificial tears may be better tolerated. Patients are advised never to overuse artificial tear products and to follow the regimen exactly. A newer medication called cyclosporine ophthalmic emulsion (Restasis) is an anti-inflammatory and immunosuppressive medication used for chronic moderate-to-severe dry eyes that are due to chronic inflammation. When artificial tear substitutes do not relieve dry eye, ophthalmic corticosteroids may be beneficial.

Anatomy and Physiology of the Ears

The ears are the organs of hearing. They have external, middle, and inner parts (see Figure 29-7). The ears also function in the sense of equilibrium (balance). Since the ears are located on each side of the head, binaural hearing, which is hearing from both sides, is possible.

EXTERNAL EAR

The outer ear consists of three parts. The outer portion is called the auricle. This is a cartilaginous flap with a fleshy lower portion commonly called the ear lobe. The external auditory canal or **external acoustic meatus** is an S-shaped tube that leads from the auricle to the middle ear. It continues inward through the temporal bone. The auricle of the ear helps to collect sound waves traveling through the air, directing them into the **eardrum** (tympanic membrane). Tiny hairs line the auditory canal; these are known as cilia, and they aid in transmitting sound waves to the inner ear. Also inside the auditory canal are modified sweat glands, known as ceruminous glands, which secrete **cerumen**. This is a thick, wax-like substance that is similar to honey in color. Commonly known as earwax, cerumen lubricates and protects the ear.

The tympanic membrane separates the external ear from the middle ear. It stretches over the auditory canal, and is a thin, semitransparent membrane. The tympanic membrane transmits sound vibrations, via the auditory ossicles, to the inner ear.

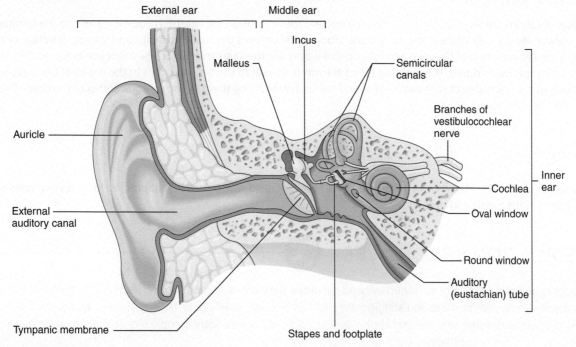

Figure 29-7 Structures of the ear.

MIDDLE EAR

The middle ear is an air-filled space that contains three small bones called **auditory ossicles**: the malleus, the incus, and the stapes. These bones transmit the sound vibrations from the tympanic membrane to the **oval window**, which leads into the inner ear. The ossicles are named for their shapes, with the malleus resembling a hammer, the incus resembling an anvil, and the stapes resembling a stirrup. The malleus is connected to the tympanic membrane. The base of the stapes fits into the oval window.

The **auditory tube** (eustachian tube) connects the middle ear to the pharynx. This tube conducts air between the middle ear and the outside of the body via the throat and mouth. It also helps to maintain equal air pressure on both sides of the eardrum, which is required for normal hearing ability. Yawning and swallowing open the auditory tube so that pressure can be equalized on either side of the eardrum.

POINTS TO REMEMBER

The auditory ossicles are the smallest bones in the body.

INNER EAR

The inner ear consists of a complex system of connected fluid-filled chambers and a tube called a **labyrinth**. The parts of the labyrinth include three **semicircular canals**, which provide a sense of equilibrium; a vestibule; and a **cochlea**, which functions in hearing. The inner ear is made up of bony structures that contain membranous structures. The bony structures are surrounded by fluid. The central portion of the inner ear is the vestibule.

The membranous structures of the inner ear include the **utricle** and **saccule**, located inside the vestibule. The utricle and saccule are membranous pouches or sacs utilized for balance. The other membranous structures are the cochlear duct, inside the cochlea, and the membranous semicircular canals inside the bony semicircular canals.

The cochlea is located slightly below the oval window. This bony structure is shaped like a snail and contains two auditory fluids: endolymph and perilymph. Both fluids aid in sound vibration transmission. The cochlea contains the **organ of Corti**, which is the true organ of hearing, and is a spiral-shaped structure. It contains tiny hair cells that are stimulated when sound vibrations are detected. Here, the vibrations are converted into nerve impulses to be interpreted by the brain. The three semicircular canals are located behind the vestibule, and they function in balance.

EAR PHYSIOLOGY

Sound vibrations are received by the auricle (pinna) and move through the external acoustic meatus to the tympanic membrane. When they strike it, the membrane vibrates. This moves the malleus, incus, and stapes. Vibration of the stapes causes vibration of the oval window. Sound waves are then transmitted to the inner ear as the endolymph and perilymph fluids ripple. This rippling effect transmits stimuli to the tiny hair cells in the organ of Corti. Nearby auditory nerve fibers detect stimulation of sound waves, transmitting them to the cerebral cortex of the brain. This is the process of hearing.

Disorders of the Ears

Hearing, as well as equilibrium, can be affected by a variety of ear disorders. In this chapter, we focus on two common conditions: otitis media and ototoxicity.

MEDICATION ERROR ALERT

Patients must be careful not to mix up eye and ear drops. If ear drops are accidentally instilled into the eyes, there is usually immediate burning and stinging, followed by redness, swelling, or blurred vision. Patients must flush the eyes out with water or saline and apply warm or cold compresses. Some people require immediate care at an emergency room or ophthalmology clinic.

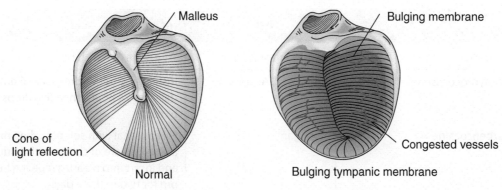

Figure 29-8 Otitis media.

OTITIS MEDIA

Otitis media is inflammation of the inner ear, which may be unilateral or bilateral. Like external otitis, it is a common cause of earaches, and both of these conditions are regularly referred to by the term "earache." Otitis media is a common childhood condition, and the most common reason children are taken to see their pediatricians. However, it also affects adults. Viruses in the nose may infect the eustachian tubes, which lead from the back of the nose to the inner ear. While acute serous otitis media may result from a viral upper respiratory infection or an allergic reaction, otitis media with effusion is caused by a collection of fluid behind the tympanic membrane, causing it to bulge (see Figure 29-8). In chronic suppurative otitis media, there is a hole in the eardrum along with an active middle ear bacterial infection.

For patients with otitis media, analgesics and decongestants may relieve pain and promote drainage. For those with suppurative otitis media, antibiotics are indicated (see Table 29-5). Severe cases or patients who do not respond to medications may require myringotomy for surgical removal of fluid to prevent permanent hearing loss, mastoiditis, or cholesteatoma. Additional medications for various ear disorders are summarized in Table 29-6.

MEDICAL TERMINOLOGY REVIEW

tympanoplasty:

tympan/o = *tympanic membrane*

-plasty = *surgical repair*

surgical repair of the tympanic membrane

Table 29-5 Medications Used to Treat Otitis Media

Generic Name	Trade Name	Average Dosage in Children
Analgesics		
antipyrine/benzocaine	Auralgan®	Solution applied into affected ear(s) q1 to 2h prn
Cephalosporins		
cefdinir	Omnicef®	PO: 14 mg/kg/day in one to two doses
ceftriaxone	Rocephin®	IM: 50 mg/kg/day in one to three doses
cefuroxime	Ceftin®	PO: 30 mg/kg/day in two divided doses
Macrolide		
azithromycin	Zithromax®	PO: 10 mg/kg/day on day one; then 5 mg/kg/day on days two to five
Penicillins		
amoxicillin	Moxatag®	PO: 90 mg/kg/day in two divided doses
amoxicillin/clavulanate	Augmentin®	PO: 90 mg/kg/day in two divided doses

Table 29-6 Additional Medications for Various Ear Disorders

Generic Name	Trade Name	Average Adult Dosage
acetic acid/hydrocortisone	VoSol HC®, Acetasol HC®	Instill three to five drops 4 to 6 times daily, for 24 hours, then five drops tid to qid
antipyrine/benzocaine	Auralgan®	Fill ear canal with solution, then moisten a small square of cotton with solution, and insert into meatus; repeat q1 to 2h prn for two to three days
benzocaine/benzethonium chloride/glycerin/polyethylene glycol 300	Americaine Otic®	Apply evenly to sufficiently lubricate ear canal
carbamide peroxide	Debrox Otic®	Instill one to five drops of 6.5% solution bid for four days
ciprofloxacin	Cetraxal®	Instill an entire single-use container's contents bid, approximately 12 hours apart for seven days
ciprofloxacin/dexamethasone	Ciprodex®	Instill four drops in affected ear bid for seven days
ciprofloxacin/hydrocortisone	Cipro HC Otic®	Instill three drops bid for seven days
polymyxin B/neomycin/hydrocortisone	Cortisporin®	Instill four drops tid to qid
triethanolamine polypetide oleate-condensate	Cerumenex®	Fill ear canal with drops and insert cotton plug; allow to remain for 15 to 30 minutes, then flush ear with lukewarm water via rubber syringe

OTOTOXICITY

Ototoxicity is drug-induced temporary or permanent hearing loss. It may exist as ear ringing or buzzing, known as *tinnitus*, and may progress to permanent damage when untreated, also affecting balance. In high doses, drugs that often cause ototoxicity include gentamicin, streptomycin, neomycin, kanamycin, amikacin, tobramycin, vancomycin, azithromycin, viomycin, cisplatin, carboplatin, ethacrynic acid, furosemide, salicylates, and quinine. Therefore, it is important that health care professionals assess each patient taking these medications on a daily basis, to ensure that treatment goals are met without any toxicity.

Anatomy and Physiology of the Nose and Sinuses

The upper respiratory system is made up of the nose, nasal cavities, pharynx, and larynx. The nose and sinuses have various physiological functions. The interior of the nose is separated into two distinct cavities by the nasal septum. They are lined by a mucous membrane that has microscopic *cilia*, which resemble tiny hairs. The mucous membrane raises the temperature of and moistens the incoming air before it can pass to the lungs. The nose is a sensory organ for smell; it also drains tears from the eyes. Since the nose and sinuses are in contact with the environment, allergens can result in allergy symptoms or infections.

Disorders of the Nose and Sinuses

Common conditions affecting the nose and sinuses include allergic rhinitis (often referred to as "hay fever") and bacterial sinusitis, which is infection of the sinuses.

ALLERGIC RHINITIS

Allergic rhinitis is irritation and inflammation of the mucous membranes that line the nasal passages. It is caused by exposure to allergens. Common symptoms include a running and itchy nose, congestion, sneezing, and postnasal drip, which is due to mucus accumulating in the back of the nose and throat. Many OTC products are able to treat these symptoms successfully. Other symptoms include watery eyes, coughing, and headache. OTC medications used to treat allergy symptoms are summarized in Table 29-7.

BACTERIAL SINUSITIS

Acute bacterial sinusitis is infection of the sinuses, with related inflammation of the nose and nasal passages. It may be secondary to an upper respiratory viral infection. Symptoms include nasal congestion and discharge, coughing, headache, sinus pressure, and fever. It is difficult to distinguish between viral and bacterial sinusitis. Since viral sinusitis improves after 7 to 10 days, acute bacterial sinusitis is diagnosed when symptoms continue for longer, or if symptoms become worse after 5 to 7 days.

Table 29-7 OTC Medications Used to Treat Allergy Symptoms

Generic Name	Trade Name	Route of Administration	Average Adult Dosage
Antihistamines (Non-Sedating)			
cetirizine	Zyrtec®	PO	5 to 10 mg once daily
fexofenadine	Allegra®	PO	60 mg bid or 180 mg once daily
loratadine	Claritin®	PO	10 mg once daily
Antihistamines (Sedating)			
chlorpheniramine	Chlor-Trimeton®	PO	4 mg q4 to 6h or extended release form: 12 mg q12h
diphenhydramine	Benadryl®	PO	25 to 50 mg q4 to 6h
Antihistamine/Mast Cell Stabilizer			
naphazoline	Clear Eyes Redness Relief®	Ophthalmic	0.012% or 0.03%: one to two drops in eye(s) up to qid
Antihistamine/Decongestant			
tetrahydrozoline	Opti-Clear®	Ophthalmic	One to two drops in each eye up to qid
Decongestants			
cromolyn	Nasalcrom®	Intranasal	One spray in each nostril tid to 6 times daily
oxymetazoline	Afrin®	Intranasal	One to three sprays in each nostril bid; do not exceed three days of use
phenylephrine	Neo-Synephrine Cold & Sinus®, Sudafed PE®	Intranasal, PO	Intranasal: two to three sprays in each nostril q4h prn; do not exceed three days of use; PO: 10 mg q4 to 6h
Mast Cell Stabilizer			
ketotifen	Zaditor®	Ophthalmic	One drop in affected eye(s) q8 to 12h (maximum two applications/day)

Summary

The eyes are made up of three primary layers: the outer sclera, the middle choroid, and the inner retina. In the sclera, the cornea helps to focus the entering light rays. In the uvea, the colored iris contains an opening called the pupil, which controls the amount of light that enters. The lens assists in focusing of images on the retina. Cones and rods differentiate colors, provide vision in bright or dim light, and function in central and peripheral vision. Disorders of eyes include conjunctivitis, glaucoma, macular degeneration, diabetic retinopathy, and retinal detachment.

The ears are also made up of three primary layers: the outer ear, the middle ear, and the inner ear. The outer ear consists of the visible auricle, the ear lobe, and the external acoustic meatus. It leads to the tympanic membrane or eardrum. The middle ear is air-filled and contains three small auditory ossicles (bones). The auditory tube connects the middle ear to the throat. The inner ear is a complex system of connected fluid-filled chambers and a tube called a labyrinth. Sound vibrations are received by the auricle, and move through the external acoustic meatus to the tympanic membrane. When the vibrations strike it, the membrane vibrates, moving the auditory ossicles. This leads to vibration of the oval window. Sound waves are transmitted to the inner ear as its fluids ripple. The rippling stimulates the tiny hair cells in the organ of Corti, and nearby auditory nerve fibers transmit the stimuli to the brain. Disorders of hearing that are discussed in this chapter include otitis media and ototoxicity. The nose is the only external organ of the respiratory system. Surrounding the nose are several cavities called sinuses. The nose and sinuses have various physiological functions. Common related disorders to the nose and sinuses include allergic rhinitis and bacterial sinusitis.

REVIEW QUESTIONS

1. Which of the following is the colored part of the eye that regulates the amount of light entering the eye?

   A. Retina
   B. Cornea
   C. Lens
   D. Iris

2. Which of the following conditions is a medical emergency?

   A. Conjunctivitis
   B. Angle-closure glaucoma
   C. Diabetic retinopathy
   D. Cataract

3. Which of the following is the deepest inner layer of the eyes?

   A. Sclera
   B. Retina
   C. Red pulp
   D. Choroid

4. Which of the following is an inflammation of the outermost layer of the eye and the inner surface of the eyelid that is commonly called "pink eye"?

   A. Glaucoma
   B. Conjunctivitis
   C. Macular degeneration
   D. Cataracts

5. Which of the following is a medication used to treat bacterial conjunctivitis?

   A. Naphazoline
   B. Azelastine
   C. Sulfacetamide
   D. Ceftin

6. Which of the following is a trade name of ciprofloxacin?

    A. Cetraxal

    B. Debrox

    C. Americaine

    D. Auralgan

7. The central portion of the inner ear is the:

    A. utricle.

    B. saccule.

    C. vestibule.

    D. cochlea.

8. Which of the following is a risk factor for retinal detachment?

    A. Diabetes mellitus

    B. Extreme nearsightedness

    C. Genetics

    D. Prolonged light exposure

9. Early treatment of which eye disorder is essential?

    A. Conjunctivitis

    B. Cataract

    C. Presbyopia

    D. Glaucoma

10. Which of the following drugs is not indicated to treat allergic conjunctivitis?

    A. Decongestants

    B. Antihistamines

    C. Adrenergic agonists

    D. Mast cell stabilizers

11. Which of the following is a trade name of azithromycin?

    A. Zithromax

    B. Ceftin

    C. Moxatag

    D. Augmentin

12. Which of the following is a first-line therapy to treat bacterial sinusitis?

    A. Doxycycline

    B. Clarithromycin

    C. Amoxicillin

    D. Trimethoprim-sulfamethoxazole

13. All of the following medications are prescribed for glaucoma, *except:*

    A. beta-adrenergic blockers.

    B. alpha$_2$-adrenergic agonists.

    C. prostaglandin analogs.

    D. cholinergic antagonists.

14. Which of the following is a trade name for tropicamide?

    A. Isopto Hyoscine®

    B. Cylogyl®

    C. Mydriacyl®

    D. Besivance®

15. Which of the following drugs may cause ototoxicity?

   A. Betaxolol
   B. Norfloxacin
   C. Azithromycin
   D. Gentamicin

CRITICAL THINKING

A 72-year-old man complains of blurred vision and says he has difficulty seeing his television and seeing words when trying to read. He had his eyeglass prescription updated about eight months ago. His physician diagnosed him with macular degeneration.

1. Define macular degeneration and the causes of this condition.

2. List the causes of blindness in the United States.

WEB LINKS

Eye Care America (American Academy of Ophthalmology): www.aao.org/eyecare-america

Eye Health Information: www.aao.org/eye-health

Hearing Loss Association of America: www.hearingloss.org

My Eye World: www.myeyeworld.com

Retina Information: maculacenter.com

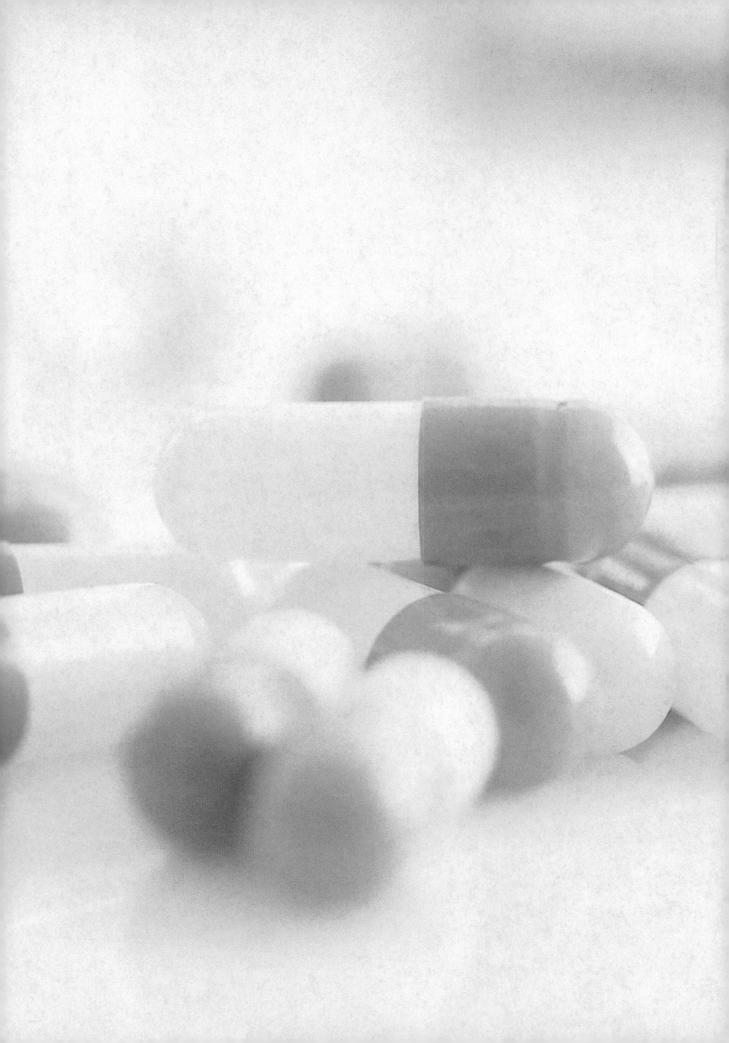

CHAPTER 30

Therapeutic Drugs for the Integumentary System

OUTLINE

OBJECTIVES

Upon completion of this chapter, the reader should be able to:

1. List the major functions of the skin.
2. Describe the structure of the layers of the skin.
3. Explain the structures of the nails.
4. Discuss the possible ways of contacting dermatitis, atopic dermatitis, and psoriasis.
5. Describe the cause of impetigo and its treatment.
6. Define herpes zoster and alopecia; discuss possible treatments.
7. Briefly explain types of skin cancers and preventions.
8. Explain the three types of burns and their effects.

9. Identify various forms of dermatophytosis.

10. Explain acne vulgaris and its treatments.

KEY TERMS

arrector pili muscle	electrodessication	onychomycosis	stratum basale
athlete's foot	epidermis	paronychia	stratum lucidum
basal cell carcinoma	keratinocytes	sebaceous glands	subcutaneous layer
comedones	lunula	sebum	sweat gland
corium	malignant melanoma	squamous cell carcinoma	tinea capitis
cryosurgery	melanin	stratified squamous epithelium	
dermis	melanocytes		

Overview

The integumentary system has several roles, including protection, regulation, and maintenance. The skin forms a barrier between the inner body and the outside environment. It is vitally important to the functioning of all other organs. It is nearly waterproof and has cells that resist harmful ultraviolet (UV) rays. The skin repels most chemicals so that they cannot harm internal functions. The skin also allows us to sweat, which is vital for regulating body temperature.

Common diseases and disorders of the skin involve infections (fungal and bacterial), inflammation, and traumatic injury. These conditions can be treated with various drugs with a primary function to relieve pain, slow or stop bacterial or fungal growth, prevent allergic reactions, relieve itching, and reduce inflammation.

Anatomy and Physiology of the Integumentary System

The integumentary system includes the skin and accessory structures (such as the nails; hair; and the sweat, ceruminous, and sebaceous glands). The integumentary system has the ability to automatically repair small cuts, rips, or burns.

MEDICAL TERMINOLOGY REVIEW

integumentary:

integument = *covering*   pertaining to covering the body

-ary = *pertaining to*

SKIN

The skin is the largest organ in the body by surface area. On an average adult, it covers more than 3000 square inches of body surface area and weighs approximately 6 lb. The skin is tough, yet flexible, and able to regenerate itself to a large degree when damaged. This is partially due to the amount of blood vessels it contains, which supply it with about one-third of the blood circulation.

The skin includes two distinct layers: the epidermis and the dermis (see Figure 30-1). The **epidermis** is the outer layer. The **dermis** is the inner layer and is thicker than the epidermis. The dermis connects the skin to fat, muscle, and other tissues beneath it. The loose connective tissue, predominately consisting of adipose (fat) tissue below the dermis, binds the skin to the underlying organs and forms the **subcutaneous layer**. The subcutaneous layer is also called the hypodermis.

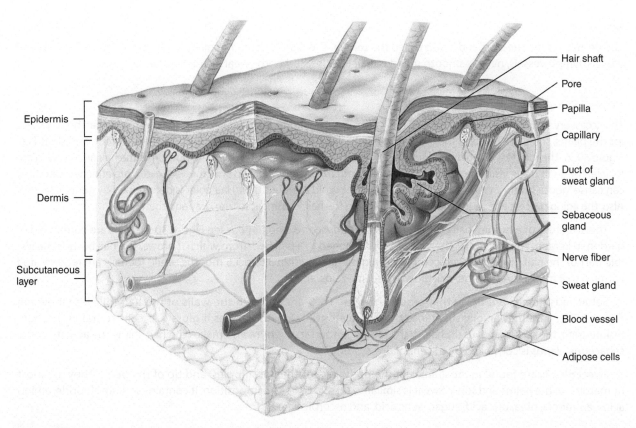

Figure 30-1 The layers of the skin and its appendages.

Epidermis

The epidermis is made up of **stratified squamous epithelium** and does not contain blood vessels. There are basically five layers of the epidermis, which include (from deepest to most superficial): stratum basale (germinativum), stratum spinosum, stratum granulosum, stratum lucidum, and stratum corneum.

- The deepest layer of the epidermis is the **stratum basale**, also known as *stratum germinativum*. It is the only layer that undergoes cell division, and pushes cells upward into all the other layers. This layer also contains **melanocytes**, which give pigmentation to the skin. These cells produce the pigment **melanin**, which helps protect the skin from damaging ultraviolet rays.

- Stratum spinosum lies under the stratum basale. It is 8 to 10 cell layers thick and contains various types of skin cells including **keratinocytes**, which are filled with a protein-like material called keratin.

- Stratum granulosum is the layer where the process of keratinization begins. This process causes the keratinocytes to lose shape and water and become hardened.

- The **stratum lucidum** is found only on the palms of the hands and soles of the feet; it is a thickened layer because of increased abrasion and the need to bear weight.

- Stratum corneum is the most superficial layer and is composed of dead cells. The cells in this layer are shed and renewed every 20 to 30 days.

MEDICAL TERMINOLOGY REVIEW

keratinocyte:

keratin/o = *hard, horny*   a hard, fibrous epidermal cell

-cyte = *cell*

Dermis

The dermis is the "true skin" and is also called the **corium**. The dermis contains collagenous fibers, elastin fibers, blood vessels, lymph vessels, nerves, smooth muscles, hair follicles, and both sweat and **sebaceous glands**.

ACCESSORY STRUCTURES

The accessory structures of the skin include the hair, nails, and various glands. Hair covers most of the human body, except for the palms, soles, and parts of the external genitalia. Each individual hair is made up of a follicle, root, and shaft (see Figure 30-2). The follicle is an epidermal tube from which the hair grows. The root is the portion of the hair anchored in the follicle. The shaft is the visible portion of the hair. Smooth muscle fibers called **arrector pili muscles** are attached, and they can cause "goose bumps" when fearful stimuli occur or in cold temperatures. Hair color is determined by genetic factors. Also, the aging process affects the amount of melanin in the hair, causing it to turn gray and then white.

The structure of a human nail consists of a root, body, edge, and **lunula** (see Figure 30-3). Nails are composed of hardened keratin. The nail root is the part of a nail attached to a nail bed, from which it grows. The nail body is the visible part of the nail. Fingernails are completely regenerated within 3.5 to 5.5 months, while toenails are regenerated within 6 to 8 months. As we age, nail growth becomes slower.

Sebaceous glands are those that produce **sebum**. They are found in the walls of the hair follicles (shown in Figure 30-2). Sebum is an oily substance that lubricates the skin and makes it glossy. As cells containing sebum disintegrate, the sebum moves up hair shafts to the skin surface. Sebum also makes the hair shiny. The activity of the sebaceous glands is controlled by the endocrine system.

Sweat glands are found in most areas of the body, except the lips, nipples, and tip of the penis. They are most numerous on the palms and soles. Sweat is similar to the blood in its composition. It contains sodium chloride, amino acids, ammonia, urea, uric acid, sugar, lactic acid, and ascorbic acid.

FUNCTIONS OF THE SKIN

The skin has four important functions: protection, sensation, secretion, and thermoregulation. Intact skin protects against pathogens entering the body. Because of skin keratinization, we are protected from losing too much water through the skin. The pH of the skin is acidic, which prevents growth of microorganisms. The sensory receptors in the dermis communicate between the external environment and nervous system to detect pain, pressure, heat, and cold. The sweat glands secrete sweat to help maintain homeostasis of the body. The sebaceous glands secrete sebum to lubricate the hair skin. The skin also produces vitamin D when it is exposed to the sun.

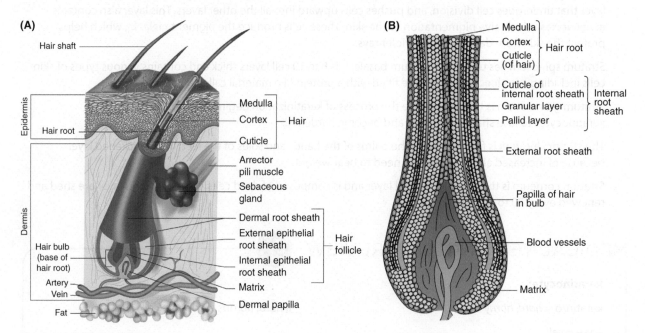

Figure 30-2 Hair structures.

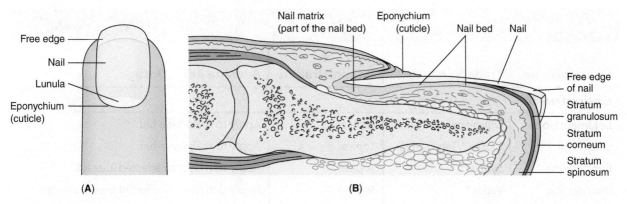

Figure 30-3 Nail structures.

Disorders of the Integumentary System

Cutaneous lesions or alterations of the skin surface commonly manifest disorders of the skin. These alterations include ulcers, fissures, macules, papules, pustules, vesicles, and nodules. Diagnosis of integumentary system diseases is often based on the appearance of a certain type of lesion or group of lesions. There are numerous disorders of the skin, hair, and nails. This chapter discusses some of the more common types of integumentary skin disorders.

POINTS TO REMEMBER

Xerodermia is a dermatologic condition characterized by rough, dry skin. It is also spelled "xeroderma."

MEDICAL TERMINOLOGY REVIEW

dermatitis:

dermat = *skin*   inflammation of the skin

-itis = *inflammation*

ATOPIC DERMATITIS (ECZEMA)

Dermatitis is an inflammation of the skin and occurs in various forms (see Figure 30-4). The more common forms include atopic dermatitis, seborrheic dermatitis, and contact dermatitis. Atopic dermatitis is a chronic or recurring skin lesion characteristic of an allergic reaction. The rash occurs in a characteristic pattern on the face, neck, elbows, knees, and upper trunk of the body. The tendency of this condition to develop is inherited, and it may occur in some infants who are sensitive to milk, orange juice, or certain other foods. The main goals in treating atopic dermatitis are to reduce the frequency and severity of eruptions, and relieve itching. The primary treatment of eczema involves topical ointments and creams containing cortisone or steroidal hormones. Two new agents, pimecrolimus (Elidel®) and tacrolimus (Protopic®), are also used. They are both classified as calcineurin inhibitor immunosuppressants.

Medications used to treat eczema are listed in Table 30-1.

SEBORRHEIC DERMATITIS

Seborrheic dermatitis is one of the most common skin conditions. Itchy, erythemic, and oily patches of skin characterize it. The lesions often shed large dandruff-like scales (see Figure 30-5). This condition is idiopathic (of unknown cause) and can occur at any age. However, it is most common during infancy, and when it occurs in infancy it is also called "cradle cap." However, heredity may predispose an individual to the condition, and emotional stress may be a precipitating factor. Low-strength cortisone or hydrocortisone creams are the most effective methods of treatment.

Table 30-1 Medications Used to Treat Atopic Dermatitis (Eczema)

Generic Name	Trade Name	Route of Administration	Average Adult Dosage
Corticosteroids			
betamethasone	Diprolene®	Topical	Apply to scalp/area bid
clobetasol	Clobex®, Temovate®	Topical	Apply to scalp/area bid
fluocinolone	Synalar®	Topical	Apply thin layer to affected area tid
fluocinonide	Vanos®	Topical	Apply thin layer to affected area bid to qid
flurandrenolide	Cordran®, Nolix®	Topical	Apply thin layer to affected area bid to tid
fluticasone	Cutivate®	Topical	Apply thin layer to affected area once daily to bid
halcinonide	Halog®	Topical	Apply sparingly bid to tid
hydrocortisone	Cortizone®	Topical	Apply thin layer to affected area bid to qid
triamcinolone	Kenalog®, Triderm®	Topical	Apply thin layer to affected area bid to qid
Calcineurin Inhibitors			
cyclosporine	Gengraf®, Neoral®, Sandimmune®	PO	2.5 mg/kg in two divided doses/day
pimecrolimus	Elidel®	Topical	Apply cream bid
tacrolimus	Protopic®	Topical	Apply ointment bid
Immunosuppressants			
methotrexate	Trexall®	PO, IM, Subcutaneous	10 to 25 mg/dose once/week
mycophenolate	CellCept®	PO	2 to 3 g/day

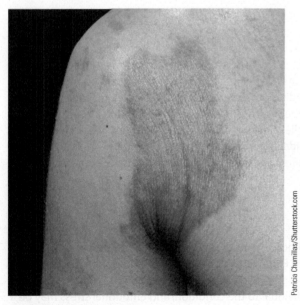

Patricia Chumillas/Shutterstock.com

Figure 30-4 Dermatitis.

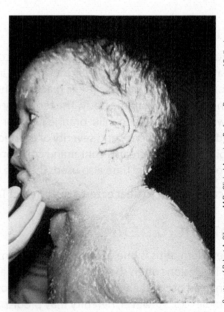

Courtesy of Robert A. Silverman, M.D., Clinical Associate Professor, Department of Pediatrics, Georgetown University.

Figure 30-5 Seborrheic dermatitis.

CONTACT DERMATITIS

Contact dermatitis is an acute inflammation of the skin. It is caused either by the action of irritants on the skin surfaces or by contact with a substance that causes an allergic reaction. A common contact dermatitis involves poison ivy, which causes vesicular eruptions that itch and burn at the site of contact. Treatment involves topical corticosteroid creams and lotions. Contact dermatitis may also be caused by poison oak or poison sumac (see Figure 30-6).

MEDICAL TERMINOLOGY REVIEW

seborrheic:

seb/o = *sebum*

-rrhea = *flow, drainage*

-ic = *pertaining to*

pertaining to secretion of sebum

PSORIASIS

Psoriasis is an inflammatory chronic, recurrent skin condition that produces silvery (raised red patches covered with white) scales (see Figure 30-7). This condition most often appears on the elbows, knees, scalp, genitalia, and trunk. Patches of psoriasis may also appear at sites of trauma. Its cause is unknown, but it seems to be genetically determined and is more common in Caucasians. Precipitating factors for the development of psoriasis include hormonal changes (such as those occurring with pregnancy), climate changes, emotional stress, and a period of generally poor health. The goal of treatment is to reduce inflammation and slow the rapid growth of skin cells that cause the condition. Treatment of psoriasis involves a combination of UV light, topical steroid creams or ointments, application of a cream containing vitamin A, coal tar preparations, antihistamines, and oatmeal baths. Injectable medications for psoriasis include etanercept (Enbrel®), adalimumab (Humira®), infliximab (Remicade®), and ustekinumab (Stelara®). A variety of medications for psoriasis are summarized in Table 30-2.

MEDICATION ERROR ALERT

Methotrexate is a medication that is used for many different conditions, including *psoriasis*. However, this drug has resulted in serious outcomes and even deaths when medication errors concerning its use occur. Methotrexate is a folic acid antagonist. Since folic acid plays a major role in cell division, its inhibition results in major toxicity to blood cells, hepatocytes, oral mucosae, lung tissue, and fetal tissue. This drug is a potent teratogen that should never be used, by women *or* men, when the woman is pregnant.

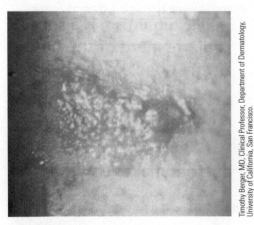

Timothy Berger, MD, Clinical Professor, Department of Dermatology, University of California, San Francisco.

Figure 30-6 Contact dermatitis.

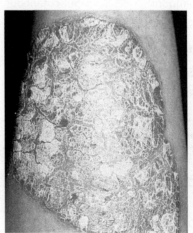

Courtesy of Robert A. Silverman, M.D., Clinical Associate Professor, Department of Pediatrics, Georgetown University.

Figure 30-7 Psoriasis.

Table 30-2 Medications Used to Treat Psoriasis

Generic Name	Trade Name	Route of Administration	Average Adult Dosage
Corticosteroids			
amcinonide	Amcort®, Cyclocort®	Topical	Apply thin layer bid to qid
betamethasone	Diprolene®	Topical spray	Apply bid, for up to 4 weeks
clobetasol	Clobex®, Temovate®	Topical	Apply bid, for up to 2 weeks
desoximetasone	Topicort®	Topical	Apply thin layer bid
fluocinolone	Derma-Smoothe/ FS Scalp®	Topical	Massage into wet or damp hair/scalp. Cover with shower cap overnight for at least 4 hours; wash with shampoo, rinse thoroughly to remove
fluocinonide	Vanos®	Topical	Apply thin layer to affected area bid to qid
flurandrenolide	Cordran®	Topical	Apply thin layer to affected area bid to tid
fluticasone	Cutivate®	Topical	Apply thin layer to affected area once/day to bid
halcinonide	Halog®	Topical	Apply sparingly bid to tid
hydrocortisone	Cortizone®	Topical	Apply thin layer to affected area bid to qid
triamcinolone	Kenalog®, Triderm®	Topical	Apply thin layer to affected area bid to qid
Antimetabolite/Antipsoriatic Agent			
methotrexate	Trexall®	PO	10 to 25 mg/dose
Psoralen			
methoxsalen	Oxsoralen-Ultra®, Uvadex®	PO	10 to 70 mg based on individual patient weight
Retinoids			
acitretin	Soriatane®	PO	25 to 50 mg once daily
tazarotene	Avage®, Tazorac®	Topical	Apply thin layer to affected area in the evening
Monoclonal Antibodies			
adalimumab	Humira®	Subcutaneous	80 mg once, then 40 mg q other week
golimumab	Simponi®	Subcutaneous	50 mg once monthly
ustekinumab	Stelara®	Subcutaneous	45 to 90 mg at week zero and 4, then q12week
Tumor Necrosis Factor (TNF) Inhibitors			
etanercept	Enbrel®	Subcutaneous	50 mg once daily or bid
infliximab	Remicade®	IV	5 mg/kg at weeks zero, two, and four; then q8week
Calcineurin Inhibitor			
cyclosporine	Gengraf®, Neoral®, Sandimmune ®	PO	2.5 mg/kg/day in two divided doses
Tree Bark Extract			
anthralin	Drithro-Creme®, Zithranol®	Topical	Apply once daily or as directed

(Continued)

Table 30-2 Medications Used to Treat Psoriasis *(Continued)*

Generic Name	Trade Name	Route of Administration	Average Adult Dosage
Vitamin D Analogue			
calcipotriene	Dovonex®	Topical	Apply thin layer bid
Coal Tar Preparation			
coal tar	DHS Tar®, Theraplex®	Topical	Body: apply at bedtime; scalp: coat lesions 3 to 12 hours before showering or shampooing

ACNE VULGARIS

Acne is a skin condition characterized by inflammation of the sebaceous glands and hair follicles (see Figure 30-8). It can occur on any skin surface and present itself at any age. Acne vulgaris is the most common type of acne, appearing on the face, upper back, and chest. It is marked by the appearance of papules, pustules, and **comedones**. Acne vulgaris primarily affects adolescents during puberty. In girls, it is usually at its worst between the ages of 14 and 17 years. In boys, it peaks in the late teenage years. This condition can cause severe scarring of the skin and results from blockage of follicles. Topical or systemic antibiotics, or both, may be used for treatment. Keratolytic agents may be appropriate for many cases of acne. Vitamin A and benzoyl peroxide gels are also effective. Table 30-3 summarizes the various medications used to treat acne vulgaris.

WHAT WOULD YOU DO?

You receive a prescription for a patient with acne vulgaris. The prescribed medication reads "tretinoin," and it is to be taken orally. You are confused because you know that tretinoin is a topical medication, but the similarly named "isotretinoin" is an oral medication. Both medications are used for acne. In this situation, what would you do?

HERPES ZOSTER (SHINGLES)

Shingles occurs in a unilateral pattern along the peripheral nerves. Pain begins after two or three days, prior to lesions appearing. Shingles may be accompanied by a fever. Eruptions begin as a rash that quickly develops into vesicles. Duration of the disease, from onset to recovery, is usually between 10 days and five weeks (see Figure 30-9). Herpes zoster is

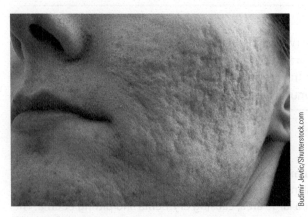

Figure 30-8 Acne vulgaris.

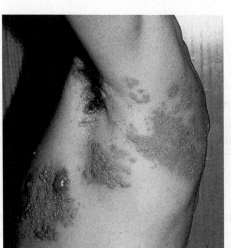

Figure 30-9 Shingles.

Table 30-3 Medications Used to Treat Acne Vulgaris

Generic Name	Trade Name	Route of Administration	Average Dosage
adapalene	Differin®	Topical	Apply once daily at bedtime
azelaic acid	Azelex®, Finacea®	Topical	Apply thin film to affected area bid
benzoyl peroxide	Clearplex V®, Neutrogena Clear Pore®	Topical	Apply sparingly once daily; slowly increase to bid or tid
clindamycin	Cleocin T®, Clindagel®, ClindaMax®	Topical	Cleocin T and ClindaMax: apply thin film bid; Clindagel: apply once daily
dapsone	Aczone®	Topical	Apply pea-sized amount daily
doxycycline	Oracea®, Vibramycin®	PO	50 to 100 mg bid
erythromycin	Ery®, Erygel®, Ery-Tab®	Topical, PO	Topical: Apply over affected area once daily or bid; PO: 250 to 500 mg bid
isotretinoin	Absorica®, Amnesteem®, Claravis®	PO	0.5 to 1 mg/kg/day in two divided doses, for 15 to 20 weeks
minocycline	Minocin®, Solodyn®	PO	50 to 100 mg bid
salicylic acid	Stri-Dex®	Topical	Apply thin layer to affected area once daily to tid
sulfamethoxazole/trimethoprim	Bactrim®	PO	One single-strength or double-strength table once daily or bid
tetracycline	Generic only	PO	1 g daily in divided doses; reduce slowly to 125 to 500 mg/day when improving
tretinoin	Retin-A Micro®	Topical	Apply once daily to lesions before bedtime

an infection caused by the varicella-zoster virus, which is the same virus that causes chickenpox. Persons who have previously had chickenpox continue to harbor the varicella-zoster virus in their nervous systems. It may emerge during times of physical stress or when the immune system is impaired. Treatments include analgesics, mild tranquilizers or sedatives, antipruritics, and steroids. Acyclovir (Zovirax®) may be administered orally, parenterally, or topically.

MEDICATION ERROR ALERT

There have been mix-ups involving the chicken pox vaccine (Varivax®) and the shingles vaccine (Zostavax®). In one documented case, a 12-month-old baby was given the Zostavax® vaccine, with the prescribing physician telling the nurse that the two vaccines were "basically the same thing." The facts do not support this statement at all because the Zostavax® vaccine contains about 14 times as much varicella antigen as the Varivax® vaccine.

CELLULITIS

Cellulitis is an acute, diffuse, bacterial infection of the subcutaneous tissue (see Figure 30-10). This condition is usually caused by an injury that pierces the outermost layer of skin and allows bacteria to reach the lower layers. Cellulitis is usually painful and is capable of spreading rapidly over a large area, causing erythema and pitting edema. The

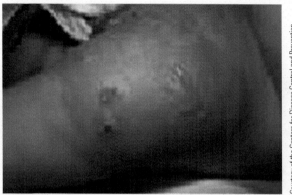

Courtesy of the Centers for Disease Control and Prevention, Public Health Image Library/Allen W. Mathies, MD.

Figure 30-10 Cellulitis.

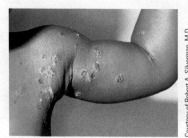

Courtesy of Robert A. Silverman, M.D., Clinical Associate Professor, Department of Pediatrics, Georgetown University.

Figure 30-11 Impetigo.

cause of cellulitis is either *Staphylococcus* or *Streptococcus*. Treatment includes immobilization and elevation of the affected body part. For discomfort, cool magnesium sulfate (Epsom salt) solution compresses may be used. Warm compresses should be applied to increase circulation. Systemic antibiotics are prescribed for the infection. Other medications include acetaminophen, aspirin, or nonsteroidal anti-inflammatory drugs (NSAIDs), alone or in combination with codeine for fever and pain.

IMPETIGO

Impetigo is a bacterial skin infection most commonly seen in children, though it is not limited only to their age group. It is highly contagious and spreads rapidly in schools where children have physical contact with each other, often during athletic events or during close play. Impetigo initially appears as a fluid-filled blister that may burst, leaving a crusty margin around the lesion (see Figure 30-11). The lesions usually develop on the legs and, less commonly, on the arms, trunk, or face. Scratching the skin may result in ulcerations, with erythema and scarring. Impetigo is caused by either *Streptococcus* or *Staphylococcus aureus*. The condition often causes intense itching that may help to spread the infection. Effective treatments include systemic antibiotics and proper cleaning of lesions two to three times per day. If mild, treatment involves gentle cleansing, removing crusts, and applying the antibiotic ointment mupirocin (Bactroban®). More severe cases, such as *bullous impetigo*, may require oral antibiotics such as penicillin derivatives (Augmentin®) or cephalosporins such as cephalexin (Keflex®). If the infection is caused by methicillin-resistant *Staphylococcus aureus* (MRSA) or other drug-resistant bacteria, antibiotics such as clindamycin or trimethoprim-sulfamethoxazole (Bactrim® or Septra®) may be needed.

MEDICAL TERMINOLOGY REVIEW

cellulitis:

cellul/o = *cell*

-itis = *inflammation*

inflammation of the cells of the skin

DERMATOPHYTOSIS

Dermatophytosis (tinea) is a chronic superficial fungal infection of the skin. It is caused by several species of fungi that can invade the skin or nails. The body regions affected classify this type of infection. The commonly used name for any type of dermatophytosis is *ringworm*. The infection causes scale-like lesions with raised edges that itch. The name "ringworm" comes from the original belief that the condition was caused by worms. It is more common in rural settings and hot, humid climates.

On the feet, ringworm is called **athlete's foot** or *tinea pedis* (see Figure 30-12). It is characterized by intense burning and stinging pruritus between the toes and on the soles of the feet. Dermatophytosis is known as *jock itch* (*tinea cruris*) when it affects the groin. Raised, red, pruritic vesicular patches on the groin area and the area surrounding it characterize this form. In children, a common form known as **tinea capitis** (see Figure 30-13) occurs on the scalp

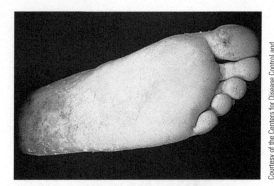

Courtesy of the Centers for Disease Control and Prevention, Public Health Image Library.

Figure 30-12 Athlete's foot.

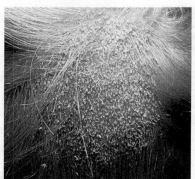

Courtesy of Robert A. Silverman, M.D., Clinical Associate Professor, Department of Pediatrics, Georgetown University.

Figure 30-13 Tinea capitis.

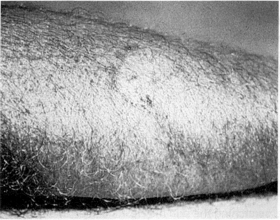

Courtesy of the Centers for Disease Control and Prevention, Public Health Image Library.

Figure 30-14 Tinea corporis.

and can cause hair loss as well as bacterial infections. Elsewhere on the body dermatophytosis is called *tinea corporis* (see Figure 30-14). Antifungal medications are used either for topical application as ointments or in an orally administered form for systemic effects. For tinea capitis, ketoconazole 2% (Nizoral shampoo®) is used. For the other types of tinea, terbinafine hydrochloride (Lamisil®), butenafine (Lotrimin Ultra®), and griseofulvin (Gris-PEG® or Grifulvin V® Oral Suspension) are used. Table 30-4 summarizes various medications used for dermatophytosis. Table 30-5 summarizes miscellaneous medications used for integumentary system disorders, and Table 30-6 gives examples of related drug terminology.

Table 30-4 Medications Used to Treat Dermatophytosis

Generic Name	Trade Name	Route of Administration	Average Adult Dosage
clotrimazole	Lotrimin®	Topical	Apply bid for two weeks
ketoconazole	Nizoral®	Topical	Apply to affected area once daily or, if shampoo form, apply once to damp skin, lather, and leave on for 5 minutes, then rinse off
miconazole	Desenex®	Topical	Apply bid for four weeks
nystatin	Nystop®	Topical	Apply to affected area bid to tid
terbinafine	Lamisil®	Topical	Apply to affected area once daily for at least one week

Table 30-5 Miscellaneous Medications Used to Treat Integumentary System Disorders

Generic Name	Trade Name	Drug Class	Uses
benzocaine	Anbesol®, Orajel®	Anesthetic	To relieve pain
dibucaine	Nupercainal®		
lidocaine	Lidoderm®		
diphenhydramine	Allerdryl®, Benadryl®	Antihistamine	To slow, stop, or prevent allergic reactions
fexofenadine	Allegra®		
loratadine	Claritin®		
bacitracin/neomycin/polymyxin B	Neosporin®	Antibacterial	To slow or stop bacterial growth
neomycin	Myciguent®		
doxepin	Zonalon®	Antipruritic	To relieve itching

Table 30-6 Drug Terminology

Drug Class	Pronunciation	Definition
alpha hydroxy acid	AL-fa hye-DROK-see	Agent added to cosmetics to improve skin appearance
anesthetic	an-es-THET-ik	Agent that relieves pain by blocking nerve sensations
antibacterial	an-tye-bak-TEER-ee-all	Agent that kills or slows the growth of bacteria
antibiotic	an-tye-bye-OT-ik	Agent that kills or slows the growth of microorganisms
antifungal	an-tye-FUN-gall	Agent that kills or slows the growth of fungi
antihistamine	an-tye-HISS-tah-meen	Agent that controls allergic reactions by blocking the effectiveness of histamines in the body
anti-inflammatory	an-tye-in-FLAH-mah-tor-ee	Agent that relieves the symptoms of inflammations
antipruritic	an-tye-proo-RIT-ik	Agent that controls itching
antiseptic	an-tye-SEP-tik	Agent that, like an antibiotic, kills or slows the growth of microorganisms
astringent	as-TRIN-jent	Agent that removes excess oils and impurities from the skin's surface
corticosteroid	kor-tih-ko-STAIR-oid	Agent with anti-inflammatory properties
emollient	eh-MOH-lee-ent	Agent that smoothes or softens skin
parasiticide	pah-rah-SIT-ih-side	Agent that kills or slows the growth of parasites

MOLES

Moles are common, usually benign skin lesions produced by groups of melanocytes. They develop in the first few years of life in many children, reaching their largest size at puberty. Sizes of moles vary greatly, and hairs may grow through them. Darkening and enlargement of a mole later in life may indicate skin cancer. Beginning at age 30, moles should be monitored for changes. If a mole is chronically irritated or infected, it should be surgically removed and examined for cancer. A mole is also referred to as a *nevus* or a birthmark.

VERRUCA VULGARIS

A verruca vulgaris is a benign growth that usually disappears on its own over time. It is commonly referred to as a wart. They are caused by the human papillomavirus, which results in uncontrolled epidermal tissue growth. Warts (verrucae) most often appear on the hands, face, neck, and knees. The virus is transmitted by direct contact. Warts may be removed with topical applications or surgery. Some forms of the human papillomavirus can cause cervical cancer in females (see Chapter 28).

VITILIGO

Vitiligo is a condition in which irregular patches of skin develop that completely lack pigmentation. The patches may enlarge, shrink, or remain the same size. This acquired disease usually affects areas of skin that are commonly exposed to the sun. Vitiligo is of unknown cause but may possibly be an autoimmune condition. It has no cure, but cosmetics may be used to cover affected skin areas. Treatment may help to stop or slow the process of depigmentation. Treatment options include topical corticosteroids, topical immunomodulators (tacrolimus or pimecrolimus), and photochemotherapy.

BURNS

Burns are disruptions or destruction of skin or tissue because of exposure to fire, UV radiation, hot water, spills, radiation, strong acids or bases, toxins, excessive heat, and electrical shocks. They may be minor and heal quickly, such as when burns are caused by sun exposure. They may also be extensive and even fatal. Burns that cause death usually do so because of fluid loss, infection, and the toxic effects of burned tissue (known as eschar). Burns are the leading causes of accidental death. They are classified into three types:

- *First-degree burns:* Involve only the epidermis; signified by redness, pain, and slight edema. These burns heal quickly and usually do not leave scars. Most sunburns are first-degree burns (see Figure 30-15A).

- *Second-degree (partial-thickness) burns:* Involve the epidermis and dermis but leave some of the dermis intact; they may appear red, tan, or white with blisters. Second-degree burns are very painful, slow healing, and may leave scars. Serious sunburns and many scaldings are second-degree burns (see Figure 30-15B).

- *Third-degree (full-thickness) burns:* The epidermis and dermis are completely destroyed, and even the deeper tissue may be damaged; the skin can repair itself only from the edges of the wound. These burns often require skin grafts, and if left to heal on their own, they may result in abnormal connective tissue fibrosis and severe disfigurement (see Figure 30-15C).

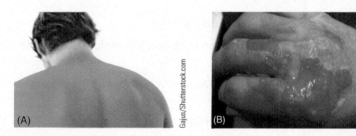
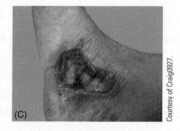

(A) Gajus/Shutterstock.com (B) Courtesy of Alcedema. (C) Courtesy of Craig0927.

Figure 30-15 Burns: (A) first-degree, (B) second-degree (partial-thickness), and (C) third-degree (full-thickness).

WHAT WOULD YOU DO?

A hospital physician ordered "5 mg morphine prn" to treat severe pain for a third-degree burn patient. A new pharmacy technician read the prescription as "50 mg" but doubted that this was correct and asked a senior pharmacy technician for her opinion. If you were the senior pharmacy technician, what would you do?

NAIL DISORDERS

Nail disorders may be signified by any unusual thickening, shape, or color, and are classified as either deformed or discolored nails. Nail deformities can be produced by many different disorders. Conditions such as psoriasis and chronic paronychia can cause the ends of the nails to separate from underlying skin. Iron deficiency anemia can cause the nails to assume a spoon-like, curved shape. Both the fingernails and toenails can experience clubbing because of congenital heart disorders or lung cancer.

Nail discoloration may be caused by various illnesses. White nail beds, for example, are caused by chronic hepatic disease. Infections of the cardiac valves, systemic lupus erythematosus, and dermatomyositis can all cause small black splinter-like areas to appear under the nails. Anemia may cause nails to appear pale in color.

Other common nail disorders include paronychia, onychomycosis, and onychocryptosis. **Paronychia** involves infection of the fold of skin at the edge of a nail (see Figure 30-16A). **Onychomycosis** is a fungal infection that causes the nails to become discolored, dry, thick, and brittle (see Figure 30-16B). Onychocryptosis is commonly known as an ingrown toenail (see Figure 30-16C). It occurs when a nail grows into the skin of the toe, resulting in inflammation.

MEDICAL TERMINOLOGY REVIEW

paronychia:

par/o = *beside, beyond, near*

onych/o = *nail*

-ia = *condition*

inflammation of the fold of skin surrounding the fingernail

MEDICAL TERMINOLOGY REVIEW

onychomycosis:

onych/o = *nail*

myc/o = *fungus*

-osis = *condition*

any fungal infection of the nails

For treatment of nail disorders, the goal is to resolve underlying causes of the illness. Nails damaged by injury usually return to normal appearance within about nine months. When a fungus causes discoloration, terbinafine HCl (Lamisil®) may be ordered.

MEDICATION ERROR ALERT

Many medications adversely affect the nail matrix by interfering with normal keratinization. If severe, this may result in horizontal depressions that often affect all fingernails and toenails, known as Beau's lines, or transverse entire-thickness sulci that split the nails apart, known as onychomadesis. Overprescribing or overuse of retinoids, such as tretinoin or isotretinoin, and antimicrobial agents are commonly linked to these conditions.

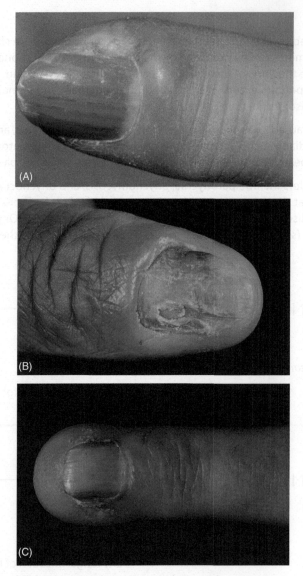

Figure 30-16 Nail diseases: (A) paronychia, (B) onychomycosis, and (C) onychocryptosis.

SKIN CANCER

Skin cancer is the most common type of cancer in the United States, particularly in areas that receive more sun. There are three different types of skin cancers: **malignant melanoma**, which is the deadliest, **basal cell carcinoma** (see Figure 30-17), and **squamous cell carcinoma** (see Figure 30-18). Melanoma is rarer than the other two types but can metastasize sooner to other parts of the body because it occurs at the base of the dermis, where it has easy access to blood and lymph vessels (see Figure 30-19). The other two types, while more common, occur in the top layer of the epidermis, and usually they do not metastasize. Basal cell and squamous cell carcinoma lesions can appear anywhere on the body. The most common sites are sun-exposed areas such as the face, scalp, ears, back, chest, arms, and backs of the hands. Malignant melanoma can appear anywhere on the skin but occurs most commonly on the backs of men and the legs of women. Treatment consists of surgical excision, **cryosurgery**, **electrodessication** and curettage, or radiation therapy.

ALOPECIA

Alopecia is commonly known as baldness (see Figure 30-20). It is the loss or absence of hair, especially on the scalp. There are several types of alopecia, including male pattern baldness, alopecia universalis, and alopecia capitis totalis. Baldness may be genetically linked, caused by hormonal conditions, malnutrition, diabetes, endocrine disorders, and may also be due to cancer chemotherapy or drug interactions. For male pattern baldness, there are a variety of drugs available such as

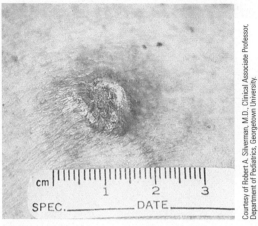

Courtesy of Robert A. Silverman, M.D., Clinical Associate Professor, Department of Pediatrics, Georgetown University.

Figure 30-17 Basal cell carcinoma.

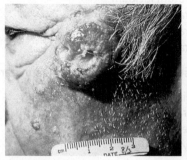

Courtesy of Robert A. Silverman, M.D., Clinical Associate Professor, Department of Pediatrics, Georgetown University.

Figure 30-18 Squamous cell carcinoma.

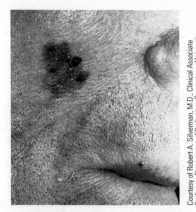

Courtesy of Robert A. Silverman, M.D., Clinical Associate Professor, Department of Pediatrics, Georgetown University.

Figure 30-19 Malignant melanoma.

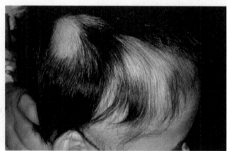

Courtesy of Robert A. Silverman, M.D., Clinical Associate Professor, Department of Pediatrics, Georgetown University.

Figure 30-20 Alopecia.

minoxidil, to regrow hair. Other treatments include various hair transplantation procedures. However, at Columbia University in New York, there have been laboratory advancements in which human hair was able to be grown from a patient's own skin tissue by producing new hair follicles. This is very promising for the future of alopecia treatment.

Summary

Pharmacy technicians must have enough knowledge about the structures, functions, and common diseases to understand appropriate treatments. The integumentary system includes the skin, nails, hair, sweat glands, ceruminous glands, and sebaceous glands. The skin forms a barrier between the inner body and the outside environment. The two distinct layers of the skin are the outer epidermis and the inner dermis. The epidermis consists of multiple layers of keratinized cells comprising stratified squamous epithelium. The dermis is the "true skin" and is also called the coreum. The structure of a nail consists of a root, body, and edge (lunula). Nails are composed of hardened keratin. Sebaceous glands produce sebum, which lubricates the skin and hair. Sweat glands are found on most body areas, but they are most numerous on the palms and soles.

The four important functions of the skin are protection, sensation, secretion, and thermoregulation. Common diseases and conditions of the integumentary system include atopic dermatitis (eczema), seborrheic dermatitis, contact dermatitis, psoriasis, acne vulgaris, herpes zoster (shingles), cellulitis, impetigo, dermatophytosis (ringworm), moles, warts, vitiligo, burns, skin cancer, alopecia, paronychia, onychomycosis, and onychocryptosis. Medications used to treat integumentary system disorders include anesthetics, antifungals, antihistamines, antibacterials, antipruritics, and anti-inflammatories (corticosteroids).

1. Which layer of the epidermis exhibits cell division?

    A.   Stratum lucidum
    B.   Stratum spinosum
    C.   Stratum granulosum
    D.   Stratum basale

2. The most abundant cells in the epidermis are:

    A.   adipocytes.
    B.   keratinocytes.
    C.   melanocytes.
    D.   erythrocytes.

3. The pale, half moon-shaped area at the base of a nail is called the:

    A.   cuticle.
    B.   eponychium.
    C.   lunula.
    D.   hyponychium.

4. Which of the following is not a function of the skin?

    A.   Production of vitamin E
    B.   Secretion
    C.   Thermoregulation
    D.   Protection

5. Which of the following infections of the skin may be contagious if it is not treated?

    A.   Psoriasis
    B.   Eczema
    C.   Impetigo
    D.   Seborrheic dermatitis

6. Herpes zoster is also called:

    A.   warts.
    B.   shingles.
    C.   gangrene.
    D.   impetigo.

7. Which of the following drugs is an antiviral?

    A.   Ciclopirox
    B.   Mupirocin
    C.   Amphotericin B
    D.   Acyclovir

8. The term for the characteristic redness of a sunburn is:

    A.   blisters.
    B.   scabs.
    C.   keloid.
    D.   erythema.

9. Severe acne vulgaris may be treated with:

    A.   diazepam (Valium®).
    B.   disopyramide (Norpace®).
    C.   isotretinoin (Accutane®).
    D.   tretinoin (Retin-A®).

10. Atopic dermatitis is not treated with which of the following?

    A. Diprolene
    B. Lamisil
    C. Cortisone
    D. Trexall

11. Manifestations of dermatophytosis include:

    A. tinea capitis, tinea pedis, tinea cruris, and tinea corporis.
    B. albinism and vitiligo.
    C. scabies and pediculosis.
    D. psoriasis and eczema.

12. The best antibiotic to use for treatment of mild impetigo is:

    A. tetracycline.
    B. metronidazole (Flagyl®).
    C. mupirocin (Bactroban®).
    D. penicillin.

13. Which of the following is the most deadly type of skin cancer?

    A. Basal cell carcinoma
    B. Squamous cell carcinoma
    C. Lipoma
    D. Melanoma

14. The patient with psoriasis may exhibit symptoms of:

    A. a large red rash, with itching.
    B. thick, flaky red patches covered with silvery white scales.
    C. firm, solid masses of cells in the skin that are larger than 0.5 cm in diameter.
    D. flat, discolored areas that are flush with the skin surface.

15. Which of the following is the trade name of dapsone?

    A. Oracea
    B. Azelex
    C. Aczone
    D. Claravis

CRITICAL THINKING

A mosquito bit a 34-year-old woman three days ago. Because of itching, she scratched the area of the bite, which was on her leg. Three days later, she developed swelling, edema, and pain. She went to see her physician, and the diagnosis was cellulitis.

1. What is the most common cause of cellulitis?

2. What is the drug of choice for cellulitis?

3. What other treatments can be offered in this condition?

WEB LINKS

American Academy of Dermatology: www.aad.org

American Burn Association: ameriburn.org

National Alopecia Areata Foundation: www.naaf.org

National Eczema Association: nationaleczema.org

National Psoriasis Foundation: www.psoriasis.org

National Rosacea Society: www.rosacea.org

The Skin Cancer Foundation: www.skincancer.org

CHAPTER 31

Complementary and Alternative Medicine

OUTLINE

History of Supplements
Dietary Supplement Regulation
Herbal Supplements
Safety and Efficacy of Dietary Supplements
Alternative Therapies

OBJECTIVES

Upon completion of this chapter, the reader should be able to:

1. Explain the terms "herb" and "botanical."
2. Describe the effects of the Dietary Supplement Health and Education Act (DSHEA).
3. Explain manufacturer recordkeeping practices for dietary supplements.
4. Identify the three types of claims allowed concerning dietary supplements.
5. Explain reasons why the FDA has issued warnings about dietary supplements.
6. Describe herbal supplements and their classification by the FDA.
7. Identify the indications for Ginkgo biloba, garcinia, and dong quai.
8. Describe the indications for black cohosh, echinacea, and St. John's wort.
9. Explain the sources and indications for glucosamine and chondroitin.
10. Identify the alternative systems of complementary and alternative medicine (CAM) therapies.

KEY TERMS

carcinogens

complementary and
alternative medicine (CAM)

dietary supplements

herbal supplement

mutagens

teratogens

Overview

Complementary and alternative medicine (CAM) involves various medical and health care practices, systems, and products that are not currently considered to be components of conventional medicine. Today, CAM has become more popular than ever before. According to the national Health Interview Survey (NHIS) of 2007, an estimated 38% of adults in the United States have used some form of CAM therapy. Natural products are the most popular form of CAM, making up about 20% of all CAM therapies. In 2014, the American Herbal Products Association (AHPA) reported that nearly one in five Americans use some form of CAM, with non-vitamin, non-mineral dietary supplements being most popular, followed by chiropractic or osteopathic manipulation, yoga, massage, meditation, and special diets. Dietary supplements are easily purchased over-the-counter (OTC) without any prescription being required. This is important to understand, since many supplements can interact with other commonly used substances, possibly leading to potentially dangerous interactions.

The use of herbal substances is focused upon restoring normal balance to the body. They usually are of lower cost and easier access than traditional medications. However, problems include herbs that come from foreign countries, which may lack adequate safety controls that ensure that they will be effective, yet harmless. Therefore, every patient using CAM must discuss treatments with a physician in order to avoid interactions with prescribed and OTC medications, as well as potential adverse effects.

History of Supplements

The terms *herb* and *botanical* have been used historically for plant products that may contain healing, flavor-enhancing, or food enhancement properties. Herbs have been used for many centuries. One of the first recorded uses occurred in 3000 BC, when garlic was prescribed to treat a medical condition. Thousands of herbs, alone or in combinations, have been used in Western and Eastern medicine.

The use of herbs started to decline in the latter years of the 1800s, as the pharmaceutical industry developed. Manufacturers found it simpler to formulate, standardize, and distribute their own drug products in comparison to natural herbal products. Many herbal products were removed from the market as regulations increased. Health care focused on treating diseases, instead of promoting wellness to prevent the eventual development of disease.

In the 1970s, there was a resurgence of interest in herbal products and alternative therapies. Today, most Americans take a few of these products regularly, or have taken them previously. With gradual aging of the population and long lifespans, many older Americans have looked for treatments that are less expensive yet more effective than standard prescription medications.

Dietary Supplement Regulation

The Dietary Supplement Health and Education Act (DSHEA) of 1994 attempted to regulate herbal supplements as part of its description of **dietary supplements**. These supplements are intended to enhance or supplement the diet. They include botanicals, herbs, vitamins, minerals, amino acids, enzymes, organ tissues, and extracts or metabolites not approved as drugs by the FDA. Various forms of supplements include tablets, capsules, gelcaps, softgels, liquids, and powders. They cannot be "represented" as actual foods or meals and must be clearly labeled as *dietary supplements*. Manufacturers are only required to notify the FDA when they intent to market a *new* dietary supplement. The manufacturer must provide the FDA with some evidence of the new supplement's safety, however. This requirement does not exist whenever a new manufacturer simply wants to release their own versions of dietary supplements that have been previously marketed by other companies. However, because of the DSHEA, the FDA can now remove a supplement that may pose a significant or unreasonable risk to the public. There have been many reports of contamination, impurities, and inconsistent amounts of ingredients.

The DSHEA also established the Office of Dietary Supplements (ODS), part of the National Institutes of Health (NIH). The ODS coordinates research on dietary supplements, publishing information about legal and regulatory issues. The National Center for Complementary and Alternative Medicine (NCCAM) is a newer part of the NIH. It coordinates research and training about CAM and publishes information about CAM to health care providers and consumers.

The Dietary Supplement and Nonprescription Drug Consumer Protection Act took effect in 2007. It required manufacturers to include contact information on labels for consumers, so that they can report adverse effects of the products. If a manufacturer is alerted to such an event, it must inform the FDA within 15 days after receiving a consumer complaint. Manufacturers must keep records of such events for at least six years, subject to FDA inspection.

The FDA requires manufacturers to evaluate the identity, potency, purity, and composition of all products, with labels accurately reflecting this information.

In 2008, a final rule for Current Good Manufacturing Practice in Manufacturing, Packaging, Labeling, or Holding Operations for Dietary Supplements became effective. It was intended to ensure acceptable manufacturing practices for dietary supplements, including consistent processing, meeting of quality standards, and acceptable identity, purity, strength, and composition. The FDA has stated that it helps prevent ingredients being present in inconsistent amounts; incorrect ingredients; contaminants such as bacteria, glass, lead, or pesticides; foreign materials, improper packaging, and mislabeling.

Even with the existing regulations, there is no real standardization in the dietary supplement industry. Manufacturers do not have to demonstrate product effectiveness before selling these supplements. The labeling is required to state that the product is not intended to diagnose, treat, cure, or prevent any disease. However, the labels can still make other claims. It is legal to state that the supplements promote healthy immune systems, reduce anxiety and stress, help maintain cardiovascular function, and reduce pain and inflammation. The labels may indicate that the product contains certain substances, but this claim may or may not be correct. The included amounts of ingredients may or may not be factual. It is important to remember that just because a supplement is described as "natural," this is no guarantee that it is safe to use.

Under the law, there are three types of claims that are allowed:

- *Health claims*—when there is a reduced risk of acquiring a disease with intake of a particular substance; for example, a product that contains calcium may state that a high-calcium diet will reduce risks for osteoporosis

- *Nutrient content claims*—allow manufacturers to describe levels of ingredient contents; for example, "low sodium" or "high fiber"

- *Structure/function claims*—describing how a substance affects normal structure or function, or how it may be helpful for deficiency, along with health maintenance, or affecting normal aging; for example, a supplement containing vitamin A may state that it "promotes better vision"; *note*: these types of claims must include the phrase: "This statement has not been evaluated by the FDA. This produce is not intended to diagnose, treat, cure, or prevent any disease."

Claims cannot state that the supplement treats specific diseases. All dietary supplement labels must include the correct supplement name, the fact that it is a supplement, manufacturer information, a complete ingredients list, and a "supplement facts" label. The FDA monitors labeling of supplements to prevent false, misleading claims. The FDA has the power to recall supplements, and the Federal Trade Commission (FTC) monitors advertising of supplements.

Patient medical histories must include complete listings of herbal supplements so that their effects and interactions can be tracked over time. These products have a potential for causing allergic reactions due to ingredients that may be either unlisted or not noticed by the consumer. Patients taking medications such as insulin, warfarin, or digoxin should be educated to avoid supplements until they have discussed them with their physicians since these drugs have great potential for interactions.

The AHPA assigns safety ratings to all herbal products in four categories:

- Class 1—may be safely consumed if used appropriately

- Class 2—carry usage restrictions, unless otherwise directed by a qualified expert:

  - 2a—for external use only

  - 2b—not to be used during pregnancy

  - 2c—not to be used during lactation and nursing

  - 2d—other specific use restrictions, as noted

- Class 3—have significant data resulting in the label, "To be used only under the supervision of an expert qualified in the appropriate use of this substance." The label of a Class 3 herbal product must include the following:

  - Dosage

  - Contraindications

- Potential adverse effects

- Potential drug interactions

- Any other relevant information related to safe use

- Class 4—Those that have insufficient data available for classification

A major difference between dietary supplements and prescription drug involves reduced post-marketing surveillance requirements. Periodic safety updates are not required for dietary supplements.

The FDA has issued many warnings for dietary supplements (see Figure 31-1). Supplements called "PC-SPES" and the manufacturer recalled "SPES" because they were found to contain alprazolam and warfarin. The supplement called "kava" received a warning because it was reported to cause liver-related injuries such as hepatitis, cirrhosis, and liver failure. A well-known warning concerned "Ephedra" and ephedrine-containing supplements, which the FDA prohibited from sale in the United States due to unreasonable risks for increased blood pressure, heart attack, and stroke. The FDA warned 23 manufacturers to stop distribution, or be sanctioned, of androstenedione-containing products since there was no evidence supporting their safety, and they could be harmful since they are converted to testosterone in the body. Several brands of "Shark Cartilage" capsules had lots contaminated with *Salmonella* recalled. "Red Yeast" products received a warning because the supplements contained lovastatin, which could lead to drug interactions. "Blue Steel" and "Hero" products were warned because of an undeclared ingredient similar to sildenafil, which could lead to unsafe decreases in blood pressure, or serious interactions with nitrates. "Viril-Ity Power Tabs" and "Xiadafil VIP Tabs" were recalled because they contained hydroxyhomosildenafil, which could lead to unsafe decreases in blood pressure or serious interactions with nitrates. Six weight loss supplements were recalled because they contained sibutramine or a similar substance, both of which were linked to heart attacks and strokes, and also contained the active ingredient in Prozac. Ten bodybuilding supplements were recalled because they contained anabolic steroids or related compounds linked to prostate cancer, aggression, and infertility.

Herbal Supplements

A **herbal supplement** may be defined as any mixture of ingredients, based on plant sources, designed for improvement of health or treatment of various conditions. Herbal supplements are not considered by the FDA to be drugs but, instead, food products. They are often used to supplement traditional medical therapies. This has led to undesired medical outcomes, interactions with drugs, and toxicity. Patients must be aware that taking herbal supplements should not occur without consulting their physician. There must be dialog about the supplements being taken, the quantities, and especially, the prescription drugs that are also being used. Since the FDA does not regulate these supplements, there is no independent verification method concerning their quality and effectiveness, or the quantity of their ingredients. Some herbs contain substances that are toxic to all body systems or, usually, to the liver. Others are **carcinogens**, **mutagens**, or **teratogens**.

Herbal supplements are available as capsules, liquids, powders, and in other forms. Since they are "natural," many people believe them to contain stronger healing properties than "synthetic" drugs. However, lack of sufficient testing means that proof of actual effectiveness is not well documented. The term *herb* is defined as a *botanical* product without stems or bark. Botanicals have been used for thousands of years to treat many different conditions.

Complementary and alternative medicine (CAM) is defined as diverse medical and health care systems, practices, and products not presently considered being part of conventional medicine. It involves healing systems and therapies, including herbal therapies, nutritional supplements, and special diets. The term *complementary* is separated from the term *alternative* by how the person uses the chosen therapy. It is considered complementary if used along with traditional medical treatments, but considered alternative if used in place of traditional medical treatments. All types of people utilize CAM, but it is most prevalent in females, of a variety of races, with higher education levels. Overall, approximately one of every three adults in the United States uses some form of CAM. Aside from dietary and herbal supplements, CAM also includes mega-vitamins, proteins, homeopathy, naturopathy, acupuncture, traditional Chinese medicine, yoga, meditation, support groups, cognitive-behavioral therapy, biofeedback, art and music therapy, chiropractic or osteopathic manipulation, massage, Reiki therapy, therapeutic touch therapy, and pulsed or magnetic field therapy.

The term *dietary supplement* may also be referred to with the terms *botanical, herbal, herbal medicine*, or *herbal therapy*. Use of the word "herbal" may be confusing since some but not all dietary supplements have plant origins.

DANGEROUS

Food and Drug Administration Says
Dietary Supplements containing BD, GBL, and GHB can kill you!

Dangerous products sold as dietary supplements for bodybuilding, weight loss, and sleep aids have been linked to deaths and severe sickness requiring hospitalization. These products are made from chemicals named:

- gamma hydroxybutyric acid (GHB),
- gamma butyrolactone (GBL),
- and 1,4 butanediol (BD).

Swallowing any of these ingredients may make you extremely sick and may even kill you.

BD, GBL, and GHB are used to make floor stripper, paint thinner, and other industrial products. FDA determined that dietary supplements containing these chemicals are really unapproved drugs because of the effect they have on the body. It is illegal to sell anything for human consumption that contains GHB, GBL, or BD. They can cause breathing problems, coma, vomiting, seizures and sometimes death. GHB, GBL and BD also increase the effects of alcohol and are even more dangerous when taken along with other drugs.

Items that contain BD include Revitalize Plus, Serenity, Enliven, GHRE, SomatoPro, NRG3, Thunder Nectar and Weight Belt Cleaner. GBL product names include: Longevity, Revivarant, G.H. Revitalizer, Gamma G, Blue Nitro, Insom-X, Remforce, Firewater and Invigorate. Previously, FDA warned consumers not to drink the products named Cherry fX Bombs, Lemon fX Drops and Orange fX Rush.

The dangerous products may list 1,4 butanediol, tetramethylene glycol, gamma butyrolactone or 2(3H)-Furanone di-hydro on the label—but some products have no label at all.

GBL-related products are listed as "party drugs" on internet sites, advertised in muscle-building magazines, and sold in health food stores as dietary supplements. Some of these products have been used as "date rape" drugs.

In 1990, FDA banned the use of GHB, but some companies switched ingredients to GBL and after warnings about GBL, switched to BD. These are all very similar chemicals which the body converts to GHB with the same dangerous effects. GBL-related products have been linked to at least 122 serious illnesses reported to FDA-- including three deaths.

For more information contact the Food and Drug Administration
at 1-888-INFO-FDA or visit the website at www.FDA.GOV

From U.S. food and drug administration, www.fda.gov.

Figure 31-1 FDA warning about dietary supplements.

Some supplements, for example, are derived from fish, minerals, and other sources. People sometimes call dietary supplements "alternative medicines" or "homeopathic medicines." However, *homeopathic medicine* actually is an individualized practice of formulating treatments and is not at all the same as the use of dietary supplements. Homeopathy, as a practice, utilizes its own compendia of medications.

There are many differences between herbal supplements and prescription or OTC drugs. Most modern drugs contain only one active ingredient that is standardized and accurately measured. This differs from many herbal supplements, which can contain a variety of active ingredients, in extremely varied quantities and strengths. They may contain large amounts of active chemicals that do not interact well for a controlled effect. There have been attempts to standardize certain herbal extracts, including ginkgo biloba and ginseng root.

As of 2016, the top 10 most commonly used dietary supplements, according to the American Botanical Council, were as follows:

- Horehound—for the common cold, coughing, digestion, inflammation
- Echinacea—for the common cold, effects of cancer treatments

- Cranberry—for urinary tract infections
- Ivy leaf—for respiratory congestion
- Turmeric—for arthritis, dyspepsia, stomach pain, intestinal problems
- Black cohosh—for premenopausal and menopausal symptoms
- Garcinia—for appetite control, weight loss, control of glucose and cholesterol
- Green tea—for protection against cancer, improving cognition, weight loss
- Ginger—for nausea, pain relief, diarrhea, improving appetite, motion sickness
- Fenugreek—for diabetes and cholesterol control, acid reflux, skin lesions

Table 31-1 lists a large amount of herbal supplements, their uses, and potential interactions.

Table 31-1 Commonly Used Herbal Supplements

Herb	Uses	Potential Interactions
Alfalfa	Cleanses the body; acts as nutritional supplement	Warfarin, contraceptives, estrogens, immunosuppressants, photosensitizing agents
Aloe	For antihistamine effects, decreases pain from burns and skin irritations; also has laxative effects	Digoxin, antidiabetes agents, various oral medications, sevoflurane, stimulant laxatives, warfarin, diuretics
Astragalus	Increases energy; promotes tissue regeneration; increases metabolism; strengthens the body; used for upper respiratory infections	Cyclophosphamide, lithium, immunosuppressants
Bilberry (only to be used for a short period of time)	Treats diarrhea, menstrual cramps, vision problems, varicose veins, and circulatory problems	Anticoagulants, antiplatelet agents, aspirin, insulin, iron, NSAIDs, oral antidiabetic agents
Black cohosh (not to be used in pregnancy, lactation, or by women with estrogen-dependent tumors)	Relieves menopausal symptoms and headaches	Antihypertensives, hormone replacement therapies, oral contraceptives, and sedatives/hypnotics
Cayenne	Boosts energy, improves digestion, increases circulation, and stimulates the heart	Cocaine, anticoagulants, antiplatelet agents, theophylline, ACE inhibitors
Chamomile (allergic reactions are common)	Used as anti-inflammatory, antispasmodic, and anxiolytic; also used for mild sedation	Warfarin, ardeparin, dalteparin, danaparoid, enoxaparin, heparin, other blood thinners
Cranberry	Used for urinary tract infections	Warfarin, cytochrome P450 2C9 (CYP2C9) substrates
Dong quai	Used for gynecological conditions such as premenstrual syndrome	Anticoagulants, antiplatelet agents, warfarin
Echinacea (use cautiously during pregnancy and lactation; may have spermicidal activity)	Enhances the immune system; acts as anti-inflammatory agent; used for upper respiratory infections	Amiodarone, anabolic steroids, ketoconazole, methotrexate, immunosuppressants

(Continued)

Table 31-1 Commonly Used Herbal Supplements *(Continued)*

Herb	Uses	Potential Interactions
Evening primrose (oil)	Source of essential fatty acids; relieves premenstrual or menopausal symptoms; relieves rheumatoid arthritis and other inflammatory conditions	Phenothiazines such as chlorpromazine
Feverfew (may alter clotting times)	Blocks inflammatory substances in the blood; used for headaches	Many different cytochrome P450 substrates, anticoagulants, antiplatelet agents
Garlic	Reduces blood cholesterol and blood pressure; acts as anticoagulant	Aspirin and other NSAIDs, warfarin, insulin, oral hypoglycemic agents, antiplatelet agents
Ginger	Treats gastrointestinal GI problems such as nausea; used for menstrual cramps; acts as anti-inflammatory agent	Aspirin and other NSAIDs, heparin, warfarin, antiplatelet agents
Ginkgo (avoid during pregnancy and lactation)	Improves memory and reduces dizziness	Anticonvulsants, aspirin and NSAIDs, heparin, warfarin, TCAs
Ginseng (*Panax ginseng* and *Siberian ginseng*) cause a variety of dangerous adverse effects and should be avoided)	Relieves stress; decreases fatigue; enhances the immune system and memory	CNS depressants, digoxin, diuretics, insulin, oral hypoglycemic agents, warfarin, antidepressants, mood stabilizers, antiestrogens, anxiolytics, antihypertensives
Golden seal (avoid during pregnancy or in young children)	Dries secretions; aids in digestion; reduces inflammation; acts as a mild antimicrobial	Cyclosporine, digoxin, various cytochrome P450 substrates, P-glycoprotein substrates
Grape seed extract (avoid during pregnancy, lactation, and in children)	Source of essential fatty acids; antioxidant; restores microcirculation to body tissues; used for allergies	Cytochrome P450 1A2 (CYP1A2) substrates, phenacetin, warfarin
Green tea	Acts as antioxidant; lowers LDL cholesterol; prevents cancer; relieves various GI problems	Antacids, bronchodilators, MAOIs, xanthines, dairy products, ephedra
Horny goat weed	Enhances sexual function	High blood pressure medications, anticoagulants, antiplatelet agents, NSAIDs, thrombolytics, ticlopidine, tirofiban, warfarin
Horse chestnut seed extract	Treats circulatory problems, varicose veins, edema, itching, cramping, and hemorrhoids	Anticoagulants, antidiabetic agents, aspirin and other salicylates, iron salts
Kelp	Used for thyroid disorders; goiter remedy (due to its high iodine content)	Digoxin, ACE inhibitors, potassium supplements, thyroid hormone, potassium-sparing diuretics
Melatonin	Acts as sedative and tranquilizer	CNS depressants, contraceptives, caffeine, fluvoxamine, antidiabetes agents, immunosuppressants, anticoagulants, antiplatelet agents, nifedipine GITS, benzodiazepines, verapamil

(Continued)

Table 31-1 Commonly Used Herbal Supplements *(Continued)*

Herb	Uses	Potential Interactions
Milk thistle	Acts as antitoxin; protects against liver disease	Drugs that are metabolized by the P-450 enzyme (such as beta-blockers and certain analgesics)
Parsley	Used for diuretic, expectorant, and laxative effects	Warfarin, diuretics, aspirin
Red clover	Treats menopausal symptoms and cancer	Anticoagulants and antiplatelet agents
Rose hips	Used for chest and nasal congestion	Aluminum-containing medications, estrogens, fluphenazine, lithium, warfarin, aspirin, choline magnesium trisalicylate, salsalate
Saw palmetto	Treats benign prostatic hypertrophy	Anticoagulants, antiplatelet agents, hormones such as estrogens, oral contraceptives, and androgens, immunostimulants, and NSAIDs
Soy	Protein, vitamin, and mineral supplementation; used for menopausal symptoms; prevents cardiovascular disease; anticancer agent	Thyroid agents (dextrothyroxine, levothyroxine, liothyronine, liotrix, thyroglobulin)
St. John's wort (use cautiously due to a variety of adverse effects)	Reduces depression and anxiety; acts as anti-inflammatory agent	CNS depressants, opioid analgesics, cyclosporine, efavirenz, indinavir, protease inhibitors, SSRIs, TCAs, antidepressants, warfarin
Tee tree oil	Used for skin disorders such as rashes; for burns	No known interactions
Valerian	Relieves stress and promotes sleep	Barbiturates, benzodiazepines, and other CNS depressants
Yohimbe	Increases male sexual potency; aphrodisiac; used for weight loss	ACE inhibitors, antihypertensives, beta-blockers, calcium channel blockers, alpha-adrenergic blockers, CNS stimulants, MAOIs, phenothiazines, SSRIs, sympathomimetics, TCAs, caffeine-containing products, and high-tyramine foods (such as wine, beer, aged cheese, liver)

Abbreviations in this table: ACE—angiotensin-converting enzyme; CNS—central nervous system; GI—gastrointestinal; LDL—low-density lipoprotein; MAOI—monoamine oxidase inhibitor; NSAID—nonsteroidal anti-inflammatory drug; SSRI—selective serotonin reuptake inhibitor; TCA—tricyclic antidepressant.

Safety and Efficacy of Dietary Supplements

Clinical trials are used to investigate the safety and efficacy of dietary supplements. The National Institutes of Health NCCAM is a large sponsor of these trials. Several reports on supplement trials are listed in this section, including information about black cohosh, echinacea, feverfew, ginkgo biloba, glucosamine–chondroitin, saw palmetto, St. John's wort, and a few miscellaneous substances.

The supplement's possible adverse effects, toxicity, purity, and likelihood of contamination during manufacturing should be considered. The reputation of each manufacturer should be evaluated, since standardization is lacking between the many different companies selling dietary supplements. There are also many different formulations for the identical dietary supplement, which may utilize different parts of the source plant or animal. Often, only certain parts of a plant, for example, are pharmacologically active. Other substances mixed into a formulation may affect its potency.

When a dietary supplement may be of uncertain safety and efficacy, there are resources that can be consulted about the manufacturer and other information. These include Consumer Labs, USP Verified Dietary Supplements, NSF Laboratories, and LabDoor. When there are concerns about a supplement, the health care provider should discourage the patient from using it. Also, the Natural Medicines Comprehensive Database can be used to identify and review all of the ingredients that may be contained. For supplements that contain multiple ingredients, there is a higher risk for adverse effects and interactions, and it is more difficult to determine which ingredient or ingredients were involved in the outcome.

Surgery patients have unique risks in relation to dietary supplements. Certain supplements may cause an increased risk for bleeding, cardiovascular instability, and sedation. Bleeding risks include epidural hematoma or excessive bleeding during surgery. Changes in heart rate and blood pressure, as well as development of ventricular arrhythmias, may occur. There can also be prolongation of anesthesia or excessive sedation. It is generally recommended that patients stop all dietary supplements two weeks before any elective surgery.

BLACK COHOSH

Black cohosh (*Actaea racemosa*) is a popular supplement, derived from a flowering plant that grows in the forests of eastern North America (see Figure 31-2). It is used for menopausal symptoms such as hot flashes. Hormone replacement therapy for these symptoms increases the risk for thromboembolic disease, cardiovascular disease, and certain

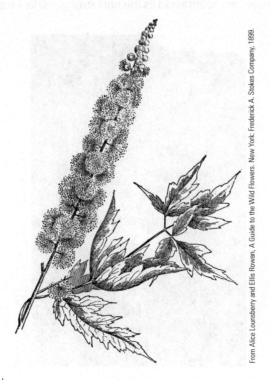

From Alice Lounsberry and Ellis Rowan, A Guide to the Wild Flowers. New York: Frederick A. Stokes Company, 1899.

Figure 31-2 Drawing of black cohosh.

types of cancer. Because of this, many women have looked for alternatives to hormone therapy. Black cohosh was investigated for this use. However, its pharmacologic actions show some amount of hormonal activity, and it is described as a selective estrogen receptor modulator (SERM). Black cohosh was compared in studies against conjugated estrogens, tibolone, and a placebo.

It appears to reduce the severity, but not the frequency, of hot flashes, insomnia, sexual problems, and vaginal dryness. It was concluded that black cohosh lacks strong evidence supporting its effectiveness against menopausal symptoms. Women with a history of breast cancer have a great need for something besides estrogen to treat hot flashes, and the standard treatment of breast cancer often results in hot flashes. Black cohosh was also studied in this group of patients, and it appeared to be only slightly helpful. Adverse reactions to black cohosh are slight but may include nausea. Liver function tests may be required.

Pregnant women because of its potential hormonal properties should not use black cohosh. It should be avoided in patients with breast cancer or a history of breast cancer. High doses may cause nausea, dizziness, visual effects, bradycardia, and increased perspiration. There have been more than 80 worldwide cases of liver damage, though the cause-and-effect relationship is not defined. Long-term use of black cohosh may cause thickening of the uterine lining, which could link to an increased risk of uterine cancer.

Echinacea

Echinacea is a group of herbaceous flowering plants of the daisy family (see Figure 31-3). They are found only in eastern and central North America. Echinacea supplements are commonly used to prevent or treat the common cold, but also for urinary tract infections, upper respiratory tract infections, herpes, and other infections. It is believed that echinacea stimulates and improves immune system function. However, various studies have shown that echinacea is not effective in preventing the common cold. It has only a slightly higher effect than placebo on treating a cold at onset.

Most adverse effects of echinacea are mild, with nausea and allergy being reported. Long-term use over more than eight weeks may actually lower immune system function. Echinacea should be avoided or used cautiously in patients with immune disorders such as rheumatoid arthritis, systemic lupus erythematosus, or leukemia. It should be avoided in any patient receiving immunosuppressants, such as corticosteroids, medications used to treat immune system disorders, or in patients receiving transplanted organs. Chronic use of technician must be avoided when receiving chemotherapy for cancer, since immune system suppression may be increased. The European Herbal Medicinal Products Committee and the U.K. Herbal Medicines Advisory Committee recommend against the use of Echinacea in children under 12 years of age. Pregnant women should avoid its use until stronger safety supporting evidence is available.

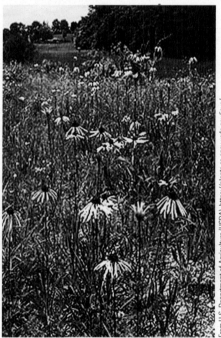

From U.S. Department of Agriculture (USDA), https://plants.sc.egov.usda.gov/java/largeImage?imageID=ecpa_1v.jpg

Figure 31-3 Echinacea.

Feverfew

Feverfew (*Tanacetum parthenium*) is a flowering plant, also in the daily family. People primarily use this to treat frequent migraine headaches. It is not used to treat the condition once the migraine occurs but is used to decrease the number of migraines that develop. In traditional herbal medicine, feverfew has been used for fever, arthritis, and digestive problems. Feverfew has a variety of pharmacologic actions in the body, but it is not known how it may prevent migraines. Most studies have not shown feverfew to have any significant action against migraines, however. This supplement has been associated with withdrawal, or a post-feverfew syndrome, following prolonged use. This causes anxiety, headache, sleeplessness, joint pain and stiffness, nervousness, and tiredness. Patients should be instructed never to chew feverfew leaves as they can cause mouth ulcerations and irritation. Other reported adverse effects include increased heart rate and gastrointestinal symptoms. The active ingredients in feverfew include *parthenolide*, which has been shown to induce apoptosis in some cancer cell lines in vitro, and possibly to target cancer stem cells. Pregnant women should not take feverfew. It can interact with blood thinners and increase risks for bleeding. It may also interact with a variety of medications metabolized by the liver.

Ginkgo Biloba

Ginkgo biloba is also commonly known as *ginkgo* or *gingko*, as well as the *maidenhair tree*. It is native to China and was first recorded as being used as a medicine in the late 15th century. In Germany, ginkgo biloba was first used medicinally in 1965. Today, it is used for memory problems, dementia such as Alzheimer's disease, and other central nervous system disorders. Many studies have been conducted on this supplement, with results showing it to be only slightly more effective than placebo. The conclusion is that there is no strong evidence to show that ginkgo biloba improves dementia or cognitive impairment.

Adverse effects include dizziness, tinnitus, angina, headache, and increased blood pressure. There are concerns about spontaneous bleeding, surgical bleeding complications, and interactions with antiplatelets and anticoagulants such as warfarin, digoxin, antihypertensive agents, aspirin, trazodone, and CNS agents. There are several reported cases of serious bleeding complications. The supplement may reduce platelet aggregation, leading to concerns about severe bleeding, especially when used with antiplatelets or anticoagulants. It should be used with caution when taking other herbs known to increase bleeding, such as garlic, ginseng, red clover, dong quai, danshen, black cohosh, saw palmetto, or ginger. Ginkgo should be avoided during lactation because of a lack of safety evidence, and it may increase bleeding time in pregnant women. Since it contains ginkgolic acids, which are extremely allergenic, the supplement may provoke allergic reactions in people who are allergic to poison ivy, mangoes, or cashew nuts.

Glucosamine–Chondroitin

Glucosamine and chondroitin are dietary supplements taken together or separately, usually for osteoarthritis. Glucosamine is an amino sugar that is a precursor for biochemical synthesis of glycosylated proteins and lipids. It is commercially produced by hydrolysis of shellfish exoskeletons, and less often from fermentation of corn or wheat. Glucosamine is sold as either a hydrochloride or sulfate form. The sulfate form has been studied more extensively. Glucosamine may help rebuild cartilage lost in joints of patients who have osteoarthritis, but this is not proven. Unlike the nonsteroidal anti-inflammatory drugs (NSAIDs), glucosamine is not believed to inhibit cyclooxygenase enzymes. Chondroitin sulfate is a glycosaminoglycan made up of a chain of alternating sugars. It is an important structural component of cartilage that provides much of its resistance to compression. It may work against osteoarthritis by preventing cartilage from being degraded within the joints. For supplements, chondroitin is obtained from animal cartilage.

Studies of glucosamine have shown a 28% improvement in pain, after two to three months of treatment, in patients with osteoarthritis. Other studies have shown a much lower improvement percentage in comparison to placebo. In comparison to ibuprofen, patients had a comparable lessening in pain within one week, meaning that glucosamine is a much slower-acting agent. Studies of these two supplements, separate and combined, have not shown significant results, and chondroitin is not recommended in the treatment of osteoarthritis. Primarily, adverse effects of glucosamine are nausea, heartburn, and diarrhea. Since glucosamine is mostly derived from shellfish exoskeletons, people who are allergic to shellfish should be warned about taking this supplement. Adverse effects of chondroitin include stomach pain and nausea. There is also a concern about possible interactions with warfarin, aspirin, and additional medications that affect blood clotting.

Saw Palmetto

Saw palmetto (*Serenoa repens*) is a small palm tree found in the Southeastern United States. It is primarily used to treat benign prostatic hyperplasia (BPH). It causes some inhibition of 5-alphareductase, which is similar to how prescription medications approved for this condition work. However, this supplement does not decrease the size of the prostate or lower hormone levels. Multiple studies have revealed that saw palmetto does have some ability to reduce the urinary symptoms of BPH.

Many men take saw palmetto because there are several adverse effects, including impotence, of the available prescription medications. Adverse effects include back pain, dizziness, upper respiratory tract infections, diarrhea, rash, and abdominal pain. Overall, most studies do not support the use of saw palmetto for treating BPH. Serious adverse effects have been slight, but included liver toxicity and bleeding associated with surgery.

St. John's Wort

St. John's wort (*Hypericum perforatum*) is a flowering plant in the family *Hypericaceae*. It is used to treat depression, and there have been a variety of studies for this use, as well as for obsessive–compulsive disorder, menopausal symptoms, smoking cessation, and various psychological disorders. For its antidepressant effects, St. John's wort may utilize reuptake of serotonin, dopamine, and norepinephrine. Its effectiveness has been documented, and it may be very close to the effects of standard antidepressants. St. John's wort has been shown to be two to six times more effective than placebo for patients with various levels of depression, except for major depression. Overall, most clinicians agree that St. John's wort is effective for mild to moderate depression, but not for severe depression. Adverse effects include anxiety, sleeplessness, restlessness, nausea, sensitivity to light, potentially life-threatening *serotonin syndrome*, withdrawal after long-term use, and sexual side effects. St. John's wort increases liver enzyme actions and causes the liver to break down medications more quickly. This results in decreased serum levels of many medications.

A large amount of drugs may interact with this supplement. These drugs include oral contraceptives, cyclosporine, digoxin, human immunodeficiency virus (HIV) drugs, cancer medications, warfarin, prescription antidepressants, and ranolazine. People should not take this supplement with bipolar disorder due to the higher risk for mania. Other agents that may interact with St. John's wort include benzodiazepines, antiarrhythmics, beta-blockers, calcium channel blockers, and statins. Outcomes of interactions between St. John's wort and various medications have included organ graft rejections, unplanned pregnancies, and decreased control of HIV. This supplement has serotonergic activity within the brain, which can cause interactions with serotonin reuptake inhibitors (SSRIs), tricyclic antidepressants, sibutramine, and serotonin agonists used for migraines. Therefore, each patient taking St. John's wort must have a thorough medication review to eliminate possible interactions.

MEDICATION ERROR ALERT

Part of the reason that herbal supplements are often used without being fully understood can be explained by this simple fact: Many herbs listed for use as herbal supplements are also listed on the FDA's Poisonous Plant Database! These include herbs such as aloe, black cohosh, chamomile, feverfew, ginkgo, milk thistle, rose hips, St. John's wort, and valerian.

Alternative Therapies

Alternative therapies focus on treating each person individually, considering the health of the whole person. They emphasize integration of mind and body, promoting disease prevention, self-care, and self-healing. Alternative therapies also recognize spirituality as part of health and healing. Research is ongoing about whether CAM therapies are

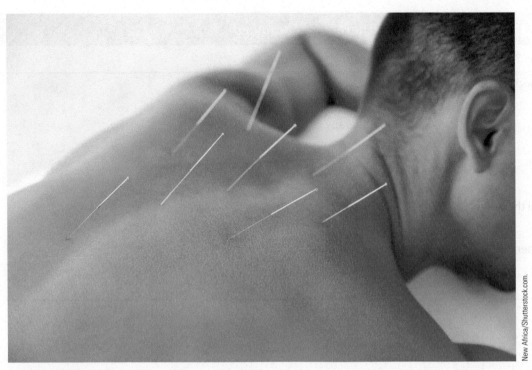

Figure 31-4 Acupuncture.

totally or partially effective, or not at all effective. Some therapies have proven effectiveness, but others do not. Therapies include specific diets, homeopathy, chiropractic, acupuncture (see Figure 31-4), massage, exercise, relaxation techniques, hypnotherapy, biofeedback, prayer, counseling, and detoxification therapies. The value of CAM therapies lies in an ability to reduce the need for medications. When drug doses are reduced, this leads to fewer potential adverse effects. Examples of CAM are listed in Table 31-2.

Health care professionals should be sensitive to patients' beliefs about CAM therapies. Advantages and limitations should be explained to patients so that they can make accurate choices about their health care. Alternative therapies can work together with pharmacotherapy to achieve successful treatment outcomes. In many cultures, home remedies and folk remedies are used alongside pharmacotherapy.

Table 31-2 Examples of CAM Therapies

Type of Therapy	Examples
Alternative systems	Chinese traditional medicine, including acupuncture and herbs
	Chiropractic
	Homeopathy
	Native American medicine, including medicine wheels, sweat lodges
	Naturopathy
Biologic therapies	Herbs
	Nutritional supplements
	Specially designed diets
Manual therapies	Hand-mediated biofield techniques
	Massage
	Physical therapy
	Pressure-point techniques

(Continued)

Table 31-2 Examples of CAM Therapies *(Continued)*

Type of Therapy	Examples
Mind–body techniques	Biofeedback
	Guided imagery
	Hypnotherapy
	Meditation
	Movement therapies such as dance and music
	Yoga
Spiritual therapies	Faith, prayer
	Shamans
Other therapies	Animal assistance
	Bioelectromagnetics
	Detoxification

Summary

Plant products, described with the terms "herb" and "botanical," have been used for various medical conditions over thousands of years. Herbal supplements, as part of the description of "dietary supplements," began to be regulated with the Dietary Supplement Health and Education Act (DSHEA) of 1994. Even with attempts at better management and control of the supplement industry, no systematic standardization is in place. It is important that patient medical records include all information about dietary supplements being taken, along with prescription and OTC medications, due to the great potential for serious interactions. There have been many FDA-issued warnings about certain dietary supplements. Complementary and alternative medicine (CAM) involves diverse systems, practices, and products that are considered "outside" of conventional medicine. Today, there are stricter controls concerning the safety and efficacy of new dietary supplements.

REVIEW QUESTIONS

1. For how long must manufacturers keep records of the adverse effects of dietary supplements?

    A.   Three months
    B.   Two years
    C.   Three years
    D.   Six years

2. Which of the following is not one of the types of claims allowed for dietary supplements?

    A.   Nutrient content claims
    B.   Prevention claims
    C.   Structure or function claims
    D.   Health claims

3. Which of the following organizations monitors advertising of dietary supplements?

    A.   FTC
    B.   FDA
    C.   EDA
    D.   CDC

4. Which of the following herbal supplements is used for depression?

   A. Ginger
   B. Garlic
   C. St. John's wort
   D. Green tea

5. Which of the following dietary supplements is used for appetite control?

   A. Garcinia
   B. Cranberry
   C. Echinacea
   D. Black cohosh

6. Which of the following dietary supplements is used for premenstrual syndrome?

   A. Echinacea
   B. Dong quai
   C. Aloe
   D. Alfalfa

7. Which of the following herbal supplements is indicated to treat benign prostatic hyperplasia?

   A. St. John's wort
   B. Ginseng
   C. Green tea
   D. Saw palmetto

8. Which of the following is an indication for Ginkgo biloba?

   A. Improving memory
   B. Lowering LDL cholesterol
   C. Reducing inflammation
   D. Boosting energy

9. Which of the following herbs is used for the relief of menopausal symptoms?

   A. Ginseng
   B. Aloe
   C. Black cohosh
   D. Ginkgo biloba

10. Which of the following is not an example of "alternative systems therapy"?

   A. Chiropractic
   B. Hypnotherapy
   C. Naturopathy
   D. Acupuncture

11. Which of the following dietary supplements is indicated for pain relief but may take longer than ibuprofen to be effective?

   A. Glucosamine
   B. Ginkgo biloba
   C. St. John's wort
   D. Saw palmetto

12. Which of the following, according to the FDA, is the major safety issue when using kava?

   A. Neurotoxicity
   B. Liver toxicity
   C. Heart attack
   D. Kidney impairment

13. Which of the following dietary supplements is used at the onset of symptoms to reduce severity of a cold?

    A.   Saw palmetto
    B.   Chondroitin
    C.   Echinacea
    D.   Ginkgo biloba

14. Which of the following is the name of the law regulating dietary supplements?

    A.   Dietary Supplement Labeling Act
    B.   Complementary and Alternative Medicine Act
    C.   Dietary Supplement Health and Education Act
    D.   Food, Drug, and Cosmetic Act

15. Which of the following refers to the meaning of "herb"?

    A.   Dietary supplements from all sources
    B.   Plant-derived dietary supplements
    C.   Animal-derived dietary supplements
    D.   Mineral-derived dietary supplements

CRITICAL THINKING

Twice in one month, a 32-year-old man complained to his physician about increasing fatigue, loss of appetite, poor sleep patterns, and an inability to concentrate at work. The physician suspected moderate depression, and offered to prescribe a selective serotonin reuptake inhibitor (SSRI), but the patient did not want it. Instead, he explained that he had heard about a dietary supplement called St. John's wort and its effective ability to treat depressive symptoms.

1. Would St. John's wort be appropriate for this patient's diagnosis?

2. What are the possible interactions regarding prescription and OTC medications?

WEB LINKS

Clinical Trials: www.clinicaltrials.gov

Consumer Lab: www.consumerlab.com

FDA Dietary Supplements: www.fda.gov/food/dietarysupplements

FDA MedWatch: www.fda.gov/safety/medwatch/safetyinformation/default.htm

LabDoor: labdoor.com

Medline Plus: medlineplus.gov/druginformation.html

Memorial Sloan-Kettering Cancer Center: www.mskcc.org/cancer-care/diagnosis-treatment/symptom-management/integrative-medicine/herbs

National Center for Complementary and Integrative Health: nccih.nih.gov

Natural Medicines Comprehensive Database: naturalmedicines.therapeuticresearch.com

NSF Laboratories: www.nsf.org/services/by-type/lab-testing

USP Verified Dietary Supplements: www.usp.org/verification-services/verified-mark

Abbreviation	Explanation
aaa	Apply to affected area
ac; a.c.; AC	Before meals
ACE	Angiotensin-converting enzyme
ADD	Attention-deficit disorder
ADH	Antidiuretic hormone
ADHD	Attention-deficit hyperactivity disorder
ADME	Absorption, distribution, metabolism, and elimination
ADR	Adverse drug reaction
AIDS	Acquired immunodeficiency syndrome
AM; a.m.	Morning
ANDA	Abbreviated New Drug Application
APAP	Acetaminophen (Tylenol®)
AphA	American Pharmacy Association
ARBs	Angiotensin receptor blockers
ASA	Aspirin
b.i.d.; BID	Twice daily
BMI	Body Mass Index
BP	Blood pressure
BUD	Beyond-use date
°C	Degrees centigrade (Celsius)
Ca++	Calcium
Cap; cap	Capsule
CDC	Centers for Disease Control and Prevention
CF	Cystic fibrosis
CHF	Congestive heart failure
CNS	Central nervous system
COPD	Chronic obstructive pulmonary disease
CPR	Cardiopulmonary resuscitation
CSP	Compounded sterile preparation

(Continued)

Abbreviation	Explanation
CV	Cardiovascular
D_5; D_5W; D5W	Dextrose 5% in water
D_5 ¼; D5 1/4	Dextrose 5% in ¼ normal saline; dextrose 5% in 0.225% sodium chloride
D_5 ⅓; D5 1/3	Dextrose 5% in ⅓ normal saline; dextrose 5% in 0.33% sodium chloride
D_5 ½; D5 1/2	Dextrose 5% in ½ normal saline; dextrose 5% in 0.45% sodium chloride
D_5LR; D5LR	Dextrose 5% in lactated Ringer's solution
D_5NS; D5NS	Dextrose 5% in normal saline; dextrose 5% in 0.9% sodium chloride
DAW	Dispense as written
D/C	Discharge
DCA	Direct compounding area
Dig	Digoxin
disp	Dispense
EC	Enteric-coated
Elix	Elixir
eMAR	Electronic Medication Administration Record
EPO	Epoetin alfa; erythropoietin
ER; XR; XL	Extended-release
°F	Degrees Fahrenheit
$FeSO_4$	Ferrous sulfate; iron
g; G	Gram
gr	Grain
GI	Gastrointestinal
GMP	Good manufacturing practice
gtt; gtts	Drop; drops
h; hr	Hour
HC	Hydrocortisone
HCTZ	Hydrochlorothiazide
HIPAA	Health Insurance Portability and Accountability Act
HIV	Human immunodeficiency virus
HMO	Health Maintenance Organization
HRT	Hormone replacement therapy
IBU	ibuprofen; Motrin
ICU	Intensive care unit
IM	Intramuscular
IND	Investigational New Drug Application
Inj	Injection
IPA	Isopropyl alcohol

Abbreviation	Explanation
ISDN	Isosorbide dinitrate
ISMO	Isosorbide mononitrate
ISMP	Institute for Safe Medication Practices
IV	Intravenous
IVF	Intravenous fluid
IVP	Intravenous push
IVPB	Intravenous piggyback
JCAHO	Joint Commission on the Accreditation of Healthcare Organizations
K; K$^+$	Potassium
KCl	Potassium chloride
kg	Kilogram
L	Liter
LAFW	Laminar airflow workbench; hood
lb	Pound
LD	Loading dose
LVP	Large-volume parenteral
Mag; Mg; MAG	Magnesium
MAR	Medication Administration Record
mcg	Microgram
MDI	Metered-dose inhaler
MDV	Multiple-dose vial
mEq	Milliequivalent
mg	Milligram
mL	Milliliter
mL/hr	Milliliters per hour
mL/min	Milliliters per minute
MMR	Measles, mumps, and rubella vaccine
MRSA	Methicillin-resistant *Staphylococcus aureus*
MOM; M.O.M.	Milk of magnesia
MVI; MVI-12	Multiple vitamin injection; multivitamins for parenteral administration
Na$^+$	Sodium
NABP	National Association of Boards of Pharmacy
NaCl	Sodium chloride; salt
NDA	New Drug Application
NDC	National Drug Code
NF; non-form	Non-formulary

(Continued)

Abbreviation	Explanation
NKA	No known allergies
NKDA	No known drug allergies
NPO; npo	Nothing by mouth
NR	No refills
NS	Normal saline; 0.9% sodium chloride
½ NS	One-half normal saline; 0.45% sodium chloride
¼ NS	One-quarter normal saline; 0.225% sodium chloride
NSAID	Non-steroidal anti-inflammatory drug
NTG	Nitroglycerin
OC	Oral contraceptive
ODT	Orally disintegrating tablet
OPTH; OPHTH; Opth	Ophthalmic
OTC	Over the counter; no prescription required
oz	Ounce
pc; p.c.; PC	After meals
PCA	Patient-controlled anesthesia
PCN	Penicillin
pH	Acid-base balance
PHI	Protected health information
PM; p.m.	Afternoon; evening
PN	Parenteral nutrition
PNS	Peripheral nervous system
PO; po	Orally; by mouth
PPE	Personal protective equipment
PPI	Proton pump inhibitor
PR	Per rectum; rectally
PRN; p.r.n.	As needed; as occasion requires
PTSD	Post Traumatic Stress Disorder
PV	Per vagina; vaginally
PVC	Polyvinyl chloride
QA	Quality assurance
q.i.d.; QID	Four times daily
QTY; qty	Quantity
RA	Rheumatoid arthritis
RDA	Recommended daily allowance
Rx	Prescription; pharmacy; medication; drug; recipe; take
sig	Signa; write on label; directions

Abbreviation	Explanation
SL; sub-L	Sublingual
SMZ-TMP	Sulfamethoxazole and trimethoprim (Bactrim®)
SNRI	Serotonin norepinephrine reuptake inhibitor
SPF	Sunburn protection factor
SR	Sustained-release
SSRI	Selective serotonin reuptake inhibitor
STAT; Stat	Immediately; now
STD	Sexually transmitted disease
subcut; SUBCUT	Subcutaneous
SUPP; Supp	Suppository
susp	Suspension
SVP	Small-volume parenteral
SW	Sterile water
SWFI	Sterile water for injection
Tab; tab	Tablet
TB	Tuberculosis
TBSP; tbsp	Tablespoon; tablespoonful; 15 mL
TDS	Transdermal delivery system
TKO; TKVO; KO; KVO	To keep open; to keep vein open; keep open; keep vein open
TNA	Total Nutrition Admixture
TPN	Total parenteral nutrition
TSP; tsp	Teaspoon; teaspoonful; 5 mL
ung	Ointment
USP	U.S. Pharmacopoeial Convention
USP-NF	U.S. Pharmacopoeia-National Formulary
UTI	Urinary tract infection
UV	Ultraviolet light
VAG; vag	Vagina; vaginally
Vanco	Vancomycin
VO; V.O.; V/O	Verbal order
w/o	Without
Zn	Zinc
Z-Pak	Azithromycin; Zithromax

Drug Class	Definition	Example
LIQUIDS		
Aerosol	A pressurized dosage form, in which solid or liquid drug particles are suspended in a gas, to be dispensed in a cloud or mist.	Proventil HFA® inhaler
Elixir	A drug that is dissolved in a solution of alcohol and water.	Tylenol® elixir
Emulsion	A mixture of oils in water.	Cod liver oil
Liniment	A drug mixed with oil, soap, alcohol, or water, and applied externally.	Camphor liniment
Lotion	An aqueous preparation containing suspended ingredients.	Nutraderm® lotion
Spirit	A drug combined with an alcoholic solution, which is volatile.	Aromatic spirit of ammonia
Spray	A fine stream of medicated vapor, used to treat the nose and throat.	Dristan® nasal spray
Syrup	A drug dissolved in a solution of sugar and water.	Robitussin® cough syrup
Tincture	An extract of a therapeutic substance in alcohol.	Tincture of benzoin
SOLIDS		
Capsule	A drug contained in a water-soluble gelatin capsule.	Benadryl® capsule
Cream	A drug combined in a generally non-greasy base, resulting in a semisolid preparation.	Aristocort® topical cream
Ointment	A drug combined with an oil based that results in a semisolid preparation.	Polysporin® ointment
Suppository	A drug mixed with cocoa butter or another firm base, designed to melt at body temperature.	Nupercainal® suppository
Tablet	Powdered medication that has been pressed into a disc shape.	Aspirin tablet

Generic Name	Trade Name
haemophilus b conjugate vaccine (tetanus toxoid conjugate)	ActHib vials
interferon gamma-1b	Actimmune vials
tetanus toxoid, reduced diphtheria toxoid, acellular pertussis vaccine adsorbed (Tdap) vaccine	Adacel vials
proparacaine	Alcaine ophthalmic solution
amoxicillin	Amoxil suspension
succinylcholine chloride	Anectine vials
aspirin	Aspirin Uniserts suppositories
lymphocyte immune globulin	Atgam vials
amoxicillin with clavulanic acid	Augmentin suspension
interferon beta-1a	Avonex syringes
azithromycin	Azasite ophthalmic solution
bacitracin	BACiiM vials
erythromycin/benzyl peroxide	Benzamycin gel
interferon beta-1b	Betaseron vials
penicillin g benzathine	Bicillin syringes
diltiazem hydrochloride	Cardizem vials
alprostadil	Caverject vials
cefuroxime axetil	Ceftin suspension
cefprozil	Cefzil suspension
fosphenytoin sodium	Cerebyx vials
ciprofloxacin	Cipro suspension
estradiol/norethindrone	Combipatch transdermal
glatiramer acetate	Copaxone syringes
desmopressin	DDAVP vials
digoxin immune fab	Digiband vials
cefadroxil	Duricef suspension
estramustine phosphate	Emcyt capsules
etancercept	Enbrel syringes
hepatitis b vaccine	Engerix-B vials

(Continued)

Generic Name	Trade Name
epoetin alfa	Epogen vials
saquinavir	Fortovase soft gels
somatropin	Genotropin cartridges
hepatitis a vaccine	Havrix syringes/vials
carboprost tromethamine	Hemabate vials
insulin lispro	Humalog pens/vials
somatropin	Humatrope vials
adalimumab	Humira syringes
regular insulin	Humulin R vials
insulin	Iletin vials
interferon alfacon-1	Infergen vials
lopinavir/ritonavir	Kaletra capsules/solution
lactobacillus acidophilus/bulgaricus	Lactinex tablets
insulin glargine	Lantus pens/vials
chlorambucil	Leukeran tablets
loracarbef	Lorabid suspension
rubella virus vaccine live	Meruvax vials
methylergonovine maleate	Methergine vials
calcitonin salmon	Miacalcin nasal spray
measles, mumps, rubella virus vaccine live	MMR II vials
aalprostadil	Muse nasal spray
nystatin	Mycostatin pastilles
pegfilgrastim	Neulasta syringes
filgrastim	Neupogen syringes/vials
gabapentin	Neurontin suspension
cisatracurium besylate	Nimbex vials
somatropin	Norditropin cartridges
ritonavir	Norvir soft gels
insulin	Novolin vials
insulin aspart	Novolog vials
pancuronium bromide	Pavulon vials
promethazine	Phenergan suppositories
pneumococcal vaccine polyvalent	Pneumovax 23 vaccine vials
conjugated estrogens	Premarin secule vials
epoetin alfa	Procrit vials
rabies vaccine	RabAvert vials

Generic Name	Trade Name
sirolimus	Rapamune solution vials
ribavirin/interferon alfa-2b	Rebetron (Rebetol with Intron A) capsules/vials
becaplermin	Regranex gel
risperidone	Risperdal Consta vial kits
octreotide acetate	Sandostatin vials
cefixime	Suprax suspension
beractant	Survanta vials
oseltamivir phosphate	Tamiflu suspension
liotrix	Thyrolar tablets
atracurium besylate	Tracrium vials
amoxicillin	Trimox suspension
penicillin v	Veetids suspension
insulin	Velosulin vials
etoposide	VePesid capsules
doxycycline	Vibramycin suspension
trifluridine	Viroptic ophthalmic solution
latanoprost	Xalatan ophthalmic solution
rocuronium bromide	Zemuron vials
azithromycin	Zithromax suspension

Source: https://pharmacytechshq.com/wp-content/uploads/2018/12/Commonly-refrigerated-drugs-medications-prescriptions.pdf

Accupril (ACE inhibitor)	Accutane (anti-acne drug)
acetazolamide (anti-glaucoma drug)	acetohexamide (oral antidiabetic drug)
Aciphex (proton pump inhibitor)	Accupril (ACE inhibitor)
Aciphex (proton pump inhibitor)	Aricept (anti-Alzheimer's drug)
Actos (oral hypoglycemic)	Actonel (bisphosphonate—bone-growth regulator)
Adriamycin (antineoplastic)	Aredia (bone-growth regulator)
albuterol (sympathomimetic)	atenolol (beta-blocker)
Aldomet (antihypertensive)	Aldoril (antihypertensive)
Alkeran (antineoplastic)	Leukeran (antineoplastic)
Alkeran (antineoplastic)	Myleran (antineoplastic)
allopurinol (anti-gout drug)	Apresoline (antihypertensive)
alprazolam (anti-anxiety agent)	lorazepam (anti-anxiety agent)
Amaryl (oral hypoglycemic)	Reminyl (anti-Alzheimer's drug)
Ambien (sedative-hypnotic)	Amen (progestin)
amiloride (diuretic)	amlodipine (calcium channel blocker)
amiodarone (anti-arrhythmic)	amrinone (inotropic agent)
amitriptyline (antidepressant)	nortriptyline (antidepressant)
Apresazide (antihypertensive)	Apresoline (antihypertensive)
Aripiprazole (antipsychotic)	Lansoprazole (proton pump inhibitor)
Arlidin (peripheral vasodilator)	Aralen (antimalarial)
Artane (cholinergic blocking agent)	Altace (ACE inhibitor)
Asacol (anti-inflammatory drug)	Avelox (fluoroquinolone antibiotic)
asparaginase (antineoplastic agent)	pegaspargase (antineoplastic agent)
Atarax (anti-anxiety agent)	Ativan (anti-anxiety agent)
atenolol (beta-blocker)	timolol (beta-blocker)
Atrovent (cholinergic blocking agent)	Alupent (sympathomimetic)
Avandia (oral hypoglycemic)	Coumadin (anticoagulant)
Avandia (oral hypoglycemic)	Prandin (oral hypoglycemic)
Bacitracin (antibacterial)	Bactroban (anti-infective, topical)
Benylin (expectorant)	Ventolin (sympathomimetic)
Brevital (barbiturate)	Brevibloc (beta-adrenergic blocker)

Bumex (diuretic)	Buprenex (narcotic analgesic)
bupropion (antidepressant; smoking deterrent)	buspirone (anti-anxiety agent)
Cafergot (analgesic)	Carafate (anti-ulcer drug)
calciferol (vitamin D)	calcitriol (vitamin D)
carboplatin (antineoplastic agent)	cisplatin (antineoplastic agent)
Cardene (calcium channel blocker)	Cardizem (calcium channel blocker)
Cardura (antihypertensive)	Ridaura (gold-containing anti-inflammatory)
Cataflam (NSAID)	Catapres (antihypertensive)
Catapres (antihypertensive)	Combipres (antihypertensive)
cefotaxime (cephalosporin)	cefoxitin (cephalosporin)
cefuroxime (cephalosporin)	deferoxamine (iron chelator)
Celebrex (NSAID)	Cerebyx (anticonvulsant)
Celebrex (NSAID)	Celera (antidepressant)
Cerebyx (anticonvulsant)	Celera (antidepressant)
chlorpromazine (antipsychotic)	chlorpropamide (oral antidiabetic)
chlorpromazine (antipsychotic)	prochlorperazine (antipsychotic)
chlorpromazine (antipsychotic)	promethazine (antihistamine)
Clinoril (NSAID)	Clozaril (antipsychotic)
clomipramine (antidepressant)	clomiphene (ovarian stimulant)
clonidine (antihypertensive)	Klonopin (anticonvulsant)
Combivir (AIDS drug combination)	Combivent (combination for COPD)
Cozaar (antihypertensive)	Zocor (antihyperlipidemic)
cyclobenzaprine (skeletal muscle relaxant)	cyproheptadine (antihistamine)
cyclophosphamide (antineoplastic)	cyclosporine (immunosuppressant)
cyclosporine (immunosuppressant)	cycloserine (antineoplastic)
Cytovene (antiviral drug)	Cytosar (antineoplastic)
Cytoxan (antineoplastic)	Cytotec (prostaglandin derivative)
Cytoxan (antineoplastic)	Cytosar (antineoplastic)
Dantrium (skeletal muscle relaxant)	danazol (gonadotropin inhibitor)
daunorubicin (antineoplastic)	doxorubicin (antineoplastic)
desipramine (antidepressant)	diphenhydramine (antihistamine)
dexamethasone (corticosteroid)	dextromethorphan (antitussive)
DiaBeta (oral hypoglycemic)	Zebeta (beta-adrenergic blocker)
digitoxin (cardiac glycoside)	digoxin (cardiac glycoside)
diphenhydramine (antihistamine)	dimenhydrinate (antihistamine)
dopamine (sympathomimetic)	dobutamine (sympathomimetic)
Doribax (antibiotic)	Zovirax (antiviral)

(Continued)

DTaP (diphtheria, tetanus toxoids, and acellular pertussis)	Tdap (tetanus toxoid, reduced diphtheria toxoid, and acellular pertussis)
Durasal (salicylate)	Durezol (corticosteroid)
Edecrin (diuretic)	Eulexin (antineoplastic)
enalapril (ACE inhibitor)	Anafranil (antidepressant)
enalapril (ACE inhibitor)	Eldepryl (anti-Parkinson agent)
Eryc (erythromycin base)	Ery-Tab (erythromycin base)
etidronate (bone-growth regulator)	etretinate (antipsoriatic)
etomidate (general anesthetic)	etidronate (bone-growth regulator)
E-Vista (antihistamine)	Evista (estrogen receptor modulator)
Femara (antineoplastic)	Femhrt (estrogen-progestin combination)
Fioricet (analgesic)	Fiorinal (analgesic)
Flomax (alpha-adrenergic blocker)	Volmax (sympathomimetic)
flurbiprofen (NSAID)	fenoprofen (NSAID)
folinic acid (leucovorin calcium)	folic acid (vitamin B complex)
Gantrisin (sulfonamide)	Gantanol (sulfonamide)
glipizide (oral hypoglycemic)	glyburide (oral hypoglycemic)
glyburide (oral hypoglycemic)	Glucotrol (oral hypoglycemic)
Hycodan (cough preparation)	Hycomine (cough preparation)
hydralazine (antihypertensive)	hydroxyzine (anti-anxiety agent)
hydrocodone (narcotic analgesic)	hydrocortisone (corticosteroid)
Hydrogesic (analgesic combination)	hydroxyzine (antihistamine)
hydromorphone (narcotic analgesic)	morphine (narcotic analgesic)
Hydropres (antihypertensive)	Diupres (antihypertensive)
Hytone (topical corticosteroid)	Vytone (topical corticosteroid)
imipramine (antidepressant)	Norpramin (antidepressant)
Inderal (beta-adrenergic blocker)	Inderide (antihypertensive)
Inderal (beta-adrenergic blocker)	Isordil (coronary vasodilator)
Indocin (NSAID)	Minocin (antibiotic)
K-Phos Neutral (phosphorus-potassium replenishment)	Neutra-Phos-K (phosphorus-potassium replenishment)
Lamictal (anticonvulsant)	Lamisil (antifungal)
Lamictal (anticonvulsant)	Ludiomil (alpha- and beta-adrenergic blocker)
Lamisil (antiviral)	Ludiomil (alpha- and beta-adrenergic blocker)
Lanoxin (cardiac glycoside)	Lasix (diuretic)
Lantus (insulin glargine)	Lente insulin (insulin zinc suspension)
Lioresal (muscle relaxant)	lisinopril (ACE inhibitor)
Lithostat (lithium carbonate)	Lithobid (lithium carbonate)

Lithotabs (lithium carbonate)	Lithobid (lithium carbonate)
Lodine (NSAID)	codeine (narcotic analgesic)
Lopid (antihyperlipidemic)	Lorabid (beta-lactam antibiotic)
lovastatin (antihyperlipidemic)	Lotensin (ACE inhibitor)
Ludiomil (alpha- and beta-adrenergic blocker)	Lomotil (antidiarrheal)
Medrol (corticosteroid)	Haldol (antipsychotic)
metolazone (thiazide diuretic)	methotrexate (antineoplastic)
metolazone (thiazide diuretic)	metoclopramide (GI stimulant)
metoprolol tartrate (beta-adrenergic blocker)	metoclopramide hydrochloride (GI stimulant)
metoprolol (beta-adrenergic blocker)	misoprostol (prostaglandin derivative)
Monopril (ACE inhibitor)	minoxidil (antihypertensive)
morphine sulfate (analgesic)	morphine sulfate extended release (analgesic)
nelfinavir (antiviral)	nevirapine (antiviral)
nicardipine (calcium channel blocker)	nifedipine (calcium channel blocker)
Norlutate (progestin)	Norlutin (progestin)
Noroxin (fluoroquinolone antibiotic)	Neurontin (anticonvulsant)
Norvasc (calcium channel blocker)	Navane (antipsychotic)
Norvir (antiviral)	Retrovir (antiviral)
Ocufen (NSAID)	Ocuflox (fluoroquinolone antibiotic)
Orinase (oral hypoglycemic)	Ornade (upper respiratory product)
Percocet (narcotic analgesic)	Percodan (narcotic analgesic)
paroxetine (antidepressant)	paclitaxel (antineoplastic)
Paxil (antidepressant)	paclitaxel (antineoplastic)
Paxil (antidepressant)	Taxol (antineoplastic)
penicillamine (heavy metal antagonist)	penicillin (antibiotic)
pindolol (beta-adrenergic blocker)	Parlodel (inhibitor of prolactin secretion)
pitavastatin (anti-cholesterol agent)	pravastatin (anti-cholesterol agent)
Pitocin (neuromodulator that induces childbirth)	Pitressin (antidiuretic hormone)
Plaquenil (antimalarial drug)	Provigil (analeptic drug for sleep disorders)
Platinol (antineoplastic)	Paraplatin (antineoplastic)
Pletal (antiplatelet drug)	Plavix (antiplatelet drug)
Pravachol (antihyperlipidemic)	Prevacid (GI drug)
Pravachol (antihyperlipidemic)	propranolol (beta-adrenergic blocker)
prednisolone (corticosteroid)	prednisone (corticosteroid)
Prilosec (inhibitor of gastric acid secretion)	Prozac (antidepressant)
Prinivil (ACE inhibitor)	Prilosec (GI drug)
Prinivil (ACE inhibitor)	Proventil (sympathomimetic)

(Continued)

Procanbid (anti-arrhythmic)	Procan SR (anti-arrhythmic)
propranolol (beta-adrenergic blocker)	Propulsid (GI drug)
Provera (progestin)	Premarin (estrogen)
Prozac (antidepressant)	Proscar (androgen hormone inhibitor)
quinidine (anti-arrhythmic)	clonidine (antihypertensive)
quinidine (anti-arrhythmic)	Quinamm (antimalarial)
quinine (antimalarial)	quinidine (anti-arrhythmic)
Regroton (antihypertensive)	Hygroton (diuretic)
risperidone (antipsychotic)	ropinirole (anti-Parkinsonism agent)
sulfadiazine (antibiotic)	sulfasalazine (anti-inflammatory agent)
tramadol (analgesic)	trazodone (antidepressant)
zolmitriptan (anti-migraine serotonin agonist)	zolpidem (hypnotic)

Choose the most correct answer for each question.

1. Which of the following is the brand name for paroxetine?

    A. Zoloft
    B. Tegretol
    C. Apokyn
    D. Paxil

2. Which of the following is the sensitivity of a class A prescription balance?

    A. 100 mg
    B. 60 mg
    C. 6.0 mg
    D. 0.6 mg

3. Which of the following types of ointment bases is contained in Aquaphor?

    A. Water-oil emulsion
    B. Absorption
    C. Oleaginous
    D. Oil-water emulsion

4. Which of the following is the meaning of the prefix *hyper-*?

    A. Slow
    B. Across
    C. Fast
    D. Above

5. Which of the following federal laws established the assignment of every drug to have a specific National Drug Code (NDC)?

    A. Orphan Drug Act
    B. Federal Privacy Act
    C. Drug Listing Act
    D. Prescription Drug Marketing Act

6. Which of the following is the generic name for Zocor?

    A. simvastatin
    B. ranitidine
    C. atorvastatin
    D. fluvastatin

7. Which of the following is the most appropriate route of insulin administration?

    A. PO
    B. ID
    C. SC
    D. IM

8. Which reference book is a compilation of package inserts?

   A. USPD2
   B. Physician's Desk Reference
   C. Drug Topics Red Book
   D. Facts and Comparisons

9. Which of the following medications is indicated for a body ache if the patient is taking warfarin?

   A. Narcotic analgesic
   B. NSAID
   C. ASA
   D. APAP

10. Which of the following is the route of administration for heparin?

    A. Oral
    B. IM
    C. IV
    D. IA

11. Which of the following is the definition of "pc"?

    A. Before meals
    B. After meals
    C. By mouth
    D. As needed

12. A manufacturer's invoice is $800.00 with terms being 4% of net. How much should be paid to the manufacturer if payment occurs within 30 days?

    A. $16.00
    B. $32.00
    C. $54.00
    D. $88.00

13. Which part of the brain controls body temperature, appetite, water balance, and emotions?

    A. Cerebellum
    B. Pons
    C. Hypothalamus
    D. Medulla oblongata

14. Which of the following is also known as a "crash cart"?

    A. Code red cart
    B. Code blue cart
    C. Code yellow cart
    D. Code black cart

15. What is the trade name for benztropine?

    A. Cogentin
    B. Parlodel
    C. Symmetrel
    D. Zonegran

16. Which of the following is NOT classified as a selective serotonin reuptake inhibitor (SSRI)?

    A. Prozac
    B. Paxil
    C. BuSpar
    D. Celexa

17. Which of the following laws established the requirement for opium to be a prescription drug?

    A.   Federal Food and Drug Act
    B.   Harrison Narcotic Act
    C.   Omnibus Budget Reconciliation Act
    D.   Comprehensive Drug Abuse Prevention and Control Act

18. Which of the following vitamins is NOT fat-soluble?

    A.   E
    B.   K
    C.   B6
    D.   A

19. Which of the following is a proton pump inhibitor?

    A.   Pantoprazole
    B.   Famotidine
    C.   Ranitidine
    D.   Sucralfate

20. In which of the following drug schedules is meperidine classified?

    A.   IV
    B.   III
    C.   II
    D.   V

21. A physician orders Hctz 50 mg for a one-month supply, 1 tab PO qod, ref x5. How many tablets should be given to the patient?

    A.   15
    B.   30
    C.   45
    D.   60

22. The prefix *osteo-* means which of the following?

    A.   Tissue
    B.   Muscle
    C.   Liver
    D.   Bone

23. Which of the following classifications of drugs is contraindicated in pregnant women?

    A.   C
    B.   X
    C.   B
    D.   A

24. Which of the following describes a total parenteral solution?

    A.   Isotonic solution
    B.   Hypertonic solution
    C.   Hypotonic solution
    D.   Dialysis solution

25. Which of the following is the minimum age to purchase pseudoephedrine?

    A.   16
    B.   18
    C.   20
    D.   21

26. Which of the following is a reference book that contains drug costs?

- **A.** White Book
- **B.** Green Book
- **C.** Blue Book
- **D.** Red Book

27. Which of the following is abbreviated as "MDI"?

- **A.** Multidose inhaler
- **B.** Metered-dose inhaler
- **C.** Medical diagnosis included
- **D.** Medical doctor under investigation

28. Which of the following is the trade name of cephalexin?

- **A.** Cedax
- **B.** Rocephin
- **C.** Keflex
- **D.** Cefzil

29. Which of the following organizations oversees Medicare and Medicaid payments?

- **A.** FDA
- **B.** CMS
- **C.** DEA
- **D.** PBM

30. How many hours of continuing education are required for a pharmacy technician to be recertified every two years?

- **A.** 10 hours
- **B.** 15 hours
- **C.** 20 hours
- **D.** 40 hours

31. Which of the following is NOT indicated for the treatment of hypertension?

- **A.** Lasix
- **B.** Tenex
- **C.** Aldactone
- **D.** Norvasc

32. Which of the following dosage forms is NOT solid?

- **A.** Elixir
- **B.** Powder
- **C.** Gelcap
- **D.** Pill

33. Which of the following is the site for an otic product to be instilled?

- **A.** Under the tongue
- **B.** In the nose
- **C.** In the eye
- **D.** In the ear

34. Which of the following forms must be filed in order to dispense controlled substances?

- **A.** Form 106
- **B.** Form 222
- **C.** Form 224
- **D.** Form 41

35. How many milligrams are equal to 4 gr?

    A. 6 mg
    B. 16 mg
    C. 160 mg
    D. 260 mg

36. Which of the following is the standard time that a patient would receive his medication that is equivalent to 0900 hours military time?

    A. 8 AM
    B. 9 AM
    C. 8 PM
    D. 9 PM

37. Which of the following is a common side effect of an antihistamine?

    A. Nausea
    B. Laryngitis
    C. Drowsiness
    D. Polyuria

38. How long must a laminar airflow hood be turned on prior to being used?

    A. 10 minutes
    B. 20 minutes
    C. 30 minutes
    D. 60 minutes

39. Which of the following is the trade name of pentazocine?

    A. Talwin
    B. Vicodin
    C. Xanax
    D. Halcion

40. Which of the following forms must be filed when a controlled substance is destroyed?

    A. Form 41
    B. Form 106
    C. Form 222
    D. Form 224

41. A physician ordered 30 capsules "1 cap tid ac." How many days would this prescription last for?

    A. 8 days
    B. 10 days
    C. 15 days
    D. 30 days

42. Which of the following is the maximum number of refills for a Schedule III drug?

    A. None
    B. One
    C. Five
    D. Unlimited

43. Which of the following types of inventory is performed before the pharmacy's first day of business?

    A. Physical
    B. Perpetual
    C. Initial
    D. Annual

44. Which of the following organizations conducts the "ExCPT" exam?

    A. Pharmacy Technician Certification Board
    B. National Pharmacy Association
    C. National Healthcareer Association
    D. American Society of Health-System Pharmacists

45. Which of the following is the abbreviation of potassium?

    A. Na
    B. K
    C. P
    D. Fe

46. Which of the following is the best time to administer a rectal drug intended for a systemic effect?

    A. Bedtime
    B. Early morning
    C. After dinner
    D. After a bowel movement

47. Which of the following is another name for antidiuretic hormone?

    A. Vasopressin
    B. Thymosin
    C. Oxytocin
    D. Androgen

48. Which of the following is the trade name of vincristine?

    A. Velban
    B. Deltasone
    C. Oncovin
    D. Rituxan

49. Which of the following terms refers to the amount of money that a patient must pay in a given period before a third party insurer can make a payment?

    A. Deductible
    B. Copayment
    C. Premium
    D. Capitation

50. Which of the following may be indicated to treat sleep disorders?

    A. Glucosamine
    B. Melatonin
    C. Ginseng
    D. Folic acid

Choose the most correct answer for each question.

1. Which of the following vitamin deficiencies may cause scurvy?

   A. Vitamin D
   B. Vitamin C
   C. Vitamin B12
   D. Vitamin A

2. For how long must controlled substance records be kept?

   A. One year
   B. Two years
   C. Three years
   D. Five years

3. What is the intravenous infusion rate in milliliters per hour if a total of 200 mL is administered over 2 hours?

   A. 50 mL
   B. 75 mL
   C. 100 mL
   D. 125 mL

4. What is the trade name of ketoconazole?

   A. Nizoral
   B. Monistat
   C. Oxistat
   D. Terazol

5. Which of the following is a federally funded reimbursement program?

   A. HMO
   B. PPO
   C. HSA
   D. Medicare

6. Which of the following sizes of capsules contains the largest quantity?

   A. 0
   B. 2
   C. 4
   D. 6

7. A prescription reads: Flexeril 10 mg, "i po tid." Which of the following is the total daily dose?

   A. 10
   B. 15
   C. 20
   D. 30

8. The word root *cardio* means which of the following?

   A. Liver
   B. Heart
   C. Skin
   D. Kidney

9. Which of the following federal laws requires a pharmacy to give consulting services for all patients?

   A. Orphan Drug Act
   B. Kefauver-Harris Amendment
   C. OBRA-70
   D. OBRA-90

10. Which of the following dosage forms consists of solid particles dispersed in a liquid vehicle?

    A. Suspension
    B. Emulsion
    C. Mixture
    D. Gel

11. How many grams of dextrose are in one liter of D5W?

    A. 50 mg
    B. 50 g
    C. 50 mcg
    D. 5.0 mcg

12. Which of the following is the maximum number of refills for a Schedule V drug?

    A. None
    B. Three
    C. Five
    D. Unlimited

13. Which of the following types of medication may cause constipation, dry mouth, and difficult urination?

    A. Beta-blockers
    B. Anticholinergics
    C. Alpha-blockers
    D. Cholinergics

14. Which of the following is an example of a cephalosporin?

    A. Suprax
    B. Monodox
    C. Edecrin
    D. Tigan

15. Which of the following is the total volume if 30 g of urea is dissolved to make a 10% solution?

    A. 30 mL
    B. 60 mL
    C. 120 mL
    D. 300 mL

16. Which of the following is the maximum number of different items that may be ordered on a DEA Form 222?

    A. 10
    B. 12
    C. 15
    D. 18

17. What is the generic name of Deltasone?

    A. Triamcinolone
    B. Dexamethasone
    C. Prednisone
    D. Cortisone

18. The abbreviation "Rx" on a prescription indicates which of the following?

    A. Signa
    B. Inscription
    C. Special labeling
    D. Take this drug

19. For how long must a patient wait to purchase another bottle of an exempt narcotic?

    A. 12 hours
    B. 24 hours
    C. 48 hours
    D. 72 hours

20. Which of the following parts of Medicare reimburses a retail pharmacy for prescription medications?

    A. Part C
    B. Part A
    C. Part D
    D. Part B

21. To mark up a product by 20%, how much would each item with this markup cost if its original cost was $3.00?

    A. $3.60
    B. $4.20
    C. $6.20
    D. $7.60

22. Which of the following types of insulin can be added to an intravenous solution?

    A. NPH insulin
    B. Regular insulin
    C. Isophane insulin
    D. Extended insulin zinc

23. Which of the following is NOT an antiviral drug?

    A. Clotrimazole
    B. Abacavir
    C. Rimantadine
    D. Foscarnet

24. Which of the following is the trade name of methadone?

    A. Duragesic
    B. Vicodin
    C. Dolophine
    D. Lortab

25. Which of the following is the most appropriate place to store a liquid ampicillin suspension?

    A. In a bedroom
    B. In a bathroom
    C. In a kitchen cabinet
    D. In a refrigerator

26. Which of the following is the most common route of administration?

    A.   Rectal
    B.   Oral
    C.   Topical
    D.   Nasal

27. Which of the following is the smallest in weight?

    A.   Milligram
    B.   Gram
    C.   Kilogram
    D.   Microgram

28. All of the following medications are used to treat osteoporosis, except:

    A.   Fosamax
    B.   Cardura
    C.   Actonel
    D.   Boniva

29. Which of the following vitamins can increase the blood coagulation when a patient takes warfarin?

    A.   Vitamin E
    B.   Vitamin C
    C.   Vitamin K
    D.   Vitamin A

30. Which of the following forms of managed care uses capitation?

    A.   PPO
    B.   POS
    C.   EPOS
    D.   HMO

31. Which of the following is a Schedule IV drug?

    A.   Dilaudid
    B.   Ativan
    C.   Ritalin
    D.   Amytal

32. Which of the following is a deficiency of glucocorticoids and mineralocorticoids?

    A.   Addison's disease
    B.   Cushing's disease
    C.   Graves' disease
    D.   Cushing's syndrome

33. How many milliliters are equivalent to two pints?

    A.   80 mL
    B.   280 mL
    C.   480 mL
    D.   960 mL

34. Which of the following dosage forms may be prepared using the wet gum method?

    A.   Suspensions
    B.   Spirits
    C.   Tablets
    D.   Emulsions

35. When counting tablets or capsules by using a spatula and a pill tray, how many multiple numbers are counted?

    A. 3
    B. 5
    C. 7
    D. 10

36. If one gram of dextrose provides 3.4 kilocalories, how many kcal will 250 mL of a 10% dextrose solution provide?

    A. 85 kcal
    B. 150 kcal
    C. 285 kcal
    D. 350 kcal

37. Which of the following dosage forms can be made by using compression?

    A. Suppository
    B. Troche
    C. Tablet
    D. Caplet

38. Which of the following medications can be given as a smoking cessation method and also as an antidepressant?

    A. Trazodone
    B. Zolpidem
    C. Bupropion
    D. Nicotine

39. All of the following agents require child-resistant packaging, except:

    A. Betamethasone
    B. Nitroglycerin
    C. Miglitol
    D. Naproxen

40. Which of the following conditions can cause goiter?

    A. Hyperparathyroidism
    B. Hypertension
    C. Hyperadrenalism
    D. Hyperthyroidism

41. How many days would 48 tablets of a medication last if the prescription is "1 tab tid"?

    A. 8 days
    B. 10 days
    C. 12 days
    D. 16 days

42. Which of the following is the classification schedule of methylphenidate?

    A. Schedule II
    B. Schedule IV
    C. Schedule III
    D. Schedule I

43. Which of the following terms refers to the name of the medication, the quantity, and its strength?

  A. Subscription
  B. Inscription
  C. Signa
  D. Superscription

44. Which of the following medications is contraindicated with vitamin K?

  A. Warfarin
  B. Glyburide
  C. Heparin
  D. Pentoxifylline

45. Which of the following means "the rules of a facility or institution"?

  A. Standard
  B. Protocol
  C. Policy
  D. Procedure

46. Which of the following drug recalls can be ordered if a drug may result in reversible harm or injury to a patient?

  A. Class IV
  B. Class I
  C. Class III
  D. Class II

47. Which of the following is also called a nonproprietary drug?

  A. OTC drug
  B. Trade name drug
  C. Generic drug
  D. Investigational drug

48. Which of the following substances is NOT found in a total nutrient admixture?

  A. Proteins
  B. Lipids
  C. Dextrose
  D. Amino acids

49. Which of the following is NOT an advantage of bar coding?

  A. It ensures the patient receives the correct dosage form
  B. It ensures that the patient can access the drug's lot number
  C. It ensures that the patient can access the drug's expiration date
  D. It ensures that the patient can access the date of manufacturing

50. Which of the following is the trade name of nadolol?

  A. Inderal
  B. Corgard
  C. Lopressor
  D. Toprol XL

A

abbreviations — Shortened forms of words.

absorption — The movement of a drug from its site of administration into the bloodstream.

accessory — Any individual who helps a person to violate the law either directly or indirectly.

acetylcholine (ACh) — A neurotransmitter released in the brain that stimulates nerve endings.

acromegaly — Abnormal growth of the bones of the face, hands, feet, and soft tissue that occurs after puberty; it is caused by hypersecretion of human growth hormone (hGH).

active acquired immunity — Immunity resulting from the development of antibodies within a person's body that renders the person immune; it may occur from exposure through a disease process or from immunizations.

additive effect — The combined effect of more than one agent, which is equal to the sum of the effects of each drug taken alone.

administrative law — Regulations set forth by governmental agencies, such as the Internal Revenue Service (IRS) and the Social Security Administration (SSA); also called regulatory law.

adulterate — Tampering with or contaminating a product or substance.

adverse reactions (adverse effects) — More severe symptoms or problems that develop due to the administration of a drug.

agent — An entity capable of causing disease.

agonist — A drug that binds to and produces a functional change in a particular cell.

agonist — A muscle performing an actual movement; it is also called a prime mover.

agranulocytes — A type of white blood cell that includes monocytes and lymphocytes; they are characterized by an absence of granules in their cytoplasm (cellular fluid).

airborne transmission — Contaminated droplets or dust particles suspended in the air are transferred to a susceptible host.

allergen — A foreign substance (such as pollen, dander, or mold) that can cause an allergic reaction in hypersensitive people.

allergy — A hypersensitive reaction to foreign substances (allergens) by the immune system.

alveolar sacs (alveoli) — The cluster-like air sacs located at the end of each alveolar duct in the lungs.

amenorrhea — Absence of menstrual periods, which may be caused by a hormonal imbalance, or may be a side effect of a drug.

amphiarthroses — Joints in which the surfaces are connected by disks of fibrocartilage, as between vertebrae.

ampule — A sealed glass container that usually contains a single dose of medicine. The top of the ampule must be broken off to open the container.

anaphylactic reaction — A severe form of allergic reaction to a drug that is life threatening. The patient develops severe shortness of breath and may even have cardiac collapse.

angina pectoris — A paroxysmal thoracic pain caused most often by myocardial anoxia, as a result of atherosclerosis or spasm of the coronary arteries.

angioplasty — A procedure used to widen vessels narrowed by stenosis or occlusions.

angiotensinogen — A serum glycoprotein produced in the liver that is the precursor of angiotensin.

antagonism — When two drugs act to decrease each other's effects.

antagonist — A muscle that opposes the actions of an agonist.

anthrax — A zoonotic disease caused by the anthrax bacillus that can infect humans in a number of ways and can be fatal.

antibiotic — Substance that has the ability to destroy or interfere with the development of a living organism.

antibodies — Proteins that develop in response to the presence of antigen in the body and react with the antigen on the next exposure. Antibodies may be formed from infections, immunization, transfer from mother to child, or unknown antigen stimulation.

antigens — Foreign substances that cause the production of specific antibodies. Also called immunogens.

antihistamines — Drugs that counteract the action of histamine.

725

antisepsis — Preventing infection by arresting or inhibiting growth and multiplication of infectious agents.

antiseptic — Substance that reduces the growth and multiplication of infectious agents.

antitoxins — Antibodies that neutralize toxins.

antitussives — Agents that relieve or prevent coughing.

anxiety — A physiological state consisting of fear, apprehension, or worry.

aortic valve — A valve in the heart between the left ventricle and the aorta.

apathy — A lack of feeling, emotion, interest, or concern.

apothecary system — An old English system of measurement.

aqueous humor — A watery fluid, such as that found in the eyes.

Arabic numbers — Standard numerical numbers.

aromatic water — A mixture of distilled water with an aromatic volatile oil.

arrector pili muscle — Bundles of smooth muscle fibers attached to the deep part of hair follicles, passing outward alongside sebaceous glands to the papillary layer of the corium; they act to pull the hairs, causing "goose bumps."

arrhythmias — Various conditions of abnormal electrical heart activity; the heart may beat too fast, too slow, or irregularly; also called dysrhythmias.

arthritis — Degenerative disease of the joints.

articulation — A fixed or movable joint between bones.

ASAP medication order — A medication required to be provided as soon as possible.

ascorbic acid — A water-soluble vitamin that is essential for the formation of collagen and fibroid tissue for teeth, bones, cartilage, connective tissue, and skin. It also aids in fighting bacterial infections, and in treating bleeding gums, bruising, nosebleeds, and anemia.

aseptic technique — Preparing and handling sterile products in a manner that prevents microbial contamination.

assay and control unit — A group with the responsibility for auditing the control system and evaluating product quality; similar to a quality control unit.

athlete's foot — A fungal infection of the foot; it usually starts between two toes and can spread to other toes. Athlete's foot is more properly called tinea pedis.

atrophy — A wasting or decrease in size of a body organ, tissue, or part because of disease, injury, or lack of use.

attenuation — The process of weakening pathogens.

auditory ossicles — Three small bones (the malleus, incus, and stapes) that transmit sound vibrations from the eardrum to the oval window of the ear.

auditory tube — The eustachian tube; the structure linking the pharynx to the middle ear.

audits — Systematic reviews and evaluations of records and other data to determine quality of services or products provided.

autism — A general term for a group of complex disorders of brain development; it is characterized by difficulties in social interaction, verbal and nonverbal communication, and repetitive behaviors.

autoclave — A sterilizing machine. An autoclave uses a combination of heat, steam, and pressure to sterilize equipment.

automated dispensing system — A drug dispensing system that is computer or robot based.

automated touch-tone response system — A system in which the patient can call in an order or refill a prescription and the system routes the refill orders to the proper pharmacy and assigns each order a place in the order-fulfillment sequence.

automation — The automatic control or operation of equipment, processes, or systems, which often involves robotic machinery controlled by computers.

autonomy — The right of an individual to make informed decisions for his or her own good.

avoirdupois — An old English system of weights.

B

bacilli — Rod-shaped bacteria that occur in chains, produce spores, and require oxygen to survive.

bactericidal — Able to destroy bacteria.

barbiturates — Drugs derived from barbituric acid, which act as central nervous system depressants.

bar coding — Placing a code on packaging to help standardize and regulate inventory control.

barrel chest — A large, rounded thorax, as in the inspiratory phase, considered normal in some stocky individuals and certain others who live in high-altitude areas. Barrel chest may also be a sign of pulmonary emphysema.

barrier precautions — Measures taken to minimize the risk of exposure to blood and body fluids.

basal cell carcinoma — Malignant epithelial (skin) cell tumor that begins as a papule and develops into a crater that crusts and bleeds.

batch repackaging — The reassembling of a specific dosage and dosage form of medication at a given time.

behind-the-counter (BTC) medications — Drugs not requiring a prescription, but requiring a pharmacist's discretion to purchase.

Bell's palsy — Paralysis of the facial nerve on one side, causing impaired function of the eye, mouth, muscle tone, and other components.

beneficiary — A person designated by an insurance policy to receive benefits or funds.

beyond use date — Date after which a product is no longer effective and should not be used.

biennial inventories — Complete lists of all products stored in a pharmacy, conducted every two years.

bioavailability — The term that indicates measurement of both the rate of drug absorption and the total amount of drug that reaches the systemic blood circulation from an administered dosage form.

bioethics — A discipline dealing with the ethical and moral implications of biological research and applications.

biohazard symbol — An image or object that serves as an alert that there is a risk to organisms, such as ionizing radiation or harmful bacteria or viruses.

biological agent — Living organisms that invade the host.

biologics — Agents that give immunity to diseases or living organisms.

biotechnology — The use of microorganisms such as bacteria or yeasts, or biological substances such as enzymes, to produce drugs, synthetic hormones, and other medical products.

biotin — A water-soluble B complex vitamin that acts as a coenzyme in fatty acid production and in the oxidation of fatty acids and carbohydrates.

biotransformation — Another name for metabolism.

blended-dose system — A drug distribution system that combines a unit-of-use medication package with a non–unit-dose drug distribution system.

B lymphocytes — Cells of the adaptive immune system that express cell surface immunoglobulins specific for an epitope on an antigen.

bolus — A soft mass of chewed food.

Bowman's glomerular capsule — A sac that collects fluids from the blood in the glomerulus of the kidney and processes them further to form urine; this process is called ultrafiltration.

brand name — A word, symbol, or device assigned to a product by its manufacturer, registered or not registered, as a trademark of its identity.

bronchioles — Structures in the lungs formed by the smallest bronchi.

bronchodilators — Agents that relax the smooth muscle of the bronchial tubes.

buccal — Pertaining to the inside of the cheek.

buffered tablet — A tablet that prevents ulceration or irritation of the stomach wall.

bulbourethral glands — Also known as Cowper's glands, they are exocrine glands that produce a mucus-like fluid called pre-ejaculate.

bursa — A fluid-filled sac that reduces friction between two surfaces.

C

calciferol — A fat-soluble vitamin chemically related to the steroids and essential for the normal formation of bones and teeth. It is important for the absorption of calcium and phosphorus from the gastrointestinal tract.

calcitonin — A hormone produced in the parafollicular cells (C cells) of the thyroid gland that participates in regulating the blood level of calcium and stimulates bone mineralization.

calcium — An alkaline earth metal element. The body requires calcium ions for the transmission of nerve impulses, muscle contraction, blood coagulation, cardiac functions, and other processes.

caplet — A tablet shaped like a capsule.

capsule — A solid dosage form in which the drug is enclosed in either a hard or soft shell of soluble material.

carbohydrates — Nutrients providing the main source of energy in the average diet.

carcinogenic — A substance that causes cancer.

carcinogens — Chemical compounds capable of causing cancer and other malignant tumors.

cartilage — A tough, elastic, fibrous connective tissue found in joints, the outer ear, larynx, and other parts of the body.

catecholamines — A group of sympathomimetic compounds, some of which are produced naturally by the body, and function as key neurological chemicals.

cation — A positively charged atom.

caustic — A substance that eats away at something.

cellulitis — An infection of the subcutaneous tissue that is often treated with intravenous antibiotics.

Centers for Medicare & Medicaid (CMS) — An organization that inspects and approves institutions that provide Medicaid and Medicare services.

central fill pharmacy — A high-volume pharmacy that fills prescriptions for a number of individual pharmacies.

centrally acting skeletal muscle relaxants — Also known as "spasmolytics," these agents alleviate musculoskeletal pain and spasms to reduce spasticity (continual muscular contraction).

central processing unit (CPU) — The part of the computer that does the computations.

certified — For a pharmacy technician, this means being granted recognition by a nongovernmental agency or association because of meeting predetermined qualifications they have specified as necessary. A certified pharmacy technician is credentialed as a "CPhT."

cerumen — The soft brownish-yellow wax secreted by ceruminous glands in the auditory canal of the external ear.

chain pharmacy — One of a group of retail pharmacies operated under the control of a specific company, with all facilities in the chain bearing the same name.

CHAMPVA — A comprehensive health care program in which the Office of Veterans' Affairs (VA) shares the cost of covered health care services and supplies with eligible beneficiaries.

chancre — A painless, highly contagious lesion or ulceration that may form during the primary stage of syphilis.

channels — Spoken words, written messages, and body language.

chemical agent — Substance that can interact with the body.

chemical name — Drug name derived from the chemical composition of the drug.

chemical sterilization — A method of cleaning equipment used for instruments that cannot be exposed to the high temperatures of steam sterilization.

chloride — An anion of chlorine. The most common form is sodium chloride (table salt).

chlorophyll — Green pigments found in plants and other photosynthetic organisms.

cholesterol — A waxy lipid found only in animal tissues. A member of a group of lipids called sterols, it is widely distributed in the body.

choroid — The thin, posterior membrane in the middle layer of the eye.

chyle — A white or pale yellow liquid product of digestion taken up by the small intestine; it consists mainly of emulsified fats.

chyme — The partially digested contents of the stomach. Chyme is composed of food, hydrochloric acid from the stomach, and digestive enzymes.

ciliary body — A thickened portion of the vascular tunic of the eye that connects the choroid with the iris.

civil law — Rules and regulations that govern the relationship between individuals within society.

Class A prescription balance — A two-pan device that may be used for weighing small amounts of drugs (not more than 120 g).

clinical — Having to do with the examination and treatment of patients.

clitoris — A small erectile organ at the anterior part of the vulva, homologous to the penis.

cocci — Spherical or semi-spherical bacteria.

coccobacilli — Short, oval-shaped bacilli.

cochlea — The auditory portion of the inner ear; made up of coiled, tapered tubes.

coinsurance — An arrangement in which the insured must pay either a fixed amount or a percentage of the cost of medical services covered by the insurer.

coitus — Sexual intercourse.

collections letter — A document that notifies a customer that his or her bill is past due.

collections — All of the activities of handling patient accounting and following up to ensure timely payments.

combining form — A root with an added vowel (known as a combining vowel) that connects the root with the suffix or the root to another root.

comedones — Small, flesh-colored, white, or dark bumps caused by acne that cause the skin to have a rough texture; they are found at the opening of sebaceous follicles.

common fraction — Represents equal parts of a whole.

communication — The sharing of information, ideas, thoughts, and feelings.

community pharmacy — A retail pharmacy in any local community area.

compensation — An unconscious mechanism by which an individual tries to make up for fancied or real deficiencies.

competencies — Unique skill sets and abilities in a particular field.

complementary and alternative medicine (CAM) — A large, diverse set of systems of diagnosis, treatment, and prevention based on philosophies and techniques outside those of conventional Western medicine.

complex fraction — The numerator, the denominator, or both as a whole number, proper fraction, or mixed number. The value may be less than, greater than, or equal to 1.

compounding slab — A plate made of ground glass with a hard, flat, and nonabsorbent surface for mixing compounds.

compound word — A word formed with two or more root words.

compromised host — A person whose normal defense mechanisms are impaired and is therefore more susceptible to a disease.

computerized physician order entry system (CPOE) — A computerized system in which the physician inputs the medication order directly for electronic receipt in the pharmacy.

computer — A piece of programmable equipment that stores, retrieves, and processes data.

cones — Specialized receptor cells in the retina that perceive colors and bright light.

confidentiality — The nondisclosure of a customer's privileged information unless the customer has given his or her consent.

conical graduates — Devices used for measuring liquids that have wide tops and wide bases and taper from the top to the bottom.

conjugation — A joining; in unicellular organisms, a form of reproduction in which there is a temporary union in order to transfer genetic material; in biochemistry, the joining of a toxic substance with a natural body substance to form a detoxified product for elimination from the body.

conjunctiva — Mucous membranes of the eyes.

conjunctivitis — An inflammation of the outermost layer of the eye and inner surface of the eyelid, usually due to an allergic reaction or an infection; commonly called "pink eye."

consumer — The person coming to you for the filling of prescriptions or the purchase of over-the-counter remedies for a wide variety of situations.

contact transmission — The physical transfer of an agent from an infected person to an uninfected person.

continuing education — Additional topics of study that must be earned in order to maintain certifications, including certified pharmacy technician status.

contract — A legally enforceable agreement.

contraindication — A factor or condition that increases the chance of a serious adverse reaction.

controlled substance medication order — An order for medication (generally narcotics) that requires monitored documentation of procurement, dispensing, and administration.

contusions — Injuries of body parts without a break in the skin.

conversion factor — Used to determine equivalents of specific units of measure.

coordination of benefits — A process in which two or more insurance companies apportion each one's share of responsibility of payment of a claim for health care services provided to an insured client.

copayment — A cost-sharing requirement of most insurance policies, under which it is the responsibility of the insured to make a payment of a specified amount (e.g., $20) at the time of treatment or purchase of a prescription. Some policies have both a copayment and coinsurance clause.

copper — A metallic element that is a component of several important enzymes in the body and is essential to good health.

corium — The layer of skin just under the epidermis; also known as the dermis.

cornea — The transparent front part of the eye covering the iris, pupil, and anterior chamber; it helps the eye to focus and is known as the "window" of the eye.

coronary artery bypass graft — An autograft consisting of a segment of the coronary artery grafted into place to replace a damaged or nonfunctioning area.

corpus albicans — A pale white spot on the surface of the ovary that arises from the corpus luteum if conception does not occur.

corpus callosum — A structure in the longitudinal fissure of the brain that connects the left and right cerebral hemispheres.

corpus luteum — A spheroid of yellowish tissue that grows within the ruptured ovarian follicle after ovulation and secretes progesterone.

corticosteroids — A group of hormones produced by the adrenal cortex that influence or control key processes of the body.

cost-benefit analysis — The systematic process of evaluating costs and benefits to identify those programs in which benefits supersede costs.

cost analysis — An evaluation of all information relating to the disbursements of an activity, department, program, or agency.

cost control — The implementation of managerial efforts to achieve cost objectives.

counter balance — A device capable of weighing large quantities of bulk products, up to about 5 kg. It is a double-pan balance.

cramps — Sudden, involuntary spasmodic muscular contractions causing severe pain, often occurring in the leg or shoulder as the result of strains or chills.

cream — A semisolid emulsion of either the oil-in-water or the water-in-oil type, ordinarily intended for topical use.

cretinism — A congenital condition characterized by severe hypothyroidism that is often associated with other endocrine abnormalities.

crime — A violation of the law.

criminal law — Rules and regulations that govern the relationship of the individual to society as a whole.

criminal — An individual who violates the law.

cryosurgery — Tissue destruction by freezing.

cryptorchidism — A developmental defect in which one or both testicles fail to descend into the scrotum and are retained in the abdomen or inguinal canal.

cyanocobalamin — A water-soluble substance that is the common pharmaceutical form of vitamin B_{12}. It is involved in the metabolism of protein, fats, and carbohydrates. Vitamin B_{12} is also involved in normal blood formation and neural function.

cyanosis — A bluish discoloration of the skin and mucous membranes, caused by an excess of deoxygenated hemoglobin in the blood.

cylindrical graduates — Devices used for measuring liquids that have narrow diameters that are the same from top to base.

cytochrome P-450 — A system of enzymes that plays a role in drug metabolism and contributes to drug interactions.

D

data — The raw facts the computer can manipulate.

days supply exceeded — A rejection of a medication refill due to an amount that has exceeded the preapproved supply for a specific period of days.

decimal fraction — A numerator that is expressed in numerals, with a decimal point placed so that it designates the value of the denominator, and a denominator, which is understood to be 10 or some power of 10; also called decimal.

decimal — A numerator that is expressed in numerals with a decimal point placed so that it designates the value of the denominator, and the denominator, which is understood to be 10 or some power of 10; also called decimal fraction.

decode — Translation of a message by the receiver into what is perceived to be said.

deductible — A specific amount of money that must be paid yearly before the policy benefits begin (e.g., $50, $100, $300, or $500). The higher the deductible, the lower the cost of the policy; and the lower the deductible, the higher the cost of the policy.

defense mechanisms — Tools an individual uses when required to deal with uncomfortable or threatening situations.

deglutition — The process of swallowing.

demand/stat medication order — An order for medication to be given in rapid response to a specific medical condition.

denial — A psychological defense mechanism in which confrontation with a personal problem or with reality is avoided by denying the existence of the problem or reality.

denominator — The number into which the whole is divided in an expression of division.

dentes — Teeth.

Department of Public Health (DPH) — An organization that oversees hospitals, including the pharmacy department.

dependents — The spouse and children of the insured who are also covered under the terms of the policy.

dermis — The inner skin layer, which is thicker than the epidermis; also known as the corium.

desk audits — An evaluation of a pharmacy or related facility that does not involve an auditor being sent out to the location; it is less intensive than a field audit.

detrusor muscle — The muscular layer of the urinary bladder that aids in urination.

diabetes mellitus — A complex disorder of carbohydrate, fat, and protein metabolism that is primarily a result of a deficiency or complete lack of insulin secretion by the beta cells of the pancreas, or *resis*tance to insulin.

diarthroses — Bone articulations permitting free motion in joints, such as those of the shoulders or hips.

diastole — The period between contractions of the atria or the ventricles, during which blood enters.

dietary supplements — Products containing one or more vitamins, herbs, enzymes, amino acids, or other ingredients, taken orally to supplement the diet, as by providing missing nutrients.

diffusion — The process by which particles in a fluid move from an area of higher concentration to an area of lower concentration, resulting in an even distribution of the particles in the fluid.

diphtheria — An acute, toxin-mediated disease caused by *Corynebacterium diphtheriae*.

diplococci — Spherical bacteria that occur in pairs.

disinfectant — Substances that destroy most microorganisms, but not highly resistant types such as certain spores and viruses.

disinfection — A process of cleaning that destroys most microorganisms, but not highly resistant types such as certain spores and viruses.

dispersal records — Lists of all drugs dispensed from a pharmacy or removed for any reason.

displacement — The transfer of impulses from one expression to another, such as from fighting to talking.

distribution — The process by which drug molecules leave the bloodstream and enter the tissues of the body.

diverticulosis — An intestinal condition characterized by the presence of pockets (diverticula) in the colon, which may result in bleeding or constipation.

diverticulum — A hollow or fluid-filled sac, many of which exist in the walls of the colon.

divisor — A number performing division.

dosage form — The makeup of a particular type of drug; the form in which it is given.

dosage strength — The amount of medication per unit of measure.

dram — A unit of weight in the apothecary system; 1 dram equals 60 grains.

drive-through — An external site at a pharmacy that can be accessed by driving up in the car.

drop rate — The number of drops at which an intravenous infusion is administered over a specific period of time.

drug control — A method used to eliminate or reduce the potential harm of the drug distributed.

drug distribution system — A safe and economical way of distributing a drug.

Drug Enforcement Administration (DEA) — A federal law enforcement agency that combats illegal drug use and smuggling both within the United States and abroad.

drug interaction — An interference of a drug with the effect of another drug, nutrient, or laboratory test.

drug label factor — The form of the drug dose with its equivalent in units.

drug order factor — The desired dose, dose on hand, and vehicle set up in an equation that helps to cancel the units to give the right answer in the right units for delivery.

dry heat sterilization — A method of sterilization that uses heated dry air at a temperature of 160°C to 180°C (320°F to 365°F) for 90 minutes to 3 hours.

dry powder inhaler (DPI) — A device used to deliver medication in the form of micronized powder into the lungs.

duodenum — The first and shortest part of the small intestine.

dwarfism — The abnormal underdevelopment of the body that occurs during childhood, commonly because of hyposecretion of growth hormone; it may be caused by many other conditions, including kidney disease and metabolic disorders.

dysmenorrhea — Pain during menstruation, often accompanied by cramps.

E

eardrum — The tympanic membrane; a structure that transmits sound from the air to the ossicles inside the middle ear—it separates the external ear from the middle ear.

edema — Swelling of any tissue when the interstitial fluid surrounds the cells.

ejection fraction — The fraction of blood contained in the ventricle at the end of diastole, which is expelled during its contraction; the stroke volume divided by end-diastolic volume, normally at 0.55.

electrodessication — Tissue destruction by heat.

electrolytes — Compounds that dissociate into ions when dissolved in water.

electronic balance — An instrument used to electronically weigh small amounts of drugs; the measurement is indicated on a digital screen.

electronic data interchange (EDI) — The structured transmission of data using electronic devices.

eligibility — The determination of the exact coverage to which the insured is entitled. The pharmacy technician may be responsible for checking on a customer's or patient's eligibility of coverage. This can be done over the telephone, via a voice-automated system, using computer software, over the Internet, or by checking an eligibility list for a managed care plan.

elixir — A clear, sweetened, hydroalcoholic liquid intended for oral use.

emergency medication order — An order for medication to be given in response to a medical emergency.

emphysema — A chronic pulmonary disease characterized by loss of elasticity of the lung tissue often caused by exposure to toxic chemicals and cigarette smoke.

emulsion — A system containing two liquids that cannot be mixed together in which one is dispersed, in the form of very small globules, throughout the other.

enamel — The substance that protects teeth from wear and acids, found on the crown of each tooth.

encephalitis — Inflammation of brain tissue that is often caused by a virus; it causes fever, convulsions, coma, and may be fatal.

endometriosis — A condition in which parts of tissues similar to the endometrium (lining of the uterus) grow in other areas of the body, resulting in inflammation, irritation, scar tissue, and adhesions.

endometrium — The mucous membrane lining the uterus; it is made up of the stratum basale, stratum compactum, and stratum spongiosum.

enteral nutrition — Feedings given through a tube passed directly into the stomach or intestine. Although normal eating qualifies as enteral nutrition, the term is usually applied to specially prepared liquid feedings.

enteric-coated tablet — A tablet covered in a special coating to protect it from stomach acid, allowing the drug to dissolve in the intestines.

e-prescribing — Electronic prescribing, in which drug prescriptions are transmitted from a prescriber's computer or smart device to a pharmacy computer system.

epidermis — The outer layer of the skin.

epididymis — A system of ductules that holds sperm during maturation and eventually forms a single coiled duct that is continuous with the vas deferens.

epiglottis — A flap of tissue that helps to prevent food from entering the trachea during swallowing.

ergonomic — The science of designing equipment to maximize productivity by lessening the discomfort and fatigue of employees.

erythema migrans — A rash often seen in the early stages of Lyme disease. The rash represents an actual skin infection with Lyme bacteria.

erythropoiesis — The process of erythrocyte production in the bone marrow, involving the maturation of a nucleated precursor (reticulocyte) into a hemoglobin-filled red blood cell. This process is regulated by the hormone erythropoietin.

erythropoietin — A glycoprotein hormone secreted by the kidneys that acts on stem cells of the bone marrow to stimulate red blood cell production.

esophageal hiatus — The aperture of the diaphragm through which the esophagus passes.

ethics — A set of standards of behavior; in a profession, a guide to correct actions that should be followed.

excretion — The process of eliminating drugs from the body.

exhalation — The act of exhaling, which is breathing out; also called expiration.

exposure control plan — A written procedure for the treatment of persons exposed to biohazardous or similar chemically harmful materials.

expressive aphasia — Inability of an individual to form language and express his or her thoughts accurately even though thought processes are intact.

extemporaneous compounding — The preparation, mixing, assembling, packaging, and labeling of a drug product based on a prescription order from a licensed practitioner for the individual patient.

external acoustic meatus — An S-shaped tube in each ear that leads inward through the temporal bone.

external noise — Physical noise such as typing or traffic that interferes with hearing a message.

externships — Also called *acting internships,* in which individuals work in actual pharmacies in order to gain practical, hands-on experience.

extremes — The two outside terms in a proportion.

F

falciform ligament — The ligament separating the two lobes of the liver.

fallopian tubes — Two very small tubes that lead from the ovaries into the uterus; the mature ovum travels down these tubes from the ovaries to the uterus.

fats — Substances composed of lipids or fatty acids and occurring in various forms.

fatty acids — Any of several organic acids produced by the hydrolysis of neutral fats.

felony — A serious crime, such as murder, kidnapping, assault, or rape, that is punishable by imprisonment for more than one year.

fermentation — A process of converting organic compounds, such as carbohydrates, to simpler compounds, such as ethyl alcohol, by using enzymes that do not require oxygen; fermentation usually results in the production of energy.

fibromyalgia — A syndrome characterized by chronic pain in the muscles and soft tissues surrounding joints, fatigue, and tenderness in various body sites.

field audits — An intensive, systematic investigation of a pharmacy or other facility's operational practices, procedures, records, inventory, and accounting.

file — A set of data or a program that has been given a name.

filiform papillae — The rough papillae at the front of the tongue that are important in licking.

filtration — The process of passing a substance through a filter to remove specific particles.

fire safety and emergency plan — A written procedure that includes fire extinguisher locations, fire alarm pull-box locations, sprinkler system location, exit signs, and clear directions to the quickest and safest exit of a building during an emergency.

first-pass effect — The process in which a drug reaches the liver and is partly metabolized before becoming available to the body for systemic effects.

fistula — An abnormal passageway between two organs or from an organ to the body surface.

floor stock system — A system of drug distribution in which drugs are issued in bulk form and stored in medication rooms on patient care units.

fluidextract — A pharmacopeial liquid preparation of vegetable drugs, made by filtration, containing alcohol as a solvent or as a preservative, or both.

fluoride — A substance that prevents tooth decay and protects against osteoporosis and gum disease.

folacin — A water-soluble vitamin essential for cell growth and the reproduction of red blood cells.

folic acid — A water-soluble vitamin essential for cell growth and the reproduction of red blood cells.

fomite — Object contaminated with an infectious agent such as instruments or dressings.

food additive — Any substance that becomes part of a food product.

Food and Drug Administration (FDA) — The agency within the U.S. Department of Health and Human Services that is responsible for assurance of the safety, efficacy, and security of drugs used for humans and pets, biological products, medical devices, cosmetics, radioactive products, and the national food supply.

formed elements — The red blood cells, white blood cells, and platelets.

formulary — A document that specifies particular drug forms and compositions.

form — The structure and composition of a drug.

fornix — The part of the vagina that surrounds the uterine cervix.

fovea centralis — A small depression in the center of the macula that has the greatest visual acuity and lies directly opposite to the pupil.

fraction — An expression of division with a number that is the portion or part of a whole.

franchise pharmacy — A pharmacy in which the owner purchases the right to use a specific pharmacy company's business model and brand for a prescribed time period.

fungi — Microorganisms that grow in single cells or in colonies.

fungicidal — Having a killing action on fungi.

fungiform papillae — The mushroom-shaped papillae in the middle of the tongue; they contain taste buds.

G

gallbladder — A pear-shaped sac-like organ located in a depression of the surface of the liver; it functions in the storage of bile.

gas sterilization — The use of a gas such as ethylene oxide to sterilize medical equipment.

gavage — Feeding with a stomach tube.

gel — A jelly or the solid or semisolid phase of a colloidal solution.

gelcap — An oil-based medication that is enclosed in a soft gelatin capsule.

generic name — The approved, nonproprietary name of a drug; generic drugs by law must have the same active ingredients as their trademarked equivalents.

genetic engineering — The scientific alteration of the structure of genetic material in a living organism that involves the production and use of recombinant DNA.

genitourinary — Referring to the reproductive organs and the urinary system.

geometric dilution — A process by which a uniform distribution of substances in a mixture is achieved. When mixing agents, the medicament is first mixed with an equal weight of diluent. A further quantity of diluent equal in weight to the mixture is then incorporated. This process is repeated until all the diluent has been mixed in.

gigantism — Abnormally large growth of body tissue due to an excess of growth hormone during childhood.

gingivae — The pink ridge that surrounds the bases of the teeth.

glomerulus — A knot of capillaries surrounded by the Bowman's glomerular capsule that receives blood from the renal circulation; each glomerulus and its surrounding capsule make up a renal corpuscle.

glottis — The opening to the larynx.

glucagon — An important hormone involved in carbohydrate metabolism; it is antagonistic to insulin.

goblet cells — Unicellular glands that secrete mucus.

gout — A disturbance of uric acid metabolism occurring mostly in males, characterized by painful inflammation of the joints, especially of the feet and hands.

grain — The basic unit of weight in the apothecary system.

Gram stain — A sequential procedure involving crystal violet and iodine solutions followed by alcohol that allows rapid identification of organisms as gram-positive or gram-negative types.

gram-negative — Microorganisms that stain red or pink with Gram stain.

gram-positive — Microorganisms that stain blue or purple with Gram stain.

gram — The basic unit for weight in the metric system.

granule — A very small pill, usually gelatin- or sugar-coated, containing a drug to be given in a small dose.

granulocytes — A type of white blood cell that includes neutrophils, eosinophils, and basophils; these cells have granules in their cytoplasm.

Graves' disease — A condition of primary hyperthyroidism; it is characterized by a diffuse goiter and exophthalmos (a bulging of the eyes anteriorly out of the eye orbits).

group purchasing — A process by which groups of buyers work together to negotiate with pharmaceutical manufacturers to get better prices and benefits based upon the ability to promise high committed volumes.

growth hormone — A hormone secreted by the anterior pituitary gland in response to growth hormone-releasing hormone. Its secretion is controlled in part by the hypothalamus.

gummas — Soft granulomas with necrotic centers and inflamed, fibrous capsules that are characteristic of tertiary syphilis.

H

Haemophilus influenzae — A gram-negative bacterium that commonly causes otitis media or bacterial meningitis in children.

half-life — The time it takes for the plasma concentration of a drug to be reduced by 50%.

hardware — The parts of the computer that you can touch.

haustra — Pouches found in the colon.

hazard communication plan — Application of warning labels for all hazardous chemicals.

headache — Pain in any region of the head, ranging from a dull ache to sharp, throbbing pain. Also called cephalgia.

health insurance — A type of contract purchased by individuals or employers that provides reimbursement for specified medical and related expenses.

hematoma — A localized mass of blood outside the blood vessels that appears to be discolored.

hematuria — The presence of blood in the urine.

hemochromatosis — Disorder caused by deposition of hemosiderin in the tissues of the body; it can cause cirrhosis of the liver, destruction of the pancreas, and heart failure.

hepatitis — Inflammation of the liver caused by microorganisms, especially viruses, or drugs such as alcohol and other poisons.

hepatopancreatic ampulla — The sac-like swelling between the liver and pancreas.

herbal supplement — A dietary supplement that contains medicinal herbs.

high-density lipoproteins (HDLs) — Lipoproteins that carry cholesterol from cells to the liver for eventual excretion.

high-efficiency particulate air (HEPA) filters — Special filters designed to trap very small particles that other filters cannot trap; they can remove nearly 100% of particles that are 0.3 micrometers or larger in diameter.

hilum — A depression at the part of an organ where vessels and nerves enter and leave.

home health care pharmacy — The practice of pharmacy that provides medications, home health care products and services, and pharmaceutical care to patients at home.

homeostasis — The body's ability to maintain stability and constancy.

hormones — Natural chemical substances secreted into the bloodstream from the endocrine glands; they regulate and control organ and tissue activity.

hospice — Originally a facility, usually within a hospital, intended to care for the terminally ill, in particular, by providing physical comfort to the patient and emotional support and counseling to the patient and the family; currently hospice care is also provided in home settings.

hospital pharmacy — The provision of pharmaceutical services within an institutional or hospital setting.

household system — System of measurement used in most homes; this is not an accurate system of measurement for medications.

hydrophobia — A fear of water; a symptom linked to difficulty in swallowing, which is caused by rabies as the disease progresses.

hyperalimentation — The administration of a nutritionally adequate hypertonic solution consisting of glucose, protein, minerals, and vitamins through an indwelling catheter into the superior vena cava.

hyperglycemia — Abnormally increased content of glucose in the blood.

hyperlipidemia — The presence of raised or abnormal levels of lipids (fatty molecules) or lipoproteins (biochemicals containing proteins and lipids) in the blood.

hyperpyrexia — Extremely high temperature, which is considered a medical emergency.

hypersensitivity reaction — A type of unpredictable reaction caused in some patients by drugs such as aspirin, penicillin, or sulfa products. This generally occurs when a patient has received a drug and his or her body has developed antibodies against it.

hypertension — High blood pressure; a chronic elevation of the blood pressure equivalent to or greater than 140/90 millimeters of mercury (mm Hg).

hypertrophy — Enlargement of an organ or body part resulting from an increase in the size of its cells.

hypervitaminosis — An abnormal condition resulting from excessive intake of toxic amounts of one or more vitamins, especially over a long period.

hypnosis — A trance-like state resembling sleep that is induced by the suggestions of one person upon another who accepts them as effective.

hypnotic — A drug that induces sleep; often used to treat insomnia and in surgical anesthesia.

hypovitaminosis — A condition related to the deficiency of one or more vitamins.

I

idiosyncratic reaction — A unique, strange, or unpredicted reaction to a drug.

ileocecal sphincter — The muscle between the ileum and cecum.

ileum — The third part of the small intestine, measuring 12 feet or 3.7 meters in length.

immunity — Protection from a disease resulting from exposure to the agent causing that disease or a closely related illness.

immunogenicity — The ability of a substance, such as an antigen, to provoke an immune response.

immunogen — An antigen.

immunoglobulins — Blood products that contain disease-specific antibodies for passive immunity.

immunology — The study of immune responses.

improper fraction — A fraction in which the numerator is greater than or equal to the denominator.

inactivated vaccines — Vaccines in which the infectious components have been destroyed by chemical or physical treatments.

independent purchasing — A process in which the director of pharmacy or buyer directly contacts and negotiates pricing with pharmaceutical manufacturers.

induration — An excessive hardening or firmness of any body site. It is one of the signs of inflammation.

influenza A — A virus causing moderate to severe illness, affecting all age groups.

influenza B — A virus causing a mild illness; usually affects only children.

influenza C — A virus causing infection of the upper respiratory tract.

infundibulum — The abdominal opening of a fallopian tube.

inhalation — The act of inhaling, which is breathing in; also called inspiration.

innate immunity — The type of immunity that involves the innate immune system, which includes anatomical barriers, inflammation, the complement system, white blood cells, coagulation, neural regulation, and pathogen specificity.

inpatient — Refers to inside a hospital or other health care institution. In relation to pharmacy, this means that the pharmacy is located in a hospital or institution in which patients stay overnight or for longer periods of time.

input devices — Any piece of equipment that allows data to be entered into the computer system.

inscription — Medication prescribed.

insulin — A hormone that extensively affects metabolism and many other body systems; it is secreted when the blood glucose level rises.

internal noise — An individual's beliefs or prejudices that interfere with decoding a message.

international units — A standardized amount of medication required to produce a certain effect.

Internet pharmacy — An established commercial website that enables a patient to obtain medications by way of the Internet.

internships — Periods of work experience, usually at the beginning of a person's career, located within organizations for a limited time period, to gain skills and experience.

interstitial fluid — An extracellular fluid that fills the spaces between most of the cells of the body and provides a substantial portion of its liquid environment.

intradermal injection — Between the layers of the skin. A dose of an agent administered between the layers of the skin.

intramuscular injection — Inside a muscle. Normally used in the context of an injection given into a muscle.

intravenous injection — Into a vein. Most commonly used in the context of an injection given directly into a vein.

intrinsic factor — A glycoprotein produced by the parietal cells of the stomach; it is required for the body's absorption of Vitamin B_{12}.

inventory control — A method of controlling the amount of product on hand to maximize the return on investment.

inventory turnover rate — A mathematical calculation of the number of times the average inventory is replaced over a period of time (usually annually).

inventory — The stock of medications a pharmacy keeps immediately on hand.

investigational medication order — An order for medication given under direction of research protocols that also require strict documentation of procurement, dispensing, and administration.

invoice — A form that describes a purchase and the amount that is due.

iodine — An essential micronutrient of the thyroid hormone thyroxine.

iron — A common metallic element essential for the synthesis of hemoglobin.

islets of Langerhans — Clusters of cells within the pancreas that produce insulin, glucagon, and pancreatic polypeptide.

J

jaundice — Yellowing of the skin and white portion of the eyes. It is caused by the presence of bilirubin and bile pigments in the skin, and it is usually a sign of liver disease.

jejunum — The second part of the small intestine, measuring 8 feet or 2.4 meters in length.

K

keratinocytes — Skin cells that produce hormone-like substances, stimulating development of T lymphocytes and defending against infection.

killer cells — Large, granular lymphocytes that appear to have the ability to destroy tumor cells.

kwashiorkor — A disease caused by extreme lack of protein.

L

labia majora — The outer folds of the vulva that surround the vestibule.

labia minora — The inner, highly vascularized connective tissue folds of the vulva that surround the vestibule.

labyrinth — A system of fluid passages in the inner ear, including the semicircular canals and the cochlea.

lacerations — Cuts or breaks in the skin.

lacteals — The tiny vessels in the villi of the walls of the small intestine through which chylomicrons are absorbed and released into the lymphatic system.

laminar airflow hood — A system of circulating filtered air in parallel-flowing planes in hospitals or other health care facilities. The system reduces the risk of airborne contamination and exposure to chemical pollutants in surgical theaters, food preparation areas, hospital pharmacies, and laboratories.

laminar flow — Air that has been passed through a high-efficiency particulate air (HEPA) filter so that it is as pure as possible for use in sterile compounding and other procedures.

larynx — Commonly known as the voice box, it is hard, rigid, and composed of cartilage.

law — A rule or regulation established by a governing body.

leading zeros — Zeros that precede decimal points; 0.2 is an example that has a leading zero.

legend drug — A medication that may be dispensed only with a prescription; also known as a prescription drug.

legibility — The degree to which something is able to be read based on its appearance.

levigate — To grind into a smooth substance with moisture.

licensed — Being granted permission by a government agency to engage in an occupation. Most states do not require pharmacy technicians to be licensed.

ligaments — Sheets or bands of tough, fibrous tissue connecting bones or cartilages at a joint or supporting an organ.

liniment — A liquid preparation for external use, usually applied by friction to the skin.

lipids — Fats.

lipoproteins — Conjugated proteins in which lipids form an integral part of the molecules; they are synthesized primarily in the liver and contain varying amounts of cholesterol, fat-soluble vitamins, phospholipids, and triglycerides.

liter — The basic unit for volume in the metric system.

lithotripsy — The use of high-energy shock waves to fragment and disintegrate renal calculi (kidney stones).

live attenuated vaccines — Vaccines containing living organisms or intact viruses that have undergone radiation or temperature conditioning to produce safe vaccinations that will help the patient become immune to a specific disease.

lobules — The basic functional units of the liver, surrounded by liver cells (hepatocytes).

long-term care pharmacy organization — An organization involving a licensed professional pharmacy or practice that provides medications and clinical services to long-term care facilities and their residents.

long-term care — A range of health and health-related support services provided over an extended period of time.

lotion — A semisolid preparation applied externally to protect the skin or to treat a dermatologic disorder.

low-density lipoproteins (LDLs) — Lipoproteins that carry blood cholesterol from all cells.

lozenge — A small, disk-shaped tablet composed of solidifying paste containing an astringent, an antiseptic, or an oil-based drug used for local treatment of the mouth or throat. It is held in the mouth until dissolved. Also known as a troche.

lumen — The tubular space or channel within any organ or structure of the body.

lunula — A pale, half-moon-shaped area at the base of a nail.

lymph nodes — Oval or bean-shaped structures organized into clusters and located primarily in the axillae (armpits), neck, mouth, lower arm, and groin. Their main function is to filter bacteria and other cells out of the lymph.

lymph — A thin, watery fluid originating in organs and tissues of the body that circulates through the lymphatic vessels, and it is filtered by the lymph nodes.

lymphatic capillaries — The networks of small lymphatic vessels that collect lymph from the intercellular fluid and constitute the beginning of the lymphatic system.

lymphatic sinuses — The channels in a lymph node crossed by a reticulum of cells and fibers and bounded by flattened, rod-like cells known as littoral cells. There are subcapsular, trabecular, and medullary sinuses.

M

macula lutea — A small yellowish area containing the fovea centralis, located near the center of the retina, at which visual perception is most acute.

macular degeneration — A condition primarily affecting older adults, wherein the macula area of the retina of the eye becomes thinner and atrophies, sometimes resulting in bleeding; it often results in loss of vision.

magnesium — A silver-white mineral element. It is the second most abundant cation of the intracellular fluids in the body and is essential for many enzyme activities.

mail-order pharmacy — A licensed pharmacy that uses the mail or other carriers (e.g., overnight carriers or parcel services) to deliver prescriptions to patients.

malignant melanoma — Aggressive tumor of bottom-layer skin cells (melanocytes), which may also affect the eyes or bowels.

malnutrition — Ingestion of nutrients inadequate to maintain health and well-being.

malpractice — Professional misconduct, or the demonstration of an unreasonable lack of skill, resulting in injury, loss, or damage to a patient.

Mantoux test — An intradermal screening for tuberculin hypersensitivity. A red, firm patch of skin at the injection site greater than 10 mm in diameter after 48 hours is a positive result that indicates current or prior exposure to tubercle bacilli.

marasmus — Severe wasting caused by lack of protein and all nutrients or faulty absorption.

master formula sheet — A list of all ingredients, lot numbers, compounding instructions, and expiration dates of a compounded substance.

means — The two inside terms in a proportion.

measles — An acute, highly contagious viral infectious disease that causes respiratory symptoms and widespread rash; it may also cause an ear infection or pneumonia and can be fatal.

mediastinum — The central compartment of the thoracic cavity within the chest.

Medicaid — A government-funded health cost assistance program that pays for health services and pharmacy expenses for enrolled U.S. citizens who cannot afford to pay for their own health care. It also covers those who are blind, disabled, orphaned, or underage parents.

medical asepsis — Complete destruction of organisms after they leave the body.

medical ethics — The discipline in which merits, risks, and social concerns are evaluated concerning the practice of medicine.

medicare advantage plan — A type of health plan providing coverage within Part C of Medicare; it pays for managed health care based on a monthly fee rather than on the basis of billing a fee for each service provided.

Medicare — A government-funded program that pays for health coverage for people over age 65, and certain other persons.

medication order — The written order for particular medications and services to be provided to a patient within an institutional setting; medication orders are written by physicians, nurse practitioners, or physician's assistants.

medication reconciliation — The process of comparing a patient's medication orders to all of the medications that the patient has been taking.

melanin — A dark pigment that provides skin and hair color and absorbs ultraviolet radiation in sunlight.

melanocytes — Cells that give the skin pigmentation.

melatonin — A substance formed by the pineal gland that is involved in the circadian rhythms.

memory — The ability of the computer to store and retrieve data.

menadione — A fat-soluble, injectable form of synthetic vitamin K3.

meningitis — Inflammation of the meninges of the brain or spinal cord due to viral or bacterial infection.

meniscus — The curved upper surface of a column of liquid in a container.

menorrhagia — Abnormally heavy or prolonged menstruation; repeated episodes of menorrhagia may be due to hormonal problems, uterine diseases, or cancer. Menorrhagia may lead to iron deficiency anemia.

menses — The monthly flow of blood and cellular debris from the uterus; it begins at puberty and stops at menopause.

mesentery — Extensions of the visceral peritoneum.

mesocolon — An extension of the visceral peritoneum of the colon.

metabolism — The process whereby drugs are acted upon by enzymes in the body and are converted to metabolic derivatives.

metered dose inhaler (MDI) — A handheld pressurized device used to deliver medications for inhalation.

meter — The basic unit for length in the metric system.

metric system — Worldwide standard system of measurement.

microorganism — Organism that is too small to be seen by the unaided eye.

microvilli — Small projections found on the free edges of villi of intestinal epithelial cells that increase the absorptive surface of the cells.

milliequivalent — A unit of measure based upon the chemical combining power of a substance.

milliunit — One thousandth of a unit.

minerals — Inorganic substances occurring naturally in the earth's crust, having a characteristic chemical composition.

minim — The basic unit of volume in the apothecary system.

minuend — A number from which another is subtracted.

misbranding — Fraudulent labeling or marking.

misdemeanor — A crime less serious than a felony, punishable by a fine or imprisonment for less than one year.

mitral valve — A bicuspid valve situated between the left atrium and left ventricle.

mixed fraction — A whole number and a proper fraction that are combined. The value of the mixed number is always greater than 1.

mixture — A mutual incorporation of two or more substances, without chemical union, in which the physical characteristics of each of the components are retained.

modem — A device used to transfer information from one computer to another.

mode of transmission — The process that bridges the gap between the portal of exit of the infectious agent and the portal of entry of the susceptible host.

modified unit-dose system — A drug distribution system that combines unit-dose medications that are "blister" packaged onto a multiple-dose card; also known as a blister card, punch card, or bingo card.

modular cassette — These cassettes contain either one-week or two-week medication strips that also contain reserve doses in a narrow plastic slide-tray design.

mons pubis — A rounded, raised area of fatty tissue above the pubic symphysis of females.

mortar — A cup-shaped vessel in which materials are ground or crushed.

multiple medication package — A medication package in which all medications to be given at a specific time of a given day are packaged together; also known as an adherence package or pouch package.

multiple sclerosis — A disease caused by progressive demyelination of nerve cells in the brain and spinal cord.

multiplicand — A number to be multiplied by another.

multiplier — A number by which another is multiplied.

mumps — An acute viral illness that begins with fever, headache, muscle aches, tiredness, and loss of appetite; it is followed by swelling of the salivary glands, and sometimes it causes orchitis, which (rarely) leads to infertility.

muscular dystrophy — A genetic disease characterized by progressive deterioration and wasting of muscle fibers.

mutagens — Chemical agents that increase rates of genetic mutation by interfering with function of nucleic acids.

myasthenia gravis — A disease characterized by progressive fatigue and generalized weakness of the skeletal muscles.

myelin — A layer of phospholipids that surrounds the axons of many neurons; it acts as an insulator to electrical impulses.

myocardial infarction (MI) — A heart attack; it results in reduction of blood flow through one of the coronary arteries, causing ischemia and necrosis.

myocarditis — Inflammation of the heart.

myometrium — The muscular layer of the wall of the uterus.

myxedema — The most severe form of hypothyroidism.

N

National Council for Prescription Drug Programs (NCPDP) — A nonprofit organization representing every sector of the pharmacy industry; it develops standards and provides education about pharmacy-related topics.

National Drug Code (NDC) — A unique and permanent product code assigned to each new drug as it becomes available in the marketplace; it identifies the manufacturer or distributor, the drug formulation, and the size and type of its packaging.

National Formulary (NF) — A database of officially recognized drug names.

natural active acquired immunity — Resistance to the causative pathogen for an infection because of the presence of antibodies and stimulated lymphocytes in individuals who have had that infection.

negligence — A type of unintentional tort alleged when a person has performed, or failed to perform, an act that a reasonable person would, or would not, have performed in similar circumstances.

neuroblastoma — A highly malignant tumor consisting of primitive ectodermal cells from the neural plate during embryonic life; it may originate in any part of the sympathetic nervous system but is most common in the adrenal medulla.

neurohormone — A type of hormone secreted by neuroendocrine cells that aids in stimulation of body functions.

neurohypophysis — Posterior lobe of the pituitary gland.

neuromuscular blocking agents — Drugs that block neuromuscular transmission at the neuromuscular junction; they cause paralysis of specific skeletal muscles.

neuron — Basic cell of the nervous system; carries nerve impulses.

neutral fats — Fats consisting of about 95% triglycerides or triacylglycerols.

niacin — A part of two enzymes that regulate energy metabolism.

nondiscretionary — Not subject or left to an individual's own discretion. For pharmacy technicians, nondiscretionary duties include typing, computer usage, reports and other documentation, and ordering of supplies.

nuclear pharmacy — A pharmacy that is specially licensed to work with radioactive materials, previously called radiopharmacy.

numerator — The portion of the whole being considered in an expression of division.

nutrient — A chemical substance found in food that is necessary for good health.

nutrition — The sum of the processes involved in the taking in of nutrients and their assimilation and use for proper body functioning and maintenance of health.

O

ointment — A semisolid preparation that usually contains medicinal substances and is intended for external application.

oligomenorrhea — Abnormally light menstrual periods.

onychomycosis — Any fungal infection of the nails.

opiates — Narcotic alkaloids found in opium.

opioids — Chemical substances that have morphine-like action in the body; commonly used for pain relief.

optic disc — A small oval-shaped area on the retina marking the site of entrance into the eyeball of the optic nerve.

oral — Pertaining to the mouth. Medication given by mouth.

orchitis — A painful condition of the testicles that may involve inflammation, swelling, and infection.

organ of Corti — The spiral-shaped organ of the inner ear that contains auditory "hair cells" that provide the sense of hearing.

orphan drug — A drug that is developed for small populations of people in need of the drug.

osteoblasts — The bone-forming cells that are derived from the embryonic mesenchyme and, during the early development of the skeleton, produce the bone matrix.

osteoclasts — Large multinucleated bone cells that absorb and remove osseous tissue.

osteocytes — Mature osteoblasts that have become embedded in the bone matrix.

osteogenic cells — The cells in the inner layer of the periosteum that develop into osteoblasts.

osteomalacia — Softening of bone tissue due to loss of calcium; sometimes called adult rickets.

osteomyelitis — Inflammation, almost always due to bacterial infection, of a bone and the marrow within it.

osteoporosis — A bone disease characterized by reduced bone mineral density, leading to an increased risk of fracture.

ototoxicity — The property of being toxic to the ears.

ounce — A unit of weight in the apothecary system; 1 ounce equals 8 drams.

outpatient — In relation to pharmacy, this means community pharmacy settings.

output devices — Any piece of equipment that allows data to exit the computer system.

oval window — A membrane-covered opening leading from the middle ear to the vestibule of the inner ear.

over-the-counter (OTC) — A medication that may be purchased without a prescription directly from the pharmacy; also known as a nonprescription drug.

overpayment — Payment by the insurer or by the patient of more than the amount due.

ovulation — The release of a mature ovum or oocyte from an ovary.

P

pacemaker — The sinoatrial node, composed of specialized nervous tissue and located at the junction of the superior vena cava and right atrium.

pain scales — Charts used to measure a patient's pain intensity level.

pantothenic acid — A member of the vitamin B complex (B5). It is widely distributed in plant and animal tissues and may be an important element in human nutrition.

papillae — Projections of the lamina propria covered with epithelium, which are present in the oral cavity on the tongue.

parenteral nutrition — A combination of amino acids, dextrose, fats, vitamins, minerals, electrolytes, and water administered intravenously. Parenteral nutrition is capable of providing all the nutrients needed to sustain life.

parenteral — Administration by some means other than through the gastrointestinal tract; referring particularly to introduction of substances into an organism by intravenous, subcutaneous, intramuscular, or intramedullary injection.

parenteral — Injected directly into body tissue through skin and veins.

paronychia — An infection of the fold of skin at the margin of a nail.

parotitis — Inflammation of the salivary glands.

passive acquired immunity — Immunity acquired from the injection or passage of antibodies from an immune person or animal to another for short-term immunity; an example is the temporary immunity acquired by an infant from its mother.

paste — A topical, semisolid formulation containing a pharmacologically active ingredient in a fatty base.

pathogenic — Capable of producing disease.

pathogen — Agent, such as a microorganism, that causes disease.

patient identification number — An individual numeric code that identifies a specific patient, used in pharmacies and other health care facilities.

patient prescription system — A system of drug distribution in which a nurse supplies the pharmacy with a transcribed medication order for a particular patient and the pharmacy prepares a three-day supply of the medication.

pepsinogen — The substance from the gastric glands that is converted into pepsin in the presence of acids.

pepsin — The protease that digests most proteins in the stomach, changing them to polypeptides; when it combines with hydrochloric acid, it is the primary active component of gastric juice.

percent — A fraction whose numerator is expressed and whose denominator is understood to be 100.

perimetrium — The peritoneum covering the fundus as well as the ventral and dorsal aspects of the uterus.

peristalsis — Successive waves of involuntary smooth muscle contractions in the gastrointestinal tract that force the contents forward.

peritonitis — Inflammation of the peritoneum (the membrane lining parts of the abdominal cavity and visceral organs).

pernicious anemia — A disorder of red blood cells that causes them to develop enlarged, misshapen forms; it is caused by the inability to absorb vitamin B_{12} from the diet.

perpetual inventory systems — Inventory control systems that allow monthly drug use reviews.

personal digital assistant (PDA) — A handheld device that runs on its own battery power so that it may be used anywhere.

pertussis — An acute infectious disease caused by the bacterium *Bordetella pertussis*; also known as whooping cough.

pestle — A solid device that is used to crush or grind materials in a mortar.

Peyer's patches — Collections of many lymphoid follicles closely packed together, forming oblong elevations on the mucous membrane of the small intestine.

phagocytosis — The ability of a cell to engulf solid particles.

pharmaceutical care — The care provided to a patient by the pharmacy, which encompasses all aspects of drug therapy from dispensing to drug monitoring.

pharmacodynamics — The study of the biochemical and physiological effects of drugs. It is also defined as the study of the mechanism of action of drugs.

pharmacokinetics — The study of the action of drugs within the body, including the mechanisms of absorption, distribution, metabolism, and excretion.

pharmacopeias — Books containing official lists of medicinal drugs and information about their preparation and use.

pharmacy compounding — The preparation, mixing, assembling, packaging, or labeling of a drug or device.

pharmacy shop — Term used to describe the first stand-alone pharmacies.

pharmacy — The art and science of dispensing and preparing medication and providing drug-related information to the public.

pheochromocytoma — A vascular tumor of the chromaffin tissue of the adrenal medulla or sympathetic paraganglia, characterized by excessive release of epinephrine or norepinephrine; it causes persistent or intermittent hypertension.

phospholipid — A phosphorus-containing lipid.

phosphorus — A nonmetallic chemical element occurring extensively in nature as a component of phosphate rock. Phosphorus is essential for the metabolism of protein, calcium, and glucose.

physical agent — Factors in the environment that interact with the body.

physiochemical — Related to physiology as well as chemistry.

piggyback — A method of adding medication from a vial to an intravenous (IV) medication by removing the contents of the vial using a syringe and injecting it into the IV bag of medication.

pill — A small, globular mass of soluble material containing a medicinal substance to be swallowed.

pipette — A long, thin, calibrated hollow tube, which is made of glass used for measuring liquids.

pituitary gland — An endocrine gland suspended beneath the brain in the sphenoid bone, supplying numerous hormones that govern many vital processes.

placebo — A simulated medication that contains no active ingredients.

plan limitations exceeded — A rejection of a medication refill in which the amount requested exceeds the amount allowed by insurance plan.

plasma cells — Differentiated B cells that secrete antibodies.

plasma — The fluid portion of blood that remains after all blood cells have been removed. Plasma consists of water and dissolved proteins, as well as amino acids, fats, electrolytes, gases, glucose, and metabolic wastes.

plaster — A solid preparation that can be spread when heated and that becomes adhesive at the temperature of the body.

pneumonia — An acute inflammation of the lungs, often caused by inhaled Streptococcus pneumoniae.

point-of-sale (POS) master — An inventory control system that allows inventory to be tracked as it is used.

policies and procedures manual — A formal document specifying guidelines for operations of an institution.

policy limitation — The exclusion of specific medical conditions or procedures from reimbursement under a health insurance policy. Some types of exclusions are acquired immunodeficiency syndrome (AIDS), attempted suicide, cancer, losses due to injury on the job, and pregnancy.

policy — Statement of the definite course or method of action selected to support goals of the overall organization.

poliomyelitis — Inflammation of the spinal cord that leads to paralysis.

polypharmacy — Meaning "many drugs"; refers to taking multiple medications for necessary or unnecessary reasons.

portal of entry — The route by which an infectious agent enters the host.

portal of exit — The route by which an infectious agent leaves the reservoir to be transferred to a susceptible host.

posting — The updating of inventory in pharmacy computer software databases, along with reconciling differences between current and new stock.

potassium — An alkali metal element. Potassium salts are necessary to the life of all plants and animals. Potassium in the body helps to regulate neuromuscular excitability and muscle contraction.

potentiation — Mechanism by which one drug prolongs the effects of another drug.

powder — A dry mass of minute separate particles of any substance.

preauthorization — Prior authorization; many private insurance companies and prepaid health plans have certain requirements that must be met before they will approve diagnostic testing, hospital admissions, inpatient or outpatient surgical procedures, other specific procedures, and specific treatment or medications. For example, most outpatient intravenous therapies require a prior approval authorization.

precaution — Specific warning to consider when medications are prescribed or administered.

preceptor — A person who guides, tutors, and provides direction aimed at a specific performance.

prefix — A part of a word structure that occurs before or in front of the word and modifies the meaning of the root.

prejudice — A preformed and unsubstantiated judgment or opinion about an individual or a group, either favorable or unfavorable.

premium — The cost of the coverage provided by an insurance policy; this may vary greatly depending on the age and health of the individual and the type of insurance protection. The premium may be paid in full or in part by the employer and/or the employee.

prescriptions — Written instructions from licensed physicians or other individuals indicating drugs, their forms, strengths, and other information that are to be dispensed to specific patients.

prime supplier — A single supplier with whom a relationship is established to obtain lower prices.

PRN (as needed) medication order — An order for medication to be given in response to a specific defined parameter or condition.

procedure — Statement of a series of steps to implement the policies of the department or organization.

product — The answer obtained by multiplying two or more quantities together.

professionalism — Behavior based on a body of knowledge and ethical standards to serve the public.

professional pharmacy services (PPS) — All of the activities that a licensed pharmacy provides.

profession — An occupation or career that requires specialized education, ongoing training, and knowledge.

programs — A set of electronic instructions that tell the computer what to do; also called software.

projection — A defense mechanism by which a repressed complex in the individual is denied and conceived as belonging to another person, such as when faults that the person tends to commit are perceived in or attributed to others.

prolactin — A hormone produced and secreted by the anterior pituitary gland; after parturition, it is essential for the initiation and maintenance of milk production.

proper fraction — A fraction in which the numerator is smaller than the denominator and designates less than one whole unit.

proportion — The relationship between two equal ratios.

prostate gland — A firm gland located at the base of the male urethra; it secretes an alkaline fluid that is a major component of ejaculatory fluid.

protected health information (PHI) — Any information about a patient's health status, provision of health care, or payment for health care.

protein — The only one of six essential nutrients containing nitrogen.

pulmonary valve — A tricuspid valve located between the right ventricle and pulmonary artery.

pulse — The surging of blood through arteries that is caused by contraction of the heart; the pulse rate is normally equal to heart rate.

pupil — The black circular center of the eye; it opens and closes when muscles in the iris expand and contract in response to light.

pyloric sphincter — The muscle that closes the pylorus, also known as the pyloric valve.

pyridoxine — A water-soluble vitamin that is part of the B complex. It acts as a coenzyme essential for the synthesis and breakdown of amino acids.

Q

quality control unit — A group with the responsibility for auditing the control system and evaluating product quality; sometimes called an assay and control unit.

quality control — In the pharmaceutical field, an organized effort of all individuals directly or indirectly involved in the production, packaging, and distribution of quality medications, which are safe, effective, and acceptable.

quotient — The answer to a division problem.

R

rabies — The only rhabdovirus that infects humans; it is a zoonotic disease characterized by fatal meningoencephalitis.

radiopharmaceutical — A drug that is or has been made to be radioactive. Although a few radiopharmaceuticals are used to treat diseases (e.g., radioactive iodine), most are used as diagnostic agents.

rationalization — A psychoanalytic defense mechanism through which irrational behavior, motives, or feelings are made to appear reasonable.

ratio — A mathematical expression that compares two numbers by division.

reagent kit — Vials containing particular compounds, usually in freeze-dried form, that are used in nuclear pharmacy.

receptive aphasia — A physical limitation after certain neurological injuries, which leaves the person incapable of understanding all that is said.

receptor — The recipient site on a cell for which a drug has an affinity.

Reed–Sternberg cell — One of a number of large, abnormal, multinucleated reticuloendothelial cells in the lymphatic system, found in Hodgkin's disease.

refill too soon — A rejection of a medication refill in which the refill has been requested too soon after a previous refill was requested.

refraction — The ability of the eye to bend light so that an image is focused on the retina.

registered — Being placed on a list of similar practicing individuals by the state board of pharmacy.

regression — An unconscious defense mechanism involving a return to earlier patterns of adaptation.

regulatory law — Regulations set forth by governmental agencies. It is also called administrative law.

renal corpuscle — A filtration unit in the kidney that consists of a knot of capillaries (the glomerulus) surrounded by the Bowman's glomerular capsule.

renal tubule — The portion of the nephron in the kidney that contains the tubular fluid filtered through the glomerulus.

renin — An enzyme secreted by the kidneys that breaks down protein and produces a rise in blood pressure, as well as stimulating the release of angiotensin II.

repression — A defense mechanism of keeping out and ejecting or banishing from consciousness an unacceptable idea or impulse.

reservoir — The place where an agent can survive.

retina — The sensitive membrane in the inner layer of the eye; it decodes light waves and transmits information to the brain.

retinol — A fat-soluble vitamin essential for skeletal growth, maintenance of normal mucosal epithelium, reproduction, and visual acuity.

Reye syndrome — A complication that occurs almost exclusively in children taking aspirin, primarily in association with influenza B or varicella zoster. Patients present with severe vomiting and confusion, which may progress to coma, due to swelling of the brain.

rheumatic fever — An acute, systemic inflammatory disease that may develop due to inadequate treatment of an upper respiratory streptococcal infection followed by joint pain and inflammation and cardiac valvular disease.

rheumatoid arthritis — A chronic disease marked by stiffness and inflammation of joints, weakness, loss of mobility, and deformity.

riboflavin — One of the heat-stable components of the B complex. It is involved as a coenzyme in the oxidative processes of carbohydrates, fats, and proteins.

rods — Specialized receptor cells in the retina that perceive dim light but not colors.

root — The main part of a word that gives the word its central meaning.

rubella — A mild, highly infectious viral disease common in childhood. Also known as German measles.

rugae — Anatomical folds or wrinkles, such as those in the stomach, which disappear as the stomach fills.

S

saccule — The smaller of the two membranous sacs in the vestibule of the inner ear.

safety data sheet (SDS) — Written or printed material concerning a hazardous chemical that includes information on the chemical's identity and physical and chemical characteristics.

sanitization — A process of cleansing to remove undesirable debris.

sarcasm — Hostile and cruel language intended to hurt someone.

scheduled intravenous (IV)/total parenteral nutrition (TPN) solution order — An order for medication given by means of an injection; these medications are to be prepared in a controlled (sterile) environment.

scheduled medication order — An order for medication that is to be given on a continuous schedule.

sclera — A thick, tough, white membrane in the outer layer of the eye.

sebaceous glands — Skin glands that secrete an oily substance called sebum.

sebum — The oily secretion of the sebaceous glands of the skin, composed of keratin, fat, and cellular debris. Combined with sweat, sebum forms a moist, oily, acidic film that is mildly antibacterial and antifungal.

sedation — The use of a sedative agent to reduce excitement, nervousness, or irritation, commonly prior to a medical procedure.

sedatives — Substances that suppress the central nervous system and induce calmness, relaxation, drowsiness, or sleep.

semen — A whitish fluid of the male reproductive tract that consists of spermatozoa suspended in secretions from the prostate and bulbourethral glands.

semicircular canals — Three interconnected tubes inside the inner ear that are filled with a fluid called endolymph; they are part of the labyrinth of the ear.

seminal vesicles — The glandular pouches that lie on each side of the male reproductive tract and secrete nutrients required by the semen into the ejaculatory duct.

seminiferous tubules — Channels in the testes where spermatozoa develop, and through which they exit.

sexual harassment — Intentional, clearly understood statements or intentional, clearly understood action that causes another to feel that his or her job is at risk if the sexual advances are rejected.

short dating — The dating of any medication that only has a short shelf life, usually 30 days or less.

side effects — Mild, but annoying, responses to a medication.

signa — Directions for patient.

skeletal muscle — A usually voluntary muscle made of elongated, multinucleated, striated muscle.

smallpox — Acute viral disease that was essentially eradicated in 1979. It causes a disfiguring rash, headache, vomiting, and fever.

sodium — One of the most important elements in the body. Sodium ions are involved in acid–base balance, water balance, transmission of nerve impulses, and contraction of muscles.

software — A set of electronic instructions that tell the computer what to do; also called programs.

solution — A liquid dosage form in which active ingredients are dissolved in a liquid vehicle.

solvent — The liquid substance in which another substance is being dissolved.

specialty mail-order pharmacy — A mail-order pharmacy that concentrates on specific areas of the prescription drug market.

specific affinity — The attraction a drug has for particular cells.

spermatic cord — The structure of the male reproductive system that includes the pampiniform plexus, nerves, vas deferens, testicular artery, and other vessels.

spermatogonia — Male germ cells that form spermatocytes early in spermatogenesis.

spirilla — Spiral-shaped bacteria, or other types of microorganisms, which require oxygen to survive.

spirit — An alcoholic or hydroalcoholic solution of volatile substances; also called an essence.

spleen — A soft, highly vascular, roughly ovoid organ situated between the stomach and diaphragm, in the left hypochondriac region of the abdomen.

spore — A resistant stage of bacteria that can withstand an unfavorable environment.

sporicidal — A substance that kills spores.

squamous cell carcinoma — Malignant tumor *of* the flat, scale-like cells of the most superficial layer of the skin, mouth, esophagus, bladder, prostate, lungs, and vagina.

standard code sets — Under HIPAA, "codes used to encode data elements, tables of terms, medical concepts, diagnostic codes, or medical procedure." A code set includes the codes and descriptors of the codes.

standards — Established by authority, custom, or general consent as a model or example; something set up and established by authority as a rule for the measure of quantity, weight, extent, value, or quality.

standing order — A physician's order that can be exercised by other health care workers when predetermined conditions have been met.

staphylococci — Spherical, gram-positive, and parasitic bacteria usually occurring in grape-like clusters.

starter kit — A group of medications provided to a hospice patient by the hospice pharmacy to provide a "start" in treatment for most urgent problems that can develop during the last days or weeks of life.

State Board of Pharmacy (BOP) — An agency that registers pharmacists and pharmacy technicians. In each state, the BOP regulates the practice of pharmacy, licenses pharmacies, imposes sanctions against those who violate the Pharmacy Act, and governs practice standards, drug storage, security, dispensing, facility requirements, internships, and continuing education.

statement — A request for payment, often covering several invoices during a specific time period.

statutes — Rules and regulations resulting from decisions by legislatures.

stent — A device or mold of a suitable material used to provide support for vessels or tubular structures that are being anastomosed.

sterile product — A substance that contains no living microorganisms.

sterilization — Complete destruction of all forms of microbial life.

stratified squamous epithelium — The skin tissue that makes up the epidermis (the outer skin layer).

stratum basale — The deepest layer of the epidermis, composed of dividing stem cells and anchoring cells; also known as stratum germinativium.

stratum lucidum — A layer of lightly staining corneocytes in the deepest level of the stratum corneum; found primarily in the thick epidermis of the palmar and plantar skin.

streptococci — Round or oval-shaped, gram-positive bacteria occurring in pairs or chains.

subcutaneous injection — The administration of medication by means of a needle and syringe into the layer of fat and blood vessels beneath the skin.

subcutaneous layer — A loose connective tissue layer beneath the dermis that binds the skin to underlying organs; it is predominantly made up of adipose tissue; also called hypodermis.

sublimation — An unconscious defense mechanism in which unacceptable instinctual drives and wishes are modified into more personally and socially acceptable channels.

sublingual — Pertaining to the area under the tongue.

subscriber — The individual or organization protected in case of loss under the terms of an insurance policy. The subscriber is known as an insured, member, policyholder, or recipient. In group insurance, the employer is known as the insured and the employees are the risks.

subscription — Dispensing directions to pharmacist.

subtrahend — A number that is subtracted from another.

suffix — A word ending that modifies the meaning of the root.

superscription — Rx symbol.

supply dosage — Refers to both the dosage strength and the form of the drug: the number of measured units per tablet of the concentration of a drug.

suppository — A small, solid body shaped for ready introduction into one of the orifices of the body other than the oral cavity (e.g., rectum, urethra, or vagina), made of a substance, usually medicated, that is solid at ordinary temperature but melts at body temperature.

surgical asepsis — The complete destruction of organisms before they enter the body.

susceptible host — A person who lacks resistance to an agent and is vulnerable to contracting a disease.

suspension — A liquid dosage form that contains solid drug particles floating in a liquid medium.

suspensory ligaments — Ligaments that support organs or body parts, such as those that hold the lenses of the eyes in place.

sustained release (SR) — A capsule that provides a controlled release of the dosage over a designated period of time.

sweat gland — A gland found in most parts of the body that secretes a clear substance to remove body wastes.

symptomatology — The study of symptoms of diseases.

synarthroses — Articulations that lack joint cavities.

synergism — The cooperative effect of two or more drugs given together to produce a stronger effect than that of either drug given alone.

synergist — A muscle that assists an agonist.

syrup — A liquid preparation in a concentrated aqueous solution of a sugar used for medicinal purposes or to add flavor to a substance.

systole — The point in the cardiac cycle when the heart muscle contracts, forcing blood out of the heart and into a blood vessel.

T

tablet triturate — Solid, small, and usually cylindrically molded or compressed tablets.

tablet — A solid dosage form containing medicinal substances with or without suitable diluents.

tachypnea — An abnormally rapid rate of breathing of more than 20 breaths per minute in adults.

tare — The weight of an empty capsule used to compare with the full capsule.

taste buds — Receptors located in fungiform papillae of the tongue that discriminate sour, sweet, salty, bitter, and umami (deliciousness) taste sensations.

tendinitis — Inflammation of a tendon.

tendons — Bands of tough, inelastic fibrous tissues that connect muscles with their bony attachments.

teratogenic — A substance that causes developmental malformation to an embryo or fetus.

teratogens — Agents that cause physical effects in developing embryos; substances that may result in birth defects.

tetanus — An acute, often fatal disease caused by an exotoxin produced by Clostridium tetani.

The Joint Commission — An organization that surveys and accredits health care organizations.

thiamin — A water-soluble, crystalline compound of the B complex, essential for normal metabolism and health of the cardiovascular and nervous systems.

third-party payer — An organization or corporation that pays medical claims for patients; third-party payers reimburse providers directly, with patients making only any required copayments.

thoracic duct — The common trunk of all the lymphatic vessels in the body, except those on the right and left sides of the head, neck, and thorax.

thymosin — A naturally occurring immunological hormone secreted by the thymus gland.

thyroxine — A hormone of the thyroid gland that stimulates the metabolic rate.

time limit — The amount of time from the date of service to the date (deadline) a claim can be filed with the insurance company. Each insurance program has specific time limits that must be adhered to or the insured party will not be able to collect from the insurance company.

tincture — An alcoholic solution prepared from vegetable materials or from chemical substances.

tinea capitis — A common form of fungal infection of the scalp.

tine test — In this test, the tuberculin antigen is injected just under the skin with a multipronged instrument. The antigen is located on the spikes (tines) that penetrate the skin. If results are positive, the skin around the injection site will be red and swollen like a mosquito bite 48 to 72 hours after the injection. It is not as accurate as the Mantoux test.

T lymphocytes — Lymphocytes that exhibit cell surface receptors that recognize specific antigenic peptide-major histocompatibility complexes.

tocopherol — A fat-soluble vitamin essential for normal reproduction, muscle development, resistance of erythrocytes to hemolysis, and various other biochemical functions.

tonsils — Small rounded masses of tissue, especially lymphoid tissue, located in the pharynx.

topical — Pertaining to a drug that is applied to the surface of the body.

tort — A civil wrong committed against person or property.

total parenteral nutrition (TPN) — An intravenous feeding that supplies all the nutrients necessary for life.

total volume — The quantity contained in a package.

touch screen — A monitor with a touch-sensitive surface, on which the touch of a finger makes a selection as a mouse pointer does.

toxemia — An abnormal condition associated with the presence of toxic substances in the blood.

toxoid — A toxin that has been treated with chemicals or heat to decrease its toxic effect but retain its antigenic powers.

trabeculae — Any of the supporting strands of connective tissue projecting into an organ and constituting part of the framework of that organ.

trade name — A drug name, followed by the registered symbol®, which indicates that the name is registered to a specific manufacturer or owner and that no one else can use it.

trailing zeros — Zeros that follow decimal points; 2.0 is an example that has a trailing zero.

transcription — The process of entering a physician's order into a computer; incorrect transcription can be a potential cause of medication errors.

TRICARE — A health care program serving active duty service members, members of the National Guard (including reserve members), retirees, their families, survivors, and selected former spouses worldwide.

tricuspid valve — A valve situated between the right atrium and right ventricle.

triglycerides — Simple fat compounds consisting of three molecules of fatty acid and glycerol. Triglycerides make up most animal and vegetable fats and are the principal lipids in the blood, where they circulate within lipoproteins.

trigone — The smooth triangular portion of the mucosa at the base of the urinary bladder.

triturate — To reduce to a fine powder by friction.

troche — A small, disk-shaped tablet composed of solidifying paste containing an astringent, antiseptic, or oil-based drug used for local treatment of the mouth or throat. It is held in the mouth until dissolved. Also known as a lozenge.

tuberculosis — A chronic granulomatous infection caused by *Mycobacterium tuberculosis*. It is generally transmitted by the inhalation or ingestion of infected droplets and usually affects the lungs.

tunica albuginea — A dense, white, fibrous sheath enclosing a body part or organ.

U

ultraviolet (UV) radiation — Invisible rays that emanate from the sun that can cause skin damage and cancer; UV radiation can also be used to effectively disinfect surfaces and air.

unit-dose drug distribution system — A system for distributing medication in which the pharmacy prepares single doses of medications for a patient for a 24-hour period.

unit-dose system — A drug distribution system that provides medication in its final unit of use form.

unit-of-use packaging — The repackaging of products from bulk containers into patient-specific containers.

unit — The amount of medication required to produce a certain effect.

United States Pharmacopeia (USP) — A nonprofit organization that sets standards for the identity, strength, quality, purity, packaging, and labeling of drug products; www.usp.org.

universal precautions — A set of guidelines for infection control.

uremia — The presence of high levels of protein waste (urea) in the blood.

urethritis — Inflammation of the urethra caused by an infection such as chlamydia.

users — The individuals who work with computers regularly.

utricle — The larger of the two membranous sacs in the vestibule of the inner ear; it is connected with the semicircular canals.

uvea — The region of the eye containing the iris, choroid membrane, and ciliary bodies.

uvula — A conical projection hanging from the posterior border of the soft palate.

V

vaccination — A small amount of toxin administered to increase one's resistance and prevent illness from higher exposure to the same toxin.

vaccination — The process of immunization for prevention of diseases.

vacuole — A clear or fluid-filled space or cavity within a cell, which occurs when a droplet of water is ingested by the cytoplasm.

vas deferens — The primary secretory duct of the testicles through which semen is carried from the epididymis to the prostatic urethra, where it ends as the ejaculatory duct.

vasopressin — A hormone that decreases the production of urine by increasing the reabsorption of water by the renal tubules; it is also called antidiuretic hormone.

vector-borne transmission — An agent is transferred to a susceptible host by animate means.

vehicle transmission — An inanimate material (solid object, liquid, or air) that serves as a transmission agent for pathogens.

venae cavae — The collective name for the superior and inferior vena cava, which are the veins that return deoxygenated blood from the body into the right atrium of the heart.

ventilation — The act of ventilating, which is to breathe in and out.

very low-density lipoproteins (VLDLs) — Lipoproteins made by the liver to transport lipids throughout the body.

vial — A small glass or plastic bottle intended to hold medicine.

villi — Small, slender processes in the body; in the digestive tract, they increase the absorptive area of the mucous membrane.

viremia — The presence of viruses in the blood.

virion — Complete RNA or DNA particles surrounded by protein shells that constitute infectious forms of viruses.

vitamin A — A fat-soluble vitamin essential for skeletal growth, maintenance of normal mucosal epithelium, reproduction, and visual acuity. This vitamin is also called retinol.

vitamin B complex — A group of water-soluble compound vitamins.

vitamin B$_{12}$ — A water-soluble substance that is the common pharmaceutical form of vitamin B$_{12}$. It is involved in the metabolism of protein, fats, and carbohydrates. Vitamin B$_{12}$ is also involved in normal blood formation and neural function. This vitamin is also called cyanocobalamin.

vitamin B$_1$ — A water-soluble, crystalline compound of the B complex, essential for normal metabolism and health of the cardiovascular and nervous systems. This vitamin is also called thiamin.

vitamin B$_2$ — One of the heat-stable components of the B complex. It is involved as a coenzyme in the oxidative processes of carbohydrates, fats, and proteins. This vitamin is also called riboflavin.

vitamin B$_3$ — Part of a coenzyme needed for energy metabolism. This vitamin is also called niacin.

vitamin B$_5$ — A member of the vitamin B complex. It is widely distributed in plant and animal tissues and may be an important element in human nutrition. This vitamin is also called pantothenic acid.

vitamin B$_6$ — A water-soluble vitamin that is part of the B complex. It acts as a coenzyme essential for the synthesis and breakdown of amino acids. This vitamin is also called pyridoxine.

vitamin B$_7$ — A water-soluble, B complex vitamin that acts as a coenzyme in fatty acid production, oxidation of fatty acids, and carbohydrates. This vitamin is also called biotin.

vitamin B$_9$ — A water-soluble vitamin essential for cell growth and the reproduction of red blood cells. This vitamin is also called folic acid or folacin.

vitamin C — A water-soluble vitamin that is essential for the formation of collagen and fibroid tissue for teeth, bones, cartilage, connective tissue, and skin. It also aids in fighting bacterial infections, and in the treatment of bleeding gums, bruising, nosebleeds, and anemia. This vitamin is called ascorbic acid.

vitamin D — A fat-soluble vitamin chemically related to the steroids and essential for the normal formation of bones and teeth. It is important for the absorption of calcium and phosphorus from the gastrointestinal tract. This vitamin is also called calciferol.

vitamin E — A fat-soluble vitamin essential for normal reproduction, muscle development, resistance of erythrocytes to hemolysis, and various other biochemical functions. This vitamin is also called tocopherol.

vitamin K — A group of fat-soluble vitamins that are essential for the synthesis of prothrombin in the liver and are involved in the clotting of blood. These vitamins are also called quinones.

vitamins — Organic substances necessary for life, although they do not independently provide energy.

vitreous humor — The semisolid fluid behind the iris of the eye. It gives the eye its firmness and shape.

vulva — The external genital organs of the female, including the mons pubis, labia majora, labia minora, clitoris, and vestibule of the vagina.

W

waiting period — The period of time that an individual must wait to become eligible for insurance coverage (e.g., 30 days), before coverage commences or for a specific benefit (e.g., an employee must wait 9 months before seeking maternity benefits); also known as an elimination period.

want book — A list of drugs and devices that routinely need to be reordered.

West's nomogram — A quick reference guide that calculates the body surface area (BSA) of infants and young children based on their height and weight.

wheal — An intensely itchy skin eruption larger than a hive.

Z

Z-track method — A method of intramuscular injection of medication in which the skin must be pulled to one side before the tissue is grasped for the injection of such medication. It is used when a drug is highly irritating to subcutaneous tissues or has the ability to permanently stain the skin.

zinc — A metallic element that is an essential nutrient in the body and is used in numerous pharmaceuticals such as zinc acetate and zinc oxide.

INDEX

O